PRIMARY CARE
PAIN MANAGEMENT

PRIMARY CARE PAIN MANAGEMENT

Charles De Mesa, DO, MPH
Associate Professor, Director of Pain Medicine Fellowship
Department of Anesthesiology and Pain Medicine
University of California, Davis School of Medicine
Sacramento, California

Samir J. Sheth, MD
Associate Volunteer Faculty
University of California, Davis School of Medicine
Sacramento, California
Interventional Pain Management Physician
Sutter Roseville Medical Center
Roseville, California

Craig Keenan, MD
Professor
Director, Internal Medicine Residency Program
Department of Internal Medicine
University of California, Davis School of Medicine
Sacramento, California

Robert M. McCarron, DO, DFAPA
Professor and Vice Chair of Education and Integrated Care
Program Director, Psychiatry Residency Program
Director, Train New Trainers Primary Care
Psychiatry Fellowship
Department of Psychiatry and Human Behavior
University of California, Irvine School of Medicine
President, California Psychiatric Association
Past President, Association of Medicine and Psychiatry
Orange, California

Joslyn John, MD
Assistant Professor
Assistant Program Director, Physical Medicine and Rehabilitation Residency
Undergraduate Medical Education Director, Physical Medicine and Rehabilitation
H. Ben Taub Department of Physical Medicine and Rehabilitation
Baylor College of Medicine
Houston, Texas

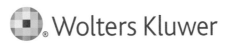

. Wolters Kluwer

Philadelphia • Baltimore • New York • London
Buenos Aires • Hong Kong • Sydney • Tokyo

Director, Medical Practice, Professional & Education: Rebecca S. Gaertner
Editorial Coordinator: Dave Murphy
Editorial Assistant: Brian Convery
Production Project Manager: Bridgett Dougherty, Sadie Buckallew
Design Coordinator: Steve Druding
Manufacturing Coordinator: Beth Welsh
Prepress Vendor: TNQ Technologies

9 8 7 6 5 4 3 2 1

Printed in China

Library of Congress Cataloging-in-Publication Data

ISBN-13:978-1-4963-7880-4

Cataloging in Publication data available on request from publisher.

---

shop.lww.com

CONTRIBUTING AUTHORS

Zar Baqai, MD
Physician
Department of Anesthesiology and Pain Medicine
University of California, Davis Medical Center
Sacramento, California

Richard Jacob Boyce, DPT
Pain Specialist/Physical Therapist
Neurology/Pain Clinic
DC VA Medical Center
Washington, DC

Nathan Bryant, PharmD
Pain Management Pharmacist
Department of Pharmacy
University of California, Davis Health
Sacramento, California

Kevin Burnham, MD
Assistant Professor
Department of Internal Medicine
University of California, Davis School of Medicine
Sacramento, California

David Copenhaver, MD
Associate Professor, Vice Chair Anesthesiology and Pain
    Medicine
University of California, Davis School of Medicine
Sacramento, California

Brian A. Davis, MD, FACSM
Professor
Department of Physical Medicine and Rehabilitation
Co-Director of PM&R Sports Medicine Fellowships
University of California, Davis Health System
Sacramento, California

Charles De Mesa, DO, MPH
Associate Professor, Director of Pain Medicine
    Fellowship
Department of Anesthesiology and Pain Medicine
University of California, Davis School of Medicine
Sacramento, California

Jeremy DeMartini, MD
Assistant Clinical Professor
Training Director Internal Medicine/Psychiatry
Residency Program
Department of Psychiatry and Behavioral Sciences
University of California, Davis School of Medicine
Sacramento, California

Anthony DiGirolamo, DO
Clinician-Physiatry and Pain Medicine
Department of Physical Medicine and Rehabilitation
The Center for Orthopedic and Neurosurgical Care and
    Rehabilitation
Bend, Oregon

Omar Dyara, DO
Assistant Professor
Medical College of Wisconsin
Milwaukee, Wisconsin

Lindsey Enoch, MD
Acting Assistant Professor
Departments of Psychiatry and Behavioral Sciences
University of Washington
Seattle, Washington

Erielle Anne P. Espina, PharmD
Pharmacist
Department of Pharmacy
University of Washington Medical Center
Seattle, Washington

Christopher Gilbert, PhD
Psychologist
Osher Center for Integrative Medicine
University of California, San Francisco
San Francisco, California

Jesse Goitia, MD
Physician
Chief Resident
Department of Internal Medicine
University of California, Davis School of Medicine
Sacramento, California

Charity Hale, PharmD
Pain Management and Palliative Care
University of California, Davis Medical Center
Sacramento, California

Shelly Henderson, PhD
Associate Clinical Professor
Department of Family and Community Medicine
University of California, Davis School of Medicine
Sacramento, California

Calvin H. Hirsch, MD
Professor of Clinical Medicine (Geriatrics) and Public
    Health Sciences
Division of General Medicine
University of California, Davis Medical Center
Sacramento, California

Mark Holtsman, PharmD
Clinical Professor
Department of Anesthesiology and Pain Medicine
University of California, Davis School of Medicine
Sacrament, California

Misty Humphries, MD, MAS, RPVI, FACS
Assistant Professor, Department of Surgery
Division of Vascular and Endovascular Care
University of California, Davis School of Medicine
Sacramento, California

Prathap Jayaram, MD
Director
Regenerative Sports Medicine
Assistant Professor
H. Ben Taub Department of Physical Medicine &
    Rehabilitation Orthopedic Surgery
Baylor College of Medicine
Houston, Texas

Joslyn John, MD
Assistant Professor
Assistant Program Director, Physical Medicine and
    Rehabilitation Residency
Undergraduate Medical Education Director, Physical
    Medicine and Rehabilitation
H. Ben Taub Department of Physical Medicine and
    Rehabilitation
Baylor College of Medicine
Houston, Texas

Mark Johnson, PhD
Clinical Psychologist
Department of Behavioral Medicine
Bay Area Pain and Wellness
San Francisco, California

Nicolas Karvelas, MD
Interventional Pain Medicine, Physical Medicine and
    Rehabilitation, Spine and Nerve Diagnostic Center
Roseville, California

Christine Kho, MD
Resident Physician
Internal Medicine and Psychiatry Program
University of California, Davis School of Medicine
Sacramento, California

Ian J. Koebner, PhD, MSc, MAOM
Director
Integrative Pain Management
Assistant Professor
Department of Anesthesiology and Pain Management
University of California, Davis School of Medicine
Sacramento, California

Paul G. Kreis, MD
Associate Chief
Department of Anesthesiology and Pain Medicine
University of California, Davis School of Medicine
Sacramento, California

Sungeun Lee, MD
Pediatric Anesthesiologist
Anesthesiology
Kaiser Permanente
Roseville, California

Joshua Lee, MD
Anesthesiologist
Department of Anesthesiology
The Permanente Medical Group
Modesto, California

Marc Lenaerts, MD, FAHS
Clinical Professor
Department of Neurology and Anesthesiology/Pain
    Management
University of California, Davis School of Medicine
Sacramento, California

Martin AC Manoukian, BS
University of California, Davis School of Medicine
Sacramento, California

Payal Mapara, PsyD
Clinical Psychologist
Assistant Clinical Professor
Department of Mental Health and Psychiatry
San Francisco VA Medical Center and University of
    California San Francisco
San Francisco, California

Robert M. McCarron, DO, DFAPA
Professor and Vice Chair of Education and Integrated Care
Program Director, Psychiatry Residency Program
Director, Train New Trainers Primary Care
Psychiatry Fellowship
Department of Psychiatry and Human Behavior
University of California, Irvine School of Medicine
President, California Psychiatric Association
Past President, Association of Medicine and Psychiatry
Orange, California

Christopher Migdal, BS
Medical Student
School of Medicine
University of California, Davis School of Medicine
Sacramento, California

Joshua Minori, DO
Pain Medicine/Physical Medicine and Rehabilitation
    Interventional Spine and Pain Management
Salt Lake City, Utah

Kathleen Nowak, PharmD, BCACP, AAHIVP
Clinical Pharmacist
Department of Outpatient Clinical Pharmacy Services
Mission Health System
Asheville, North Carolina

Morgan O'Connor, MD
Fellow, Pain Medicine
Department of Physical Medicine and Rehabilitation
University of California
Los Angeles School of Medicine
Los Angeles, California

John Onate, MD
Associate Clinical Professor
Department of Psychiatry
University of California, Davis School of Medicine
Sacramento, California

Catherine Platt, MD
Pain Management Specialist
Desert Orthopedics
Bend, Oregon

Ravi Prasad, MD
Clinical Professor
Department of Anesthesiology and Pain Medicine
University of California, Davis School of Medicine
Sacramento, California

Amir Ramezani, PhD
Phycologist
Associate Clinical Professor
Department of Physical Medicine and Rehabilitation
University of California
Sacramento, California

Matthew Reed, MD, MSPH
Assistant Dean for Student Affairs
Department of Psychiatry
University of California
Irvine, California

Damoon Rejaei, MD
Department of Pain Medicine
Woodland Health Clinic
Woodland, California

Kathryn Schopmeyer, DPT
PT Program Coordinator, Pain Management
Department of Rehabilitation Services
San Francisco VA Healthcare System
San Francisco, California

Arjun Sharma, MD
Anesthesiologist and Pain Management Specialist
VAMC Anesthesia Department
VA Medical Center
San Francisco, California

Samir J. Sheth, MD
Associate Volunteer Faculty
University of California, Davis School of Medicine
Sacramento, California
Interventional Pain Management Physician
Sutter Roseville Medical Center
Roseville, California

Naileshni Singh, MD
Associate Professor
Department of Anesthesiology and Pain Medicine
University of California, Davis School of Medicine
Sacramento, California

Karen Snider, DO
Professor
Neuromusculoskeletal Medicine/Osteopathic
    Manipulative Medicine
Assistant Dean for Osteopathic Principles and Practice
    Integration
Department of Family Medicine, Preventive Medicine,
    and Community Health
A.T. Still University - Kirksville College of Osteopathic
    Medicine
Kirksville, Missouri

Joseph Solberg, DO
Assistant Professor
Director Daniel and Jane Och Spine Hospital
Department of Rehabilitation and Regenerative
    Medicine
Columbia University
New York, New York

Scott Stayner, MD, PhD
Pain Management Specialist
ThedaCare Orthopedic Care
Appleton, Wisconsin

Ami Student, PsyD
Staff Psychologist
Department of Behavioral Health
Boise Veterans Affairs Medical Center
Boise, Idaho

Efrain Talamantes, MD, MBA, MS
Assistant Professor
Associate Director, Center for Reducing Health
 Disparities
Associate Director, Internal Medicine Residency
 Program
UC Davis School of Medicine
Clinical and Translational Science Center (CTSC)
Sacramento, California

Shweta Teckchandani, DO
Pain Management Fellow
Department of Pain Medicine
University of Washington Medical Center
University of Washington
Seattle, Washington

Amode Tembhekar, BS
Medical Student
School of Medicine
University of California, Davis School of Medicine
Sacramento, California

Brian Toedebusch, MD
Assistant Professor
Department of Physical Medicine and Rehabilitation
University of Missouri
Columbia, Missouri

Hunter Vincent, DO
Resident Physician
Department of Physical Medicine and Rehabilitation
University of California, Davis School of Medicine
Sacramento, California

Rebecca Vogsland, PT, DPT
Assistant Director
Comprehensive Pain Center
Department of Physical Medicine and Rehabilitation
Minneapolis VA Health Care System
Minneapolis, Minnesota

Dustin Ward, MD
Pain Management Physician and Anesthesiologist
Maple Grove, Minnesota

Rachel Worman, PT, DPT, MPT
Sacramento, California

Jon Zhou, MD
Assistant Clinical Professor
Department of Anesthesiology and Pain Medicine
University of California, Davis School of Medicine
Sacramento, California

FOREWORD

Few areas of primary care medicine pose as many daunting challenges as the management of chronic nonmalignant pain.

The prevalence of chronic nonmalignant pain is widespread, and the burden of suffering endured by patients is enormous. Although management of pain is assumed to be within the domain of primary care clinicians, performing a proper comprehensive assessment of chronic pain can be time-consuming for busy health care professionals who are often overwhelmed by their schedules.

The voices of multiple stakeholder groups including patient advocacy groups, professional societies, public and private purchasers of care, the media, State Medical and Pharmacy Boards, the Drug Enforcement Administration, the Food and Drug Administration, the Centers for Disease Control, and law enforcement are growing louder and more forceful. To complicate matters, the regulatory environment addressing opioids is rapidly changing, making it difficult to stay fully informed, thus creating considerable legal peril for providers.

As health care professionals we are charged with doing what is in the best interest of our patients. In *Crossing the Quality Chasm: A New Health System for the 21st Century*, the IOM's Committee on the Quality of Health Care in America asserted that "Americans should be able to count on receiving care which meets their needs based on the best scientific knowledge."

And yet, how is the busy health care professional to heed the many loud voices, navigate the differing values and balance the conflicting expectations so prevalent in the management of chronic pain? What is the best way to effectively allocate valuable time to comprehensively evaluate chronic pain? Where do they find the time to spend with patients in order to individualize treatment and determine the best way to address the needs of a patient with chronic nonmalignant pain? How are they to assimilate the latest research evidence based in treatment plans? Who helps provide guidance regarding the right balance between effective treatment and patient safety?

The authors of *Primary Care Pain Management*, based on their comprehensive training and collective years of patient care and academic experience, provide busy health care professionals with a pragmatic, highly readable individualized approach to managing patients with pain.

Using a methodical approach, the reader is informed how to comprehensively evaluate pain, assess risk factors, establish realistic therapy goals, discuss with patients the potential benefits and known risks of various treatment options, maximize the safety and efficacy of pain treatment, and understand when or when not to use various pharmacologic agents, including opioids.

Above all else, *Primary Care Pain Management* advocates for a compassionate, patient-centered approach to the management of pain. This is, at its heart, the essence of primary care.

Kurt J. Slapnik, MD
Diplomate, American Board of Family Medicine
Medical Director, UC Davis Health Network

ACKNOWLEDGMENTS

We would like to thank the authors for their tireless efforts and creative support for pain education and training, which we believe will transform clinical care. We acknowledge key individuals who assisted with the editing process including Robert McCarron, DO, Craig Keenan, MD, and Joslyn John, MD, Rakshitha Mohankumar, BS, Rob Izar, BS, and Indu Dornadula, MD. For illustrative support, we are grateful for the contributions from Taysia De Mesa, Dylan De Mesa, and Tai Diep. Finally, we would like to thank our associates from Wolters Kluwer including Dave Murphy, Kristina Oberle, and Bridgett Dougherty as well as Ramkumar Soundararajan, Project Manager at TNQ Technologies. It has been a pleasure working with you. We are very grateful to you for all your help.

PREFACE

We are pleased to introduce you to *Primary Care Pain Management*, the clinical resource for educating primary care providers on safe and effective treatments for chronic pain conditions. This book helps to fill in the gaps for understanding chronic pain and offers evidence-based recommendations in the care of patients with chronic pain as well as supplements and updates the already expansive knowledge of primary care providers. It would be an understatement to say that the opioid epidemic has changed the landscape of medicine. It has forced many providers to change the way they practice and it has put many primary care providers and pain management specialists into uncomfortable situations with their patients and has also made many primary care providers feel vulnerable. While the opioid epidemic has certainly been very troubling, it has also forced us to revisit and reevaluate potentially safer and more effective treatment options for chronic pain patients.

Broad improvements in education are delivered through the chapters, which summarize the multiple causes and effects of pain, the range of treatments available, and the fundamental understanding of treating chronic pain through the biopsychosocial model.

Furthermore, strategies included in the text focus on ways to improve care for the populations disproportionately affected by and undertreated for pain. The chapters also include important information on Addiction and Behavioral Medicine, which aims to improve the learner's knowledge and skills that are necessary for the comprehensive pain assessment and treatment in a very difficult patient population.

Primary Care Pain Management represents 17 UC Davis–Interprofessional and Departmental disciplines including primary care, specialty, and subspecialty teams. It also represents collaboration with our University of California partners in San Francisco and Los Angeles, and other private University Medical Institutions as well as the United States Veterans Affairs Health Care System.

Primary Care Pain Management was written because the authors and editors believe that the primary care providers on the front line of medicine have a substantial impact on reducing suffering and improving quality of life through multidisciplinary efforts, safe and effective pain assessment, appropriate referrals, and individualized treatment and that these refined treatment plans will lead to improved health outcomes.

Charles De Mesa, DO, MPH
Associate Professor
Director of Pain Medicine Fellowship
Department of Anesthesiology and Pain Medicine
University of California, Davis School of Medicine
Sacramento, California

Samir J. Sheth, MD
Associate Volunteer Faculty
University of California, Davis School of Medicine
Sacramento, California
Interventional Pain Management Physician
Sutter Roseville Medical Center
Roseville, California

CONTENTS

SECTION II

Psychiatric Disorders and Pain   49

SECTION III

Fundamentals of Pain History, Physical Exam and Assessment   83

SECTION IV

Chronic Pain Treatment 191

BASIC PRINCIPLES

Part 1

BASIC PRINCIPLES OF CHRONIC PAIN IN THE PRIMARY CARE SETTING

1

ESSENTIAL TOOLS OF PRIMARY CARE PAIN MEDICINE

Catherine Platt, MD, Samir J. Sheth, MD, Ian J. Koebner, PhD, MSc, MAOM, Anthony DiGirolamo, DO and Charles De Mesa, DO, MPH

INTRODUCTION

Pain is a major public health concern. The National Academy of Medicine estimates that 100 million Americans suffer from chronic pain, more than those who suffer from heart disease, cancer, and diabetes combined.[1] The annual cost of chronic pain is over $600 billion, and in a given year 126 million adults experience some pain with about one-third (40 million adults) experiencing severity.[2] Pain is one of the most common reasons individuals seek primary medical care, yet pain care is routinely inadequate and without comprehensive assessment or treatment plan.[3] Furthermore, pain is associated with poor general health, health-related disability, and increased health care utilization.[3] According to national estimates, back pain, joint pain, neck pain, and headaches are among the most common types of pain experienced by US adults (see Table 1-1).[4-6]

The prevalence of common painful conditions has remained stable despite improved understanding of the mechanisms of pain syndromes and the development of novel medications and medical devices (see Table 1-1). A focus on treatment rather than prevention has contributed to the epidemic of chronic pain. One of

the treatments continues to be the use of opioid medications. Morbidity and mortality from opioid-related overdose has increased with the rise in opioid prescriptions. In 2015; 12.5 million people in the United States misused opioid medications, and 33,000 died from complications associated with opioid overdose.[7,8] In fact, at the time of this publication, opioid overdose is now the leading cause of accidental death in the United States.[8] Therefore, emphasis on pain education, assessment, and knowledge of pain medications is central to improving the health of the person.

TREATMENT STRATEGIES

Chronic pain management requires treatment strategies tailored to each person and not overly reliant on single modalities. In addition to the various treatments, management also requires patients to be participants in their own care, which often begins with fostering a healthy lifestyle. The cells of our body need nutrients, oxygen, and healthy sleep to recover, repair, and perform activities of daily living. A predominantly plant-based, whole-food diet delivers a balance of vitamins, minerals and antioxidants. Anti-inflammatory diets high in fruits, vegetables, nuts, whole grains, fish, and healthy oils such as the Mediterranean diet or purely plant-based diets, such as a Vegan diet, are associated with decreased pain and improved mood. Decreased pain and improved mood further promote healthy choices.[9,10]

Similarly, consistent moderate aerobic exercise promotes healthy weight with associated decreased pain, improved general conditioning, and increased function. Cardiovascular health enhances oxygen and nutrient delivery to the cells supporting tissue function, recovery,

TABLE 1-1 Age-Adjusted Percentages of Selected Health Conditions Among US Adults, NHIS 2002, 2007, 2012

HEALTH CONDITION	2002[4]	2007[5]	2012[6]
Low back pain past 3 mo	26.4%	25.4%	27.6%
Arthritis	20.9%	20.3%	20.6%
Neck pain past 3 mo	13.8%	12.8%	13.9%
Severe headache or migraine past 3 mo	15.0%	12.3%	14.1%

Adapted from Nahin RL, Boineau R, Khalsa PS, Stussman BJ, Weber WJ. Evidence-based evaluation of complementary health approaches for pain management in the United States. Mayo Clin Proc. 2016;91(9):1292-1306. Copyright © 2016 Elsevier. With permission.

and repair, and the endorphins associated with cardiovascular exercise also improve mood and healthy choices.

Along with maintenance of a home exercise routine, patients should be reminded of the deleterious effects smoking has on bone mineral content and the small blood vessels, which then impair oxygen delivery to intervertebral disks.[11,12] Smoking accelerates degenerative disk disease—one of the most common sources of chronic low back pain.[13-16] Depression and chronic pain levels are also greater in smokers compared with nonsmokers.[17]

Finally, poor sleep is associated with chronic widespread pain. This is seen regularly in fibromyalgia.[18] Restorative sleep is predictive of improvement or resolution of chronic pain.[19-22]

As defined by the International Association for the Study of Pain (IASP), "Pain is an unpleasant sensory *and* emotional experience that is associated with actual or potential tissue damage or described in such terms." Psychosocial stressors, both internal turmoil and external conflict, exacerbate chronic pain. The ability to regulate affective experience, including negative emotion and pain, influences physical and mental health. Chronic pain and depression are associated with structural and functional changes in the brain with maladaptive neuroplasticity. Mindfulness and meditation have the ability to relieve pain by strengthening our ability to modulate our affective pain experience, fostering adaptive neuroplastic changes, and promoting return to healthier brain structure and function. Just as mindfulness and meditation promote psychologic health from within, healthy social relationships with others are important for mental and physical well-being.[13]

BIOPSYCHOSOCIAL MODEL

The Biopsychosocial Model introduced by George Engel, MD, in the 1970s adapted below illustrates the interrelationships of biologic, psychologic, and social factors contributing to the pain experience and suffering. The ensuing chapters will further explain specific pain states and management strategies while also emphasizing the importance of the model when developing impressions and recommendations. As primary care providers, meaningful chronic pain management begins with you. The challenges are communicating and successfully motivating for healthy lifestyle and long-term pain management strategies.

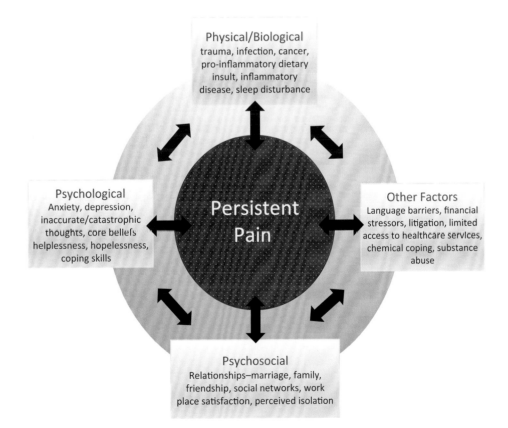

CONCLUSION

Treating chronic pain is a humbling experience, but the benefits from both an individual and societal level are far-reaching. We, as the authors of this book, aim to make the primary care provider a frontline pain management specialist.

REFERENCES

1. Gaskin DJ, Richard P. The economic costs of pain in the United States. *J Pain.* 2012;13(8):715-724.

2. Nahin RL. Estimates of pain prevalence and severity in adults: United States, 2012. *J Pain.* 2015;16(8):769-780.

3. Research., I.o.M.C.o.A.P. *Relieving Pain in America: A Blueprint for Transforming Prevention, Care, Education, and Research.* National Academies Press; 2011.

4. Lethbridge-Cejku M, Schiller JS, Bernadel L. Summary health statistics for U.S. adults: National Health Interview Survey, 2002. *Vital Health Stat 10.* 2004;(222):1-151.

5. Pleis JR, Lucas JW. Summary health statistics for U.S. adults: National Health Interview Survey, 2007. *Vital Health Stat 10.* 2009;(240):1-159.

6. Blackwell DL, Lucas JW, Clarke TC. Summary health statistics for U.S. adults: National Health Interview survey, 2012. *Vital Health Stat 10.* 2014;(260):1-161.

7. Tice P, Adams KT, Adams T, et al. *Reports and Detailed Tables From the 2015 National Survey on Drug Use and Health (NSDUH).* 2016 March 7, 2018; Published September 7, 2016. Available from: https://www.samhsa.gov/sam-hsa-data-outcomes-quality/major-data-collections/reports-detailed-tables-2015-NSDUH.

8. Rudd RA, Seth P, David F, Scholl L. Increases in drug and opioid-involved overdose deaths – United States, 2010–2015. *MMWR Morb Mortal Wkly Rep.* 2016;65(5051):1445-1452. doi:10.15585/mmwr.mm655051e1.

9. Bosma-den Boer MM, van Wetten ML, Pruimboom L. Chronic inflammatory diseases are stimulated by current lifestyle: how diet, stress levels and medication prevent our body from recovering. *Nutr Metab (Lond).* 2012;9(1):32.

10. Kiecolt-Glaser JK. Stress, food, and inflammation: psychoneuroimmunology and nutrition at the cutting edge. *Psychosom Med.* 2010;72(4):365-369.

11. Abate M, Vanni D, Pantalone A, Salini V. Cigarette smoking and musculoskeletal disorders. *Muscles Ligaments Tendons J.* 2013;3(2):63-69.

12. Shi Y, Weingarten TN, Mantilla CB, Hooten WM, Warner DO. Smoking and pain: pathophysiology and clinical implications. *Anesthesiology.* 2010;113(4):977-992.

13. Cacioppo JT, Cacioppo S. Social relationships and health: the toxic effects of perceived social isolation. *Soc Personal Psychol Compass.* 2014;8(2):58-72.

14. Bastian LA, Driscoll MA, Heapy AA, et al. Cigarette smoking status and receipt of an opioid prescription among veterans of recent wars. *Pain Med.* 2017;18(6):1089-1097.

15. Behrend C, Schonbach E, Coombs A, Coyne E, Prasarn M, Rechtine G. Smoking cessation related to improved patient-reported pain scores following spinal care in geriatric patients. *Geriatr Orthop Surg Rehabil.* 2014;5(4):191-194.

16. Behrend C, Prasarn M, Coyne E, Horodyski M, Wright J, Rechtine GR. Smoking cessation related to improved patient-reported pain scores following spinal care. *J Bone Joint Surg Am.* 2012;94(23):2161-2166.

17. Hooten WM, Shi Y, Gazelka HM, Warner DO. The effects of depression and smoking on pain severity and opioid use in patients with chronic pain. *Pain.* 2011;152(1):223-229.

18. Moldofsky H, Scarisbrick P, England R, Smythe H. Musculoskeletal symptoms and non-REM sleep disturbance in patients with "fibrositis syndrome" and healthy subjects. *Psychosom Med.* 1975;37(4):341-351.

19. Ancoli-Israel S. The impact and prevalence of chronic insomnia and other sleep disturbances associated with chronic illness. *Am J Manag Care.* 2006;12(8 suppl):S221-S229.

20. Kupfer DJ, Reynolds CF. Management of insomnia. *N Engl J Med.* 1997;336(5):341-346.

21. Davies KA, Macfarlane GJ, Nicholl BI, et al. Restorative sleep predicts the resolution of chronic widespread pain: results from the EPIFUND study. *Rheumatology (Oxford).* 2008;47(12):1809-1813.

22. National Heart, L.a.B.I. *Your Guide to Healthy Sleep.* Bethesda, MD: National Institutes of Health; 2005.

PAIN ANATOMY AND PHYSIOLOGY

Damoon Rejaei, MD and Samir J. Sheth, MD

FAST FACTS

- Pain transmission and sensation is a complex phenomenon composed of multiple components including nociceptor activation, ascending spinal tracts, descending spinal tracts, and higher brain centers.
- Various nociceptors and chemical mediators are involved in experiencing different pain sensations from thermal, mechanical, or chemical stimuli.
- Chronic pain can result from peripheral sensitization, central sensitization, or both.

INTRODUCTION

Although pain is experienced by nearly the entire human species, defining and detecting pain in humans can be elusive. For millennia, describing and defining pain has been of great interest. Indeed, Aristotle (384-322 BC) argued that pain was an emotion and associated it with the heart. In contrast, Galen (AD 130-201) emphasized the brain as the organ of feeling and placed pain into the realm of the mind.[1] In 1906, Sir Charles Sherrington explicitly distinguished between the complex human experience of pain and that of nociception by defining nociception as the sensory detection of a noxious event or a potentially harmful environmental stimulus.[2] The

ability to detect noxious stimuli is fundamental to the survival of an organism, as witnessed by the early death of people who carry rare recessive genotypes rendering them congenitally insensitive to pain. In modern times, a more comprehensive view is upheld on the definition of pain. The International Association for the Study of Pain defines pain as "an unpleasant sensory and emotional experience associated with actual or potential tissue damage."[3]

The pain system grossly spans the entire neuraxis. This is evidenced by the fact that both the peripheral destruction of tissue and the psychological distress of trauma can often lead to similar patient reports of pain. The fundamental mechanisms behind these similar experiences, however, must be different. Moreover, despite the termination of an acutely painful stimulus, the patient with chronic pain continues to live with an "unpleasant sensory and emotional experience." This chapter attempts to elucidate the fundamental anatomy and physiology responsible for chronic pain. Grossly, the pain system can be divided into the following components:

Nociceptors: Peripheral nerve fibers that detect noxious stimuli (i.e., thermal, mechanical, or chemical).

The spinal cord and ascending nociceptive tracks: Projection neurons that carry pain signals from the dorsal horn of the spinal cord to higher centers of the central nervous system (CNS), such as the brain.

Higher centers in the CNS and descending inhibitory tracts: These pathways allow for the modulation of pain from higher CNS structures to the spinal cord.

NOCICEPTORS

Nociceptors are a population of peripheral neurons responsible for detecting painful stimuli. Their cell bodies are located in the dorsal root ganglion (DRG) for the body and in the trigeminal ganglion for the face. As such, in the body, nociceptors have their cell bodies located in the peripheral nervous system (PNS), whereas in the face their cell bodies are located in the CNS. Interestingly, nociceptors are pseudounipolar, meaning their axonal projections divide to travel both centrally to the spinal cord (and from there to higher brain centers) and peripherally to the skin and other organs (Figure 2-1). Classically one imagines information in neurons to travel in one direction with a clear linearity between dendritic input of information to the cell body and the axonal output of neurotransmitters. However, the pseudounipolar nature of nociceptors allows for the bidirectional travel of information. This is significant because therapeutic

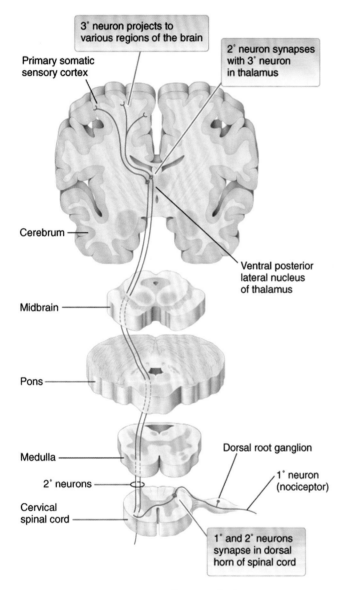

FIGURE 2-1 Pain pathways. Primary (1°) nociceptors have cell bodies in the dorsal root ganglion and synapse with secondary (2°) afferent neurons in the dorsal horn of the spinal cord. Primary afferents use the neurotransmitter glutamate. The 2° afferents travel in the lateral areas of the spinal cord and eventually reach the thalamus, where they synapse with tertiary (3°) afferent neurons. The processing of pain is complex, and 3° afferents have many destinations, including the somatosensory cortex (localization of pain) and the limbic system (emotional aspects of pain). Reprinted with permission from Golan DE. Principles of Pharmacology. 4th ed. Philadelphia, PA: Wolters Kluwer; 2016.

drugs can target the peripheral axonal terminal (i.e., anti-inflammatory medication) to prevent nociceptor activation and/or the central axonal terminal (i.e., intrathecal drug delivery) of nociceptors to prevent neurotransmitter release at the level of the spinal cord.[4,5]

There are 2 major classes of nociceptors: medium-diameter thinly myelinated Aδ neurons and small-diameter unmyelinated C fiber neurons.[6] Both Aδ and C fiber afferents are further subdivided into other classes, which is beyond the scope of this chapter. These afferent nerves can detect thermal, mechanical, or chemical environmental stimuli. Aδ and C fibers are only a subset of sensory fibers present in the PNS (Table 2-1). Given their thin and myelinated axons, Aδ fibers mediate acute and precisely localized pain. In contrast, C fibers mediate poorly localized and delayed pain.

Nociceptor Activation

Nociceptors are activated by a variety of environmental stimuli, including thermal, mechanical, and various chemical stimuli. The pain threshold for heat activation of nociceptors in both Aδ and C fibers has been found to typically rest around 43°C.[7] The transient receptor potential (TRP) group of ion channels are activated by heat. One of the most studied members of this family of ion channels is the TRPV1 receptor, which was identified as the molecular target for capsaicin, the pungent component of "spicy" or "hot" chili peppers. Indeed, mice that genetically lack this TRPV1 receptor show significant impairment in their ability to detect noxious heat stimuli.[8] Under normal physiological conditions, heat or acidosis can lead to the transient opening of TRPV1 channels, which in turn leads to calcium and sodium influx into the cell and action potential propagation into the spinal cord. Interestingly, in contrast to transient activation of the TRPV1 channel, high concentrations or repetitive exposure to capsaicin can cause persistent opening of the TRPV1 channel. This in turn, leads to a large influx of calcium into the cell, leading to activation of calcium-dependent proteases and cytoskeleton breakdown (i.e., receptor inactivation). This is how topical capsaicin formulations are used to treat a variety of pain conditions (i.e., postherpetic neuralgia).[9]

A variety of chemical mediators and environmental toxins can trigger nociceptor activity. TRPA1, another member of the TRP group of ion channels, has been found to respond to a variety of environmental compounds such as allyl isothiocyanate (from the wasabi plant) or allicin (from garlic). Acrolein, an environmental toxin found in vehicle exhaust and tear gas, can also activate the TRPA1 channel, leading to pain in the eyes and airways. This can have a more severe impact in patients suffering from respiratory diseases (i.e., asthma).[10] To highlight the role of TRPA1 channels, mice lacking the TRPA1 gene show significantly reduced reactivity to the aforementioned chemicals.[11]

As a result of tissue damage and inflammation, certain endogenous chemical mediators can also contribute to the pain process. These chemicals are often termed to be the "chemical milieu of inflammation." In the event of tissue damage, a variety of cells such as mast cells, basophils, platelets, macrophages, and neutrophils infiltrate

TABLE 2-1 Fibers of the Peripheral Nervous System

FIBER TYPE	PHYSIOLOGIC ROLE	PAIN QUALITY	FUNCTION	MYELINATED	AVERAGE DIAMETER (μm)	AVERAGE CONDUCTION VELOCITY (m/s)
A α	Motor		Muscle spindle, motor to skeletal muscle	Yes	15	100
A β	Sensory		Proprioceptive, touch, pressure	Yes	8	50
A γ	Motor		Skeletal muscle tone	Yes	6	20
A δ	Sensory	Rapid, sharp, localized	Nociceptive, touch, temperature	Yes	2	15
B	Sympathetic		Preganglionic, controls vascular smooth muscle	Yes	3	9
C	Sensory	Slow, diffuse, dull	Nociceptive, touch, temperature, also postganglionic, controls viscera and afferent relay to skin	No	1	1

Adapted from Cousins MJ, Bridenbaugh PO. Neural Blockade in Clinical Anesthesia and Management of Pain. 3rd ed. Lippincott Williams and Wilkins; 1998:44-45 and Wainger B, Brenner GJ. Mechanisms of chronic pain. In: Longnecker DE, Mackey SC, Newman MF, Sandberg WS, Zapol WM, eds. Anesthesiology. McGraw-Hill Education; 2018:1441-1455

the injured area. These cells release a variety of chemicals such as neurotransmitters, peptides (substance P, CGRP, bradykinin), lipids (prostaglandins, leukotrienes, endocannabinoids), and cytokines. These chemicals can then bond to certain receptors (such as TRPV1, TRPA1) on the nociceptors and hence lead to their activation. A variety of drugs such as nonsteroidal anti-inflammatory drugs (i.e., ibuprofen and aspirin) reduce this inflammatory pain by inhibiting prostaglandin synthesis through cyclooxygenase 1 and 2 inhibition.

Various nerve fibers in the PNS detect different mechanical stimuli of varying intensity as shown in Table 2-1. However, unlike the nociceptive receptors activated by thermal or chemical stimuli, those activated by mechanical stimuli are not yet clear. Part of the challenge in elucidating these receptors is limitations in developing accurate experimental models to study noxious mechanical insults. Nonetheless, studies involving the worm *Caenorhabditis elegans* have identified a group of sodium channels located on the epithelium named acid-sensing ion channels (ASICs) as potentially involved in mechanical activation of nociceptors. However, studies on mice lacking functional ASICs did not show significant deficits in mechanical nociception, rendering the involvement of these channels questionable.[12]

Pain Signal Conduction

Once the aforementioned thermal, chemical, or mechanical stimuli activate the Aδ or C fiber afferent terminal, an electrical signal is made, which is transmitted through the activity of various ion channels throughout the neuron. Various voltage-gated sodium and potassium channels are responsible for signal propagation throughout the neuron. Indeed, local anesthetics block pain transmission through targeting these ion channels.

The neuronal sodium channels have 2 functional gates: an outer m gate and an inner h gate. These gates, depending on their "open" or "closed" status, allow the influx or outflow of sodium from the neuron. In the resting state, the outer m gate is closed, whereas the inner h gate is open. On nerve stimulation, the sodium ionophore is activated with opening of the m gate and hence the rapid inward flux of sodium and action potential propagation down the neuron. Local anesthetics are able to enter the neuron across the lipid membrane or through the channels themselves. Once inside the neuron, they bind and block the sodium ionophore from within the cell and therefore prevent propagation of the axonal action potential.[13] To further highlight the role of sodium channels in signal conduction and pain perception, humans with loss of function of the Nav1.7 subtype of sodium channels are unable to detect noxious stimuli.[14]

Voltage-gated calcium channels, although not involved in electrical signal propagation through the neuron, do play a key role in neurotransmitter release to the spinal cord from nociceptor terminals. These voltage-gated calcium channels are composed of 4 pore-forming subunits. The gabapentinoid anticonvulsants, gabapentin and pregabalin, act by blocking the α2δ subunit of calcium channels thereby preventing neurotransmitter release from the nociceptor terminals at the level of the spinal cord, a treatment now widely used to treat neuropathic pain.[15]

Peripheral and Central Sensitization

Peripheral sensitization can occur when local inflammatory changes cause diminished threshold to nociceptor activation due to increased firing from hyperexcitable neurons. Briefly, neurons become excitable with the release of various chemicals such as calcitonin gene-related peptide (CGRP) and substance P from nociceptors, which in turn increase vascular permeability and edema, which allows for influx of bradykinin, cytokines, and growth factors. Increase in ectopic activity along nerves can also result in hyperexcitable neurons.[16] These changes lead to decreased perception threshold for pain signals peripherally.

In certain cases, persistent peripheral pain signal conduction can similarly lead to a process called central sensitization. There is no single mechanism responsible for central sensitization. Central sensitization refers to various neuronal changes in the CNS that render it overtly sensitized, with the end result of increased pain perception. In the face of repetitive noxious stimuli, or in the event of particularly intense noxious stimuli, the threshold for the activation of the nociceptive system decreases so that further noxious stimuli are even more amplified. With time, the nociceptive system returns to its normal baseline. However, certain neuronal changes can cause this state of "heightened awareness" to persist, leading to chronically painful conditions. When this occurs, pain perception is no longer a protective defense mechanism. Instead, normally innocuous stimuli can become painful (allodynia), there can be a prolonged and intensified response to noxious stimuli (hyperalgesia), or the painful sensation can spread beyond the site of injury (secondary hyperalgesia).[17]

Glutamate is the primary neurotransmitter released by peripheral nociceptors onto their second-order neurons. It binds to several different types of receptors, including amino-3-hydroxy-5-methyl-4-isoxazole propionate (AMPA), *N*-methyl-ᴅ-aspartate (NMDA), and kainate receptors. The NMDA receptor is a key player in the central sensitization process. Under normal circumstances, the NMDA receptor is at rest and is blocked by a single magnesium ion sitting at its pore. Repetitive or particularly intense noxious stimuli lead to a continuous release of glutamate (and other neuropeptides such as substance P and CGRP), causing magnesium to relieve the block, and subsequently calcium is allowed to flow into the cell. As a result of the increased intracellular calcium, various signaling pathways and calcium-dependent kinases are activated. These signaling pathways lead to increased synaptic efficacy and cause phosphorylation of NMDA and AMPA receptors, which increases their activity, conductance, and density on the lipid membrane, causing postsynaptic hyperexcitability.[17]

Central sensitization also contributes to allodynia and neuropathic pain. As a result of peripheral nerve damage, sensory neurons in the DRG develop certain changes in their gene expressions, effecting approximately 1000 transcripts, including ion channels, receptors, transmitters, and axonal regeneration. Moreover, peripheral nerve injury causes degeneration of C fibers in lamina II. Together, this combination of decreased afferent C fiber input with the increased regenerative gene expression, creates the molecular environment for myelinated Aβ fibers to grow synapses into lamina I and II and create new nociceptive inputs.[17-19] As a result, Aβ fibers, which were originally involved only in light touch and pressure sensations, are then transmitting nociceptive information as well.

Glial Cell Interactions

The traditional view that chronic pain states emerge solely from neuronal damage that results in activation of ascending pain pathways or from changes in neuronal function has been challenged by a growing body of evidence that demonstrates remarkable regulation of neuronal activity by the immune system.[20] Glial cells (astrocytes and microglia) represent the most abundant cells in the CNS and under normal circumstances function as resident macrophages.[21] Research in the last decade has found painful syndromes to be associated with glial cell upregulation and activation, leading to a new paradigm that considers some chronic pain conditions to be, at least partially, a state of "gliopathy."[22] Within hours of a peripheral nerve injury microglia accumulate in the dorsal horn of the spinal cord where they release a variety of signaling molecules including cytokines (i.e., TNF-alpha, interleukin-1beta and 6), which promote central sensitization. This is also illustrated by the observation that injection of activated microglia into the cerebral spinal fluid can reproduce behavioral changes seen with nerve injury.[4,23]

THE SPINAL CORD AND ASCENDING NOCICEPTIVE TRACKS

As mentioned earlier, nociceptors send axonal projections to the spinal cord. Specifically, these axonal projections enter the gray matter of the spinal cord's dorsal column. Here they synapse onto second-order neurons, which then travel cephalad toward the brain. Not all nociceptor axons, however, terminate on second-order neurons at the same level as their own cell body is located in the DRG—some traverse caudally or rostrally 1 or 2 spinal segments before synapsing in what is termed Lissauer's dorsolateral tract.[24]

The gray matter of the spinal cord is divided into 10 organized laminae (Rexed laminae I-X). Various peripheral nerves (including nociceptors) terminate on specific laminae where they communicate with their respective second-order neurons. In regards to nociceptors, C fibers terminate onto laminae I and II (lamina II is also called substantia gelatinosa based on its physical appearance), whereas Aδ fibers terminate on lamina I and V. Interestingly, the second-order neurons in lamina I and V form the multiple ascending pathways that project to the brain, whereas the C fibers terminating in lamina II mostly synapse predominantly with interneurons, which then project deeper to lamina V and its ascending neurons. Moreover, lamina V also receives input from visceral afferent as well as Aβ fibers that mediate cutaneous light touch and pressure. As such, one can see that lamina V neurons receive various noxious and nonnoxious inputs, leading to them being called wide dynamic range neurons[18,24] (Figure 2-2).

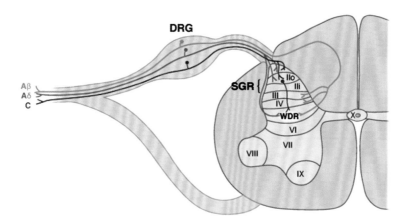

FIGURE 2-2 Schematic representation of the spinal projections of primary afferent fibers. In general, unmyelinated C fibers synapse with the interneurons in laminae I (marginal layer) and II (substantia gelatinosa of Rolando [SGR]). Cutaneous Aδ fibers usually project to laminae I, II, and V, and Aβ fibers primarily terminate in laminae III, IV, and V in the dorsal horn. Large-diameter myelinated fibers innervating muscles, joint, and viscera may also terminate in laminae I, IV-VII and the ventral horn. Second-order wide dynamic range (WDR) neurons are located in lamina V and receive input from nociceptive and nonnociceptive neurons. DRG, dorsal root ganglia. Reprinted with permission from Flood P, Rathmell JP, Shafer S. Stoeltings Pharmacology and Physiology in Anesthetic Practice. 5th ed. Philadelphia, PA: Wolters Kluwer; 2015.

The main nociceptive output from the dorsal column of the spinal cord that travels to the brain is composed of second-order neurons from laminae I and V. These cephalad projections of second-order neurons together form the spinothalamic and spinoreticulothalamic tracts that cross to the spinal cord to synapse on contralateral thalamic and brainstem nuclei as illustrated in Figure 2-3. Specifically, the spinothalamic tract projects to the ventral posterolateral thalamic nucleus and relays discriminative information about the nature of a noxious stimulus. In contrast, the spinoreticulothalamic tract projects to various brainstem nuclei before projecting to the medial thalamus. As such, the spinoreticulothalamic tract contributes to the negative affective components of pain perception that involve the amygdala and limbic system[24] (Table 2-2).

INHIBITORY TRACTS

Various inhibitory neurons and descending pathways play a significant role in pain modulation. This concept was first introduced by Melzack and Wall in 1965 who hypothesized the "gate control theory" of pain by postulating that loss of inhibitory interneurons in the dorsal horn can contribute to pain. Today we know the dorsal horn is in fact densely populated by these inhibitory interneurons, which use gamma-amino butyric acid (GABA) and glycine as their neurotransmitters to inhibit pain. Experiments in rodents have shown that intrathecal administration of GABA and glycine antagonists produce hypersensitivity behaviors similar to that observed after peripheral nerve injury.[4] In contrast, the intrathecal administration of GABA agonists, such as midazolam, has been shown to produce analgesia. Peripheral nerve injury may cause a reduction in GABA interneuron

density, adding disinhibition as a contributing factor to chronic neuropathic pain development following peripheral nerve injury.[24]

In addition to the inhibitory interneurons of the spinal cord, various descending supraspinal tracts also contribute to dorsal horn nociceptive transmission. The periaqueductal gray (PAG) and the rostral ventromedial medulla (RVM) form the PAG-RVM-DH (dorsal horn) descending inhibitory pathway. The PAG and RVM receive input from various centers of the brain, including the hypothalamus, amygdala, and prefrontal cortex. The inhibitory neurons then terminate in the dorsal horn predominantly in laminae I and II, and also in other laminae, including IV, V, VI, and X, to modulate nociceptive transmission.[2,18,25]

The RVM is composed of both serotonergic neurons (from the nucleus raphe magnus) and noradrenergic neurons (from the nucleus reticularis gigantocellularis), which receive input from the opioid receptor–rich PAG. PAG and RVM receptors are primary sites of action of systemic opioids. Stimulation of the PAG or RVM leads to the release of serotonin in the spinal cord, which can inhibit or promote the excitability of spinothalamic neurons depending on the type of serotonin receptor activated.[25]

Descending noradrenergic pathways originating from the pontine region of the brain have antinociceptive effects at the level of the dorsal horn. These pathways elicit their effect by activating α2 receptors on primary afferent nociceptors. It is through these descending inhibitory pathways and their neurotransmitters that various medications, such as tricyclic antidepressants and serotonin-norepinephrine reuptake inhibitors, are thought to exert their mechanism of action in the treatment of neuropathic pain[25] (Figure 2-3).

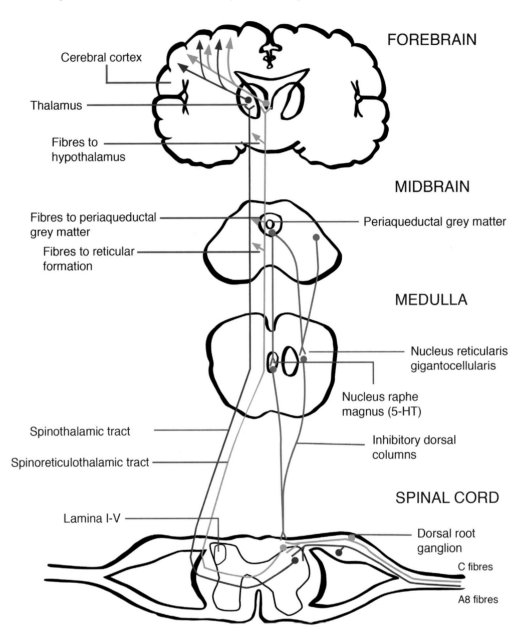

FIGURE 2-3 Illustration depicting the role of descending inhibitory tracts in modulating the pain response (blue). The descending noradrenergic (NE) and serotonergic (5-HT) pathways originating from the brainstem are involved in pain modulation at the level of the dorsal horn.

TABLE 2-2 Brain Regions Involved With Pain and Brief Description of Some of the Proposed Functions

BRAIN REGION	FUNCTIONS
Anterior cingulate cortex	Affective, emotional component to pain; suffering and coping behaviors
Insular cortex	May play a role in negative affective pain processing
Prefrontal cortex	Memory retrieval, decision making, and attention processing in relation to pain
Primary and secondary somatosensory cortices	Localization of pain; pain discrimination
Nucleus accumbens	Placebo analgesia
Amygdala and limbic system	Emotional events surrounding painful stimuli; fear response to pain
Hippocampus	Storage of past painful events

Reproduced from Cohen SP, Mao J. Neuropathic pain: mechanisms and their clinical implications. BMJ. 2014;348:f7656. With permission from BMJ Publishing Group Ltd.

CONCLUSION

Pain anatomy and physiology involves complex anatomical and biochemical systems. Significant progress has been made in understanding the basic functioning of nociceptors as well as fundamental ascending and descending pain pathways. However, the underlying mechanism of various chronic pain states remains to be elucidated. Much progress must still be made in understanding the mechanisms through which nervous system pathology results in chronic hyperexcitable states.

Persistent and intense pain can lead to neuroplastic changes within the nervous system, rendering the basic science of pain physiology even more challenging. Novel neuroanatomical techniques (i.e., functional magnetic resonance imaging and positron emission tomography) are being used to further investigate in vivo brain activity in the chronic pain state. As our understanding of pain anatomy and physiology evolves, so will our therapeutic drugs and interventional procedures. Having an up-to-date understanding of our current knowledge in chronic pain medicine, while also being cognizant of the many limitations the basic science of chronic pain holds, will help providers in selecting appropriate treatments for the patient with chronic pain.

REFERENCES

1. Dallenbach KM. Pain: history and present status. *Am J Psychol.* 1939;52:331-347.
2. Brenner GJ. The Massachusetts General Hospital Handbook of pain management. In: Ballantyne JC, ed. *The Massachusetts General Hospital Handbook of Pain Management.* Lippincott Williams & Wilkins; 2006:3-18.
3. Merskey H, Bogduk N. Classification of chronic pain. *IASP Pain Terminol.* 1994. doi:10.1002/ana.20394.
4. Basbaum AI, Bautista DM, Scherrer G, Julius D. Cellular and molecular mechanisms of pain. *Cell.* 2009;139:267-284.
5. Basbaum AI, Jessell TM. Principles of neural science. *Neurology.* 2000. doi:10.1036/0838577016.
6. Meyer RA, Ringkamp M, Campbell JN, Raja S. Peripheral mechanisms of cutaneous nociception. In: *Wall and Melzack's Textbook of Pain.* 2006:3-34. doi:10.1016/B978-0-7020-4059-7.00001-2.
7. Cesare P, McNaughton P. A novel heat-activated current in nociceptive neurons and its sensitization by bradykinin. *Proc Natl Acad Sci USA.* 1996;93:15435-15439.
8. Caterina MJ. Impaired nociception and pain sensation in mice lacking the capsaicin receptor. *Science.* 2000;288:306-313.
9. Anand P, Bley K. Topical capsaicin for pain management: therapeutic potential and mechanisms of action of the new high-concentration capsaicin 8 patch. *Br J Anaesth.* 2011;107:490-502.
10. Bautista DM, Jordt SE, Nikai T, et al. TRPA1 mediates the inflammatory actions of environmental irritants and proalgesic agents. *Cell.* 2006;124:1269-1282.
11. Caceres AI, Brackmann M, Elia MD, et al. A sensory neuronal ion channel essential for airway inflammation and hyperreactivity in asthma. *Proc Natl Acad Sci USA.* 2009;106:9099-9104.
12. Page AJ, Brierley SM, Martin CM, et al. The ion channel ASIC1 contributes to visceral but not cutaneous mechanoreceptor function. *Gastroenterology.* 2004;127:1739-1747.
13. Columb MO, MacLennan K. Local anaesthetic agent. *Anaesth Intensive Care Med.* 2007;8:159-162.
14. Cox JJ, Reimann F, Nicholas AK, et al. An SCN9A channelopathy causes congenital inability to experience pain. *Nature.* 2006;444:894-898.
15. Davies A, Hendrich J, Van Minh AT, et al. Functional biology of the alpha(2)delta subunits of voltage-gated calcium channels. *Trends Pharmacol Sci.* 2007;28:220-228.
16. Cohen SP, Mao J. Neuropathic pain: mechanisms and their clinical implications. *BMJ.* 2014;348:f7656.
17. Latremoliere A, Woolf C. Central sensitization: a generator of pain hypersensitivity by central neural plasticity. *J Pain.* 2010;10:895-926.
18. Wainger B, Brenner GJ. Mechanisms of chronic pain. In Longnecker DE, Mackey SC, Newman MF, Sandberg WS, Zapol WM, eds. *Anesthesiology.* McGraw-Hill Education; 2018:1441-1455.
19. Maratou K, Wallace VC, Hasnie FS, et al. Comparison of dorsal root ganglion gene expression in rat models of traumatic and HIV-associated neuropathic pain. *Eur J Pain* 2009;13:387-398.
20. Watkins LR, Maier SF. The pain of being sick: implications of immune-to-brain communication for understanding pain. *Annu Rev Psychol.* 2000;51:29-57.
21. Gosselin RD, Suter MR, Ji RR, Decosterd I. Glial cells and chronic pain. *Neuroscience.* 2010;16:519-531.

22. Ji RR, Berta T, Nedergaard M. Glia and pain: is chronic pain a gliopathy? *Pain.* 2013;154.

23. Coull JAM, Beggs S, Boudreau D, et al. BDNF from microglia causes the shift in neuronal anion gradient underlying neuropathic pain. *Nature.* 2005;438:1017-1021.

24. Hudspith MJ. Anatomy, physiology and pharmacology of pain. *Anaesth Intensive Care Med.* 2016;17:425-430.

25. Kwon M, Altin M, Duenas H, et al. The role of descending inhibitory pathways on chronic pain modulation and clinical implications. *Pain Pract.* 2014;14:656-668.

3

TARGETED PAIN INTERVIEW

Charles De Mesa, DO, MPH and Dustin Ward, MD

INTRODUCTION

Communication is key in the interview process. Listen and pause to gain a sense of the context of the pain within the individual's life. Check for understanding by summarizing the patient's history of present illness. This offers opportunity for clarification, eliminating any impediment treatment progress. Essential elements of a pain interview will help create a comprehensive and individualized treatment plan. These include the following:

- Chief complaint
- Pain diagram
- Mechanism of injury
- Onset
- Location
- Duration
- Characteristics
- Aggravating/alleviating factors
- Radiation
- Treatments (including psychological treatments, physical therapy, acupuncture, acupressure, chiropractic and/or osteopathic treatments, essential oils, medical cannabinoids in States where it is legal)
- Legal issues
- Surgical, medical, social, and family history
- Substance abuse history

To determine the chief complaint, you may ask "What is the main problem for which you are seeking treatment here today?" Using a pain diagram that enables the patient to mark or shade the areas that are painful (see Fig. 3-1). Next ascertain the onset and duration of pain by asking the following questions: "When did your current pain start? Can you briefly describe how your current pain started?"

MEDICATIONS

Verify current pain medications, dosages, and frequency to determine therapeutic benefit. Obtain a list of previous medications (including psychopharmacologic and over-the-counter drugs), dosages, and frequency including the reasons for discontinuation. This will help identify adequate trial of medications. Determine whether the patient had previous injection therapies, when the injections were performed, and whether any pain relief was attained. For instance, ask "What percentage of pain relief did you derive from the injection(s)?" "How long did your pain relief last following the injection?" Different types of injections may include cervical or lumbar epidural steroid injections, neural blockade procedures, facet (z-joint) blocks, radiofrequency ablations, and joint injections. Previous physical therapy (PT) participation, the specific type of PT, when treatments took place, duration, and whether benefit was derived should also be discussed. For instance, the patient may have participated in a PT program with a focus on acute pain therapeutic modalities rather than functional restoration therapies while concomitantly learning active self-management strategies for chronic pain. In this scenario, successful PT was limited based on approach.

DIAGNOSTIC STUDIES

Previous diagnostic studies including the approximated date and results if known are important. These may include X-rays, CT scans, or MRI imaging. These can be helpful to track changes or detect interval development of a new pain problem. Electromyography (EMG) and nerve conduction studies (NCSs) help to identify abnormalities of peripheral nerves, muscle, and neuromuscular junction (NMJ) function. They can provide information on location of pathology, chronicity, and severity. EMG and NCSs also help determine the progression of abnormalities or

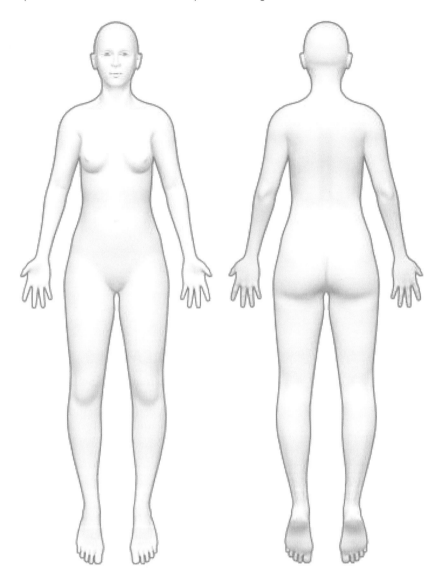

FIGURE 3-1 Example of a pain body diagram which can be marked to communicate the painful area.

recovery from abnormal function. Laboratory studies such as elevated sedimentation rate (ESR) and C-reactive protein (CRP) are helpful in determining associated inflammatory or infectious process requiring further workup. B_{12}, vitamin D, autoimmune-specific labs should be obtained if history and physical examination are concerning for rheumatologic disease.

Identifying other pain problems provides opportunity to address other pain complaints in subsequent visits longitudinally. You may ask, "Do you have other pain problems? Where is your other pain located?" "We will focus on your back pain today because that is worst. On our subsequent visit let's spend time addressing your elbow pain."

PAST HISTORY

Legal issues will have implications in predicting decline in pain and improved function. For example, patients involved in litigation related to pain with associated worker's compensation claim or legal issues may interfere with response to treatments. These individuals may not experience decline in pain and/or improvement in function. Therefore, such information is best known ahead of time.

Psychological treatment should be investigated. Questions may include "Have you ever had psychiatric, physiological, or social work evaluations or treatments for your current problem?" Allow the patient to expand on these. Have him or her elaborate on types of psychological types of treatments that may be relevant (i.e., biofeedback, pain psychologist, mindfulness, meditation).

The effect of pain on employment status should also be determined. Has the employment status been affected by the present pain condition and is the current unemployment because of the present pain condition? If the patient is unemployed, how long has he or she been off work because of pain.

Careful history of past surgical, medical, social, and family history should be acquired. With regard to tobacco use, determining current smoking history, whether the individual ever smoked and the amount smoked (in pack-years), provides an overall assessment. Determine if and when the individual quit smoking and since when can be useful information which can be applied during motivational interviewing (see Chapter 4).

History of alcohol use establishes how many cans or bottles of beer, glasses of wine, and shots of hard liquor are consumed per week. History of alcoholism and whether the patient attended Alcoholics Anonymous program is clinically useful.

Obtaining drug use history should be explicit. For example, rather than asking "Do you use drugs?" it is best to ask "Do you have a history of heroin, cocaine, or amphetamine abuse?" "Do you have addiction to other substances? If so which ones?" Have you ever been in a detoxification program for drug abuse? Do you attend or have you attended Narcotics Anonymous? If you are clean and sober, how long have you been abstinent? "Does anyone in your family have a history of addiction to substances? If so, what is the family relationship?"

Employment history whether full-time, part-time, temporarily disabled, permanently disabled, unemployed, retired, or unemployed because of pain provides insight into the degree to which work is affected from pain. Any history of prior temporary disability or military disability is also helpful.

ASSESSMENT

Common validated outcome measures such as the pain disability index (PDI) assess the extent to which aspects of the patient's life are disrupted by chronic pain.[1] Another rapid measure is a 3-item scale assessing pain intensity and interference known at the PEG scale.[2] It is an ultrabrief pain measure that is perfect for the primary care setting. Such scales can be used to track the effect of interventions for relieving pain and improving function.

PEG: A 3-Item Scale Assessing Pain Intensity and Interference

1. What number best describes your pain on average in the past week?

0   1   2   3   4   5   6   7   8   9   10

No pain   Pain as bad as you
                                     can imagine

2. What number best describes how, during the past week, pain has interfered with your enjoyment of life?

0   1   2   3   4   5   6   7   8   9   10

No pain   Pain as bad as you
                                     can imagine

3. What number best describes how, during the past week, pain has interfered with your general activity?

0   1   2   3   4   5   6   7   8   9   10

No pain   Pain as bad as you
                                     can imagine

To compute the PEG score, add the 3 responses to the questions above, and then divide by 3 to get a final score out of 10.

The final PEG score can mean very different things to different patients. The PEG score, like most other screening instruments, is most useful in tracking changes over time. The PEG score should decrease over time after therapy has begun.

CONCLUSION

Because pain is subjective and therefore an untestable hypothesis, the goal of a targeted pain interview is to listen carefully, ask the right questions, assess function, monitor treatment, and connect with patients so that progress is achieved and healing takes place for all involved.[3]

REFERENCES

1. Tait RC, Chibnall JT, Krause S. The pain disability index: psychometric properties. *Pain.* 1990;40(2):171-182.
2. Krebs EE, Lorenz KA, Bair MJ, et al. Development and initial validation of the PEG, a three-item scale assessing pain intensity and interference. *J Gen Intern Med.* 2009;24(6):733-738.
3. Fishman S. *Listening to Pain.* Waterford Life Sciences; 2006:12-13.

4

MOTIVATIONAL INTERVIEWING

Shelly Henderson, PhD and Amir Ramezani, PhD

FAST FACTS

- Motivational interviewing (MI) is more than the use of a set of techniques or strategies. It is characterized by a particular "spirit" or clinical "way of being" that is the context or interpersonal relationship within which the techniques are employed.
- The spirit of MI is based on 3 key elements: collaboration between the provider and the patient; evoking or drawing out the patient's ideas about change; and emphasizing the autonomy of the patient.
- There are 4 principles that guide the practice of MI: (1) Express Empathy, (2) Support Self-Efficacy, (3) Roll with Resistance, and (4) Develop Discrepancy.

PRIMARY CARE AND CHRONIC PAIN

Primary care providers are on the front lines of managing essential care for individuals experiencing chronic pain. With pain affecting 100 million Americans, 25 million of whom report chronic daily pain,[1] at an estimated economic cost of $560 to 635 billion/year,[2] chronic pain is one of the most important issues in population health and primary care. Yet providers and patients are often dissatisfied with treatment processes and outcomes.[3] Motivational interviewing (MI) promotes self-management and assists patients in moving toward health-related behaviors that aid in chronic pain management.

MI, with its roots in the addiction field, offers an evidence-based approach to address the behaviors related to chronic pain and opiate addiction. MI has been shown to outperform traditional advice giving in the treatment of behavioral problems and diseases related to alcohol abuse, drug addiction, smoking cessation, weight loss, poor treatment adherence, physical inactivity, asthma, and diabetes.[4] Individuals experiencing chronic pain also present with many of the lifestyle-related conditions mentioned above.[5] Pain and its associated symptoms can be modified by behavioral changes. An MI approach has been shown to be successful in relieving pain, improving function, and enhancing the use of self-management skills for people with pain.[6]

Miller and Rollnick (2002) describe MI as a "directive, patient-centered counseling style for enhancing intrinsic motivation to change by exploring and resolving ambivalence."[7] MI is more than the use of a set of techniques or strategies. It is characterized by a particular "spirit" or clinical "way of being" that is the context or interpersonal relationship within which the techniques are employed. That is, the effectiveness of MI depends on the fundamental aspect of how the provider relates to the patient.

SPIRIT OF MOTIVATIONAL INTERVIEWING

The spirit of MI is based on 3 key elements: collaboration between the provider and the patient; evoking or drawing out the patient's ideas about change; and emphasizing the autonomy of the patient.

Collaboration (vs. confrontation) is a partnership between the provider and the patient, grounded in the point of view and experiences of the patient. This contrasts with the traditional biomedical model where the physician is the expert and the patient is passive. Collaboration builds rapport and facilitates trust in the helping relationship, which can be challenging in a more hierarchical relationship. This does not mean that the provider automatically agrees with the patient about the nature of the problem or the changes that may be most appropriate. Although the provider and patient may see things differently, the therapeutic process is focused on mutual understanding, not the provider being right or the patient dictating treatment.

Using MI, the provider draws out the individual's own thoughts and ideas, rather than imposing his or her opinion. This tends to increase the patient's motivation, as commitment to change is most powerful and sustainable when it comes from the patient. Lasting change occurs when the patient discovers his or her own reasons and determination to change. The provider's job is to "draw out" the person's own motivations and skills for change, not to tell him or her what to do or why he or she should do it, no matter how scientifically valid or clinically convincing the provider's reasons may be.

The final element is based on the bioethical principle of autonomy. Unlike the traditional biomedical model that emphasizes the clinician as an authority figure, MI recognizes that the true power for change rests within the patient. Ultimately, the patient is responsible to make a behavioral change that improves his or her health and pain management. This empowers the patient and increases his or her sense of responsibility to take action in his or her pain management care. Providers reinforce that there is no single "right way" to change and that there are multiple ways in which change can occur. In addition to deciding whether they will make a change, patients are encouraged to take the lead in developing a "menu of options" as to how to achieve the desired change.

PRINCIPLES OF MOTIVATIONAL INTERVIEWING

There are 4 principles that guide the practice of MI: (1) Express Empathy, (2) Support Self-Efficacy, (3) Roll with Resistance, and (4) Develop Discrepancy (Table 4-1).

Empathy involves seeing the world through the patient's eyes, thinking about things as the patient thinks about them, and feeling things as the patient feels them to share in the patient's experiences. This approach provides the basis for patients to be heard and understood, and in turn, patients are more likely to honestly share his or her experiences in depth.

For example, a patient tells the primary care provider that he cannot go to work because of his pain and is worried about his finances. The provider mentally places herself in the patient's life and states the following:

- "I imagine not being able to work and worrying about finances is scary."
- "I would feel sad if I could no longer do the things I use to do, particularly at work."

In the above scenarios, the provider communicates to the patient the core emotion that another would feel if they "put him/herself in their shoes." Ultimately, the patient feels emotionally heard. This opens the door to the initial stages of building mutual trust.

Regarding **Self-Efficacy**, MI promotes a strengths-based approach. This means that patients have within themselves the capabilities to change successfully. A patient's belief that change is possible (i.e., self-efficacy) is needed to instill hope about making those difficult changes. Patients often have previously tried and been unable to achieve or maintain the desired change, creating doubt about their ability to succeed. In MI, providers support self-efficacy by focusing on previous successes and highlighting skills and strengths that the patient already has. For example, the provider may state the following to promote self-efficacy:

- "You were successful in coming here today and voicing how you want to improve your health."
- "You have made positive changes in your life."

TABLE 4-1 Motivational Interviewing Principles			
MI PRINCIPLE	**RATIONALE**	**SKILLS/TOOLS**	**AS COMPARED TO …**
Express empathy	• Demonstrate acceptance and understanding of patient ambivalence	• Reflective listening • Open-ended questions • Summary	• Providing data and statistics to convince patient of need for change
Support self efficacy	• Build patient's confidence in his or her ability to change	• Affirmations • Reflect change talk • Identify patient's strengths	• Getting too far ahead of patient (misalignment with stage of change) • Focusing on what's going wrong rather than patient's attempts to change
Roll with resistance	• Refrain from confronting or arguing about patient's behavior • Use as opportunity to learn about patient's experience	• Reflective listening • Open-ended questions	• Engaging in power struggle • Arguing with patients about why they should change • Giving ultimatums
Develop discrepancy	• Evoke/illuminate discrepancy between patient behavior and patient's beliefs/values	• Use decisional balance • Use change rulers • Reflective listening • Open-ended questions • Summary	• Arguing for healthy behavior based on provider's values • Pointing out inconsistencies in patient behavior

- "Managing pain takes time and energy just like you dedicated time and energy in the past when you stopped your alcohol use."
- "Your value of living a healthy life with your daughter helped you to stop smoking in the past; I can see you really care for your daughter. Let's keep this value in mind as we discuss your pain management."

"Rolling with Resistance" means slowing down and reflecting back the patient's concerns. From an MI perspective, resistance in treatment occurs when the patient experiences a conflict between their view of the "problem" or the "solution" and that of the clinician or when the patient experiences their freedom or autonomy being impinged upon. These experiences are often based on the patient's ambivalence about change, which is a normal part of the change process. In MI, providers avoid eliciting resistance by not confronting the patient, and when resistance occurs, they work to de-escalate and avoid a negative interaction, instead "rolling with it." Actions and statements that demonstrate resistance remain unchallenged especially early in the treatment relationship. The MI value on having the patient define the problem and develop his or her own solutions leaves little for the patient to resist. A frequently used metaphor is "dancing" rather than "wrestling" with the patient. In exploring patient concerns, health care providers invite patients to examine new points of view and are careful not to impose their own ways of thinking. A key concept is that providers avoid the "righting reflex," a tendency born from concern, to ensure that the patient understands and agrees with the need to change and to solve the problem for the patient. An example of rolling with resistance includes the following:

A primary care provider wants to lower the patient's opioids because she is feeling sedated with oxycodone.

- Patient: "I need my medication, I don't want to stop it. It helps me go to work!"
- Provider: "It's stressful to even think about changing the oxycodone. You need it to go to work." (Complex Reflection). "I wonder if we can brainstorm some solutions? How do you think we can provide you with pain relief at work but with less sedating effects of the oxycodone?"

This empathetic and reflective response builds rapport and trust between the patient and provider allowing for further conversation. If resistance continues, the provider may respond, "I see that work and pain relief are important to you. Can I have your permission to return to opioid medications at later time? I really want for us to spend a good amount of time thinking about pain management options that are right for you and that I feel comfortable with."

Motivation for change occurs when people perceive a mismatch between "where they are and where they want to be." Providers practicing MI work to develop this by helping patients examine the discrepancies between their current behavior and their values and future goals. When patients recognize that their current behaviors place them in conflict with their values or interfere with accomplishment of self-identified goals, they are more likely to experience increased motivation to make important life changes. It is important that the provider using MI does not use strategies to develop discrepancy at the expense of the other principles (such as empathy and self-efficacy). The provider aims to gradually help patients to become aware of how current behaviors may lead them away from, rather than toward, their important goals. For example, providers may highlight the discrepancy by stating the following:

- For the patient who is ambivalent about taking antidepressants: "You mentioned that your goal is to return to work. How do your current problems with your mood fit into that plan?"
- For the patient who is ambivalent about physical therapy: "Your goal is to wean off pain pills. How does physical therapy fit in with that goal?"
- For the patient who is ambivalent about dietary changes for weight loss: "You want to lose weight as a way to manage your back pain. How does your soda intake fit with that goal?"

The practice of MI involves the skillful use of certain techniques for bringing to life the "MI spirit," demonstrating the MI principles and guiding the process toward eliciting patient change talk and commitment for change. Change talk involves statements or nonverbal communications indicating the patient may be considering the possibility of change. We will return to change talk and go through specific examples in an upcoming section of this chapter.

SKILLS OF MOTIVATIONAL INTERVIEWING

Often called microcounseling skills, OARS[8] is a brief way to remember the basic approach used in MI: open-ended questions, affirmations, reflections, and summaries are core provider behaviors employed to move the process forward by establishing a therapeutic alliance and eliciting discussion about change.

Open-ended questions are not easily answered with a "yes/no" or short answer containing only a specific, limited piece of information. Open-ended questions invite elaboration and thinking more deeply about an issue. Although closed questions have their place and are at times valuable (e.g., when collecting specific information in an assessment), open-ended questions create forward momentum used to help the patient explore the reasons for and possibility of change. For example, the provider suspects depression with his patient. The provider may ask a patient with chronic pain the following open-ended questions to better learn about the relationship of pain and depression:

- "What role does pain play in the way you feel emotionally?"
- "How does stress impact your pain?"
- "How do you cope with depression and pain?"
- "What are the advantages of treating depression when it comes to managing pain?"
- "What are the things you would do in your life if pain and depression were not in the picture?"

Affirmations are statements that recognize patient strengths. They assist in building rapport and in helping the patient see himself or herself in a different, more positive light. To be effective they must be congruent and genuine. The use of affirmations can help patients feel that change is possible even when previous efforts have been unsuccessful. Affirmations often involve reframing behaviors or concerns as evidence of positive patient qualities. Affirmations are a key element in facilitating the MI principle of Supporting Self-Efficacy. For instance, a provider helps a patient to recognize the positive aspects of depression and pain by stating the following:

- "I appreciate you being honest with me and yourself about how much physical therapy you actually did last week."
- "I want to thank you for your openness and trust in me to talk about the sadness you are experiencing because of the pain. This helps me to better address all aspects of your life."
- "You showed courage and strength when you stopped smoking in the past. I can see your courage and strength now, too, as we work together to help you with pain and opioid management."
- "I can see that your concern about how pain interferes with work and finances reflects how much you care about your family."

Reflections (also called reflective listening) are perhaps the most crucial skill in MI. They have 2 primary purposes. First is to bring to life the principle of Expressing Empathy. By careful listening and reflecting responses, the patient comes to feel that the provider understands the issues from his or her perspective. Beyond this, strategic use of reflective listening is a core intervention toward guiding the patient toward change, supporting the goal-directed aspect of MI. In this use of reflections, the provider guides the patient toward resolving ambivalence by a focus on the negative aspects of the status quo and the positives of making change. There are several levels of reflection ranging from simple to more complex. Different types of reflections are skillfully used as patients demonstrate different levels of readiness for change. For example, some types of reflections are more helpful when the patient seems resistant and others more appropriate when the patient offers statements more indicative of commitment to change. Examples of reflections were noted when discussing the principle of developing discrepancies. **Summaries** are a special type of reflection where the provider recaps what has occurred in all or part of a health care visit. Summaries communicate interest, understanding, and call attention to important elements of the discussion. They may be used to shift attention or direction and prepare the patient to "move on." Summaries can highlight both sides of a patient's ambivalence about change and promote the development of discrepancy by strategically selecting what information should be included and what can be minimized or excluded.

CHANGE TALK

Change talk is defined as statements by the patient revealing consideration of, motivation for, or commitment to change. In MI, the provider seeks to guide the patient to expressions of change talk as the pathway to change. Research indicates a clear correlation between patient statements about change and outcomes. This means that the more someone talks about change, the more likely they are to change. Different types of change talk can be described using the mnemonic DARN-CAT.[9]

- **D**esire (I want to change)
- **A**bility (I can change)
- **R**eason (It is important to change)
- **N**eed (I should change)
- **C**ommitment (I will make changes)
- **A**ctivation (I am ready, prepared, and willing to change)
- **T**aking Steps (I am taking specific actions to change)

Commitment, activation, and taking steps are examples of implementing change talk and are the most predictive of a positive outcome.

STRATEGIES FOR EVOKING CHANGE TALK

There are specific therapeutic strategies that are likely to elicit and support change talk in MI. The following is a list of 10 tools that can be used in any given patient encounter.[8]

1. Ask Evocative Questions: Ask an open-ended question, the answer to which is likely to be change talk.
2. Explore Decisional Balance: Ask for the pros and cons of both changing and staying the same.
3. Good Things/Not-So-Good Things: Ask about the positives and negatives of the target behavior.
4. Ask for Elaboration/Examples: When a change talk theme emerges, ask for more details. "In what ways?" "Tell me more?" "What does that look like?" "When was the last time that happened?"
5. Look Back: Ask about a time before the target behavior emerged. How were things better, different?
6. Look Forward: Ask what may happen if things continue as they are (status quo). Try the miracle question: If you were 100% successful in making the changes you want, what would be different? How would you like your life to be 5 years from now?
7. Query Extremes: What are the worst things that might happen if you do not make this change? What are the best things that might happen if you do make this change?
8. Use Change Rulers: Ask: "On a scale from 1 to 10, how important is it to you to change [the specific target behavior] where 1 is not at all important, and a 10 is extremely important? Follow-up: "And why are you at ___and not _____ [a lower number than stated]?" "What might happen that could move you from ___ to [a higher

number]?" Alternatively, you could also ask "How confident are that you could make the change if you decided to do it?"

9. Explore Goals and Values: Ask what the person's guiding values are. What does he or she want in life? Ask how the continuation of target behavior fits in with the person's goals or values. Does it help realize an important goal or value, interfere with it, or is it irrelevant?

10. Come Alongside: Explicitly side with the negative (status quo) side of ambivalence. "Perhaps _____ is so important to you that you won't give it up, no matter what the cost."

STAGES OF CHANGE

Assessing readiness to change is a critical aspect of MI. Motivation, which is considered a state not a trait, is not static and thus can change rapidly from day to day. If providers know where patients are in terms of their readiness to change, they will be better prepared to recognize and deal with a patient's motivation to change. The Stages of Change model[10] shows that, for most people,

a change in behavior occurs gradually, with the patient moving from being uninterested, unaware, or unwilling to make a change (precontemplation), to considering a change (contemplation), to deciding and preparing to make a change (preparation) (Table 4-2). Genuine, determined action is then taken (action) and, over time, attempts to maintain the new behavior occur (maintenance). Relapses are almost inevitable and become part of the process of working toward life-long change.

A simple and quick way to assess stage of change is to use a Readiness to Change Ruler.[8] This scaling strategy conceptualizes readiness or motivation to change along a continuum and asks patients to give voice to how ready they are to change using a ruler with a 10-point scale where 1 = definitely not ready to change and 10 = definitely ready to change. Depending on where the patient is, the subsequent conversation may take different directions. The central dilemma for most people who are confronting health behavior change is ambivalence. Ambivalence is a state of having simultaneous, conflicting feelings toward both a current behavior and a new behavior. Ambivalence is most prominent during the contemplative stage.

TABLE 4-2 Intervention for Stage of Change	
STAGE OF CHANGE	**MI INTERVENTION**
Precontemplation The patient is not yet considering change or is unwilling or unable to change.	• Establish rapport, ask permission, and build trust • Elicit the patient's perceptions of the problem • Provide personalized feedback about assessment findings • Express concern and keep the door open

Contemplation
The patient acknowledges concerns and is considering the possibility of change but is ambivalent and uncertain.
	• Normalize ambivalence
	• Help the patient "tip the decisional balance scales" toward change by:
	  • Eliciting and weighing pros and cons of behavior
	  • Examining the patient's personal values in relation to change
	  • Emphasizing patient autonomy

Preparation The patient is committed to and planning to make a change in the near future but is still considering what to do.	• Clarify the patient's own goals and strategies for change • Offer a menu of options for change or treatment • With permission, offer expertise and advice • Consider and problem-solve barriers to change • Explore treatment expectancies and the patient's role • Elicit from the patient what has worked in the past
Action The patient is actively taking steps to change but has not yet reached a stable state	• Support a realistic view of change through small steps • Normalize difficulties for the patient in early stages of change • Help the patient identify high-risk situations and develop appropriate coping strategies to overcome these • Assist the patient in finding new support for positive change
Maintenance The patient has achieved initial goals such and is now working to maintain gains.	• Affirm the patient's resolve and self-efficacy • Affirm the use of new coping strategies to avoid a return to old behavior • Maintain supportive contact • Develop a "fire escape" plan if the patient resumes old behavior
Relapse The patient has experienced a recurrence of symptoms and must now cope with consequences and decide what to do next.	• Help the patient re-enter the change cycle and commend any willingness to reconsider positive change • Explore the meaning and reality of the relapse as a learning opportunity • Assist the patient in finding alternative coping strategies • Maintain supportive contact

When using MI in the primary care setting, it is essential to focus on 1 behavior at a time. Once the provider and patient have agreed upon an agenda for the visit and the patient has identified a behavior of concern, the provider can use a 3-step process to frame the conversation. Elicit-Provide-Elicit is a simple approach that is congruent with MI. The steps are as follows: (1) Determine what the patient already knows, (2) Reflect what they know and add information to help them understand more fully, and (3) Ask what they want to know more about. For example, after determining that a patient is ambivalent about exercise, the provider may elicit from the patient:

- "Tell me what you know about the impact of exercise on back pain?"
- "What do you think would be the benefits of more regular exercise?"
- "What would you be most interested in knowing about exercise for back pain?"

After listing to the patient's perspective and understanding, the clinician asks for permission before offering advice. This increases the likelihood that the patient will not be resistant to the suggestions offered. The clinician provides information:

- "I am aware of some strategies other people have found helpful. Would you like to hear about some of these?"

"I wonder what you will think about this...." "See which of these you think might apply to you..." Lastly, the provider follows with open-ended questions to check in with the patient and elicit his or her feedback:

- "What else would you like to know?"
- "What do you think is the next step for you?"
- "So what do you make of that?"
- "What do you think about that?"
- "What does all of this mean to you?"
- "How does that apply to you?"

Cases Example

A 56-year-old woman with obesity, sleep apnea, depression, and chronic lumbar radiculopathy is focused on taking Norco 10 to 325 mg 6 times per day. She reports "this medication is not working. I can't go to work and I definitely can't exercise – it hurts too much." She describes low motivation and depression. The primary care provider decides to utilize principles of MI. The following is the conversation between the provider and the patient:

Provider: I appreciate you bringing the issue of your medications to the front of our appointment. Would you like to make this the focus of our meeting today? (Support Self-Efficacy, inviting the patient to develop an agenda and increase participation and responsibility).

Patient: Yes the Norco has not been working; I cannot go to work. I feel like I just use the Norco to slow down my thoughts and relax. I need to stop taking it because my whole life is centered around Norco, but I get nervous if I stop it.

Provider: The Norco is not working, and you are feeling like you want to stop but you feel nervous. I can see that could be stressful. Have you ever stopped any medication or substance in the past? (Reflection, Self-Efficacy, Express Empathy).

Patient: Yes, I stopped smoking. It was really hard but I did it!

Provider: What allowed you to successfully quit? (Open-ended question).

Patient: I stopped because my mother died of a heart attack and I don't want to die like she did; I want to be around for my daughter.

Provider: You value living a full life and not letting your life be shortened by a medical condition. You want to be around for your daughter. (Complex Reflection; Supporting Self-Efficacy).

In the above scenario, the provider affirms and reflects back the values that helped the patient make a change in the past (e.g., values of living life, health, and being a mother for her daughter). In the future, the provider can use the patient's self-efficacy to plant the seed to make the same health-related change when it comes to managing the detrimental effects of high-dose opioid use. The following is the continuation of the dialog between the provider and patient:

Patient: Yes I love my daughter, she is very important to me.

Provider: You want to be present for her. (Complex Reflection).

Patient: The pain keeps me from spending time with her.

Provider: I imagine not being able to spend time with your daughter feels like you are missing out. (Reflection and Expressing Empathy).

Patient: I don't feel like myself anymore. I lost who I was because of the pain; I just want to go to work and be a mother again.

Provider: What are some solutions we can think about together? I am specifically thinking about solutions when it comes to managing the Norco so it is not too sedating? What are some ways to better help you function at work without sedation? What are some solutions to help you spend more time with your daughter?

CONCLUSION

Repeatedly educating our patients about the dangers of various therapeutic options, such as opiate use, and the importance of health behavior change for chronic pain management is not always successful and can become frustrating for the primary care provider and patient. A feeling of failure, especially when repeated, may cause patients to give up and avoid contact with their provider or avoid treatment altogether. Patients who fail are often labeled "noncompliant" or "unmotivated." Labeling a patient in this way places responsibility for failure on the patient's character and ignores the complexity of the behavior change process.

MI is an evidence-based communication style that brings patients and their primary care providers into a partnership and prevents the stalemate that so often plagues difficult interactions around chronic pain management and health behavior change. These principles and techniques are foundational concepts that are at the root of any therapeutic relationship that intends to bring about change in health-related behaviors.[11] The markers of a productive MI encounter are the following:

- The patient does most of the talking and the work.
- The patient accepts the possibility of change.
- The patient accepts responsibility for change.
- The visit feels like dancing, not wrestling.

REFERENCES

1. Nahin RL. Estimates of pain prevalence and severity in adults: United States, 2012. *J Pain.* 2015;16(8):769-780.
2. Gaskin DJ, Richard P. The economic costs of pain in the United States. *J Pain.* 2012;13(8):715-724.
3. Upshur CC, Luckmann RS, Savageau JA. Primary care provider concerns about management of chronic pain in community clinic populations. *J Gen Intern Med.* 2006;21(6):652-655.
4. Rubak S, Sandbaek A, Lauritzen T, Christensen B. Motivational interviewing: a systematic review & meta-analysis. *Br J Gen Pract.* 2005;55(513):305-312.
5. Ang DC, Kaleth AS, Bigatti S, et al. Research to Encourage Exercise for Fibromyalgia (REEF): use of motivational interviewing design and method. *Contemp Clin Trials.* 2011;32(1):59-68.
6. Turk DC, Gatchel RJ. *Psychological Approaches to Pain Management: A Practitioner's Handbook.* 2nd ed. New York: Guilford; 2002.
7. Miller WR, Rollnick S. *Motivational Interviewing: Preparing People for Change.* 2nd ed. New York: Guilford Press; 2002.
8. Miller WR, Rollnick S. *Motivtional Interviewing: Helping People Change.* 3rd ed. NewYork: Guilford Press; 2013.
9. Rollnick S,Miller W, Butler C. *Health Behavior Change: A Guide for Practitioners.* Edinburgh: Churchill Livingstone; 1999.
10. Prochaska JO, DiClemente CC, Norcross JC. In search of how people change. *Am Psychol.* 1992;47:1102-1104.
11. Ramezani A, Rockers DM, Wanlass RL, McCarron RM. Teaching behavioral medicine professionals and trainees an elaborated version of the Y-Model: implications for the integration of cognitive-behavioral therapy (CBT), psychodynamic therapy, and motivational interviewing. *J Psychother Integr.* 2016;26(4):407-424.

5

RATIONAL ANALGESIC POLYPHARMACOTHERAPY: A NOVEL TREATMENT APPROACH IN PAIN MANAGEMENT

Joseph Solberg, DO and Hunter Vincent, DO

OVERVIEW
PAIN GENERATORS
  Neuropathic Pain
  Nociceptive Pain
  Cancer Pain
    References

FAST FACTS

1. Rational analgesic polypharmacotherapy (RAPP) is a novel multidimensional approach to combination drug therapy, which places greater emphasis on a patient's comorbid medical conditions, medication side effect profile, and drug mechanism of action to provide safer and more efficacious pain management.
2. If a combination of 2 medications does not deviate significantly from the individual dose response curve, then the drugs are considered additive. However, if the addition of a second drug creates a larger pain-relieving effect, they are considered supra-additive or synergistic.

Any treatment algorithm for managing pain is often met with significant barriers owing to the subjective nature of pain, variable intensity, and biopsychosocial factors that influence the patient experience. Although a multimodal approach to pain management is often efficacious, it is important to understand the role of pharmacotherapy. Identifying the cause of a painful condition, whether it be mechanical, neuropathic, inflammatory, cancer-related, or a combination of these is integral in determining which pharmacologic intervention is most applicable. Research has investigated a pharmacologic strategy known as combination drug therapy (CDT), which in theory involves the use of additive or synergistic drugs to achieve more effective pain relief.[1] However, because of our incomplete understanding of pain mechanisms, a paucity of clinical research, and vast medication options, most applications of CDT are largely based on clinical experience and anecdotal evidence. A safer and more appropriate approach to pharmacologic intervention with CDT is termed rational analgesic polypharmacotherapy (RAPP). This incorporates a multidimensional perspective of a patient's unique clinical history and pain symptoms (see Figure 5-1).

RAPP is a novel multidimensional approach to CDT, which places greater emphasis on a patient's comorbid medical conditions and medication side-effect profile. This approach utilizes scientific principles to create a more individualized multidrug pain management regimen tailored to each individual patient. When utilizing RAPP, it is important to understand the therapeutic interactions between medications. By definition, if a combination of 2 medications does not deviate significantly from the individual dose response curve, then the drugs are considered additive. However, if the addition of a second drug creates a larger pain-relieving effect, they are considered supra-additive or synergistic.[1] The pain-relieving effects of this multidrug approach can be achieved via drugs of the same class with differing pharmacokinetics, drugs of different drug classes, or different combinations of drugs with different routes of administration. RAPP also uses strategies such as medication cycling, which limits consistent exposure to 1 specific medication or combines drugs at lower doses to reduce overall side effects of individual medications. In this chapter, we will discuss the principles of RAPP

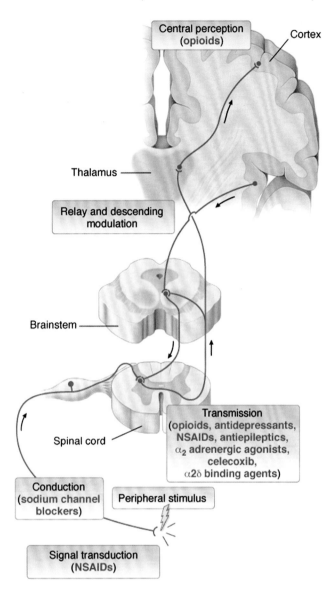

FIGURE 5-1 Summary of the sites of action of the major drug classes used for pain management. Analgesics target various steps in pain perception, from the initiation of a pain stimulus to the central perception of that pain. Nonsteroidal anti-inflammatory drugs (NSAIDs) modulate the initial membrane depolarization (signal transduction) in response to a peripheral stimulus. Sodium channel blockers decrease action potential conduction in nociceptive fibers. Opioids, antidepressants, NSAIDs, antiepileptic drugs (anticonvulsants), and α2-adrenergic agonists all modulate transmission of pain sensation in the spinal cord by decreasing the signal relayed from peripheral to central pain pathways. Opioids also modulate the central perception of painful stimuli. The multiple sites of action of analgesics allow a combination drug approach to be used in pain management. For example, moderate pain is often treated with combinations of opioids and NSAIDs. Because these drugs have different mechanisms and sites of action, the combination of the drugs is more effective than one drug alone. Reprinted with permission from Golan DE. *Principles of Pharmacology.* 4th ed. Philadelphia, PA: Wolters Kluwer; 2016.

in the context of different pain generators, which will form a preliminary framework for a safe and novel pharmacologic algorithm.

PAIN GENERATORS

Determining the pain generators will help in the choice of most appropriate analgesic classes. For example, a combination including opioid medications may be appropriate for a patient with pain due to malignancy but not for chronic nonmalignant low back pain. Therefore, we will discuss RAPP approaches in different clinical scenarios, with the understanding that there very well may be multiple concurrent pain generators (i.e., nociceptive, neuropathic, cancer pain).

Neuropathic Pain

Neuropathic pain can be caused by a variety of conditions both centrally and peripherally mediated, allowing for multiple target treatment areas.[2] Pharmacotherapy is a fundamental part of multimodal therapy in the treatment of neuropathic pain, with drug classes encompassing antiepileptic, antidepressant, gabapentanoid, and opioid analgesics, which all have multiple routes of administration. However, many of these medications have dose-related side effects as well as other contraindications. In addition, the overall efficacy of many neuropathic medications for chronic nonmalignant pain has been called into question.[3,4] Initiating a pharmacologic regimen for neuropathic pain with a single agent as opposed to multiple medications simultaneously allows for observation of medication side effects and tolerability. The European Federation of Neurological Societies published guidelines in 2010 on neuropathic pain pharmacotherapy, which recommended using single drugs at relatively high doses (up to 150 mg for tricyclic antidepressants, 3600 mg of gabapentin, 400 mg of tramadol) as the first and second lines of treatment, whereas combination therapies are recommended for patients who show only partial response to drugs administered alone.[5] It is not uncommon for patients suffering from neuropathic pain to need multiple medications to provide analgesia. If there is inadequate response to a single agent, the principles of RAPP apply.

When determining which medications to initiate for combination therapy under the RAPP approach, a stepwise decision process should be used (see Figure 5-2). It is important to first evaluate the patient's medical history/comorbidities, current medication regimen, as well as allergies. For example, a tricyclic antidepressant is not the ideal choice in a patient with cardiac arrhythmia because of potential cardiotoxic, proarrhythmic side effects. In addition, it could potentially cause worsening mental status and sedation. Likewise, duloxetine would not be a good first choice in a patient already on a selective serotonin and/or norepinephrine reuptake inhibitor such as sertraline or venlafaxine owing to the medication's serotonergic effects and the potential to cause serotonin syndrome. It is also important to identify

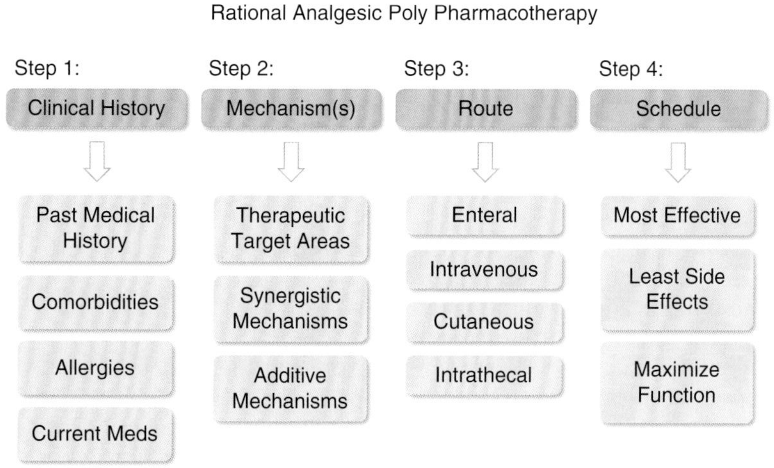

Rational Analgesic Poly Pharmacotherapy

FIGURE 5-2 Rational analgesic polypharmacotherapy (RAPP) places emphasis on a patient's comorbid medical conditions and medication side-effect profile and creates an individualized medication treatment plan.

risk factors such as renal disease, liver disease, and previous adverse reactions, which can all place a patient at higher risk for side effects or negative outcomes.[1]

After thoroughly examining a patient's clinical history and risk factors, one can safely investigate the best pharmacotherapy for the individualized patient. Potential mechanisms of neuropathic pain medications include sodium channel blockers, calcium channel blockers, N-methyl-D-aspartate antagonists, serotonin/norepinephrine reuptake inhibitors, central alpha-2 agonists, and opioid receptor agonists/partial agonists. When combining medications, it is important to assess whether the medications have similar or different mechanisms of action and whether or not the mechanisms have additive or synergistic effects on specific target areas (see Figure 5-1 for specific target areas). An example would be a combination of pregabalin and duloxetine, which are medications that act on different receptors. Pregabalin acts on the alpha-2 delta voltage-gated calcium channels, whereas duloxetine acts as a selective serotonin and norepinephrine reuptake inhibitor. If a patient is nonresponsive, or has side effects, to conventional dose monotherapy with pregabalin or duloxetine, it is reasonable to consider combination therapy.[6] This may allow for reduced doses and decreased side effects from each individual medication. A Cochrane review from 2012 concluded that combination therapies for neuropathic pain may in fact provide synergistic analgesia and reduce overall side effects, although no specific combination was recommended.[7] Combinations that included opioids did show increased efficacy; however, frequent side effects. Although opioid medications may be helpful in acute neuropathic pain, their use in chronic neuropathic pain conditions is unlikely to provide sustained benefit and the initiation of opioid medications should be avoided or used with caution.[8]

Combination pharmacotherapy is not limited to the oral route, and often topical applications can be beneficial. Topical medications have the advantage of being primarily locally acting, reducing side effects, and may especially be helpful in peripheral neuropathic

conditions such as diabetic peripheral neuropathy or postherpetic neuralgia. Topical medications may be used in conjunction with oral therapies, in combination with other topical medications, or in a compounded formulation. An example would be a combination of capsaicin, which acts at the transient receptor potential vanilloid type 1 (TRPV-1) receptor, and lidocaine/prilocaine, which are sodium channel blockers. Although both act on different target areas via different mechanisms, their combination could potentially be synergistic in neuropathic pain relief.[9] Please see chapter 34 *Compounding and Topical Medications* for further discussion.

Many neuropathic agents have significant side-effect profiles, and patient tolerance should be monitored closely. Sedation is one side effect that can diminish the overall level of patient's functioning. As such, when prescribing neuropathic pain medications that commonly cause sedation, such as gabapentanoids, tricyclics, and sodium channel blockers, it is important to consider a dosing schedule that minimizes the impact of a drug's potential side effects and does not sedate the patient during the daytime if possible. Alternatively, some medications such as serotonin/norepinephrine reuptake inhibitors tend to be more activating and may be administered in the morning instead of evening, which may lead to poor sleep.

Nociceptive Pain

Nociceptive pain can be either acute or chronic, typically described as aching, sharp, throbbing, and usually initiated by tissue damage. The role of combination pharmacotherapy for the treatment of acute versus chronic nociceptive pain differs significantly. Acute nociceptive pain can be from any event causing tissue damage such as a fracture, kidney stones, or postsurgical pain. Most patients with acute nociceptive pain will not need combination medical therapy because the pain is self-limited. However, combination therapy may be beneficial in postoperative pain, acute headache, and in certain populations at risk for medication side effects. In these populations, applying the principles of RAPP is still important, because the medical condition, type of surgery, or postoperative treatment plan may dictate the specifics of a pain regimen. Although opioid medications may be indicated for acute nociceptive pain, practitioners should set expectations with patients for the duration of treatment with these medications, as chronic opioid therapy should be avoided in most cases.

Regarding chronic nociceptive pain management, a risk-benefit analysis of selected medications is essential to ensure patient safety, as these medications will be taken for longer durations. Long-term use of medications such as nonsteroidal anti-inflammatory drugs (NSAIDs), benzodiazepines, and opioid poses significant risk to patients and should be avoided or used with caution. As an example, opioid medications are unlikely to be of significant long-term benefit in treatment of chronic nociceptive pain owing to patient tolerance, dose escalation, and medication side effects.[8] In addition, NSAID use is associated with kidney damage, gastrointestinal (GI) bleeding and cardiovascular risk.[10] However, there are multiple classes of NSAIDs and certain medications may be better tolerated in certain patients. Some NSAIDs, such as celocoxib and meloxicam (at 7.5 mg daily dosing), have fewer GI side effects. Naprosyn may have fewer cardiovascular-related events, and sulindac may cause less kidney damage. Refer to chapter 32 *NSAIDs*, which summarizes the different classes of NSAIDs, their mechanism of action, and clinical differences.[11] A potential option to mitigate some of the side effects of NSAIDs is to rotate the medications throughout the week. For example, alternating daily between an NSAID and paracetamol. This will decrease the long-term exposure of NSAIDs and may reduce the risk of GI bleeding and kidney damage.

Because of the broad nature of nociceptive pain, there are several factors to be considered before starting a nociceptive pain regimen. Whether acute or chronic, identifying the cause of the nociceptive pain is essential in formulating an appropriate regimen. With a multitude of causes for nociceptive pain, it is best to identify a primary pain source through patient's history and physical examination before starting pharmacotherapy. Second, when starting a medication for chronic nociceptive pain, carefully consider the long-term implications of the therapy. Third, when prescribing medications, one must take into account the central sensitization that can occur and understand that there is some overlap with neuropathic medications.

Let us use a clinical example to illustrate these general considerations for nociceptive pain. If a practitioner wants to establish a pain regimen for an elderly patient with a history of cardiac disease and chronic myofascial pain, he or she might consider combining a topical medication, such as 5% lidocaine cream, with a muscle relaxer, such as baclofen, which provides both localized treatment to the area of myofascial pain as well as systemic muscle relaxation. Baclofen may be best suited for this individual because of the patient's cardiac disease and potentially may have a more desirable side-effect profile than other muscle relaxers in this population. In contrast, using carisoprodol as first-line treatment of chronic

muscle spasticity may not be the best option because of potential long-term ramifications with dependence, addiction, and side effects such as respiratory depression when combined with other medications. Furthermore, adding medications with mechanisms involving modulation of central sensitization such as serotonin/norepinephrine or gabapentanoids may be a safe and effective supplement, an option that many practitioners do not consider.[12]

Cancer Pain

Applying the principles of RAPP is equally important in pain due to malignancy. One must recognize the many challenges in managing this type of pain, which may result from tumor burden or surgery or occur post radiation and during or post chemotherapy. There are likely to be both nociceptive and neuropathic pain generators. In patients with terminal cancer, the World Health Organization (WHO) stepladder is the standard of care (see Figure 5-3). Taking this into account, combination pharmacotherapy may provide improved analgesia, decreased side effects, and improvement in quality of life for patients with malignancy.

For patients with chronic pain in malignant tumor in remission, the therapeutic regimen becomes a challenging question. Because this situation is now considered chronic pain, a long-term pain strategy applies and the WHO stepladder is unlikely to be safe. For reasons already presented, a nonopioid regimen should be employed because opioid medications are unlikely to provide lasting benefit at a given dose and often require

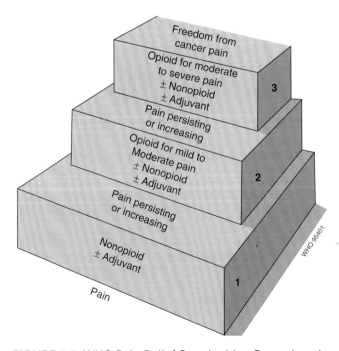

FIGURE 5-3 WHO Pain Relief Step Ladder. Reproduced with permission from the World Health Organization. *Cancer Pain Relief.* 2nd ed. Geneva, Switzerland: World Health Organization; 1996.

medication escalation. However, opioid medications with partial agonist/antagonist mechanisms, such as buprenorphine, may be appealing in this population and are further discussed in the *Buprenorphine Use in the Primary Care Setting* chapter. If opioid medications are used, it is critical to evaluate the risks in the setting of the individual patients' comorbidities.

In some cases, more invasive techniques may be required. Intrathecal drug therapy involves the implantation of a catheter and pump to facilitate the delivery of medication directly to the intrathecal space, which minimizes the systemic side effects of medications. Currently, the only analgesic medications that are approved by the US Food and Drug Administration for intrathecal delivery are baclofen, morphine, and ziconotide. Other intrathecal medications and combinations are used and can be beneficial for neuropathic and cancer-related pain. However, this topic is beyond the scope and purpose of this chapter. Nevertheless, it is essential to know that this therapy exists for patients with significant medication side effects or escalation of analgesic medications. An ideal candidate for intrathecal drug therapy is a patient suffering from pain due to malignancy who responds to oral opioid medications but has significant side effects of sedation. Patients should have a minimum life expectancy of 3 months and a successful catheter trial and be able to tolerate anesthesia/surgery before pump and catheter implantation. Initial randomized trial data included patients with a visual analog scale for pain of at least 5/10 and taking greater than or equal to 200 mg of oral morphine equivalents at the time of implant.

The purpose of this discussion is to introduce the concept of RAPP and provide perspective on the importance of evaluating each individual's specific clinical situation, understanding the mechanisms of action, and creating a risk-benefit analysis before initiating a therapeutic pain regimen. As you explore in further details the intricacies of pain management in the coming chapters, identifying types of pain, whether nociceptive, neuropathic, cancer related, or a combination of these, is an important step in determining the appropriate medication regimen. The patient's age, current medications, allergies, and comorbidities all need to be taken into consideration and are equally important for optimizing an individual's therapeutic plan. Key strategies for RAPP include using medications that target different receptors that provide additive or synergistic effects; using 2 or more medications at a lower dose, which may decrease side effects; alternating medications to prevent consistent exposure

and using different routes of administration. Although current trends in CDT focus on applications rooted in a clinician's experience or anecdotal evidence, we highly recommend the use of the aforementioned framework to establish a more comprehensive and stepwise approach to utilizing polypharmacy in your clinical practice.

REFERENCES

1. Mao J, Gold MS, Backonja MM. Combination drug therapy for chronic pain: a call for more clinical studies. *J Pain.* 2011;12(2):157-166.

2. Eisenberg E, Suzan E. Drug combinations in the treatment of neuropathic pain. *Curr Pain Headache Rep.* 2014;18:463.

3. Malik KM, Nelson AM, Avram MJ, et al. Efficacy of pregabalin in the treatment of radicular pain: results of a controlled trial. *Anesthesiol Pain Med.* 2015;5:e28110.

4. Alviar MJM, Hale T, Dungca M. Pharmacologic interventions for treating phantom limb pain. *Cochrane Database Syst Rev.* 2016;10:CD006380. doi:10.1002/14651858. CD006380.pub3.

5. Attal N, Cruccu G, Baron R, et al; European Federation of Neurological Societies. EFNS guidelines on the pharmacological treatment of neuro-pathic pain: 2010 revision. *Eur J Neurol.* 2010;17:1113-1188.

6. Tesafaye S, Wilhelm S, Lledo A, et al. Duloxetine and pregabalin: high-dose monotherapy or their combination? The "COMBO-DN study" – a multinational, randomized, double-blind, parallel-group study in patients with diabetic peripheral neuropathic pain. *Pain.* 2013;154:12:2616-2625.

7. Chaparro LE, Wiffen PJ, Moore RA, Gilron I. Combination pharmacotherapy for the treatment of neuropathic pain in adults (review). *Cochrane Database Syst Rev.* 2012;(7):CD008943.

8. Chou R, Turner JA, Devine EB, et al. The effectiveness and risks of long-term opioid therapy for chronic pain: a systematic review for a National Institutes of Health Pathways to Prevention Workshop. *Ann Intern Med.* 2015;162:276-286.

9. Sommer C, Crucco G. Topical treatment of peripheral neuropathic pain: applying the evidence. *J Pain Symptom Manage.* 2017;53(3):614-629.

10. Rainsford KD, Velo GP. *Side-Effects of Anti-Inflammatory Drugs–4.* Dordrecht: Kluwer Academic Publishers; 1992.

11. Hoque I, Chatterjee A, Bhattacharya S, Biswas R, Auddy S, Mondal K. A review on different types of the non steroidal anti-inflammatory drugs (NSAIDs). *Int J Adv Multidiscip Res.* 2016;(9):41-51.

12. Patel R. Dickenson A. Mechanisms of the gabapentinoids and α 2 δ-1 calcium channel subunit in neuropathic pain. *Pharmacol Res Perspect.* 2016;4(2):e00205.

SPECIAL POPULATIONS

6

HEALTH DISPARITIES IN PAIN MANAGEMENT

Efrain Talamantes, MD, MBA, MS

FAST FACTS

- African Americans are subject to racial health disparities, but there is increasing evidence that Asian and Hispanic populations are at risk.
- Women more often report pain but do not necessarily get assessed for their pain complaints.
- The racial health disparities that are prevalent in adults are also present when treating chronic pain in the pediatric population.
- Geriatric patients often underreport pain, but a large percentage of the elderly population have chronic pain.

INTRODUCTION

The Institute of Medicine (IOM) defines health disparities as differences in treatment provided to members of different racial (or ethnic) groups that are not justified by the underlying health conditions or treatment preferences of patients.[1] Pain management varies and is commonly tailored to the patient's individual pain condition and needs. However, when pain management differences are not justified by the underlying pain condition or treatment preference of a patient, this contributes to health disparities.[2] Disparities in pain management have been well documented and not limited to racial or ethnic minorities and may include other characteristics such as gender, sexual identity, age, disability, religion, socioeconomic status, geographic location, and other social determinants. This chapter identifies some of the most common health disparities in pain management.

BACKGROUND

Nearly 100 million American adults suffer from chronic pain, and disparities in pain management may occur because of a variety of patient-, provider- and system-level factors.[3] Differences in pain management commonly occur in the setting of an uncertain diagnosis and limited treatment options. In addition, a patient's background, identity, or affiliation and other characteristics may limit a clinician's ability to develop a comprehensive patient-centered pain evaluation and treatment plan. For example, a clinician may not able to communicate effectively with a patient with low health literacy or limited English proficiency, not have the training or allied staff support to adequately develop a treatment plan, and these challenges can result in suboptimal pain management.[4] Reducing pain management disparities for all patients will ensure those most vulnerable receive optimal pain management evaluation and treatment.

RACE AND ETHNICITY

Racial-ethnic disparities are often solely attributed to lack of access to health care. However, even racial-ethnic minority patients with access to health care still receive lower quality of care. Patient race-ethnicity influences physician interpretation of patients' complaints and clinical-decision making, such as treatment or procedure referrals.[5,6] Racial-ethnic minorities consistently receive less adequate treatment for acute and chronic pain when compared with non-Hispanic whites, even when controlling for age, gender, and pain intensity.[7] These pain management disparities may occur when there is pain intensity underreporting and/or clinicians have a limited awareness of their own cultural beliefs and stereotypes regarding pain, racial-ethnic minorities, and the use of opiate analgesia. For example, a study of primary care physicians (PCPs) in 12 academic medical centers across the United States found that the PCP's underestimated pain scores of African American patients by greater than 2 points on an 11-point numeric pain rating scale 47% of the time compared to 33.5% of the time for non-African Americans. In addition, systemic literature reviews consistently show African Americans are more likely to experience undertreatment of pain when compared to non-Hispanic whites.[8–10] Racial-ethnic differences in pain reporting and treatment are increasingly documented in other groups such as Hispanic- and Asian Americans.[11] Recent studies are exploring racial bias as possible cause of pain management disparities and early results suggest clinicians may hold false beliefs about biological differences between racial-ethnic groups.[12]

SEX AND GENDER

Sex refers to biologically based differences, whereas gender refers to a socially based identity.[13] These terms are not interchangeable. Most basic science pain research has included male subjects only and few have explored sex differences.[14] Clinically the prevalence of pain reporting is higher among women compared to men.[3,15,16] The most concerning pain management disparity in women is the gap between them reporting pain and not receiving an appropriate evaluation and treatment.[3,17] While psychosocial research supports the cultural stereotype that women are more willing to report pain than men,[18] biological differences such as fluctuations in estrogen during menses and pregnancy have been linked to migraine and temporomandibular pain conditions.[19,20] In addition, the impact of these biological differences on opioid response have been contradictory and unclear.[13,21] Further research is needed to further characterize sex and gender differences in pain and pain management. Training should also include education on how clinicians can provide culturally and clinically appropriate care for lesbian, gay, bisexual, and transgender (LGBT) people.[22]

CHILDREN AND ADOLESCENTS

Suboptimal pain management has also been described in children and adolescents. Overall pain is undertreated in acute pain conditions such as appendicitis, sickle cell crisis, fractures, and burns, and these disparities in pain management may be more pronounced in racial-ethnic minorities.[23–25] For example, approximately 57% of almost 1 million children evaluated in the emergency department diagnosed with appendicitis received analgesia, and black children were less likely to receive opioid analgesia than white children.[23] Latino children undergoing adenoidectomy or tonsillectomy have also been found to receive less opioid medication than non-Latino children.[26] Reservations with adequately treating pain, specifically with opioids, may be the concern of adverse outcomes including addiction. These concerns, however, are not consistent across all racial-ethnic groups and are further complicated by access to pediatric pain specialists. Children located in rural compared with urban hospitals may not have access to pediatric pain specialists resulting in limited availability of nerve blocks.[27]

OLDER ADULTS

The prevalence of musculoskeletal, neuropathic, and cancer pain increases with age.[28] However, as patients age, pain management is complicated by increasing comorbidities, including declining organ function and polypharmacy.[29] For example, despite demonstration that the World Health Organization's (WHO) 3-level ladder approach is appropriate and effective in relieving cancer pain in more than 90% cases, pain management is inadequate.[30] Up to 40% of elderly patients with cancer experience daily pain.[31] No physiologic changes in pain perception in the elderly have been demonstrated.[32] Underreporting may be complicated by depression, sensory impairment, and dementia. Pain management disparities in the elderly will persist in context of limited medication options with less side-effect profiles, including opioids and concern for addiction or misuse/abuse. Additional research and education is needed to advance individualized approach to prescribing medications tailored to patients' health status and risk factors.

SUMMARY

This chapter has summarized some of the most common pain management health disparities. Demographic changes in education, socioeconomic status, race-ethnicity, gender, and age will require continued education, training, and research to eliminate pain management health disparities and improve care. Eliminating pain management disparities is further challenged with increasing concern for opioid addiction and abuse.

TABLE 6-1 Common Pain Management Health Disparities, Potential Causes, and Recommendations for Reduction

SPECIFIED GROUP/ CHARACTERISTICS	POTENTIAL CAUSES	RECOMMENDATIONS
Racial-ethnic minorities	**Patient-level:** Pain intensity underreporting **Provider-level:** Limited cultural awareness, biases, and stereotypes **System-level:** Patient-physician racial concordance, improved patient-physician communication support	**Patient-level:** Encourage patient to accurately report pain intensity levels **Provider-level:** Cultural awareness, bias, and barriers to pain management training **System-level:** Patient-centered pain management interventions, culturally appropriate educational interventions
Sex and gender	**Patient-level:** Estrogen levels are linked to pain conditions in females **Provider-level:** While women report more pain, they are less likely to receive treatment compared with men **System-level:** Limited inclusion of women in research studies and inadequate training in diagnosis and treatment of pain disorders more common in women	**Patient-level:** Ensure women's pain complaints are thoroughly evaluated and treated **Provider-level:** Avoid sex- or gender-specific pain interventions **System-level:** More research is needed that includes females and women in studies
Children and adolescents	**Patient-level:** Access to pain specialists in rural areas **Provider-level:** Undertreatment of acute pain conditions **System-level:** Concern with opioid addiction, misuse, or abuse	**Patient-level:** Ensure pain of children and adolescents is thoroughly evaluated and treated **Provider-level:** Consistent assessment of pain conditions across all age groups **System-level:** Patient-centered pain management interventions, culturally appropriate educational interventions
Older adults	**Patient-level:** Decline in organ function, including sensory impairment and dementia **Provider-level:** Undertreatment of pain conditions due to opioid side effects **System-level:** Concern with opioid addiction, misuse, or abuse	**Patient-level:** Ensure older patients are thoroughly evaluated and treated **Provider-level:** Account for comorbidities and polypharmacy, slower titration of pain medication **System-level:** Patient-centered pain management interventions, opioid treatment training

While the causes of health disparities are multifactorial, knowledge of how clinicians can minimize these discrepancies in pain management is critical to providing all patients with high quality and safe care. Table 6-1 summarizes common pain management health disparities, the potential patient-, provider-, and system-level causes, and recommendations to mitigate these disparities.

REFERENCES

1. Smedley BD, Stith AY, Nelson AR. Unequal treatment: confronting racial and ethnic disparities in health care. *J Natl Med Assoc.* 2005;97:303. Available from: http://www.nap.edu/catalog/10260/unequal-treatment-confronting-racial-and-ethnic-disparities-in-health-care.

2. McGuire TG, Alegria M, Cook BL, Wells KB, Zaslavsky AM. Implementing the Institute of Medicine definition of disparities: an application to mental health care. *Health Serv Res.* 2006;41(5):1979-2005.

3. Pizzo PA, Clark NM, Carter Pokras O. *Relieving Pain in America: A Blueprint for Transforming Prevention, Care, Education, and Research.* Institute of Medicine; 2011. Available from: http://www.nap.edu/download/13172.

4. Devraj R, Herndon CM, Griffin J. Pain awareness and medication knowledge: a health literacy evaluation. *J Pain Palliat Care Pharmacother.* 2013;27(1):19-27. Available from: http://www.ncbi.nlm.nih.gov/pubmed/23379354.

5. van Ryn M, Burke J. The effect of patient race and socio-economic status on physicians' perceptions of patients. *Soc Sci Med.* 2000;50(6):813-828. Available from: http://www.sciencedirect.com/science/article/pii/S027795369900338X%5Cnhttp://www.sciencedirect.com/science?_ob=ShoppingCartURL&_method=add&_udi=B6VBF-46FPT4T-6&_acct=C000050221&_version=1&_userid=10&_ts=1312558794&md5=a2f0b9f-22977a1781290720048c106ce%5Cnh.

6. van Ryn M. Research on the provider contribution to race/ethnicity disparities in medical care. *Med Care.* 2002;40(1 suppl):I140-I151.

7. Mossey JM. Defining racial and ethnic disparities in pain management. In: *Clinical Orthopaedics and Related Research.* 2011:1859-1870.

8. Cintron A, Morrison RS. Pain and ethnicity in the United States: a systematic review. *J Palliat Med.* 2006;9(6):1454-1473.

9. Ezenwa MO, Ameringer S, Ward SE, Serlin RC. Racial and ethnic disparities in pain management in the United States. *J Nurs Scholarsh.* 2006;38(3):225-233.

10. Meghani SH, Byun E, Gallagher RM. Time to take stock: a meta-analysis and systematic review of analgesic treatment disparities for pain in the United States. *Pain Med.* 2012;13:150-174.

11. Rowell LN, Mechlin B, Ji E, Addamo M, Girdler SS. Asians differ from non-Hispanic Whites in experimental pain sensitivity. *Eur J Pain.* 2011;15(7):764-771.

12. Hoffman KM, Trawalter S, Axt JR, Oliver MN. Racial bias in pain assessment and treatment recommendations, and false beliefs about biological differences between blacks and whites. *Proc Natl Acad Sci.* 2016;113(16):201516047. Available from: http://www.pnas.org/content/113/16/4296.abstract.

13. Greenspan JD, Craft RM, LeResche L, et al. Studying sex and gender differences in pain and analgesia: a consensus report. *Pain.* 2007;132.

14. Mogil JS, Chanda ML. The case for the inclusion of female subjects in basic science studies of pain. *Pain.* 2005;117(1–2). Available from: http://journals.lww.com/pain/Fulltext/2005/09000/The_case_for_the_inclusion_of_female_subjects_in.1.aspx.

15. LeResche L. Defining gender disparities in pain management. *Clin Orthop Relat Res.* 2011;469:1871-1877.

16. Fillingim RB, King CD, Ribeiro-Dasilva MC, Rahim-Williams B, Riley JL. Sex, gender, and pain: a review of recent clinical and experimental findings. *J Pain.* 2009;10(5):447-485. Available from: http://www.sciencedirect.com/science/article/pii/S1526590008009097%5Cn, http://www.ncbi.nlm.nih.gov/pubmed/19411059%5Cn and http://www.pubmedcentral.nih.gov/articlerender.fcgi?artid=PMC2677686.

17. Chen EH, Shofer FS, Dean AJ, et al. Gender disparity in analgesic treatment of emergency department patients with acute abdominal pain. *Acad Emerg Med.* 2008;15:414-418.

18. Robinson ME, Riley JL, Myers CD, et al. Gender role expectations of pain: relationship to sex differences in pain. *J Pain.* 2001;2(5):251-257. Available from: http://www.ncbi.nlm.nih.gov/pubmed/14622803.

19. Marcus DA. Interrelationships of neurochemicals, estrogen, and recurring headache. *Pain.* 1995;62:129-139.

20. LeResche L, Sherman JJ, Huggins K, et al. Musculoskeletal orofacial pain and other signs and symptoms of temporomandibular disorders during pregnancy: a prospective study. *J Orofac Pain.* 2005;19(3):193-201. Available from: http://search.ebscohost.com/login.aspx?direct=true&db=ddh&AN=36831098&lang=pl&site=ehost-live%5Cn-http://content.ebscohost.com/ContentServer.asp?T=P&P=AN&K=36831098&S=R&D=ddh&EbscoContent=dGJyMNLr40SeprE4y9fwOLCmr02eprFSs6a4T-bOWxWXS&ContentCustomer=dGJyMPG.

21. Cairns BE, Gazerani P. Sex-related differences in pain. *Maturitas.* 2009;63:292-296.

22. Daniel H, Butkus R. Lesbian, gay, bisexual, and transgender health disparities: executive summary of a policy position paper from the American College of Physicians. *Ann Intern Med.* 2015;163(2):135-137. Available from: http://annals.org/article.aspx?doi=10.7326/M14-2482.

23. Goyal MK, Kuppermann N, Cleary SD, Teach SJ, Chamberlain JM. Racial disparities in pain management of children with appendicitis in emergency departments. *JAMA Pediatr.* 2015;169(11):1-7. Available from: http://archpedi.jamanetwork.com/article.aspx?doi=10.1001/jamapediatrics.2015.1915.

24. Brown JC, Klein EJ, Lewis CW, Johnston BD, Cummings P. Emergency department analgesia for fracture pain. *Ann Emerg Med.* 2003;42(2):197-205.

25. Selbst SM, Clark M. Analgesic use in the emergency department. *Ann Emerg Med.* 1990;19(9):1010-1013. Available from: http://www.ncbi.nlm.nih.gov/pubmed/2393166.

26. Jimenez N, Seidel K, Martin LD, Rivara FP, Lynn AM. Perioperative analgesic treatment in Latino and non-Latino pediatric patients. *J Health Care Poor Underserved.* 2010;21(1):229-236. Available from: http://www.pubmedcentral.nih.gov/articlerender.fcgi?artid=4011632&tool=pmcentrez&rendertype=abstract.

27. Chiao FB, Wang A. An examination of disparities in pediatric pain management centered on socioeconomic factors and hospital characteristics. *J Racial Ethn Heal Disparities.* 2017;1-5. Available from: http://dx.doi.org/10.1007/s40615-017-0343-3.

28. Savvas SM, Gibson SJ. Overview of pain management in older adults. *Clin Geriatr Med.* 2016;32(4):635-650. Available from: http://www.sciencedirect.com/science/article/pii/S0749069016300507.

29. Guerriero F. Guidance on opioids prescribing for the management of persistent non-cancer pain in older adults. *World J Clin Cases.* 2017;5(3):73-81. Available from: http://www.ncbi.nlm.nih.gov/pmc/articles/PMC5352962/.

30. Zech DF, Grond S, Lynch J, Hertel D, Lehmann KA. Validation of World Health Organization Guidelines for cancer pain relief: a 10-year prospective study. *Pain.* 1995;63(1):65-76.

31. Bernabei R, Gambassi G, Lapane K, et al. Management of pain in elderly patients with cancer. *Jama J Am Med Assoc.* 1998;279(23):1877-1882. Available from: http://jama.ama-assn.org/cgi/content/abstract/279/23/1877.

32. Kwentus JA, Harkins SW, Lignon N, Silverman JJ. Current concepts of geriatric pain and its treatment. *Geriatrics.* 1985;40(4):48-54, 57. Available from: http://www.ncbi.nlm.nih.gov/pubmed/3884442.

7

GERIATRIC PATIENTS

Calvin H. Hirsch, MD and Samir J. Sheth, MD

FAST FACTS

- Chronic pain in the elderly is very common and exacerbated by age-related physiologic changes.
- Geriatric pain assessment taking into account cognitive ability of the patient should be integrated into routine care.
- Opioids are subject to potentially serious drug interactions due to the polypharmacy in older adults with multiple comorbidities.
- Age-related changes in drug metabolism compound the challenge of pain pharmacotherapeutics.
- Pain reduction is a means to an end: in geriatric patients, emphasis should be placed on optimization

of functional status and psychosocial well-being through a multimodal approach involving pain relief, physical therapy, exercise, and counseling.

INTRODUCTION

Chronic pain is extremely common as we get older, and therefore it is very important to understand the various presentations of chronic pain in geriatric patients. Age-related physiological changes not only make the body susceptible to chronic pain states, but also cause various issues surrounding pharmacological management of pain in the elderly (fall risk, drug-drug interactions, etc.) which can make therapeutic options limited. Awareness of nonpharmacological options to treat chronic pain in the geriatric population allows the provider to offer a more comprehensive and potentially a more effective treatment plan. As such, this chapter will describe safe, rational, and multidisciplinary approaches for geriatric pain management.

NATURE AND SIGNIFICANCE
Epidemiology

Chronic pain disproportionately affects older adults and adversely impacts physical functioning and quality of life. Among adults age 65 and older living in the community, the prevalence has been estimated between 25% and 76%, with the wide variability reflecting differences in the surveyed population and study methodology. In long-term-care settings, the overwhelming majority (83%-93%) of older adults report chronic pain.[1] In a population-based survey in Sweden, the prevalence of pain lasting 3 or more months rose from 39% in the age group 65-74 to 48% among adults age 85 and older, with an estimated 5.4% annual increase in pain prevalence after age 65.[2] However, an increase in prevalence with advancing old age has not been found in all epidemiological studies.[1] Most studies have found a higher prevalence of chronic pain in older women compared to older men.[1,2] In the Swedish survey, the average severity of chronic pain was moderate and caused moderate interference in daily activities, remaining fairly stable across old-age groups. Problems with mobility predicted the onset of chronic pain 12 months later. In women, but not men, pain duration, pain in more than 1 location, and pain severity predicted the persistence of chronic pain at 24 months of follow-up.[2] The most frequently reported sites for chronic pain include the back, the lower extremities (hip, knee), and other joints.[1]

Multimorbidity and Chronic Pain

In older adults, chronic pain generally occurs in the context of multimorbidity. In the multicenter MultiCare Cohort study of 3189 older primary-care patients in Germany (mean age 74 years), men and women each had an average of 7 chronic conditions. Seventy percent of men and 85% of women reported chronic pain, which moderately or severely limited their functioning in 15% and 22%, respectively. Of importance, different combinations of comorbidities were associated with a significantly different prevalence of chronic pain. For example, in women with chronic low-back problems, the addition of gastroesophageal reflux disease (GERD) was associated with a 63% prevalence of chronic pain, compared to 47% in women without GERD. Men who had chronic low-back problems plus ischemic heart disease had a 38% prevalence of chronic pain, compared to 28% of men with back problems but no heart disease.[3] The mechanism by which combinations of morbidities influence the perception of pain remains unknown.

Depression and anxiety: Significant depressive symptoms, which commonly co-occur with anxiety, are found in 10%-20% of adults age 65 and older, depending on the population surveyed and the screening instruments used.[4–6] The prevalence of depression rises to 27% among institutionalized older adults.[7] Based on data from a continuing-care retirement community, it has been estimated that roughly 13% of older adults suffer from comorbid depression and chronic pain.[8] Chronic pain and depression strongly influence each other. In patients with chronic pain, the odds ratio (OR) of having more severe and more disabling chronic pain increases in the presence of depression and anxiety. In the Netherlands Study of Depression and Anxiety, after adjusting for age, gender, chronic disease, antidepressant use, and other demographic factors, adults with depression and anxiety were 3 times more likely to experience mild, nondisabling pain than nondepressed, nonanxious adults, but they were 30 times more likely to have severe and disabling pain (95% CI 12.68-72.23). The association of depression or anxiety with pain is graded, with more severe depression and more severe anxiety more likely to be associated with higher pain grades. Compared to not being depressed, having moderate depressive symptoms increased the likelihood of having severely disabling and limiting pain 3-fold, but having severe depression increased the OR of severely disabling pain nearly 8-fold. Similarly, compared to no anxiety, moderate or severe anxiety increased the OR of severely disabling and limiting pain approximately 7 and 13 times, respectively.[9]

The physiological basis for the interrelationship between depression and the perception of pain remains unclear, but single nucleotide polymorphisms in the functional promoters of serotonin-receptor genes have been associated with chronic pain.[10]

Aging also appears to facilitate the dynamic interaction of depression and pain. It is generally accepted that abnormalities in serotonergic (5-hydroxytriptamine [5-HT]) neurotransmission play an important role in depression. In the rat brain, regional 5-HT levels change with aging and are accompanied by regional alterations in the brain density of 5-HT$_{1A}$ children and young adults; older humans also show regional differences in 5-HT$_{1A}$ and 5-HT$_{2A}$ receptor density,[12] with significant increases in receptor density in brain regions (in the absence of known depression) that are qualitatively similar to the increased receptor density seen in depressed, middle-aged adults.[13] The serotonergic system, along with the noradrenergic system, plays a role in pain modulation through a complex set of descending pathways that receive input from the cortex, thalamus, and amygdala and feed into the midbrain, brain stem, and spinal cord,[14] which may help explain the efficacy of the serotonin-noradrenergic reuptake inhibitor, duloxetine, in neuropathic and osteoarthritic pain.[15]

Chronic Pain, Central Sensitization, and Aging

With aging, there is a decline in both structure and function of peripheral sensory nerves, in particular, the A∂ fibers, corresponding to an unchanged or reduced sensitivity to pain-producing stimuli in older patients. However, once the pain is perceived, the perception of pain is often greater than that experienced by younger patients responding to an identical stimulus.[16] To this aging phenomenon is added the pain amplification of nociceptive stimuli (pain hypersensitivity) that commonly accompanies chronic pain states. Among patients referred to a Swiss pain clinic, central pain hypersensitivity (determined by the threshold for a withdrawal reflex) was found in 80% (mean age = 50 years).[17] In chronic joint pain, the poor association between radiologic abnormalities and perceived pain suggests an important role for central sensitization. Given the prevalence of musculoskeletal pain in older adults and the frequency of arthroplasties in this population, it is notable that chronic postoperative pain after knee replacement ranges from 10% to 24% and from 7% to 23% after total hip arthroplasty.[18] In degenerative joint disease, patients commonly experience joint hyperalgesia that progresses to regional pain; this is believed to reflect central sensitization. Patients who experience general pain sensitization *around* (not just in) the knee after knee replacement tend to report higher levels of pain, greater disability, and worse quality of life.[19]

Aging predisposes to central sensitization through abnormalities in mast cell and glial function that amplifies and perpetuates the pain response through a state of neuroinflammation. Mast cells are strategically located near nerve endings and the vasculature, allowing mast cell mediators such as bradykinin, histamine, and prostaglandins to stimulate a nociceptive response. In the central nervous system, mast cells are found in the spinal cord and are particularly concentrated in the thalamus. In older adults, mast cells are more likely to degranulate in response to inflammation, theoretically promoting an inflammatory response in peripheral tissues. Brain mast cells directly and indirectly (through somatosensory neurons) stimulate microglia and astrocytes to release proinflammatory cytokines. In old age, microglia exist primarily in a primed, rather than quiescent, state, resulting in more robust and prolonged production of proinflammatory cytokines.[16] In this setting, dysfunctional modulation of chronic nociceptive stimuli can occur and offers a physiologic explanation for the prevalence of central sensitization and the burden of chronic pain in older patients.

CHALLENGES IN PAIN MANAGEMENT IN OLDER ADULTS

Under-Recognition of Pain

Physicians commonly under-recognize pain in their older patients. On the patient's side, it is not uncommon to under-report pain because of a belief that pain is normal in old age, culturally or socially mediated stoicism, language barriers, fear of becoming addicted to pain medications, or fear that admission of pain will result in a loss of independence.[20] Moderate to severe cognitive impairment impairs communication of pain. Despite the movement to include pain as the "fifth vital sign," an absence of pain during the vital-sign check may result in the provider's failure to inquire about pain experienced during daily activities or at night. Pressure to assess multiple chronic conditions and review medications during a short outpatient visit may limit the ability to assess chronic pain. The patient's impaired hearing can lead to misleading answers and result in an inaccurate or incomplete assessment of symptoms. Family informants may have poor insight into the patient's pain or pain-related changes in behavior. Disease-focused and time-pressured health care providers also may miss important visual clues that should elicit questions about pain, such as use of a cane, a severely kyphotic spine, or limited range of motion of the neck.

Clinicians' fear of drug complications or causing addiction often results in the pharmacological *undertreatment* of older patients' acute and chronic pain.[1,21,22] The misuse of opioids does occur in older patients and is more likely to occur in the presence of underlying comorbid psychiatric conditions, principally depression and a history of substance misuse.[23,24] Most misuse in the elderly involves opioids that are legitimately prescribed. However, prescribing too low a dose of opioid in moderate to severe pain may result in inadequately treated pain and repeated requests from the patient for more opioids, suggesting addictive behavior. When the physician does not increase the dose, the patient may resort to taking supplementary opioids from a friend or relative,

reinforcing the appearance of addiction. Cessation of the opioid-seeking behavior when the physician increases the dose may reflect the phenomenon of "pseudoaddiction," that is, opioid-seeking behavior for the purpose of pain relief, not opioid craving. Unfortunately, in clinical practice, pseudoaddiction can be difficult to differentiate from true addiction, worsening of the underlying condition and opioid-induced hyperalgesia.

Pain is commonly undertreated in older patients in institutional settings. Evaluation of 387 consecutive patients admitted to geriatric units in 8 acute-care Italian hospitals revealed that two-thirds of patients had at least moderate pain. Only one-third of patients reporting the severest level of pain received a strong opioid. Over 50% of all patients with moderate or more severe pain experienced no or only mild pain relief.[22] In a study of 12 Austrian nursing homes, pain prevalence among cognitively impaired but verbally responsive patients was high (over two-thirds) but comparable to cognitively intact patients. However, approximately 80% of nonverbal, cognitively impaired patients were found to have pain using observational methods. Nearly 20% of nonverbal patients with pain did not receive analgesics, compared to 6% of cognitively intact patients.[25]

Atypical Presentation of Acute Pain in the Older Adult

Although this chapter focuses on chronic pain, a discussion of atypical presentations of *acute* pain conditions is necessitated by their frequency in older patients and their ability to delay diagnosis and adversely affect outcomes. Atypical presentation of abdominal pain and chest pain has the potential to cause the most serious consequences to the patient. Abdominal pain is the fourth most common complaint of older patients presenting to the emergency department (ED),[26] but the presenting symptoms may be vague and not include all components of the "classic" presentation and therefore may not point to the diagnosis. Among patients age 80 and older presenting with abdominal pain and requiring emergent surgery, only 30% have a fever >35.5°C and a white cell count >15,500/mm^3.[27] The "typical" presentation of small-bowel obstruction includes diffuse abdominal pain, nausea, vomiting, distention, and constipation/obstipation. However, in older patients, the full constellation of symptoms may not be present early on, and diarrhea may be present. More than half of older patients with acute cholecystitis initially fail to exhibit the combination of nausea, vomiting, and fever, and leukocytosis is absent in up to 40%. With acute pancreatitis, older patients may present with vague upper abdominal pain *without* radiation to the back, with or without nausea and vomiting. Only 17% of older patients with acute appendicitis with perforation present with the "typical" triad of right lower quadrant pain, fever, and leukocytosis,[26] the pain often is vague and may begin as loss of appetite or diffuse abdominal pain. In an older patient, rebound tenderness may be absent in acute peritonitis. Reasons for the atypical presentations largely remain unknown. Age-related changes to peripheral nerves may change the characteristics of the pain. Concomitant use of non-steroidal anti-inflammatory drugs (NSAIDs) or opioids may blunt the pain and delay presentation.

Acute myocardial infarction without chest pain is more likely to occur in patients over the age of 70 (and particularly over the age of 80), as well as in women.[28] Older patients with urinary tract infection are more likely than younger patients to present atypically with loss of appetite, malaise, delirium, or falls rather than dysuria. Because of atypical presentations, any acute abdominal or chest pain in the older patient should be taken seriously.

Assessment of Pain

Given the high prevalence of chronic pain, its assessment should be integrated into the routine review of systems (ROS) for older patients:

- How often do you experience pain?
- Where and when do you experience it?
- What is the average severity of the pain?
  - How tolerable is this average level of pain?
  - What makes it worse or better?
- Do you experience acute worsening of the pain?
  - How often?
  - When and where?
  - How tolerable are these exacerbations?
  - How long do they last?
  - What makes them worse or better?
- Does pain affect what you can do or how you do it?
- Does the pain affect your sleep?
- What do you take or do to reduce the pain?
- How well do these interventions work?

To facilitate pain assessment, a pain questionnaire, developed and validated for older patients, can be substituted for the pain ROS, such as the office-friendly 12-item version of the Geriatric Pain Measure,[29] whose use is not copyrighted (Table.7-1).

Although self-report of pain loses its sensitivity and accuracy as cognitive impairment worsens, it can provide an important clue to the existence of pain and serves as a starting point for observing the patient and asking the caregiver questions that may help to localize the pain and determine its etiology. Table 7-2 summarizes clues to the presence of pain in patients with advanced dementia.

From the caregiver, ascertain whether there has been a change in activities or behavior. For example, does the patient now refuse to walk? Is there new agitated behavior or a change in sleep patterns? Does the patient resist being moved during routine caregiving? Severe pain in demented patients can present as withdrawal or involution, with reduced communication, reduced movement, clenched fists, grimacing, eyes tightly closed, and/or refusal to eat or open the mouth. On physical examination, does the patient exhibit any of these characteristics? Does he or she rub or hold any part of the body or guard a body part such as an arm or leg when he or she moves? Does he or she resist being touched generally or in a specific location? Does the patient grimace during a physical-exam maneuver such as sitting the patient up

to auscultate the lungs? If the source of discomfort can be localized and appears musculoskeletal, the caregiver should be asked about recent trauma, and the patient should be inspected for signs of trauma such as ecchymoses or splinting during the lung examination, suggesting a broken rib. The physician should be mindful of the caregiver's reaction to physical indicators of trauma; indifference or effusive denial of culpability should raise concern about elder mistreatment. A commonly overlooked source of pain in cognitively impaired patients is a dental abscess. The mouth should be inspected; if resistance is encountered, a panoramic dental roentgenogram or facial computerized tomography can be helpful to rule out dental abscesses.

Chronic pain can be more difficult to identify in patients with dementia, as there may not be an acute change in function or behavior to raise concern. Behaviors such as pacing and rocking, or refusing to eat or drink, commonly occur in advanced dementia. In this advanced dementia, subtle changes in behavior can offer clues to chronic pain. For example, does the patient now limp when walking? Does the patient want to spend more time in bed? Does he regularly rub his knee? An important rule of thumb when evaluating these patients is to assume that conditions that *could* cause pain *are* causing pain. If the patient shows signs of osteoarthritis, with malformed knees, or has significant kyphosis from osteoporotic fractures, the patient may be suffering from pain related to these conditions. In such cases, a trial of a scheduled, safe analgesic such as acetaminophen (paracetamol) may be indicated.

Nursing assistants in skilled nursing or residential-care facilities provide most hands-on care and have the ability to offer important insight about function and behavioral changes related to pain. However, formal documentation of distress may be limited or absent, and a caregiver who has observed distress may not be present to talk with the primary-care provider during scheduled rounds. In these instances, implementation of standardized pain assessments completed by nursing assistants can facilitate pain evaluation by the clinician during scheduled rounds. These range from the quick Wong-Baker FACES Pain Rating Scale[30] to slightly longer but more informative instruments such as the Pain Assessment in Advanced Dementia Scale (PAINAD),[31] which is accessible without copyright restrictions through the University of Iowa School of Nursing *geriatricpain.org* website.[32] Herr et al. provide a detailed description of the most valid and clinically useful observational pain scales.[33]

CHALLENGES OF TREATING CHRONIC PAIN IN THE OLDER ADULT

Basic Principles

The objectives of interventions to reduce chronic pain target 3 domains: *palliation* (minimizing suffering), *physical functioning* (the ability to perform basic, instrumental, and advanced activities of daily living), and *psychosocial function* (the emotional and social factors enabling the

	TABLE 7-1 Geriatric Pain Measure Short Form		
	ITEM	**YES (SCORE = 2)**	**NO (SCORE = 0)**
1.	Do you currently have pain with or have you stopped moderate activities such as moving a heavy table, pushing a vacuum cleaner, bowling, or playing golf because of pain?		
2.	Do you currently have pain with or have you stopped climbing more than 1 flight of stairs because of pain?		
3.	Do you currently have pain with or have you stopped walking more than 200 yards (183 m) because of pain?		
4.	Do you currently have pain with or have you stopped walking 200 yards (183 m) or less because of pain?		
5.	Because of pain, have you cut down the amount of time you spend on work or other activities?		
6.	Because of pain, have you been accomplishing less than you would like to?		
7.	Because of pain, have you limited the kind of work or other activities you do?		
8.	Because of pain, does the work or activities you do require extra effort?		
9.	Because of pain, do you have trouble sleeping?		
10.	Does pain prevent you from enjoying any other social or recreational activities (other than religious services)?		
		Score 0-10	
11.	On a scale of 0-10, with 0 meaning no pain and 10 meaning the worst pain you can imagine, how severe is your pain today?		
12.	In the last 7 days, on a scale of 0-10, with 0 meaning no pain and 10 meaning the worst pain you can imagine, how severe has your pain been on average?		
	Total score = sum of all items		
	Transformation to a 0-100 scale: multiply total score by 2.5		

From Blozik E, Stuck AE, Niemann S, et al. Geriatric pain measure short form: development and initial evaluation. J Am Geriatr Soc. 2007;55(12):2045-2050. Copyright © 2007 Journal of the American Geriatrics Society. Reprinted by permission of John Wiley & Sons, Inc.

TABLE 7-2 Identifying Chronic Pain in the Cognitively Impaired Patient

Has there been a change in activities or behavior?

• Stopped walking? Groaning while weight-bearing?
• New agitated behavior?
• Change in sleep patterns?
• Resistance to being moved?

In advanced dementia, severe pain can present very differently and therefore assess if patient has:

• Reduced communication, reduced movement
• Clenched fists, grimacing, tightly closing eyes
• Refusal to eat, drink, even open mouth

Does patient rub or guard a body part or brace themselves during movement?

individual to have satisfying roles and relationships within the home, work place, and community). Medications can play an essential role in treating chronic pain, but in older adults it can cause unanticipated adverse reactions and poor outcomes if not thoughtfully and carefully managed as part of a broad strategy.

As in younger adults, pharmacologic management of chronic pain requires a step-wise approach that selects analgesics most appropriate for the type of pain (e.g., neuropathic vs. nonneuropathic) and begins with the safest analgesics and builds upward as needed based on the severity of pain and the effectiveness of the treatment. Adjunctive treatments, both pharmacologic and nonpharmacologic, are utilized to minimize opioid requirements and reduce the risk of opioid dependence. What differentiates older from younger chronic-pain patients is the greater relative risk of experiencing adverse reactions from the analgesics due to age-related changes in drug metabolism and sensitivity as well as from drug-drug, drug-nutrient, and drug-disease interactions that turn the tripartite objectives of palliation, physical function, and psychosocial function into a challenging balancing act of benefits vs. harms.

Age-Related Changes in Drug Metabolism and the Hazards of Polypharmacy

The multimorbidities prevalent in older adults carry with it a high burden of polypharmacy (defined as 5 or more routinely taken medications), with an associated risk of adverse drug events (ADE) and potentially harmful drug interactions. In a study of U.S. Veterans Administration hospitals, over 90% of ADE-related admissions occurred in veterans taking 5 or more medications.[34] The number of prescribed medications tends to rise with age as a result of more chronic illnesses.

The metabolism of many drugs is altered due to age-related changes in pharmacokinetics and pharmacodynamics. With aging, lean body mass (primarily muscle) and total body water decline, increasing concentrations of hydrophilic drugs, whereas the higher proportion of body fat increases the volume of distribution and serum half-life of lipophilic drugs. Drugs eliminated by the kidney can have a longer serum half-life because of the age-related decline in renal blood flow and glomerular filtration rate. The mass of the liver declines, slightly reducing phase I metabolism of drugs consisting of cytochrome P450 (CYP) oxidation, reduction, and hydrolysis, whereas phase II metabolism (glucuronidation, acetylation, and sulfation) does not appreciably change. For CYP-metabolized drugs, the possibility of serious drug interactions, including drug-opioid interactions, exists, and this possibility increases as the number of administered drugs increases. Certain hepatically metabolized drugs that are taken concurrently can interfere with the CYP metabolism of a given opioid and further increase its serum half-life, duration, and potential side-effects; whereas other CYP-metabolized drugs may induce metabolism of the opioid, reducing its effectiveness. CYP3A4, the phase I metabolic pathway for tramadol, can be induced by statins and anticonvulsants such as divalproate, and its serotonergic effects increased by selective serotonin reuptake inhibitors, all increasing the risk of seizures at otherwise therapeutic doses. Methadone and oxycodone both undergo phase I metabolism by CYP3A4 and CYP2D6, increasing the potential for adverse drug interactions. Commonly prescribed opioid analgesics interact with numerous other drugs that clinicians routinely give for arrhythmias, coronary heart disease, depression, gastroesophageal reflux disease, and other acute and chronic conditions prevalent in older adults Table 7-3.

Despite similar pharmacokinetics between men and women, oxycodone and hydromorphone achieve up to 25% higher maximal serum concentrations in women than men, irrespective of age. Ethnicity also can affect opioid metabolism.[35] In addition, many medications show age-related alterations in the type and extent of pharmacologic actions. For example, morphine (which

TABLE 7-3 Metabolic Pathway/Enzyme Involvement		
OPIOID	**PHASE 1 METABOLISM**	**PHASE 2 METABOLISM**
Morphine[12]	None	Glucuronidation via UGT2B7
Codeine[13]	CYP2D6	None
Hydrocodone[14]	CYP2D6	None
Oxycodone[11]	CYP3A4	None
	CYP2D6	
Methadone[15]	CYP3A4	None
	CYP2B6	
	CYP2C8	
	CYP2C19	
	CYP2D6	
	CYP2C9	
Tramadol[16]	CYP3A4	None
	CYP2D6	
Fentanyl[10]	CYP3A4	None
Hydromorphone[17]	None	Glucuronidation via UGT2B7
Oxymorphone[18]	None	Glucuronidation via UGT2B7

From Smith HS. Opioid metabolism. Mayo Clin Proc. 2009;84(7):613-624.

may have a lower half-life in the elderly due to decreased renal clearance) has an overall mg/kg greater analgesic effect in the elderly. Benzodiazepines and benzodiazepine-GABA receptor agonists such as zolpidem increase postural sway and fall risk relatively more in older compared to younger adults. Because very old individuals tend to be excluded from clinical drug trials, the recommended starting dose of most medications is geared to the nonelderly. A maxim of geriatric prescribing is to start at a low dose, often below the published starting dose, and slowly titrate upward as needed to achieve the desired effect. Older patients especially require cautious dosing of opioids. Potential drug interactions should be examined before prescribing any new medication.

Drugs and Cognitive Impairment

All opioids, including tramadol, can impair cognition and precipitate delirium in the elderly, compounding the negative impact that moderate to severe pain already has on memory and executive functioning.[36] Numerous other psychoactive medications that are commonly prescribed to older adults also affect cognition. Benzodiazepines affect both cognition and balance, and the highest prevalence of long-term use occurs in the elderly,[37,38] whose dependence on sedative-hypnotics for sleep or chronic anxiety may have started years earlier. Benzodiazepines can add to the pharmacodynamic effects of opioids, increasing the risk of excess sedation and respiratory depression, in addition to confusion. Medications with centrally acting anticholinergic properties can impair cognition and cause delirium and are ubiquitous in the geriatric pharmacopoeia. They include bladder antispasmotics (e.g., oxybutynin); first-generation (H_1) antihistamines; H_2 blockers with H_1 overlap for peptic ulcer and gastroesophageal reflux disease (e.g., ranitidine); phenothiazine derivatives used for nausea (e.g, perchlorperazine); opioids; and tricyclic antidepressants. Numerous common medications have weak to moderate anticholinergic properties at normal therapeutic doses (e.g., furosemide, digoxin, atenolol, metoprolol, warfarin, isosorbide, chlorthalidone, bupropion, paroxetine), but when prescribed to the same patient can cause substantial additive anticholinergic activity that contributes to the risk of confusion,[39] especially in the presence of opioids.

Drugs and Falls in the Elderly

Numerous medications have been associated with falls through a variety of putative mechanisms, including nonspecific dizziness, orthostatic hypotension (antihypertensives), bradycardia (beta-blockers, acetylcholinesterase inhibitor cognitive enhancers), cerebellar dysfunction (anticonvulsants), volume depletion (diuretics), and nonspecific CNS effects that include inattention, somnolence, and loss of balance (benzodiazepines, opioids).[40]

Opioids have been associated with as high as a 5-fold increased risk of fracture, compared to users of NSAIDs, after adjustment for other potential risk factors. This risk rises with increasing dose.[41] Both tricyclic antidepressants and anticonvulsants such as gabapentin, carbamazepine, and pregabalin have independently been associated with falls, as have virtually all classes of antidepressants.

Toward a Systematic Approach to the Management of Chronic Pain in the Elderly

A basic approach to pain management is illustrated in Figure 7-1.

It is helpful to focus the discussion with the patient and/or caregiver on the real goals of pain management: the realistically achievable maintenance or improvement of physical functioning and psychosocial well-being, to which ends palliation of pain is being sought. This calculus does not need to change when the patient enters formal palliative care (hospice) since many patients want to preserve physical independence as long as possible and to maintain clear thinking in order to enjoy hobbies and interactions with family and friends. The patient or surrogate decision maker thus will guide the extent to which symptom control takes precedence. In patients with severe cognitive impairment, the presence of distressful behaviors (moaning, rocking, grimacing, etc.) must guide the intensity of pain management.

Based on the pain assessment, the clinician must decide whether *pro re nata (prn)* analgesia or continuous pain reduction is appropriate for the average level of pain, followed by the choice for a prn analgesic for acute exacerbations. An in-depth discussion of specific

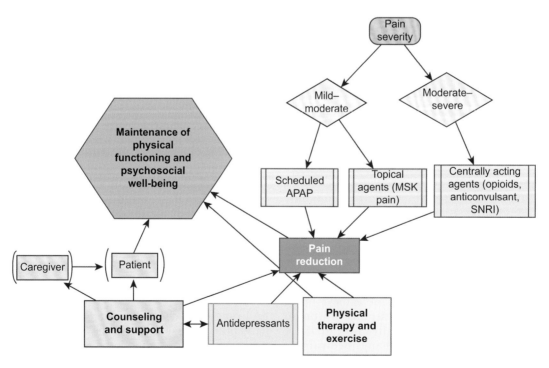

FIGURE 7-1 A systematic approach to the management of chronic pain in the elderly. APAP, acetaminophen, paracetamol; MSK, musculoskeletal; SNRI, selective norepinephrine reuptake inhibitor.

analgesic modalities is beyond the scope of this chapter. Pain treatment should utilize the least potentially toxic modalities first, before adding an opioid. For mild to moderate continuous pain, topical agents may be appropriate for localized musculoskeletal pain. Scheduled acetaminophen (APAP, paracetamol) can be utilized for any mild-moderate pain in the absence of significant liver dysfunction. Chronic NSAIDs are relatively contraindicated in older adults because of their adverse effect on renal function and the increased risk of gastrointestinal bleeding.

The clinician should base the decision to add a centrally acting agent as monotherapy or adjunctive analgesia in part on the balance between its potential benefits and its potential for adverse effects, including drug toxicity and harmful drug-drug interactions that may increase the risk of cognitive dysfunction and falls. This requires a careful review of other prescribed medications and, in some cases, changes in the selection or doses of drugs being given for other conditions. The clinician should perform an assessment of the patient's cognition, gait, and balance before prescribing long-term centrally acting analgesics.

- Has the patient fallen in the past 6 months or does he or she feel unsteady on his or her feet?
- Does he or she use a walking aid?
- Does he or she have difficulty arising from a low chair?

At a minimum, the patient should be asked to stand from his or her chair with hands folded on the chest. If he or she cannot rise without pushing off or must rock back and forth to gain momentum, his or her quadriceps muscles are weak, increasing fall risk. Next, the clinician should ask the patient to stand with his or her feet together and eyes closed, and he or she should be nudged in the chest to cause the back to sway backward (Romberg test). If he or she loses his or her balance, or cannot balance with feet together, he or she is at risk of falling. Next, the patient should be observed walking and turning 180°. Turning very slowly, using multiple steps, swaying, grasping at the wall, and/or an unsteady gait demonstrate increased risk of falling. Orthostatic hypotension occurs in up to 30% of persons >70 years of age[42]; orthostatic vital signs therefore should be obtained.

As the prevalence of mild cognitive impairment and dementia rises exponentially after the age of 75, patients age 75 and older should undergo a baseline mental status screen using a validated office-friendly instrument that includes a test of executive function, such as the Montreal Cognitive Assessment,[43] available for download at http://www.mocatest.org.[44] Given the age-associated increase in the prevalence of depressive symptoms and the close interrelationship between chronic pain and depression, the clinician should also screen for depression with a validated instrument such as the 15-item Geriatric Depression Scale (https://web.stanford.edu/~yesavage/GDS.english.short.score.html).[45]

Comorbid conditions can influence the selection of analgesics. When depression is present, choosing an SNRI such as duloxetine for the treatment of neuropathic pain may be more appropriate than prescribing a gabapentinoid. (Of note, tricyclic antidepressants are relatively contraindicated in the elderly because of their cardiac and anticholinergic side effects.) An SNRI, however, may trigger hypomania in patients with bipolar disorder and would not be the first choice for neuropathic pain. Yet adding a gabapentinoid when they already may be taking an anticonvulsant mood stabilizer may increase the risk of falls. Thus, the selection of an analgesic regimen often becomes a challenging exercise in balancing competing risks.

Physicians can inadvertently contribute to misuse by *overprescribing* an opioid for an acute pain episode, increasing the potential for diversion or misuse. For example, 67% of patients who received opioids following urological surgery at a university hospital reported that they had opioids left over from the initial prescription after their pain had resolved.[46] The instructions on the label can either guide safe use or promote excessive consumption. It is not uncommon for the *signetur (sig)* of an opioid prescription to read, "Take 1 tablet every 6 hours as needed for pain." In ignorance, the patient could take oxycodone every 6 hours for even minor pain related to the surgery or some other painful condition. Patients also may be prescribed too high a dose of the opioid. The polypharmacy experienced by older patients generally correlates with having multiple specialists, who often prescribe for the illness on which they have been consulted, without considering the patient's other conditions or medications. This can result in unintended drug-drug interactions or the prescription of medications that are inappropriate for the patient's pain management, underscoring the importance of careful medication reconciliations at each visit.

Opioid-induced hyperalgesia (OIH): The pharmacotherapy of moderate to severe pain traditionally has required opioids, which can be complicated by *opioid-induced hyperalgesia* in short-term as well as chronic use. OIH is a state of paradoxically increased pain sensitivity caused by opioids and due, in part, to alterations in the interconnected dopaminergic (antinociceptic) and GABA-ergic (pronociceptive) pathways within the mesolimbic system, midbrain, and thalamus that modulate not pain perception as well as mood and pleasure.[47–49] Brains in OIH show microglial activation and neuroinflammation that are similar to that seen in chronic pain states.[47] OIH among patients receiving chronic opioids, even low dose, appears to be common. In a study of patients with chronic joint pain awaiting orthopedic surgery, those taking low-dose opioids displayed significant hyperalgesia, compared to patients not receiving opioids.[50] Among patients undergoing elective total hip arthroplasty (mean age = 55 years), those taking opioids prior to surgery required higher postoperative morphine equivalents for analgesia, were more likely to be taking opioids at 6 weeks and at final follow-up (average = 58 months), and, most importantly, had worse functional outcomes than matched opioid-naive control patients.[49]

The Role of Nonpharmacologic Interventions in the Elderly

Optimization of physical and psychosocial functioning represents 2 of the 3 core objectives of pain management for which pain reduction alone cannot be assumed to be sufficient to address adequately.

Physical therapy and exercise: Exercise interventions for knee osteoarthritis, particularly quadriceps strengthening, have demonstrated small to moderate improvements in both self-reported pain and physical function. Although individual clinical trials have been small, meta-analysis of these studies, involving a total of 3537 subjects, provides high-quality evidence that exercise can produce reductions in pain and improvements in physical function after 2 to 6 months that are sustained for at least an additional 6 months after study completion. These changes are comparable to corresponding improvements with NSAIDs.[51] Exercise interventions for chronic pain in general are difficult to assess in the aggregate because of the heterogeneous nature of the sources of pain and the interventions used. Small sample sizes and short follow-up compromise the quality of some studies. Overall, there were variable effects of exercise on pain severity, physical function, and quality of life, but the low risk of adverse effects and the potential for meaningful benefit still make exercise an important adjunctive treatment.[52] The physician should consider an exercise prescription for most chronic-pain patients, starting, if necessary, with a referral to physical and occupational therapy to learn exercises appropriate for the patient's chronic pain and the underlying condition.

Psychosocial support: Clinicians should aggressively treat comorbid depression. An SNRI can address both depression/anxiety and serve as an alternative or adjunct to opioids, particularly for musculoskeletal and neuropathic chronic pain. For patients who are intolerant of SNRIs, selective serotonin reuptake inhibitors (SSRI) can be tried although evidence for their efficacy in chronic pain is less robust, and they share with SNRIs the potential of inappropriate antidiuretic hormone stimulation and resulting hyponatremia. The anticholinergic and potentially cardiotoxic effects of tricyclic antidepressants make them relatively contraindicated in the elderly although these agents have demonstrated efficacy for neuropathic pain.[1] Other classes of antidepressants may help with depression or anxiety, but may not have concurrent efficacy against the underlying pain.

Psychotherapy also can be useful as an adjunct for treating depression/anxiety and may provide benefits for patients unresponsive to or intolerant of antidepressants. Multiple, small-scale studies have evaluated the short-term efficacy of operant treatments for a variety of chronic-pain etiologies; the best-studied is chronic low-back pain. Overall, these approaches demonstrate some short-term efficacy for improving pain and/or function in chronic low-back pain and have been used in the elderly.[53] Compared to usual care, a randomized trial of short-term psychotherapy in 342 adults aged 20 to 70 years with chronic low-back pain demonstrated that cognitive behavioral therapy (CBT) but not

mindfulness-based stress reduction (MBSR) slightly but significantly reduced reported disability from low-back pain out to 1 year and reduced pain bothersomness out to 6 months.[54] Although not reducing cost related to low-back pain, MBSR has been shown to reduce overall health care costs over 1 year of follow-up.[55]

For older chronic-pain patients living in the community, caregiver counseling may be helpful. Caregivers at times can be "enablers" of their family member's pain, providing sympathy and support that reinforces maladaptive behaviors such as staying in bed or avoiding responsibilities. Operant conditioning seeks to modify this rewarding behavior by the caregiver. Education by the primary-care clinician may help the caregiver understand the magnitude and limitations caused by chronic pain, for which there may not be external manifestations.

SUMMARY

Pain in the geriatric population is highly prevalent and complicated by multiple factors. However assessment and therapeutic approaches are more difficult based on physiological and cognitive changes that occur with aging. An emphasis on function and quality of life should be factored when developing recommendations for this population. Finally, using a careful, deliberate approach to develop a comprehensive, multidisciplinary treatment plan should be used for all geriatric pain patients whenever possible.

REFERENCES

1. Abdulla A, Adams N, Bone M, et al. Guidance on the management of pain in older people. *Age Ageing.* 2013;(42 suppl 1):i1-i57.
2. Larsson C, Hansson EE, Sundquist K, Jakobsson U. Chronic pain in older adults: prevalence, incidence, and risk factors. *Scand J Rheumatol.* 2017;46(4):317-325.
3. Scherer M, Hansen H, Gensichen J, et al. Association between multimorbidity patterns and chronic pain in elderly primary care patients: a cross-sectional observational study. *BMC Fam Pract.* 2016;17:68.
4. Schulz R, Beach SR, Ives DG, Martire LM, Ariyo AA, Kop WJ. Association between depression and mortality in older adults: the cardiovascular health study. *Arch Intern Med.* 2000;160(12):1761-1768.
5. Weyerer S, Eifflaender-Gorfer S, Kohler L, et al. Prevalence and risk factors for depression in non-demented primary care attenders aged 75 years and older. *J Affect Disord.* 2008;111(2-3):153-163.
6. McDougall FA, Kvaal K, Matthews FE, et al. Prevalence of depression in older people in England and Wales: the MRC CFA study. *Psychol Med.* 2007;37(12):1787-1795.
7. McDougall FA, Matthews FE, Kvaal K, Dewey ME, Brayne C. Prevalence and symptomatology of depression in older people living in institutions in England and Wales. *Age Ageing.* 2007;36(5):562-8.
8. Zis P, Daskalaki A, Bountouni I, Sykioti P, Varrassi G, Paladini A. Depression and chronic pain in the elderly: links and management challenges. *Clin Interv Aging.* 2017;12:709-720.

9. de Heer EW, Gerrits MM, Beekman AT, et al. The association of depression and anxiety with pain: a study from NESDA. *PLoS One.* 2014;9(10):e106907.

10. Lebe M, Hasenbring MI, Schmieder K, et al. Association of serotonin-1A and -2A receptor promoter polymorphisms with depressive symptoms, functional recovery, and pain in patients 6 months after lumbar disc surgery. *Pain.* 2013;154(3):377-384.

11. Rodriguez JJ, Noristani HN, Verkhratsky A. The serotonergic system in ageing and Alzheimer's disease. *Prog Neurobiol.* 2012;99(1):15-41.

12. Marinova Z, Monoranu CM, Fetz S, Walitza S, Grunblatt E. Region-specific regulation of the serotonin 2A receptor expression in development and ageing in post mortem human brain. *Neuropathol Appl Neurobiol.* 2015;41(4):520-532.

13. Kaufman J, Sullivan GM, Yang J, et al. Quantification of the serotonin 1A receptor using PET: Identification of a potential biomarker of major depression in males. *Neuropsychopharmacology.* 2015;40(7):1692-1699.

14. Ossipov MH, Dussor GO, Porreca F. Central modulation of pain. *J Clin Invest.* 2010;120(11):3779-3787.

15. Moore RA, Cai N, Skljarevski V, Tolle TR. Duloxetine use in chronic painful conditions–individual patient data responder analysis. *Eur J Pain.* 2014;18(1):67-75.

16. Paladini A, Fusco M, Coaccioli S, Skaper SD, Varrassi G. Chronic pain in the elderly: the case for new therapeutic strategies. *Pain Phys.* 2015;18(5):E863-E876.

17. Curatolo M, Muller M, Ashraf A, et al. Pain hypersensitivity and spinal nociceptive hypersensitivity in chronic pain: prevalence and associated factors. *Pain.* 2015;156(11):2373-2382.

18. Beswick AD, Wylde V, Gooberman-Hill R, Blom A, Dieppe P. What proportion of patients report long-term pain after total hip or knee replacement for osteoarthritis? A systematic review of prospective studies in unselected patients. *BMJ Open.* 2012;2(1):e000435.

19. Arendt-Nielsen L, Skou ST, Nielsen TA, Petersen KK. Altered central sensitization and pain modulation in the CNS in chronic joint pain. *Curr Osteoporos Rep.* 2015;13(4):225-234.

20. Kress HG, Ahlbeck K, Aldington D, et al. Managing chronic pain in elderly patients requires a CHANGE of approach. *Curr Med Res Opin.* 2014;30(6):1153-1164.

21. Yang M, Qian C, Liu Y. Suboptimal treatment of diabetic peripheral neuropathic pain in the United States. *Pain Med.* 2015;16(11):2075-2083.

22. Gianni W, Madaio RA, Di Cioccio L, et al. Prevalence of pain in elderly hospitalized patients. *Arch Gerontol Geriatr.* 2010;51(3):273-276.

23. Edlund MJ, Sullivan M, Steffick D, Harris KM, Wells KB. Do users of regularly prescribed opioids have higher rates of substance use problems than nonusers? *Pain Med.* 2007;8(8):647-656.

24. Levi-Minzi MA, Surratt HL, Kurtz SP, Buttram ME. Under treatment of pain: a prescription for opioid misuse among the elderly? *Pain Med.* 2013;14(11):1719-1729.

25. Bauer U, Pitzer S, Schreier MM, Osterbrink J, Alzner R, Iglseder B. Pain treatment for nursing home residents differs according to cognitive state – a cross-sectional study. *BMC Geriatrics.* 2016;16:124.

26. Leuthauser A, McVane B. Abdominal pain in the geriatric patient. *Emerg Med Clin North Am.* 2016;34(2):363-375.

27. Potts FE, Vukov LF. Utility of fever and leukocytosis in acute surgical abdomens in octogenarians and beyond. *J Gerontol A Biol Sci Med Sci.* 1999;54(2):M55-M58.

28. Coventry LL, Bremner AP, Williams TA, Celenza A, Jacobs IG, Finn J. Characteristics and outcomes of MI patients with and without chest pain: a cohort study. *Heart Lung Circ.* 2015;24(8):796-805.

29. Blozik E, Stuck AE, Niemann S, et al. Geriatric pain measure short form: development and initial evaluation. *J Am Geriatr Soc.* 2007;55(12):2045-2050.

30. Wong-Baker FACES Foundation. Available from: http://wongbakerfaces.org.

31. Warden V, Hurley AC, Volicer L. Development and psychometric evaluation of the Pain Assessment in Advanced Dementia (PAINAD) scale. *J Am Med Dir Assoc.* 2003;4(1):9-15.

32. *University of Iowa College of Nursing Csomay Center of Gerontological Excellence.* 2017. Available from: https://geriatricpain.org.

33. Herr K, Zwakhalen S, Swafford K. Observation of pain in dementia. *Curr Alzheimer Res.* 2017;14(5):486-500.

34. Marcum ZA, Amuan ME, Hanlon JT, Aspinall SL, Handler SM, Ruby CM, et al. Prevalence of unplanned hospitalizations caused by adverse drug reactions in older veterans. *J Am Geriatr Soc.* 2012;60(1):34-41.

35. Smith HS. Opioid metabolism. *Mayo Clin Proc.* 2009;84(7):613-624.

36. van der Leeuw G, Eggermont LH, Shi L, et al. Pain and cognitive function among older adults living in the community. *J Gerontol A Biol Sci Med Sci.* 2016;71(3):398-405.

37. Airagnes G, Pelissolo A, Lavallee M, Flament M, Limosin F. Benzodiazepine misuse in the elderly: risk factors, consequences, and management. *Curr Psychiatr Rep.* 2016;18(10):89.

38. Kurko TA, Saastamoinen LK, Tahkapaa S, et al. Long-term use of benzodiazepines: definitions, prevalence and usage patterns - a systematic review of register-based studies. *Eur Psychiatry.* 2015;30(8):1037-1047.

39. Carnahan RM, Lund BC, Perry PJ, Pollock BG, Culp KR. The anticholinergic drug scale as a measure of drug-related anticholinergic burden: associations with serum anticholinergic activity. *J Clin Pharmacol.* 2006;46(12):1481-1486.

40. Shoair OA, Nyandege AN, Slattum PW. Medication-related dizziness in the older adult. *Otolaryngol Clin North Am.* 2011;44(2):455-471.

41. O'Neil CK, Hanlon JT, Marcum ZA. Adverse effects of analgesics commonly used by older adults with osteoarthritis: focus on non-opioid and opioid analgesics. *Am J Geriatr Pharmacother.* 2012;10(6):331-342.

42. Ricci F, De Caterina R, Fedorowski A. Orthostatic hypotension: epidemiology, prognosis, and treatment. *J Am Coll Cardiol.* 2015;66(7):848-860.

43. Nasreddine ZS, Phillips NA, Bedirian V, et al. The montreal cognitive assessment, MoCA: a brief screening tool for mild cognitive impairment. *J Am Geriatr Soc.* 2005;53(4):695-699.

44. Nasreddine ZS. MoCA: Montreal Cognitive Assessment 2017. Available from: http://www.mocatest.org.

45. Yesavage G. Mood Scale (Short Form) 2017. Available from: https://web.stanford.edu/~yesavage/GDS.english.short.score.html.

46. Bates C, Laciak R, Southwick A, Bishoff J. Overprescription of postoperative narcotics: a look at postoperative pain medication delivery, consumption and disposal in urological practice. *J Urol.* 2011;185(2):551-555.

47. Cahill CM, Taylor AM. Neuroinflammation-a co-occurring phenomenon linking chronic pain and opioid dependence. *Curr Opin Behav Sci.* 2017;13:171-177.

48. Chang G, Chen L, Mao J. Opioid tolerance and hyperalgesia. *Med Clin North Am.* 2007;91(2):199-211.

49. Pivec R, Issa K, Naziri Q, Kapadia BH, Bonutti PM, Mont MA. Opioid use prior to total hip arthroplasty leads to worse clinical outcomes. *Int Orthopaed.* 2014;38(6):1159-1165.

50. Hina N, Fletcher D, Poindessous-Jazat F, Martinez V. Hyperalgesia induced by low-dose opioid treatment before orthopaedic surgery: an observational case-control study. *Eur J Anaesthesiol.* 2015;32(4):255-261.

51. Fransen M, McConnell S, Harmer AR, Van der Esch M, Simic M, Bennell KL. Exercise for osteoarthritis of the knee. *Cochrane Database Syst Rev.* 2015;1:Cd004376.

52. Geneen LJ, Moore RA, Clarke C, Martin D, Colvin LA, Smith BH. Physical activity and exercise for chronic pain in adults: an overview of cochrane reviews. *Cochrane Database Syst Rev.* 2017;1:Cd011279.

53. Henschke N, Ostelo RW, van Tulder MW, et al. Behavioural treatment for chronic low-back pain. *Cochrane Database Syst Rev.* 2010;(7):CD002014.

54. Cherkin DC, Sherman KJ, Balderson BH, Cook AJ, Anderson ML, Hawkes RJ, et al. Effect of Mindfulness-based stress reduction vs cognitive behavioral therapy or usual care on back pain and functional limitations in adults with chronic low back pain: a randomized clinical trial. *JAMA.* 2016;315(12):1240-1249.

55. Herman PM, Anderson ML, Sherman KJ, Balderson BH, Turner JA, Cherkin DC. Cost-effectiveness of mindfulness-based stress reduction vs cognitive behavioral therapy or usual care among adults with chronic low-back pain. *Spine.* 2017;42.

PEDIATRIC PATIENTS

Sungeun Lee, MD

FAST FACTS

- Pain in children can be difficult to gauge. The use of validated scales can better help to assess pain in children.
- Perioperative management of pain involves raising awareness to parents and medical professionals involved in the care of the pediatric patients regarding anxiety and how to manage it.
- Chronic pain in pediatric patients often presents as headaches and abdominal pain. It is important to recognize that conservative management is usually the best course of treatment after ruling out any "red flags."

INTRODUCTION

The overall approach to pain in children has come a long way in the last several decades. Not very long ago, it was believed that very young children did not experience pain, and even if they did, there was no memory of it. Thus, pain in young patients was not regularly or assertively treated. We now know that the neural mechanisms that encode pain perception and that shape our responses to pain develop early in life. Pain systems develop and function as early as 23 weeks of gestation.[1]

Proper management of pediatric patients with pain is essential as there are consequences of untreated pain in the young. Similar short- and long-term sequelae to adults can occur, such as wind up, hyperalgesia, and allodynia.[2] In children, tissue damage during certain critical periods

of development may have a lasting effect, even into adulthood. In addition, there are behavioral, psychological, and social ramifications of untreated pain in children that can carry on to adulthood and chronic pain conditions.

This chapter does not cover all the details of every pain-causing condition in children and their treatment options. Unique aspects of taking care of pain in this population will be highlighted, along with reminders of when referrals to pediatric specialists should be considered.

PAIN ASSESSMENT IN CHILDREN

As with pain assessment in all patients, the approach to pain assessment in children should be multidimensional, with attention to assessment of functionality. This involves gathering information from a variety of sources: patients (if they are able), parents, and/or caregivers. These reports should focus not just on the facets of the pain or primary pain complaint itself but also on other related areas such as school performance/attendance, social relationships, sleep, and mood disturbances. Direct observation of behavior and physiologic measurements should also be used in the assessment of pediatric patients with pain. If interventions are performed, careful monitoring of responses to therapeutic trials can keep track of progress. This broad approach to assessment allows a natural opportunity to plan and set expectations. Early conversations about goals of therapy and equipping the patient and family with knowledge, assurance, and coping skills will establish a positive relationship for all involved.

There are multiple validated scales for pain measurement in children. If a child is old enough and can understand a self-report scale, this should be the main tool used to measure and keep track of pain over time. Self-reported scales can be the simple 0-10 scale, which is useful in children old enough to understand a numerical scale. The FACES scale is the most commonly used self-reported scale for children who may not be able to reliably use a numerical scale. The scale shows a series of FACES ranging from a happy face at 0, or "no hurt," to a crying face at 10, which represents "hurts like the worst pain imaginable." Based on the faces and written descriptions, the child chooses the face that best describes his or her level of pain. In younger patients unable to use a self-report tool, there are observational scales, such as the FLACC scale. These utilize an observer's assessment of things such as Facial expression, Leg movement, Activity, Crying, and Consolability. The acronym FLACC facilitates recall of these elements. Age ranges vary for these scales, so it is essential to use clinical judgment regarding appropriateness for pain assessment. Regardless of the scale used to assess a child's pain, the key is to be as consistent as possible. This includes not only the scale used to assess but also the frequency in which it is assessed, and in what setting.

It is important to briefly note here that as in any assessment of pain causes or sources, the "red flag" list of serious illness processes must be considered. If the child's young age or presentation prevents a complete consideration by the primary care physician, the child should be referred to a pediatric specialist who can complete the workup to ensure that an undiagnosed major illness is not the source of the patient's pain.

ACUTE PAIN MANAGEMENT IN CHILDREN

Approach to nociceptive pain in children does not differ significantly from the approach used in adults. Mild to moderate pain is often treated with oral nonsteroidal anti-inflammatory drugs. Moderate pain may require the addition of an oral opioid. Moderate to severe pain may require the use of intravenous opioids to achieve rapid titration and control of the pain (Table 8-1).

There are some practical concepts when approaching opioid analgesia in children. With severe pain, intravenous administration is often effective quickly. However, each child may respond differently to a given opioid and may have differing respiratory reserve and other complicating medical conditions. Titrating to effect is important in these situations and to give time for a dose to take effect before another dose. This of course, must occur in a proper setting with personnel, monitoring, and support. Oral opioids are not ideal to titrate to effect in these situations because their peak effects may not be seen for hours and repeat oral dosing in a short interval can lead to respiratory depression and other unwanted side effects.

Table 8-2 outlines the opioid options for managing acute pain. There is a notable drug not included in this table. Codeine should not be one of the opioid options used in children. The US Food and Drug Administration placed a black boxed warning on codeine in 2013. Its use is specifically contraindicated in children undergoing adenotonsillectomy with obstructive sleep apnea. This came about after cases of death and serious adverse events in children.[3] There was evidence in some of these children that they were ultrafast metabolizers of codeine, a genetic variant of the liver enzyme pathway that turns codeine into its active form, morphine in the body. It is not readily possible to know which patients are ultrafast metabolizers of this drug, and therefore, caution should be used when prescribing this drug or other opioids that are metabolized in a similar manner.

When using medications from Tables 8-1 and 8-2, it is important to note that there are combination drugs with an opioid and acetaminophen or ibuprofen. The maximum daily dose, appropriate for the patient's age, needs to be adhered to with specific instructions to parents and caregivers about these limits.

Approaches to minimize opioid use whenever possible in children have been widely adopted in the perioperative setting. Strategies to incorporate peripheral nerve blocks, local anesthetic infiltration, and multimodal analgesic techniques can be successful. An example of this success is related to the contraindication of using codeine in children with obstructive sleep apnea after adenotonsillectomy. Many practices have converted to an approach of alternating acetaminophen and ibuprofen around the clock and opioid as a rescue if needed. Many studies have shown effective pain management with no increase in postoperative bleeding complications, which was the reason for not using ibuprofen as readily for this procedure in the past.[4]

PREPARING CHILDREN FOR INVASIVE PROCEDURES AND SURGERY

Children often show fear-related distress before an impending painful event. Often the anticipation exacerbates the anxiety, and the actual painful event and the distress surrounding it are indistinguishable to the

TABLE 8-1 Acute Pain Management in Children: NSAIDs				
DRUG	**DOSE**	**MINIMUM INTERVAL**	**MAX DAILY DOSE**	**COMMENTS**
Acetaminophen	Neonates, infants, children: 10-15 mg/kg ORAL 12 y old and older: 325-500 mg ORAL	Neonates: 6 h Infants, children: 4 h	Neonates: 60 mg/kg/d Infants and children: 75 mg/kg/d up to 3 g/d >12 y old: 3 g/d	
Ibuprofen	10 mg/kg ORAL	6 h	40 mg/kg/d, up to 1200 mg/d	
Naproxen	5-10 mg/kg	8 h	20 mg/kg/d	
Ketorolac	0.5 mg/kg IV 1 mg/kg ORAL	6 h	IV: Lesser of 2 mg/kg/d or 120 mg/d PO: 40 mg/d	Combined IV and PO max: 5 d of therapy or total 20 doses

IV, intravenous; NSAID, nonsteroidal anti-inflammatory drug; PO by mouth.

TABLE 8-2 Acute Pain Management in Children: Opioids

DRUG	DOSE	INTERVAL	COMMENTS
Morphine, ORAL	0.3 mg/kg	3-4 h	
Morphine, IV bolus	Infants: 25 µg/kg	2-3 h	3× more potent than oral morphine
	Children: 25-50 µg/kg	2-3 h	
Hydromorphone, ORAL	Infants and children: 20-40 µg/kg	4 h	4-7× more potent that oral morphine
Hydromorphone, IV bolus	Infants and children: 5-10 µg/kg	3-4 h	20× more potent than oral morphine
Oxycodone, ORAL	0.1 mg/kg	4 h	1.5× more potent than oral morphine
Hydrocodone, ORAL	0.1 mg/kg	4 h	1.5× more potent than oral morphine

From Opioid Conversion. Palliative Care: Education & Training. Available at https://palliative.stanford.edu/opioid-conversion/. Published April 19, 2013. Accessed 15 August 2018. Used with permission from Stanford University School of Medicine.

young patient. Inadequately managed procedural pain may result in long-term adverse consequences, including heightened pain sensitivity and posttraumatic stress symptoms.[5] In this regard, both distress and pain are important to assess, prevent, and relieve.

Up to 60% of children who undergo surgery in the United States experience significant preoperative anxiety.[6] Children with high presurgical anxiety were 3.5 times more likely to develop negative postsurgical behavioral reactions such as temper tantrums, separation anxiety and sleep disturbances, increased emergence delirium, and greater need for analgesia.[7]

The variables that predict a child's anxiety and pain experience can be divided as malleable and nonmalleable.

Nonmalleable

- younger age (decreases after about age 7 years)
- negative temperament
- high level of distress during prior procedures
- avoidant coping style

Malleable

- children's training in the use of coping skills
- behaviors of parents and medical staff

The malleable factors are the ones where prior education and training can have significant impact on the child's experience. Children who seek information are employing a helpful coping style and this should be encouraged to an appropriate level, as these children have better outcomes than those who avoid information.[8]

Another key effective strategy is distraction. Using this strategy is associated with lower levels of pain in a variety of painful procedure settings. The incorporation of electronics to serve as distraction during brief painful procedures or during the immediate preoperative period has made a tremendous impact on helping children cope during these stressful times. Children's hospitals commonly provide tablets, video games, and other age-appropriate electronics to patients.

Distraction is different from information avoiding in that it is deliberate or prompted refocusing of attention from the threatening situation to more pleasing thoughts, images, objects, and events.

Children who use effective coping behaviors before and during procedures have less anticipatory anxiety and subsequent pain and distress than those who do not.[8]

Educating and training children and their families to use these methods can be done before the day of the procedure by primary care physicians. A small amount of caution should be exercised when giving a lot of detailed information about the procedure to children because with too much time (more than a week or so), children can overthink and build up their anticipatory anxiety further. Studies have shown that a week is sufficient time for a child to process the information without too much anticipatory waiting time. Too little time can be to the child's detriment if they are not given sufficient time to process and understand the information.[8]

Parental anxiety is also predictive of greater child distress.

Three types of distress-promoting parent or staff behaviors[9]

1. Reassuring statements, apologies, and empathetic statements—these are emotion-focusing statements and have the effect of directing the child's attention on his or her own distress and pain, as well as on the threatening aspects of the medical procedure. Focusing on these aspects exacerbates children's anxiety and pain.
2. Giving control to the child.
3. Reassurance just before painful event.

Educating families and staff about these behaviors ahead of time may reduce their contribution to the child's distress.

Pharmacologic approaches to this issue have been employed in children for several decades. The most extensive experience is with the anxiolytic effects of oral midazolam. This is an effective approach employed immediately before the procedure in a setting equipped with proper personnel and monitoring.[10]

Many parents and caregivers inquire about parent present induction of anesthesia (PPIA), or being present for the entirety of the procedure itself. This is an opportunity to inform families about realistic expectations for the day of the procedure. There may be specific scenarios where PPIA is appropriate and possible. However, that is determined by the anesthesiologist and most centers do not practice PPIA commonly as studies have shown them to be not as effective as midazolam premedication.[10]

PEDIATRIC CHRONIC PAIN

Unfortunately, persistent and recurrent pain exists in the pediatric population as well. Some estimate that as much as 35% of children and adolescents around the world have chronic pain.[11] This category of pain includes children with chronic medical conditions, such as sickle cell disease, and pain that is the disorder itself, such as functional abdominal pain.

Comprehensive is the critical word in the assessment and treatment of chronic pain in children. Considerations should include, but not be limited to, biological, psychological, and sociocultural factors, all within the considerations of a developing child.

The best strategy for treatment is an early and multidisciplinary approach. The goal of treatment should be delineated and arrived at with the patient and family whenever possible. Focus should be to improve function and quality of life, paying attention to incorporate cognitive behavioral therapy and providing education and resources for caregivers. A referral to a pediatric pain program should be considered for children with complex pain.

Common chronic pain in the pediatric population include abdominal pain and headaches, which are discussed here briefly.

As much as 20% of school-aged children present to their primary care physician with persistent or recurrent abdominal pain.[12] It is more common in girls and in adolescents. The diagnosis of chronic abdominal pain requires 3 episodes of pain within a 3-month period that impairs the patient's activities of daily living. Accompanying symptoms such as weight loss or fever indicate a full workup to rule out other illnesses for the source of pain. Once this has been done, the pain is categorized as a functional disorder, which varies greatly in symptoms and severity but without an identifiable cause.

Definition of functional abdominal pain is symptoms at least once a week for at least 2 months, or continuously for more than 4 to 6 weeks with no evidence of an organic cause. Functional abdominal pain includes different types of abdominal pain, including functional dyspepsia and irritable bowel syndrome. The primary goal in these patients is to minimize the effects of the abdominal pain on the quality of life. Reassurance that outcome is good is important to emphasize. Depending on the history, the child may benefit from alterations in the diet and avoiding any possible identifiable stressors that trigger the abdominal pain. Some children may benefit from medications if there is significant impairment to their activities of daily living. Antispasmodics, laxatives, or acid-suppressing medications may help depending on the child's symptoms. Equipping the child and family with coping aides can be tremendously helpful to managing symptoms, such as behavioral therapy, relaxation exercise, and hypnosis. Fortunately, overall outcome is very good, with almost 50% of patients improving within a few weeks to months.[13]

Headaches present in children with similar features as in adults. Tension headaches are the most common, but patients also present with migraines. It is imperative that the patients are screened for signs and symptoms of increased intracranial pressure. Patients with undiagnosed intracranial mass can present with headaches to their primary care physician, with their only complaint being headaches. The treatment plan for tension headaches and migraines should incorporate a wide range of issues. Sleep hygiene, regular exercise, and healthy lifestyle are integral to improving function for these patients. Identifying exacerbating triggers such as caffeine, stress, and drugs and minimizing or eliminating them as much as possible is also important. Behavioral techniques can be highly effective, as well as alternative therapies such as acupuncture.[14,15]

Strategies for the management of the pediatric patient with chronic pain is multidisciplinary as discussed earlier. However, pharmacologic therapy is usually the minor component of the comprehensive approach. Centers with the resources to provide education and support, physical and occupational therapy, cognitive behavioral therapy, and child psychiatry are ideal places for children with these complex conditions.

In summary, it is important to consider the key differences in the pediatric patients who present with pain. There are often more complex factors contributing to the cause and delayed treatment. Equipping patients and families to better understand and prepare for painful experiences can make an immense difference for the child and have a positive impact on their future painful experiences. As in most scenarios, it is important to rule out most threatening organic causes of pain and to safely approach managing the pain. When a patient's young age or accompanying medical illness are beyond a primary care provider's expertise, consultation or referral to a pediatric specialist is recommended.

REFERENCES

1. Anand KJS, Aranda JV, Berde CB, et al. Summary proceedings from the neonatal pain-control group. *Pediatrics.* 2006;117:S9-S22.
2. Fitzgerald M. The development of nociceptive circuits. *Nature Rev Neurosci.* 2005;6:507-520.
3. Ciszkowski C, Madadi P, Phillips MS, Lauwers AE, Koren G. Codeine, ultrarapid-metabolism genotype and postoperative death. *N Engl J Med.* 2009;361:827-828.
4. Baugh R, Archer S, Mitchell R, et al; American Academy of Otolaryngology—Head and Neck Surgery Foundation. Clinical practice guideline: tonsillectomy in children. *Otolaryngol Head Neck Surg.* 2011;144(suppl 1):S1-S30.
5. Young KD. Pediatric procedural pain. *Ann Emerg Med.* 2005;45:160-171.
6. Wright KD, Stewart SH, Finley GA, Buffett-Jerrott SE. Prevention and intervention strategies to alleviate preoperative anxiety in children: A critical review. *Behav Modif.* 2007;31:52-79.
7. Kain ZN, Wang SM, Mayes LC, Caramico LA, Hofstadter MB. Distress during the induction of anesthesia and postoperative behavioral outcomes. *Anesth Analg.* 1999;88:1042-1047.
8. Blount RL, Piira T, Cohen LL, Cheng PS. Pediatric procedural pain. *Behav Modif.* 2006;30:24-49.

9. Blount R, Piira T, Cohen LL. Management of pediatric pain and distress due to medical procedures. In: Roberts MC, ed. *Handbook of Pediatric Psychology.* 3rd ed. New York: Guilford; 2003:216-233.

10. Kain ZN, Caldwell-Andrews AA, Mayes LC, et al. Family-centered preparation for surgery improves perioperative outcomes in children: A randomized controlled trial. *Anesthesiology.* 2007;106:65-74.

11. King S, Chambers CT, Huguet A, et al. The epidemiology of chronic pain in children and adolescents revisited: A systematic review. *Pain.* 2011;152(12):2729-2738.

12. Malaty HM, Abudayyeh S, O'Malley KJ, et al. Development of a multidimensional measure for recurrent abdominal pain in children: Population-based studies in three settings. *Pediatrics.* 2005;115:e210-e215.

13. Khan S. *Functional Abdominal Pain in Children.* American College of Gastroenterology Patient Education and Resource Center; 2012.

14. Lewis DW, Ashwal S, Dahl G, et al. Practice parameter: evaluation of children and adolescents with recurrent headaches: report of the Quality Standards Subcommittee of the American Academy of Neurology and the Practice Committee of the Child Neurology Society. *Neurology.* 2002;59:490-498.

15. Roth-Isigkeit A, Thyen U, Stoven H, et al. Pain among children and adolescent: Restrictions in daily living and triggering factors. *Pediatrics.* 2005;115:e152-e162.

II

PSYCHIATRIC DISORDERS AND PAIN

9

THE GENERAL MEDICAL PSYCHIATRIC INTERVIEW

Robert M. McCarron, DO, DFAPA, Jeremy DeMartini, MD and John Onate, MD

A 30-year-old woman with a history of chronic low back pain and intermittent headaches and tobacco use presents to transfer care from another provider with the following opening statement, "That horrible doctor ignored my pain and wanted me to suffer! I heard you are the best doctor in town. I can already tell we are going to be great friends!" The woman's speech is loud and somewhat fast. When the provider suggests she try physical therapy instead of an opioid medication, she yells, "Why don't you just kill me now?" The provider wonders if the patient is bipolar and whether she needs to be psychiatrically hospitalized.

Clinical Highlights

- The mental status examination for a psychiatric evaluation is analogous to the physical examination for a general medical assessment.
- The AMPS screening tool (Figure 9-1) includes 4 primary clinical dimensions of the psychiatric review of systems: **A**nxiety, **M**ood, **P**sychosis, **S**ubstance use. This approach can be easily used in the primary care setting as a starting point to develop a reasonable differential diagnosis for common psychiatric disorders.
- The psychiatric interview places an emphasis on psychosocial function and should give a personalized description of the patient from a biopsychosocial perspective.
- One helpful time-saving strategy is the use of the Supplemental Psychiatric History Form to help gather a preliminary psychiatric history. A patient should complete this form either before the first clinic visit or during later visits, if a psychiatric illness is suspected.

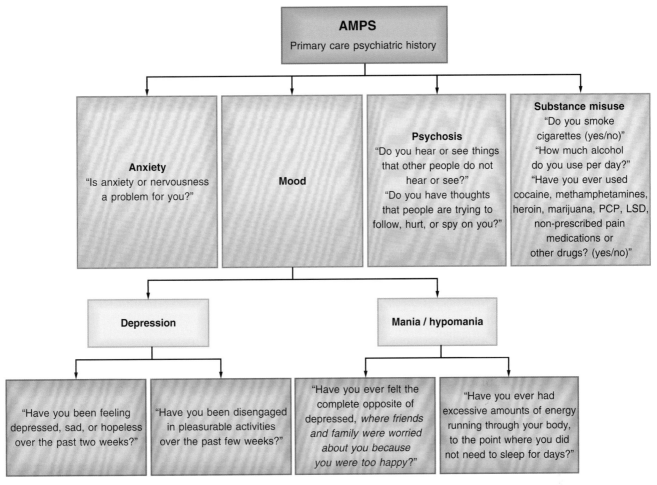

FIGURE 9-1 Psychiatric review of systems: AMPS screening tool. Reprinted with permission from McCarron RM. *Primary Care Psychiatry*. 2nd ed. Philadelphia, PA: Wolters Kluwer; 2018.

CLINICAL SIGNIFICANCE

Up to 75% of all mental health care is delivered in the primary care setting.[1] Unfortunately, reimbursement constraints and limited psychiatric training in most primary care curricula often discourage full exploration and thorough workup of mental illness.[2] Owing to the stigma of psychiatric conditions, patients are often reluctant to present to mental health settings and may not seek treatment.[3] However, most nonemergent or severe psychiatric conditions can be treated successfully in general medical care settings. The ability of the primary care clinician to carefully screen for and evaluate psychiatric symptoms is paramount to accurately diagnose and effectively treat the underlying psychiatric disorder.[4] Also, management of chronic general medical conditions, such as chronic physical pain, is usually much easier if psychiatric conditions are addressed.

Clinical assessment relies heavily on both obtaining the medical history and completing a physical examination for general medical conditions. A similar approach is taken for psychiatric disorders with 2 main differences. First, the psychiatric interview places additional emphasis on psychosocial stressors and overall level of functioning. Second, the mental status examination is analogous to the physical examination for a general medical workup and is the cornerstone for the psychiatric evaluation. Both of these tasks may be accomplished effectively with improved organization and practice. This chapter divides the psychiatric assessment into 3 sections: (1) the psychiatric interview, (2) the mental status examination, and (3) time-saving strategies.

THE PSYCHIATRIC INTERVIEW

The initial interview is important as it sets the tone for future visits and will influence the initial treatment.[5,6] Although the information obtained from the interview is critical to establish a diagnosis, a collaborative, therapeutic relationship is a key component to a successful treatment plan. Therefore, the clinician should try to balance the urgency to obtain information with the need to establish a positive, trusting therapeutic alliance with the patient. Similar in style and complementary to the general medical history, the psychiatric interview is outlined in Table 9-1.

TABLE 9-1 Outline of the Primary Care Psychiatric Interview	
Chief complaint and history of present illness	• For the first few minutes, just listen to better understand the chief complaint(s) and start the mental status examination • Make note of changes in social or occupational function • Use the AMPS screening tool for psychiatric symptoms
Past psychiatric history	• Ask about past mental health providers and hospitalizations • Inquire about whether the patient has ever thought of or attempted suicide
Medication history	• Ask about medication dosages, duration of treatment, effectiveness, and side effects
Family history	• The clinician might ask, "Did your grandparents, parents, or siblings ever have severe problems with depression, bipolar disorder, anxiety, schizophrenia, or any other emotional problems?"
Social history	***Socioeconomic status*** "How are you doing financially and are you currently employed?" "What is your current living situation and how are things at home?" ***Interpersonal relationships*** "Who are the most important people in your life and do you rely on them for support?" "How are these relationships going?" ***Legal history*** "Have you ever had problems with the law?" "Have you even been arrested or imprisoned?" ***Developmental history*** "How would you describe your childhood in one sentence?" "What was the highest grade you completed in school?" "Have you ever been physically, verbally, or sexually abused?"

Chief Complaint and History of Present Illness

The vast majority of physicians interrupt before patients can share their opening concerns.[7] By starting with open-ended questions and allowing the patient to share their perspective, the interviewer can establish rapport and start their mental status examination. Of course, this investment of time may temporarily take away from discussion of other medical conditions, but it is generally well worth the time. Reflective statements may be used to clarify and summarize particular problems (e.g., "You are telling me that you feel your previous physician did not care about your pain as he stopped your opiate medication."). Clarification may also be used (e.g., "Can you explain to me why you think your previous physician stopped the opiate medication?"). Gentle confrontation can be used to point out inconsistencies or bring topics to the forefront that a patient is avoiding or expressing ambivalence about (e.g., "When I started asking you about physical therapy you said you want me to kill you, but later you insisted that you are not suicidal, can you explain this to me?").

It is important to organize the sequence of events with each problem individually, giving the most time to the problem with the highest priority. For patients with multiple chronic problems, setting an agenda at the beginning of the encounter will also help them to understand and conceptualize their medical problems. The history of present illness should include the duration, severity, and extent of each symptom along with exacerbating and ameliorating factors. Patients vary greatly in their recall of historical material and often vague or contradictory material surfaces. Once consent is obtained from the patient, it is important to follow up on any inconsistencies with the patient and gather collateral information by speaking with family members and other treatment providers.

Psychiatric Review of Systems: AMPS Screening Tool

A thorough review of the major psychiatric dimensions (or "review of systems") should be completed for patients who present with even a single psychiatric symptom. In the time-limited primary care setting, this can be a difficult but critically important task. The most commonly encountered primary care psychiatric disorders involve 5 major clinical dimensions and can be remembered by the **AMPS** mnemonic: **A**nxiety, **M**ood, **P**sychosis, **S**ubstance use disorders (Figure 9-1). We recommend incorporating the AMPS screening tool into your daily practice, but especially when a patient has an established psychiatric disorder (including personality and eating disorders) or presents with psychiatric complaints, such as depression, anxiety, insomnia, and unexplained physical complaints. When a particular dimension is present and causing distress, further exploration is indicated (Table 9-2).

Anxiety

Anxiety is common in the primary care and pain medicine settings and often comorbid with mood, psychotic, and substance misuse disorders. It is sometimes the main catalyst for a depressive or substance use disorder, and the secondary condition(s) will not remit unless the

TABLE 9-2 The AMPS Screening Tool for Common Psychiatric Conditions

	SCREENING QUESTIONS	FOLLOW-UP QUESTIONS	DIAGNOSTIC AND TREATMENT INSTRUMENTS[a]
Anxiety	"Is anxiety or nervousness a problem for you?"	• "Please describe how your anxiety affects you on an everyday basis." • "What triggers your anxiety?" • "What makes your anxiety get better?"	Generalized Anxiety Disorders Scale (GAD - 7)
Mood	Depression[b] **1.** "Have you been feeling depressed, sad, or hopeless over the past 2 weeks?" **2.** "What do you usually like to do for fun and have you stopped doing this over the past few weeks?" Mania/hypomania **1.** "Have you ever felt the complete opposite of depressed, *when friends and family were worried about you because you were too happy?*" **2.** "Have you ever had excessive amounts of energy running through your body, to the point where you did not need to sleep for days?"	• "What is your depression like on an everyday basis?" • "How does your depression affect your daily life?" • "When did this last happen, and please tell me what was going on at that time." • "How long did this last?" • "Were you using any drugs or alcohol at the time?" • "Did you require treatment or hospitalization?"	Patient Health Questionnaire (PHQ-9) Mood Disorder Questionnaire (MDQ)
Psychosis	**1.** "Do you hear or see things that other people do not hear or see?" **2.** "Do you have thoughts that people are trying to follow, hurt, or spy on you?" **3.** "Do you ever get messages from the television or radio?"	• "When did these symptoms start?" • "What triggers your symptoms?" • "What makes your symptoms get better?"	None recommended for the primary care setting
Substance use	**1.** "How much alcohol do you drink per day?" **2.** "Have you been using any cocaine, methamphetamines, heroin, marijuana, PCP, LSD, ecstasy, or other drugs?"	If yes: • "How often do you use?" • "As a result of the use, did you experience any problems with relationships, work, finances, or the law?" • "Have you ever used any drugs by injection?" If no: • "Have you ever used any of these drugs in the past?"	• CAGE[c] • CAGE-AID (adapted to include drugs) • Alcohol Use Disorders Identification Test (AUDIT-C)
[d]Suicide	**1.** "Do you ever wish you could go to sleep and not wake up?" **2.** "Do you have any thoughts of wanting to hurt or kill yourself or somebody else?"	• "Have you ever tried to hurt or kill yourself in the past?" • "Do you have guns or other items you could use to harm yourself?"	

[a]*These are suggested instruments that could be considered. More details about relevant instruments are available in the corresponding chapters.*
[b]*If either of these 2 questions is answered affirmatively, follow-up questions should be asked and a PHQ-9 should be administered.*
[c]*See Chapters 6 and 7 for details.*
[d]*Suggest asking about suicide if one of the AMPS questions is positive.*

primary anxiety disorder is treated. Anxiety is also a significant acute risk factor for suicide that is commonly underappreciated and poorly screened (see Chapter 14). The quickest and most effective way to screen for an anxiety disorder during the interview is to simply ask, "Is anxiety or nervousness a problem for you?" If the patient reports feeling anxious, it is advisable to say, "Please describe how your anxiety affects you on an everyday basis." Depending on the answer, follow-up questions (e.g., "What type of situations or events trigger your anxiety") will help develop a reasonable differential diagnosis. Also, if anxiety is a problem, it may be helpful to ask the patient if it is a "big problem, small problem, or somewhere in between." A numerical scale may also be used to quantify the level of anxiety.

Mood

The best way to understand a patient's mood is to ask, "How would you describe your mood or emotions over the past few weeks?" The self-reported mood is also an important part of the mental status examination and should be rated as either congruent or incongruent with the corresponding affect. The 2 main components of mood (depression and mania) should be fully assessed during each primary care psychiatric interview.

Depression is often secondary to and comorbid with primary anxiety, sleep, substance use, and other psychiatric disorders. Depression may worsen with those who have severe and treatment-refractory chronic pain. Depressive symptoms should always be discussed with the patient when treating another psychiatric condition(s), even if the chief complaint is not depression. The 2 screening questions for a current major depressive episode are: (1) "Have you been feeling depressed, sad, or hopeless over the past two weeks?" and (2) "Have you had a decreased energy level in pleasurable activities over the past few weeks?" An alternative way to ask this second screening question is, "What do you normally like to do for fun and have you been doing that over the last few weeks?" The sensitivity and specificity for the detection of a major depressive episode using these screening questions are 96% and 57%, respectively.[6] If the answer to either of these 2 questions is positive, the clinician should have a high index of suspicion for a depressive disorder and probe further. An open-ended approach would be to ask, "What is your depression like on an everyday basis?" or "How does your depression affect your daily life?" In most cases, depressed patients will discuss their troubling symptoms and there will be no need to go through the entire "checklist" for depression (e.g., changes in appetite, energy, sleep, concentration). The Patient Health Questionnaire (PHQ-9) is a 9-item patient self-report form that can be used in the primary care setting to screen for depression or quantify changes in the severity of depression over the course of treatment. *All depressed patients should be asked about suicidal thoughts, plans, and intent, and a clear assessment of acute suicide risk should be included in the progress note.*

Not all depression is related to a major depressive episode. After screening for depression, one should search for evidence suggestive of a past or current manic or hypomanic episode, as discrete depressive episodes may be related to bipolar spectrum illness. It is important to screen for bipolar disorder, as the comorbidity with some psychiatric disorders is more than 50% to 80% (e.g., attention deficit hyperactivity disorder and substance use disorders). Hypomanic and manic episodes should be considered in most patients with depression, anxiety, irritability, and insomnia. Also, it is important to screen for bipolar disorder when starting an antidepressant, as unopposed antidepressants may increase the risk of inducing a manic episode and will often be ineffective

in treating bipolar depression. Once a patient has had one clearly defined hypomanic or manic episode, the lifelong diagnosis of his or her mood disorder becomes a bipolar spectrum disorder with the appropriate specifier for each mood episode (e.g., "bipolar disorder, most recent episode depressed," rather than "major depressive disorder").

On examination, it may be obvious when a manic episode is present. However, it can be quite a challenge to elicit manic symptoms from the past. Asking questions such as "Have there been times when you have had a lot of sex or shopped excessively?" or "Have you ever felt on top of the world?" may confuse the patient and can lead to diagnostic uncertainty. It is preferable to include the opinions of the patients' family and friends, as they may have different perspectives. If collateral history from friends and family is not available, the practitioner can ask, "Have you ever felt the opposite of sad or depressed, *where friends and family were worried your mood was too elevated or irritable for days to the point of needing medical attention?*" or "Have you ever had excessive amounts of energy running through your body, to the point where you did not need to sleep for days?" With the last question, it is important to differentiate primary insomnia from a lack of need for sleep due to a manic episode. If the patient answers yes to either question, the follow-up questions should be "When did this last happen?" "What was going on at that time?" and "Were you using any substances such as amphetamines or cocaine?" Most patients will be able to relive that event with you and provide specific information that will help narrow the differential diagnosis.

Psychosis

Psychotic symptoms such as disorganized speech and behavior, paranoid delusions, and hallucinations do not commonly present in the primary care setting. These symptoms are, however, important to assess, as they are often associated with mood disorders and substance misuse disorders or are secondary to a general systemic medical condition. The following questions can be used to evaluate psychosis: (1) "Do you hear or see things that other people do not hear or see?" and (2) Do you have thoughts that people are trying to follow, hurt, or spy on you?" These questions will identify a history of hallucinations or delusions (also known as positive symptoms), whereas disorganized speech or behavior will usually be evident during the mental status examination and during collection of the collateral history. In general, persistent psychotic symptoms of unclear cause warrant further psychiatric consultation and evaluation for schizophrenia.

Substance Use

Comorbid substance use, abuse, and dependence are common in primary care and chronic pain management patients presenting with psychiatric symptoms. Alcohol misuse disorders are particularly common in the United States. Substance use disorders mimic nearly all psychiatric symptoms, especially anxiety, depression, insomnia, hyperactivity, irritability, and hallucinations. Misuse of opioids has become increasingly more problematic and is now considered one of the most common causes for accidental deaths among adults. Clues to substance use may include social factors such as inability to maintain employment, interpersonal and financial problems, repeated legal offenses, and poor adherence to treatment. Key aspects of a substance abuse history include specific substance(s) used; quantity; frequency; total duration; means of getting the drug; impact of drug use on personal, family, and work functioning; and previous sobriety and treatment history. Priority should be placed on active drug use, especially that which negatively affects medical treatment and adherence.

Because nonpathologic use and misuse of alcohol are both widely encountered, we recommend assuming most patients may use alcohol on a daily basis and screen with this in mind. When asking about use of other substances, it will likely be perceived as less judgmental to avoid words such as "recreational," "illicit," or "illegal" when asking the patient about use of nonprescription substances. We recommend listing each substance when inquiring about use (e.g., "Do you use cocaine, heroin, acid, speed, ecstasy, marijuana, or nonprescribed pain medications?").

Suicidal Ideation

Almost half of those patients dying by suicide have seen their primary care provider within 1 month before their death, whereas fewer than one-quarter have seen a mental health professional.[8] Many practitioners are uncomfortable with discussing suicide, but there is no evidence that discussing suicide increases risk.[9] Asking about suicide should not be limited to patients with major depressive disorder, as substance use disorders and schizophrenia have a similar risk of suicide and anorexia nervosa has a substantially higher risk of suicide.[10] As this can be a sensitive topic for both providers and patients, it is important to both establish rapport and provide empathic rationale for asking questions related to suicide (e.g., "Sometimes when patients are in severe pain, they start to think about going to sleep and not waking up, or even killing themselves, has this happened to you?"). If a patient responds yes to a screening question, follow up with questions about intent (e.g., "How likely on a scale from 0 to 10 are you to kill yourself"), plan (e.g., "Have you thought about how you would kill yourself?), prior attempts, and access to guns or other lethal means of suicide. A provider should document suicide risk, differentiating between acute and chronic risk, whether there are any modifiable risk factors (such as removing guns from the home or stopping alcohol), and if the patient is at moderate or high acute risk to get an emergency mental health professional consult or call 911 before the patient leaves the office.

Past Psychiatric and Medication History

The structure and content of the psychiatric history is essentially the same as the medical history. Past diagnoses, treatments, hospitalizations, and mental health providers comprise the main categories. Frequency of psychiatric hospitalization may reveal severity and chronicity of the psychiatric condition. It is important to describe medication dosage, duration, response, side effects, and adherence. Obtaining prior medical records is helpful when developing a differential diagnosis and treatment plan.

Family History

Psychiatric disorders are based on both genetic and environmental factors. Patients with a family history of a first-degree relative with major depressive disorder, bipolar disorder, substance dependence, or schizophrenia have up to a 10-fold increased chance of having a mental illness.[11] Patients who have family members with psychiatric illness often have some understanding of these conditions and may have a better knowledge about treatment and available resources.

Social History

The social history lends important information on how the patient functions outside of the clinical setting. Although the information may be detailed and complex, it is most helpful to focus on the patient's level of psychosocial functioning. The social history can be divided into 4 areas: socioeconomic status, interpersonal relationships, legal history, and developmental history. The 4 areas with sample questions to prompt dialogue in these areas are illustrated in the subsequent text.

Socioeconomic Status

A quick way to determine one's socioeconomic status is to ask the following questions: "How are you doing financially and are you currently employed?" "What is your current living situation and how are things at home?" A patient's ability to secure such basic necessities as food and shelter is an important priority. For a homeless patient, gathering more detail on the factors that led to homelessness often reveals important diagnostic information. Frequent job changes or loss of employment can be clues to occult substance use or mood disorders. A patient who is seeking disability compensation versus one who must return to school or work immediately may have different urgencies about improving his or her situation.

Interpersonal Relationships and Sexual History

To explore a patient's ability to initiate and maintain relationships with family, friends, and coworkers, the clinician might ask, "Who are important people in your life and do you rely on them for support?" or "How are these relationships going?" This is also a good time to ask about sexual history. Sexual history includes gender identity, sexual orientation, current and past sexual activity, sexual performance, history of sexually transmitted infections, and the use of contraceptives. Perspectives of the patient's family, friends, and cultural group on mental illness should also be considered, because stigma about treatment and nontraditional approaches may influence treatment attitude and outcomes.

Legal History

Open-ended questions such as "Have you ever had problems with the law?" or "Have you ever been arrested or imprisoned?" are easy ways to broach the topic of legal history. Legal history provides information about psychosocial functioning as well as previous experience with violence and crime. Patients who are recently released from prison and are still on parole or have a felony record may have difficulty finding employment and suffer from stigma. Moreover, those who have been imprisoned for many years often find it difficult to reassimilate into a less structured lifestyle on release from prison. These stressors can increase the risk for substance abuse and exacerbate psychiatric symptoms, which can be a cause for nonadherence to medical care.

Developmental History

The developmental history has multiple components and can be a challenge to obtain in one encounter. Suggested questions include (1) "How would you describe your childhood in one sentence?" (2) "What was the highest grade you completed in school?" and (3) "Have you ever been physically, verbally, or sexually abused?" These questions may bring out long-standing stressors and illustrate the patient's most developed (and underdeveloped) coping strategies. Chaotic and unstable childhood development and a history of abuse are often important issues to address as part of a comprehensive psychosocial treatment plan.

MENTAL STATUS EXAMINATION

The Mental Status Examination (MSE) is an observation and report of the present cognitive, emotional, and behavioral state. The MSE is the "physical examination" of psychiatry and is meant to paint a picture of the patient. Much of the MSE is gathered as the interview unfolds. An accurate and concise description of the MSE also facilitates consultation with mental health professionals. Similar to a comprehensive neurologic examination, an in-depth cognitive assessment is not feasible (or necessary) for most clinical encounters in the primary care setting. The following summarizes high-yield, salient components of the MSE (Table 9-3).

Appearance

Appearance is a description of the overall hygiene, grooming, and dress of the patient and whether they appear their biologic age. For example, a patient who is malodorous or wearing clothing inappropriate to weather (3 jackets in summer or a tank-top in winter)

TABLE 9-3 Key Features of the Mental Status Examination (MSE)

Appearance	• What is the status of the hygiene and grooming and are there any recent changes in appearance?
Attitude	• How does the patient relate to the clinician? • Is the patient cooperative, guarded, irritable, etc., during the interview?
Speech	• What are the rate, rhythm, and volume of speech?
Mood	• How does the patient describe his or her mood? • This should be reported as described by the patient.
Affect	• Does the patient's facial expressions have full range and reactivity? • How quickly does the affect change (lability)? • Is the affect congruent with the stated mood, and is it appropriate to topics under discussion?
Thought process	• **How** is the patient thinking? • Does the patient change subjects quickly, or is the train of thought difficult to follow?
Thought content	• **What** is the patient thinking? • What is the main theme or subject matter when the patient talks? • Does the patient have any delusions, obsessions, compulsions, or suicidal or homicidal thoughts?
Perceptions	• Does the patient have auditory, visual, or tactile hallucinations?
Cognition	• Is the patient alert? • Is the patient oriented to person, place, time, and the purpose of the interview?
Insight	• Does the patient recognize that there is an illness or disorder present? • Is there a clear understanding of the treatment plan and prognosis?
Judgment	• How will the patient secure food, clothing, and shelter in a safe environment? • Is the patient able to make decisions that support a safe and reasonable treatment plan?
Reliability	• Is the patient able to provide information that is consistent and accurate with other sources?

may be gravely disabled (unable to secure adequate food, clothing, or shelter) because of a severe mental illness, such as schizophrenia, major depressive disorder, or bipolar disorder. A patient who is wearing revealing clothing, excessive jewelry, or makeup could have mania or a personality disorder. Likewise, a patient who appears much older than expected by age may have had a long history of homelessness, severe mental illness, and/or substance abuse.

Attitude

Attitude is the manner in which the patient responds to or interacts with the interviewer. The attitude can be cooperative in a typical patient; avoidant in a patient with history of trauma; intrusive, hostile, or passive-aggressive in a patient with a personality disorder; or guarded and distrustful in a patient who is paranoid. A patient's attitude and level of engagement help also in evaluating the reliability of the patient.

Speech

Speech is described by rate (e.g., slow, rapid, or pressured), volume, articulation (e.g., dysarthric, garbled), and rhythm (e.g., stuttering, stammering). Normal speech is generally described as "regular rate, rhythm, and volume." Dysarthric speech may be due to a cerebral vascular accident, medication side effects, and alcohol or substance intoxication. Rapid or pressured speech may indicate intoxication, corticosteroid-induced mania, anxiety, or bipolar mania. Increased speech latency may point to schizophrenia, dementia, or depression with related psychomotor retardation.

Mood

Mood is a description of the overall pervasive, subjective, and sustained emotional state and can be assessed by simply asking, "How would you describe your mood?" Mood should be ideally noted in the patient's own words, using quotation marks. Mood generally ranges from *depressed* to *euphoric*, with a normal or *euthymic* mood as the reference point. Other common states include empty, guilty, anxious, angry, and irritable mood.

Affect

Affect is the expressed emotional state or degree of emotional responsiveness and is inferred from the patient's collective facial expressions. Components of affect include congruency, range, reactivity, rate of change (lability), and intensity. Under normal circumstances, there should be congruency between the patient's mood and affect. If the affect and mood are incongruent and difficult to reconcile, the clinician should consider an active psychotic disorder, malingering, or factitious disorder. For example, a psychotic patient who is depressed may laugh rather than show a mood-congruent affect. A *restricted* range of affect describes limited expression of emotional states. Reactivity describes the degree of affective change in response to external cues. For example, a depressed patient may have an affect that is restricted to depressive expressions and decreased reactivity to the interviewer. A patient who is manic or intoxicated with a stimulant may exhibit a *labile* and expansive affect. A *blunted* affect is defined as a low-intensity affect with decreased reactivity, often seen in patients who have major depressive disorder or schizophrenia. A *flat* affect is not commonly encountered, has little to no emotional or facial expression, and is often found in those who have advanced Parkinson disease or catatonia.

Thought Process

Thought process describes the organization of thoughts or *how* one thinks. A normal thought process is described as *logical, goal directed,* or *linear,* which means the patient is able to complete a train of thought in reasonable depth. Although no single abnormality of thought process (also referred to as formal thought disorders) is pathognomonic for a specific disorder, this information is critical to the development of an accurate differential diagnosis. A *concrete* thought process may be logical but lacks depth. *Circumstantial* thinking refers to the painstaking movement of thoughts from the origin (point A) to the goal (point B) with excessive focus on insignificant details. A patient who exhibits *tangential* thinking will quickly change the focus of the conversation in a way that ultimately deviates from the main topic (e.g., "I know it is important to take my medications so my schizophrenia can get better. My neighbor is on a medication for his headaches; do you know which one it might be?"). *Looseness of association* is an abrupt change of focus where the thoughts are numerous and disconnected. A *disorganized* thought process refers to disconnected topics or irrelevant answers to questions posed. *Limited* (or *paucity of*) thoughts occur in patients with severe depression, those with profound negative symptoms (e.g., catatonia), or those who are internally preoccupied with delusions or hallucinations.

Thought Content

Thought content is a description of the main themes and preoccupations expressed by the patient. Simply put, the thought content is *what* the patient is thinking. Depressed patients will usually present with themes of poor self-esteem, worthlessness, or hopelessness. Patients with a somatoform disorder often focus almost exclusively on physical symptoms. *Obsessions* are intrusive thoughts that are the focus of constant and nearly involuntary attention but are by definition nonpsychotic in nature (e.g., "What if I accidently left the oven on and my house burns down?"). *Delusions* are fixed, false beliefs and are characterized by a lack of insight. Common delusional themes are paranoid (e.g., "The FBI is trying to kill me."), grandiose (e.g., "I own oil companies and rule five states!"), erotic (e.g., "I know the governor loves me."), and bizarre (e.g., "The Martians have tattooed me and that is why the police always bother me in the park."). *Illusions* are misinterpretations of sensory information (e.g., mistaking a chair for a person). *Hallucinations* are sensory perceptions in the absence of any stimuli and typically are auditory, visual, or tactile. Hallucinations are found in many psychiatric disorders not limited to schizophrenia. Suicidal or violent content should be explored in all patients with severe mental illness, especially those with *command hallucinations* (wherein the hallucination directs the patient's behavior).

Cognition

Cognitions are higher-order brain functions and include orientation, concentration, calculation, memory, and executive function. Orientation to person, location, date, and purpose should be queried. If the clinician has a high index of suspicion for a cognitive deficit, further assessment can be initiated in the primary care setting. Asking the patient to repeatedly subtract 7 starting from 100 (serial 7's) or spell "world" backward can assess concentration or attention span. Impairment in the level of alertness or consciousness is characteristic of delirium, alternatively termed encephalopathy (by neurologists) or less specifically called altered mental status (by most health professionals). Long- and short-term memory problems may become evident if the patient is unable to provide clear and organized historical data. Whenever there is a concern for cognitive deficits, the Mini-Mental State Examination (MMSE) or Montreal Cognitive Assessment (MoCA), familiar to most primary care providers, should be performed to screen for dementia and other neurocognitive disorders.

Insight

Insight describes the degree by which the patient understands his or her diagnosis, treatment, and prognosis. A patient who denies a problem that clearly exists or minimizes the severity of symptoms has poor insight. Chronic illness and suboptimal insight often lead to poor outcomes. Restoration of insight is usually a key component to the long-term treatment plan.

Judgment

Judgment is the ability to make reasonable decisions that result in safe, desirable, and socially acceptable outcomes. The ability to weigh benefits versus risks and recognize consequences of behavior is a core part of judgment. Examples of questions that assess "real-time" capacity for judgment include, "How might napping during the day affect your sleep at night?" and "What steps can you take to decrease the chance you will binge drink?"

Reliability

Reliability is an assessment of the accuracy of the history that the patient provides. Sometimes patients recount events with such inconsistency that they cannot be readily trusted. For example, a depressed patient may be asking to be discharged after being brought to the emergency room (ER) for a tranquilizer overdose. She may initially recall swallowing breath mints and later may report taking sleeping pills, but did not realize she took more than one. In other instances, the interviewer will need to verify the patient's story by obtaining collateral information (with permission) from the patient's family, friends, or health records.

PHYSICAL EXAMINATION

The physical examination gives the clinician another opportunity to build rapport and obtain historical information. Unexplained tachycardia, diaphoresis, tremors, or hyperreflexia should alert the provider about possible stimulant intoxication or alcohol-sedative withdrawal. A careful inspection of the extremities and skin revealing tattoos, burns, bruises, scars, or other injuries should

be followed up with inquires about their origins. For patients with severe mental illnesses (e.g., schizophrenia) and unstable housing, inspection of hair and skin for parasites and teeth for decay or abscesses is important, because these patients may not have routine access to medical care or may place other needs at a higher priority. Similarly, a diabetic patient with severe mental illness may not have the insight to self-monitor for foot ulcers. Therefore, the primary care provider may use the physical examination as another opportunity to gauge an individual's functional status by his or her ability to maintain activities of daily living independently and to manage his or her medical disorders.

Not to Be Missed

- A complete primary care psychiatric assessment should always include the AMPS screening tool. It is also good to consider asking about thoughts of suicide in the context of assessing mood, anxiety, psychosis, and substance misuse.

- The mood and affect should be assessed and recorded as important parts of the mental status examination. Mood is the overall internal emotional state, whereas affect is the expressed emotional state that is manifested by changes in facial expression.

- Disorders of speech and behavior are often found in those with severe mental illness and should be monitored carefully. Thought process describes *how* one thinks, and thought content describes *what* one thinks.

- A social history should be obtained on all patients who are being treated for a psychiatric illness. The main components of a primary care psychiatric social history include socioeconomic status, interpersonal relationships, legal history, and developmental history.

TIME-SAVING STRATEGIES

We recommend the following *time-saving strategies* when completing a primary care psychiatric biopsychosocial assessment.

1. Obtaining the social history is one of the most important pieces of the primary psychiatric interview. There is much to cover, and it can certainly be time intensive if not done properly. Although it is not all-encompassing, we suggest the following "starter questions" to help the clinician collect the necessary information for a social history.

Socioeconomic status
"How are you doing financially and are you currently employed?"

"What is your current living situation and how are things at home?"

Interpersonal relationships
"Who are the most important people in your life and do you rely on them for support?"
"How are these relationships going?"

Legal history
"Have you ever had problems with the law?"
"Have you even been arrested or imprisoned?"

Developmental history
"How would you describe your childhood in one sentence?"
"What was the highest grade you completed in school?"
"Have you ever been physically, verbally, or sexually abused?"

2. If you could only pick three questions during a primary care psychiatry interview, the following are suggested:
"What is your number one biggest problem that we can work on together?"
"Currently, how are you dealing with your problem?"
"Is there someone in your life who you can go to if you need help?"

3. We highly recommend using the Supplemental Psychiatric History form (Figure 9-2) for all new patients or for those who you think have significant psychiatric symptoms. This form is easy for a patient or clinician to complete and covers the pertinent psychosocial history as well as the AMPS screening questions. The clinician can quickly glance at this form and tailor further assessment accordingly. All "yes" answers should raise concern and prompt further questioning. More in-depth disorder-specific assessments are discussed in the chapters to follow.

PRACTICE POINTERS

CASE 1: The Primary Care Psychiatric Interview

A 30-year-old woman with a history of chronic low back pain and tobacco use presents to transfer care to your practice with the chief complaint, "That horrible doctor ignored my pain and wanted me to suffer! I heard you are the best doctor in town. I can already tell we are going to be great friends!" The woman's speech is loud and somewhat fast. When the provider suggests she try physical therapy instead of an opioid medication, she yells, "Why don't you just kill me now?" The provider wonders if she is manic and needs to be psychiatrically hospitalized.

The AMPSS screening questions reveal that the patient has struggled with "mood swings" since her childhood. It is clarified that she does not stay in any one mood state for several days or weeks on end, but rather fluctuates from happy to sad to anxious to irritable to irate in a matter of a few hours. The triggers for these episodes tend to be interpersonal conflicts, especially when she feels a threat of being abandoned. When she is stressed, she will occasionally have an out-of-body experience or hear a voice that is derogatory and self-critical, but these disturbances do not occur when she is calm and happy. She has a history of binge drinking alcohol as well as misusing several different prescription painkillers and tranquilizers (trading pills with friends, using the medications more frequently then prescribed, and seeking prescriptions from multiple providers), but she has never been hospitalized or suffered legal consequences because of substance use. She does not endorse any current desire to harm herself and denies access to firearms. She is looking forward to going to her mother's 60th birthday party next week.

The patient has tried several antidepressant medications but has never taken any one for more than a few days owing to vague and atypical side effects. She has never been prescribed a traditional mood stabilizer such as lithium or valproic acid. As a teenager she saw a counselor for a couple of months and briefly tried going to Alcoholics Anonymous (AA), but she has never tried an evidence-based psychotherapy such as dialectical behavior therapy (DBT). She has had numerous ER visits and a couple of short inpatient psychiatric hospitalizations for suicidal ideation and intentional overdoses. Her mother struggled with depression, and her father died of complications related to alcohol abuse. The patient experienced significant trauma, including physical abuse and neglect. She has had numerous romantic relationships with whom she has cohabitated. She is currently living with her mother, whom she feels is well supported by, and her fiancé of 3 months, whom she states is her soulmate.

After consent is obtained, a phone call is made to the patient's mother. The mother confirms the patient's psychiatric history and agrees that she tends to wear a large amount of jewelry when she leaves the house and that she has had fast and loud speech since she was a child. She also denies that the patient has had periods of hypomania or mania that lasted days or weeks or has any access to firearms.

On mental status examination, the patient appears her chronological age and has a plethora of brightly colored jewelry and noticeable makeup. She is generally cooperative but quickly changes to hostile when alternatives to opiates are suggested. Speech is loud with an increased rate, but she is interruptible. Her mood is irritable overall and her affect range is wide but appropriate to thought content. Her thought process is linear and thought content is negative for suicidal or homicidal ideation but includes themes of chronic emptiness and suffering, fears of abandonment, and splitting. She has no perceptual disturbances and is fully alert and oriented without obvious cognitive deficits. Her insight into her substance misuse is poor and judgment is fair at best. Her reliability is fair to good.

AMPS Behavioral Health History Form

Name: _____ **Date:** _____

Reason for Appointment: _____

Past Psychiatric Diagnoses (circle if applicable):

- Anxiety
- Depression
- Bipolar disorder
- Schizophrenia
- Schizoaffective disorder

- Alcohol misuse
- Drug misuse
- Borderline personality disorder
- Insomnia
- Other Mental health diagnosis

Have you ever been treated by a psychiatrist or other mental health provider?	Yes / No
Have you ever been a patient in a psychiatric hospital?	Yes / No
Have you ever tried to hurt or kill yourself?	Yes / No
Have you ever taken a medication for psychiatric reasons?	Yes / No

If yes, please list the most recent medication(s) below:

#1: _____ Did you have any problems with this medication?	Yes / No
#2: _____ Did you have any problems with this medication?	Yes / No
#3: _____ Did you have any problems with this medication?	Yes / No
#4: _____ Did you have any problems with this medication?	Yes / No
#5: _____ Did you have any problems with this medication?	Yes / No

Family Psychiatric History: Did your grandparents, parents, or siblings ever have severe problems with depression, bipolar disorder, anxiety, schizophrenia, or any other emotional problems? Yes / No

Social and Developmental History:
Socioeconomic Status
Are you currently unemployed?	Yes / No
Are you having any problems at home?	Yes / No

Interpersonal Relationships
Are you having any problems with close personal relationships?	Yes / No

Legal History
Have you ever had problems with the law?	Yes / No

Developmental History
Have you ever been physically, verbally, or sexually abused?	Yes / No
What was the highest grade you completed in school?	_____

Anxiety Symptoms, Mood Symptoms, Psychotic Symptoms, Substance Use
Is anxiety or nervousness a problem for you?	Yes / No

Mood Symptoms
• Have you been feeling depressed, sad, or hopeless over the past two weeks?	Yes / No
• Have you had a decreased interest level in pleasurable activities over the past few weeks?	Yes / No
• Have you ever felt the complete opposite of depressed, *when friends and family were worried about you because you were too happy?*	Yes / No
• Have you ever had excessive amounts of energy running through your body, to the point where you did not need to sleep for days?	Yes / No
• Do you have any thoughts of wanting to hurt or kill yourself or someone else?	Yes / No

Psychotic Symptoms
Do you hear or see things that other people do not hear or see?	Yes / No
Do you have thoughts that people are trying to follow, hurt, or spy on you?	Yes / No

Substance Use
How many packs of cigarettes do you smoke per day?	_____
How much alcohol do you drink per day?	_____
Have you ever used cocaine, methamphetamines, heroin, marijuana, PCP, LSD, Ecstacy, or other drugs?	Yes / No

FIGURE 9-2 Supplemental psychiatric history form. Reprinted with permission from McCarron RM. *Primary Care Psychiatry.* 2nd ed. Philadelphia, PA: Wolters Kluwer; 2018.

Discussion

This case illustrates a challenging scenario to many providers. In addition to having chronic pain, the patient most likely has an opioid use disorder as well as borderline personality disorder. However, caution is advised before making a personality disorder diagnosis based on an initial evaluation in a busy primary care setting. The provider likely does not have time to obtain collateral information during every intake appointment, and it would be best to observe for a persistent pattern of maladaptive traits over a series of appointments. The provider should consider bipolar disorder based on the patient's extravagant jewelry; loud, fast speech; and affective instability; however, in this case, these are chronic and persistent, not episodic in nature. When in doubt the provider may want to consider a psychiatric consultation before starting an antidepressant medication.

Although the patient does make a flagrant comment to the provider, "Why don't you just kill me now?", this appears to be a manipulative attempt to obtain opioids. The patient is at higher chronic risk of suicide owing to her history of impulsive behavior and prior attempts; however, she is not at an elevated acute risk as she is future-oriented, feels well supported, denies any intent or plan to die, and does not have access to firearms.

The complete biopsychosocial assessment helps the clinician to provide a comprehensive treatment plan. In addition to initiating a multimodal treatment of chronic pain, a plan for psychotherapy such as DBT (which has been shown to decrease suicidal thoughts and impulsive behaviors) should be considered. The clinician might say, "Chronic pain can cause high levels of stress on the body and mind, which may make it harder to deal with mood swings as well as increase the chance that you act impulsively or even harm yourself. DBT has been shown to help patients manage stress and it does not have the risk of side effects that medications may have." The patient should also be encouraged to revisit the idea of attending AA meetings, because impulsivity and chronic pain are associated with higher risk of relapse. An antidepressant that also works on descending spinal pain pathways, such as duloxetine or amitriptyline, may be useful, although the clinician should take care to start at a low dose given the patient's history of multiple antidepressant intolerances as well as provide psychoeducation and a follow-up plan if the patient experiences any hypomania or mania.

Finally, it is important to understand why the patient has recently changed primary care providers. The therapeutic connection between the patient and the clinician is paramount. In this case, the provider might be compelled to focus exclusively on "opioid-seeking behavior". However, the provider could take this as an opportunity to focus on building rapport and better understand the patient's defenses, including catastrophizing and splitting, which may contribute to fragmented care and worse outcomes. Short and somewhat frequent office visits may be indicated over the next few months to address his many concerns and maintain a biopsychosocial treatment approach.

Practical Resources

The MacArthur Initiative on Depression and Primary Care: http://www.depression-primarycare.org/

Substance Abuse and Mental Health Services Administration: http://www.samhsa.gov/index.aspx.

American Psychiatric Association Practice Guidelines: http://www.psych.org/MainMenu/PsychiatricPractice/PracticeGuidelines_1.aspx.

National Institute of Mental Health: http://www.nimh.nih.gov/health/publications/depression-a-treatable-illness.shtml.

National Alliance on Mental Illness: www.nami.org.

REFERENCES

1. Reiger DA, Boyd JH, Burke JD, et al. One month prevalence of mental disorders in the United States. *Arch Gen Psychiatry.* 1988;45:977-986.
2. Onate J. Psychiatric consultation in outpatient primary care settings: should consultation change to collaboration? *Primary Psychiatry.* 2006;13(6):41-45.
3. Kessler RC, Demler O, Frank RG, et al. Prevalence and treatment of mental disorders, 1990 to 2003. *N Engl J Med.* 2005;352(24):2515-2523.
4. Katon W, Roinson P, Von Korff M, et al. A multifaceted intervention to improve treatment of depression in primary care. *Arch Gen Psychiatry.* 1996;53(10):924-932.
5. Vergare MJ, Binder RL, Cook IA, et al. American Psychiatric Association practice guidelines for the psychiatric evaluation of adults second edition. *Am J Psychiatry.* 2006;163(6 suppl):3-36.
6. Whooley MA, Simon GE. Managing depression in medical outpatients. *N Engl J Med.* 2000;343(26):1942-1950.
7. Beckman HB, Frankel RM. The effect of physician behavior on the collection of data. *Ann Intern Med.* 1984;101(5):692-696.
8. Luoma JB, Martin CE, Pearson JL. Contact with mental health and primary care providers before suicide: a review of the evidence. *AM J Psychiatry.* 2002;159:909-916.
9. Dazzi T, Gribble R, Wessely S, Fear NT. Does asking about suicide and related behaviours induce suicidal ideation? What is the evidence? *Psychol Med.* 2014;44(16):3361-3363.
10. Chesney E, Goodwin GM, Fazel S. Risks of all-cause and suicide mortality in mental disorders: a meta-review. *World Psychiatry.* 2014;13(2):153-160.
11. Hales RE, Yudofsky SC, Gabbard GO. *The American Psychiatric Publishing Textbook of Psychiatry.* 5th ed. Washington, DC: American Psychiatric Association; 2008.

10

SOMATIZATION DISORDERS

Matthew Reed, MD, MSPH and Amir Ramezani, PhD

FAST FACTS

- Somatization is commonly encountered in the outpatient setting and often requires a long-term treatment plan.
- Psychiatric disorders, such as depression and anxiety, frequently coexist with somatic symptom and related disorders. We suggest using the anxiety, mood, psychotic and substance use disorders (AMPS) screening tool (inquiring about anxiety, mood, psychotic, and substance use disorders, see Chapter 2) when assessing the psychiatric review of systems. The prognosis of someone with a somatic symptom disorder will usually improve when comorbid psychiatric illness is promptly identified and treated.
- Although most patients with a somatic symptom and related disorder may benefit from psychiatric consultation, they often initially refuse to see a psychiatrist. Therefore, primary care practitioners play a key role in the treatment of these disorders.
- The CARE MD treatment plan (see Table 10-1) may be a useful approach for patients who have somatic symptom and related disorders.

A 32-year-old man with no previous medical history presents to an urgent care clinic complaining of "gas in the stomach," shortness of breath, and squeezing back pain that prevents him from working. Other symptoms include a "jumping sensation in the legs" and "poor circulation in the hands and feet." He is unsure about what condition he might have. He is so concerned about his health that he has been sleeping in his car near the hospital for the past few days. He has seen numerous doctors over the past 6 months and, after an extensive medical workup, has been told there are no obvious medical problems.

CLINICAL SIGNIFICANCE

Primary care practitioners encounter unexplained and perplexing somatic complaints in up to 40% of their patients.[1,2] However, medical explanations for common physical complaints such as malaise, fatigue, abdominal discomfort, and dizziness are found only 15% to 20% of the time.[3] Patients and primary care practitioners alike can become frustrated when symptoms persist without a clear cause or when symptoms seem out of proportion for any of the patient's known medical conditions. Frustration is compounded when treatments targeting the symptoms are only partially effective. Abnormal thoughts, feelings, and behaviors may develop in response to somatic symptoms and can significantly disrupt daily life. This process of developing abnormal thoughts, feelings, and behaviors in relation to bothersome somatic symptoms is loosely termed somatization. Although it is difficult to reliably determine the prevalence of somatization because of changing definitions, most studies estimate a prevalence of 16% to 20% in primary care settings.[4]

The common occurrence of somatization carries a large financial burden. A retrospective review of over 13,000 psychiatric consultations found that somatization resulted in more disability and unemployment than any other psychiatric illness.[5] Moreover, patients with somatization in

TABLE 10-1 CARE MD—Treatment Guidelines for Somatic Symptom and Related Disorders

CBT/ Consultation	• Follow the CBT treatment plan
Assess	• Exclude general medical causes and treat comorbid psychiatric disorders
Regular visits	• Schedule short frequent visits with focused • Discuss recent stressors and healthy coping strategies • Over time, excessive health care utilization will decrease
Empathy	• "Become the patient" for a brief time • During visits, spend more time listening and acknowledge patient's reported discomfort
Med-psych interface	• Help the patient self-discover the connection between physical complaints and emotional stressors ("the mind-body" connection) • Avoid comments which may be perceived as condescending or judgmental such as, "your symptoms are all psychological" or "there is nothing wrong with you medically"
Do no harm	• Avoid unnecessary diagnostic procedures • When possible, minimize unnecessary requests for referral to medical specialists

Adapted from McCarron R. Somatization in the primary care setting. Psychiatric Times. 2006;23(6):32-34.
CBT, cognitive-behavioral therapy.

the primary care setting have more than twice the outpatient utilization and overall medical care costs when compared with patients without somatization. The direct costs related to the management of unexplained physical symptoms approach 10% of medical expenditures or over $100 billion annually in the United States.[6]

DIAGNOSIS

Disorders involving somatization are defined in the Diagnostic and Statistical Manual of Mental Disorders, 5th edition (DSM-5) under the category of "somatic symptom and related disorders."[7] There are 5 key disorders from this category, including somatic symptom disorder, illness anxiety disorder, conversion disorder (functional neurological symptom disorder), psychological factors affecting other medical conditions, and factitious disorder. Prior editions of the DSM included a requirement that general medical conditions be excluded before diagnosing a somatic symptom disorder. With the release of DSM-5, this requirement has been eliminated.

To meet criteria for any of these disorders, one must have distressing somatic symptoms in addition to abnormal thoughts, feelings, and behaviors in response to the symptoms. These symptoms must also result in a significant disruption of daily life (For details please see Diagnostic and Statistical Manual of Mental Disorders 5th edition (DSM-5) pages 309-327).

PATIENT ASSESSMENT

Other than completing a thorough history and physical examination with indicated laboratory or radiographic tests, there are no specific diagnostic protocols for patients who have a somatic symptom disorder. It is important to review collateral history from other health care providers and family to help confirm the diagnosis and reduce redundant and unnecessary medical evaluations or interventions.

DIFFERENTIAL DIAGNOSIS

The differential diagnosis for unexplained physical symptoms seen in the primary care setting is extensive. It is important to keep in mind that "unexplained" somatic symptoms may be due to (1) a medical condition that has not yet been diagnosed; (2) a medical condition that is present but not yet known to the medical community at large; (3) a psychiatric condition such as malingering, factitious disorder, or one of the somatic symptom and related disorders; or (4) both a general medical condition and one of the above-mentioned psychiatric conditions. Somatic symptom disorder is no longer a "diagnosis of exclusion," but is instead based on the presence of distressing somatic symptoms plus abnormal thoughts, feelings, and behaviors in response to those symptoms. Patients may have a chronic medical condition with somatic symptoms, but their abnormal thoughts, feelings, and behaviors related to those symptoms may qualify them for an additional diagnosis of somatic symptom disorder.

Before establishing the diagnosis of a somatic symptom disorder, one should attempt to rule out the intentional production of physical or psychological symptoms. A patient with malingering is focused on feigning illness to gain external incentives such as financial compensation, controlled substances, shelter, or escape from occupational duty or criminal prosecution. Factitious disorder involves the purposeful and sometimes elaborate self-report of somatic complaints with the objective of assuming the "sick role." People with factitious disorder have no obvious external secondary gain. When treating either condition, it is important to obtain collateral history (particularly from other area hospitals and providers), conduct a focused physical examination, and consider both as diagnoses of exclusion. People who are malingering are not usually "antisocial." Instead, they are often emotionally troubled and under so much psychological stress that they engage in maladaptive and deceitful coping strategies, with resultant isolation from family, friends, and medical providers. Once a diagnosis of malingering is established, one should attempt to confront the patient in a supportive and reassuring way while trying to problem solve using a multidisciplinary team approach. Assisting malingerers with urgent stressors and attempting to find appropriate ways to meet their needs can be effective and a psychiatric referral is not normally indicated. However, if a diagnosis of factitious disorder is made, psychiatric consultation is strongly advised because this disorder can be difficult to treat and carries a poor long-term prognosis.

TABLE 10-2 Diagnosis to ICD-10 Crosswalk	
DSM-5 DIAGNOSIS	**ICD-10 CODE**
Somatic symptom disorder	F45.1
• With predominate pain	F45.42
Illness anxiety disorder	F45.21
Conversion disorder	
• With weakness or paralysis	F44.4
• With abnormal movement	F44.4
• With swallowing symptoms	F44.4
• With speech symptoms	F44.4
• With attacks or seizures	F44.5
• With anesthesia or sensory loss	F44.6
• With special sensory symptom (e.g., visual, olfactory, or hearing disturbance)	F44.6
• With mixed symptoms	F44.7
Psychological factors affecting other medical conditions	F54
Factitious disorder	F68.10
Other specified somatic symptom and related disorder	F45.8
Unspecified somatic symptom and related disorder	F45.9

ICD-10, International Classification of Diseases 10th revision.

BIOPSYCHOSOCIAL TREATMENT

The treatment approach to somatic symptom and related disorders exemplifies the "art of medicine." Because these disorders occur on a wide-ranging diagnostic continuum, with elusive causes, it is difficult to apply a strict, evidence-based approach to treatment.[8,9] We propose a simplified treatment plan that is described by the acronym CARE MD (Table 10-1).[10] This approach encourages patients to be active participants in their care and serves as a guide to help primary care practitioners effectively work with people who have somatoform disorders. Additionally, we provide a "crosswalk" reference to help practitioners achieve the correct ICD-10 diagnosis from the DSM-5 diagnosis (Table 10-2). This facilitates use of appropriate medical coding for compliance with health information privacy, billing and medical documentation.

COGNITIVE-BEHAVIORAL THERAPY/CONSULTATION

Consultation with mental health professionals and use of cognitive-behavioral therapy (CBT) has been shown to decrease the severity and frequency of somatic preoccupations.[11,12] Kroenke and Swindle, in 2000, reviewed 31 controlled studies and concluded that CBT is an effective treatment of patients with somatization. Group therapy using CBT with an emphasis on education has also been found to be beneficial.[13] CBT generally consists of 10 to 20 one-hour psychotherapy sessions with the goal of teaching patients how to take an active role in their treatment and developing skills that last a lifetime. This type of psychotherapy is based on the premise that negative, automatic, or "dysfunctional thoughts" are predominant in patients with somatic symptom and related disorders. Examples of such thoughts are "I will always be sick and never get better," "No one understands or believes my pain," and "Everyone thinks it's all in my head." Through a variety of mechanisms, patients learn to recognize and reconstruct dysfunctional thought patterns with resultant decreased somatic complaints. Patients should be encouraged to use a daily dysfunctional thought record (DTR) to self-monitor depressive or anxious emotions and associated negative thoughts.

In collaboration with the therapist, primary care providers can learn to use brief cognitive behavioral techniques and quickly review a DTR during office visits. In addition, we recommend that patients with somatic symptom, depressive, or anxiety disorders, as well as treating mental health and primary care practitioners, learn the basics of CBT. One of many practical resources includes the book *Feeling Good: The New Mood Therapy* by Davis Burns, MD.[14] The first 80 pages of this book are practical and teach the patient how to recognize dysfunctional thought patterns and complete "homework" that will reverse cognitive distortions, decrease somatization, and improve mood (Figure 10-1).

ASSESS MEDICAL AND PSYCHIATRIC COMORBIDITIES

Assessing patients on each visit for general medical problems that might explain troublesome physical complaints is essential. This is particularly important for patients who have a long history of somatic preoccupation and present with a new complaint or a worsening of existing symptoms. Up to 25% to 50% of patients with conversion disorder eventually have an identifiable, nonpsychiatric disease that explains their symptoms.[15] It is also important to screen for other

Emotions	Automatic Thoughts	Rational Response	Outcome
Rate feelings 1-10 (where 10 is most intense)	"What is running through your head" (Not an emotion or feeling)	Why is the automatic thought inaccurate (Be specific)?	Rate your feeling again on a scale of 1-10
"Sad" 8/10	"My pain will *never* go away."	"Not true –I am working hard with my doctor so my pain will get better over time." "Never is a strong word to use."	"Sad" 5/10
"Angry" 9/10	"*Everyone* thinks I am faking my pain."	"My doctor listens to me and everyone is a lot of people!" "I know my family is trying to understand my pain and depression."	"Angry" 3/10
"Anxious" 9/10	"*Nobody* will ever figure out what is wrong with me and there's no reason to go on living."	"I know I have somatic symptom disorder and doing my CBT homework will only help me." "Sometimes I feel like dying, but I know I want to live."	"Anxious" 4/10

FIGURE 10-1 Sample dysfunctional thought record.

common psychiatric diagnoses. Up to 50% of patients with somatic symptom and related disorders have concurrent anxiety or depressive disorders.[16,17] The number of unexplained somatic symptoms is highly predictive of comorbid mood and anxiety disorders as well as functional disability. Primary care clinicians can address frequently co-occurring depression by using the Patient Health Questionnaire (PHQ-9), a patient self-report tool that reliably screens for depression in the primary care setting (see Chapter 2). All patients with a score greater than 5 should be assessed for a possible major depressive disorder.

REGULAR VISITS

Regular visits with a single clinician are critical to the management of somatic symptom and related disorders. Short, frequent appointments or telephone encounters have been shown to decrease outpatient medical costs while maintaining patient satisfaction.[18] These encounters should include a brief but focused history and physical examination followed by open-ended questions such as "How are things at home?" "What is your number one, biggest problem?" or, if the patient is exposed to CBT, "Tell me about your most frequent negative thoughts since your last visit." Over time, patients can replace excessive emergency room visits or frequent calls to the clinic with this supportive, caring patient-provider interaction. Longer, less frequent visits can be reserved for assessment and treatment of other general medical disorders and health care maintenance. In sum, spending most of the time during the shorter, frequent visits on worrisome psychosocial stressors will provide an outlet for patients to better cope with somatic preoccupation.

EMPATHY

Empathy or briefly "becoming the patient" is important for developing a strong therapeutic alliance between the patient and the health care provider. The use of empathy can also minimize negative feelings or countertransference from providers. True empathic remarks such as "This must be difficult for you" or "It must be very hard to cope with what you are experiencing" are often therapeutic. Modeling empathic communication when frustrated family and friends are present may also help improve patient-family interactions outside of the clinic. Although there are clear benefits associated with an empathic communication style, it can at times be emotionally taxing for medical providers. To mitigate potential frustration or even burnout, we recommend the utilization of Balint groups or regularly scheduled, candid, and confidential discussions about challenging patient encounters with colleagues who experience similar clinical situations.

MEDICAL-PSYCHIATRIC INTERFACE

Patients diagnosed with a somatic symptom disorder should be educated about how emotions and stressors have a direct effect on their body. Understandably, many patients will not accept explanations for their unexplained physical symptoms with statements (or indirect communications) such as "It's all in your head," "There is nothing medically wrong with you," or "A psychiatrist will have to take care of your complaints." Instead, primary care practitioners should provide a diagnosis and, if necessary, arrange for a psychiatric consultation while remaining the primary point of contact for all medical issues. During short but frequent office visits, patients should be asked if their unexplained symptoms worsen as a primary stressor intensifies or if the symptoms improve as a primary stressor lessens. If the answer is affirmative to both questions, allow the patient to gradually make the connection by asking an open-ended question such as "Do you have any thoughts on why this might be?" Essentially, it is best to help the patient self-discover the connection between the unresolved conflict or emotional stress and the somatic symptoms.

DO NO HARM

Doing no harm by avoiding unnecessary procedures or consultations is the most important part of treating patients with somatic symptom and related disorders. Providers should not deviate from clinical best practices to appease a patient or minimize their own frustration. Although unnecessary invasive procedures should be avoided, routine health care maintenance should be emphasized and offered when indicated. These routine studies may be offered over time, rather than completing every test in one visit. Doing so will help keep to the principle of "short and frequent" visits. After taking reasonable steps to rule out general medical cause for the symptoms, make the appropriate somatic symptom disorder diagnosis and treat accordingly.

PHARMACOTHERAPY

Although antidepressants may be considered for the treatment of somatic symptom disorders, we generally do not recommend starting such medications, especially on the first encounter. In our clinical experience, offering psychotropic medications for a somatic symptom disorder too quickly may reinforce the idea that the symptoms are exclusively psychiatric in nature and may impair the development of a trusting therapeutic relationship. On the other hand, antidepressants should be considered when comorbid depressive or anxiety disorders are discovered and treatment is accepted by the patient. Even with a receptive patient, a significant amount of effort is typically required to educate about the potential psychiatric contribution to their unexplained physical ailment. The provider should only start psychotropic medications after establishing full collaboration with the patient.

When to Refer

- Patients with significant social or occupational dysfunction directly related to a somatic symptom (and related) disorder should be referred to a psychiatrist.
- Patients with comorbid psychopathology such as psychosis or suicidal ideation should receive an urgent psychiatric referral.
- In cases where a psychiatric referral is placed for somatization, the primary care provider should receive input from the psychiatrist but remain the primary care provider.

CASE-BASED LEARNING

CASE 1

A 32-year-old man with no previous medical history presents to an urgent care clinic complaining of "gas in the stomach," shortness of breath, and squeezing back pain that prevents him from working. Other symptoms include a "jumping sensation in the legs" and "poor circulation in the hands and feet." He is unsure about what condition he might have. He is so concerned about his health that he has been sleeping in his car near the hospital for the past few days. He has seen numerous doctors over the past 6 months and, after an extensive medical workup, has been told there are no obvious medical problems. He does not take any medications. He smokes occasionally and denies illicit drug use. He is currently unemployed. Both parents are healthy with no family history of heart disease or cancer. The physical examination reveals an anxious and somewhat dramatic man who uses frequent hand gestures. He repeatedly states, "There is something wrong with my heart." The laboratory studies, including complete blood count, basic chemistry panel, and thyroid studies, are normal. Two weeks later, the patient returns to inquire about his laboratory tests. During this visit, he reports vague physical complaints and recalls that a neurologist had suggested that he might have problems in his spine. He admits to a history of depression more than 3 years ago, which improved on its own. He denies current

depressed mood and states, "There is nothing wrong with my head." In fact, he becomes quite upset when the physician suggests that his symptoms could be related to depression or anxiety. He does concede that things have been stressful for him over the last few months and that he noticed a temporal correlation between the stress and the symptoms. He is motivated to get better and has no desire to collect disability. His physical examination was normal.

Which of the following is the most appropriate diagnosis for this patient?

A. Somatoform disorder
B. Illness anxiety disorder
C. Somatic symptom disorder
D. Malingering

(Answer: C)

Discussion

This patient exhibits several symptoms that are vague, are seemingly disconnected, and do not suggest any obvious general medical cause. This patient describes numerous somatic symptoms that are distressing and debilitating. His behavior is excessive as evidenced by repeated doctor visits and sleeping in his car near the hospital. He demonstrates a persistently high level of anxiety about his symptoms and has devoted excessive time and energy to doctor visits and medical workups. His symptoms have persisted for at least 6 months. He meets criteria for somatic symptom disorder. There is no reason to think he is intentionally feigning the symptoms for either external (e.g., financial) or internal (e.g., assuming the "sick role") gain, and therefore, he does not meet criteria for malingering or factitious disorder. He is not preoccupied with a specific illness or diagnosis, so does not have illness anxiety disorder. Treatment should begin with the development of a supportive, nonjudgmental, and collaborative relationship. It is important that the provider spend sufficient time to understand the patient's symptoms and consequent suffering. The provider may explain to the patient that, although the current symptoms may not point to a clear medical condition, continued monitoring is indicated. It is important to point out the dangers of unnecessary diagnostic tests and procedures as they can lead to false-positive results and increased morbidity. We recommend close attention to health care maintenance and general counseling about diet, exercise, and smoking cessation. After a therapeutic alliance has been established, psychoeducation regarding unexplained physical symptoms could be introduced. Subsequent exploration of possible psychosocial precipitants of the distressing physical symptoms should be attempted. Assessment of concurrent psychiatric conditions using the AMPS screening tool should be ongoing. Referral to a mental health professional may also be considered. CBT is a well-studied first-line intervention for somatic symptom and related disorders. It is advisable for medical providers to become familiar with CBT principles and the use of a DTR, as this is an evidence-based approach studied in primary care settings.

CASE 2

A 22-year-old woman with a history of insomnia, progressive fatigue, and poor concentration is brought to the emergency department by family for the third time in 7 days to see the "on-call neurologist" for "seizures." The patient recently lost her job and reluctantly reports feeling severely depressed without suicidal ideation. When asked to recall what happens during a seizure she states, "I feel confused and try to talk to people around me, but just keep shaking." There is no loss of consciousness, tongue biting, injuries, bowel or bladder incontinence, or postictal disorientation. She is unable to recall any emotional trigger before these episodes. When asked about any history of abuse, she pauses for some time but eventually denies any abuse. She has no other pertinent medical history and denies any illicit drug or alcohol use. Owing to financial difficulties she recently moved in with her family. Her mother reports that this is very uncharacteristic of her daughter.

Which of the following is the most appropriate diagnosis for this patient?

A. Epilepsy
B. Conversion disorder
C. Somatic symptom disorder
D. Malingering

(Answer: B)

Discussion

Given her description of the seizures, it is unlikely she has a true seizure disorder. This young woman underwent a recent stressor (job loss) followed by the development of a nonintentional motor abnormality most consistent with psychogenic nonepileptic seizures, a *conversion disorder*. It is often challenging to differentiate psychogenic nonepileptic seizures from epileptic seizures without the use of video-electroencephalography. Also consider that up to 30% of patients with psychogenic nonepileptic seizures have concomitant documented epilepsy, underscoring the importance of thorough evaluation and consultation with specialists. Further evaluation and potential treatment of her depressive symptoms with an antidepressant and/or CBT is indicated. There is generally a stressful event that precedes the development of conversion disorders. Identifying and addressing the emotional event may be helpful. In this case, further

exploration of physical, sexual, or emotional abuse should be attempted in a private and safe environment and without the presence of family members. It is not helpful to challenge the patient with statements such as, "your problem is strictly psychiatric" or "you do not have a medical problem." It is helpful to direct the patient toward functional recovery through the development of coping techniques and better anxiety management strategies. CBT is an evidence-based intervention that may help reduce the number of episodes and improve psychosocial function.

CASE 3

A 44-year-old man with no past medical history is seen in an emergency room with complaint of "I cannot feel my face ... I think I'm having a stroke." He can talk on the phone and eat solid and liquid foods without difficulty. He does not give permission to obtain collateral history from his family or friends. A nurse overhears him on the phone say, "It's cold out there and you better let me back in the house." When confronted, he admits his wife separated from him recently and that he is homeless. He also laments, "My face is paralyzed, and I need to be hospitalized." A neurologic examination and brain imaging are both normal. All laboratory values, including blood alcohol and toxicology screens, are also normal. The patient's response to reassurance from the emergency department physician is, "You better admit me ... at least for tonight."

Which of the following is the most appropriate diagnosis for this patient?

A. Factitious disorder
B. Conversion disorder
C. Somatic symptom disorder
D. Malingering

(Answer: D)

Discussion

In this case, a thorough diagnostic workup was done, and it is likely the patient is malingering to obtain shelter (external, secondary gain). Unlike those who have a somatic symptom disorder, patients who malinger intentionally report inaccurate information to realize a predetermined goal. Although it is often challenging, practitioners should try to empathize with patients who are malingering and focus on a solution to the actual problem. In this case, a discussion about housing options that do not include the hospital should be addressed with the patient in an assertive and nonpunitive manner. Collaboration with social workers and knowledge about local resources is important. The clinician can point out that admitting the patient to the hospital will not solve his housing problem or financial problems. Lastly, malingering should always be a diagnosis of exclusion and made only after a thorough history and physical examination have been completed. Factitious disorder should also be considered in this case. This diagnosis would apply if the patient was intentionally feigning symptoms to assume the "sick role" and gain medical attention from various health care practitioners. Patients with factious disorder are often resistant to participate in psychiatric evaluations and psychotherapy. The most important part of treatment is to recognize the disorder and do no harm by avoiding unnecessary procedures and consultations. These patients should be fully assessed for general medical, neurologic, and highly comorbid psychiatric disorders. It is important to note that, unlike malingering, somatic symptom and related disorders often originate from unconscious and unhealthy coping mechanisms to life stressors.

Practical Resources

1. Merk Manual Online. Somatic Symptom and Related Disorders. http://www.merckmanu-als.com/professional/psychiatric-disorders/somatic-symptom-and-related-disorders/overview-of-somatization.
2. Medscape. Somatic Symptom and Related Disorders. https://emedicine.medscape.com/article/294908-overview.

REFERENCES

1. Katon W, Ries RK, Kleinman A. The prevalence of somatization in primary care. *Compr Psychiatry*. 1984;25(2):208-215.
2. Kroenke K. Symptoms in medical patients: an untended field. *Am J Med*. 1992;92(1A):3S.
3. Kroenke K, Mangelsdorff AD. Common symptoms in ambulatory care: incidence, evaluation, therapy, and outcome. *Am J Med*. 1989;86(3):262-266.
4. de Waal MW, Arnold IA, Eekhof JA, et al. Somatoform disorders in general practice: prevalence, functional impairment and comorbidity with anxiety and depressive disorders. *Br J Psychiatry*. 2004;184:470-476.
5. Thomassen R, van Hemert AM, Huyse FJ, et al. Somatoform disorders in consultation–liason psychiatry: a comparison with other mental disorders. *Gen Hosp Psychiatry*. 2003;25:8-13.
6. Neimark G, Caroff S, Stinnett J. Medically unexplained physical symptoms. *Psychiatry Ann*. 2005;35(4):298-305.
7. American Psychiatric Association. *Diagnostic and Statistical Manual of Mental Disorders*. 5th ed. Washington, DC: American Psychiatric Association; 2013.
8. Simon GE, Gureje O. Stability of somatization disorder and somatization symptoms among primary care patients. *Arch Gen Psychiatry*. 1999;56:90-95.
9. Allen LA, Escobar JI, Lehrer PM, et al. Psychosocial treatments for multiple unexplained physical symptoms: a review of the literature. *Psychosom Med*. 2002;64:939-950.
10. McCarron R. Somatization in the primary care setting. *Psychiatric Times*. 2006;23(6):32-34.
11. Speckens AE, van Hemert AM, Spinhoven P, et al. Cognitive behavioural therapy for medically unexplained physical symptoms: a randomised controlled trial. *BMJ*. 1995;311:1328-1332.
12. Warwick HM, Clark DM, Cobb AM, et al. A controlled trial of cognitive behavioural treatment of hypochondriasis. *Br J Psychiatry*. 1996;169:189-195.
13. Kroenke K, Swindle R. Cognitive-behavioral therapy for somatization and symptom syndromes: a critical review of controlled clinical trials. *Psychother Psychosom*. 2000;9:205-215.
14. Burns D. *Feeling Good: The New Mood Therapy*. 2nd ed. New York: Avon Books; 1999.
15. Sadock BJ, Sadock VA. *Synopsis of Psychiatry*. Philadelphia: Lippincott Williams & Wilkins; 2015.
16. Allen L, Gara M, Escobar J. Somatization: a debilitating syndrome in primary care. *Psychosomatics*. 2001;42(1).
17. Kroenke K, Spitzer R, Williams J, et al. Predictors of psychiatric disorders and functional impairment. *Arch Fam Med*. 1994;3:774-779.
18. Smith C, Monson R, Ray D. Psychiatric consultation in somatization disorder. *Engl J Med*. 1986;14:1407-1413.

11

SUPPORTIVE PSYCHOTHERAPY AND CHRONIC PAIN PRIMARY CARE

Lindsey Enoch, MD, Robert M. McCarron, DO, DFAPA and Christine Kho, MD

OVERVIEW

Patients present to their primary care doctors with many complex problems such as chronic physical pain. Among the most challenging patient encounters include those with comorbid and psychiatric or psychosocial concerns. Many providers feel they lack the resources, time, or skills necessary to address these kinds of issues. Yet with so many patients unable to access mental health specialty care, primary care doctors are often first-line in treating mental illness and guiding their patients through everyday conflict and distress.

In this chapter, we will introduce the principles and techniques used in supportive therapy. These techniques, which can be learned and applied over just a few appointments, are effective in managing a variety of complex issues seen in primary care. By learning these skills, primary care providers can provide substantial and effective treatment to patients unable to access other forms of mental health care or social support. They are also incredibly useful for patients with mental illness who refuse, fail, or have contraindications to psychotropic medications. Moreover, supportive psychotherapeutic techniques can also be utilized in the busy primary care setting.

Conditions that can be addressed with supportive therapy techniques:

- Depression
- Anxiety
- Chronic pain
- Problems with relationships, employment, housing, and other social stressors
- Grief
- Substance abuse
- Recurrent hospitalizations or noncompliance
- Stress related to general medical problems
- Difficulties adhering to the treatment of general medical problems

First, we will review the evidence and core principles in supportive therapy, with particular focus on building coping skills. Next, we will provide a practical approach, showing how to structure appointments so that you can use these tools effectively in just 2 to 4 visits. Lastly, we will go over a case vignette that illustrates how and when to use supportive psychotherapy.

EVIDENCE

Historically, supportive therapy has been considered a nonstandardized form of therapy, making it difficult to reproduce and study against other forms of treatment. Although large randomized trials are lacking, there is evidence that it can be effective for a variety of patients. In a recent meta-analysis by Cuijpers et al., authors found that supportive therapy was as effective for treating depression as medications and other types of therapy.[1] In another study looking at treatment of depression in primary care, authors found that problem-solving therapy and interpersonal therapy, which use many of the same techniques and principles as supportive therapy, were more effective for treating depression than medications and other types of therapy.[2]

There is also evidence that some of these therapeutic techniques can benefit patients after just a few visits, and even when provided by non–mental health professionals. In a systematic review by Nieuwsma et al., authors found that even brief therapy was effective for the treatment of depression in primary care. Many studies included used protocols with only six 30-minute sessions provided by non–mental health professionals.[3] **Though this study excluded supportive therapy, these findings suggest that primary care doctors can effectively learn and use therapeutic techniques to treat depression in the context of chronic pain, even when delivered in a busy general medical setting.**

CORE PRINCIPLES

Broadly speaking, supportive therapy works by helping patients increase healthy coping skills and decrease unhealthy coping skills. Put another way, providers can help patients self-identify and utilize existing healthy coping strategies, while encouraging patients to recognize maladaptive coping mechanisms and replace with new strategies to address life stressors. By learning and applying healthier coping skills, patients can manage problems more effectively and with greater sense of control. This leads to increases in function and higher self-esteem. Also, these valuable skills can be used for a lifetime.

The acronym "PARENTS" will help you remember the core principles and skills needed to provide effective supportive therapy. First, we describe the theory behind each core principle, followed by the tools you will need to apply them.

PARENTS

Problem focused
Ally with patient
Recognize emotions
Enhance coping
Normalize
Teach
Self-esteem

Problem Focused

In supportive therapy, it is important to first identify a specific problem to treat. When patients come in with broad complaints such as "life is awful," it is important to identify a more specific problem contributing to this belief. When there are numerous, or large, complex problems, break things into smaller pieces and address whatever is most pressing. Focus on the details of the *specific* problem, noting any contributing factors, associated symptoms, etc. In addition to understanding the problem better, asking for details like this will help patients "connect the dots" between symptoms, problems, or other key factors. Be sure to ask for the patient's goals for addressing the problem, which is what your supportive therapy and their coping skills will be working toward. Help them identify a goal, making sure it is realistic and could be achieved after the next few visits.

Tools to Use:

Socratic questioning
- Ask open-ended questions.
- Identify triggers, symptoms, and associated dysfunction.

Example of provider response: "You're really struggling with your anxiety. Tell me how that's affected your life and your back pain?"

Determine a goal
- Make it realistic, concrete, and time-limited.

Example: If a patient says the goal is to be "pain free" (which may be unrealistic), it is better to identify a functional goal, such as getting back to work (concrete). You might say, "Getting your pain under control is really important. What would you like to do if you could be pain free? It sounds like work is important to you, and something we could work toward accomplishing over the next few visits. I think that would help you feel better in a lot of ways. What do you think?"

Summarize
- Confirm your understanding.
- Make connections they may not have seen.
- Use this approach as redirection when patient getting off topic.

Example of provider response: "You're having a lot of pain and trouble just getting through the day. There are a lot of different stressors weighing on you, and you'd like better pain control so you can go back work."

Ally with Patient

Supportive techniques are most akin to being a "good parent." Listen, empathize, and advise when necessary, but without directly providing an answer or solution. It is usually more effective to lead the patient to self-discovery of a workable solution. Ask about the problem, and try to listen to the patient without initial interruption. Although listening can sometimes seem too passive to be effective, many patients lack a safe place to express their feelings and concerns. In many clinical situations, silence on the part of the provider is therapeutic and, although likely foreign to patients, will often be welcomed and is evidence of genuine interest and investment of time for the patient by the provider. Building rapport and expression of interest in a patient with high levels of psychosocial stress will take time but will most often yield positive results, including improved adherence to mutually agreed-upon treatment plans.

Tools to Use:

"2 ears, 1 mouth rule"

- For at least 5 minutes, try to listen without interruption.

Show support

- Show interest with engaging body language (e.g., nodding in agreement, making eye contact, avoid crossing arms).

Be empathic

- "Become the patient" or understand the emotional state and life circumstances as best as you can.
- Demonstrate genuine empathic remarks.

Example of provider response: "You've endured a lot with your husband, and you've really tried your best. I'm glad you're telling me this."

Recognize Emotion

Oftentimes when people are distressed, they disconnect and misidentify their feelings. In almost every condition we listed above, patients have trouble recognizing, accepting, or articulating their emotions. Any emotion can become debilitating and difficult to manage when not clearly understood. In supportive therapy, the task is to help patients recognize and understand their emotions and connect them to the problem being discussed. With better emotional awareness, patients can cope more effectively and appropriately, which will lessen their distress. You can help the patient develop this valuable skill by inviting them to reflect on their emotions in the specific problem being discussed.

Tools to Use:

"And how did that make you feel?"

- Ask and ask again. People have lots of emotions and often need a few chances to recognize them.
- Use this approach when patients get overly focused on what happened (rather than why it is bothering them).

Example of provider response: "Did you have other feelings about this? Like what? What else?"

Name the emotion

- Suggest a "normal" emotional response when applicable (e.g., grief reaction).
- Ask patients to identify the emotion when challenging for them to do so.
- Use this approach to clarify and simplify complicated experiences.

Example of provider response: "Wow, it sounds like you were really scared!"

Objective interpretation

- Suggest a more accurate emotion or interpretation when applicable.
- Use when:

- patient's feeling/interpretations differ significantly from your understanding of the problem
- their "misinterpretation" is interfering with resolution of the problem

Example of provider response: "You feel lonely and like nobody cares about you, but from what you're telling me, multiple people have reached out to you in the past week. You mentioned 6 people called you and asked how you were doing. It seems like people do care about you."

Summarize

- Connect emotions to the problem being discussed.
- Use diagrams and list of key emotions and problems—provide to the patient as a reference.

Example: A patient wants to address her chronic pain with opiates, but has agreed to work with you in learning more about triggers and possible treatments. You might summarize: "Your pain is very severe, and it's making it hard for you to do many things, including exercise, sleep, and taking care of your kids. You're feeling pretty angry, sad, and disappointed. This seems like important stuff to discuss. Can we talk a bit more about how you're handling all this?"

Enhance Coping

One of the main goals of supportive therapy is to increase patients' use of healthy coping skills. It is important to explain this concept to patients, and that together, you will be coming up with ways (coping skills) for them to improve their problem, or relieve symptoms. Emphasize that everyone needs ways to manage problems, and healthier coping skills are simply skills that are more effective ways of reaching goals and controlling symptoms.

Start by learning about which coping skills the patient already has. Ask about how they have managed difficult situations in the past. As their provider, you may know of some qualities and strengths they have used to overcome previous conflicts or illnesses. Point these out. The goal is to help them utilize and expand on these to help them cope with the problem at hand.

Because patients usually cannot articulate how they cope, it is important to be able to identify healthy and unhealthy coping skills in the various ways they come up. This requires a bit more understanding about defense mechanisms. Coping skills and "defense mechanisms" are essentially the same thing: they are the way people handle problems. Once you are able to pick out a few of the patient's coping strategies, you can use your supportive techniques to help them build their healthy skills and decrease their unhealthy coping skills. Because this is such an essential part of supportive therapy, we have included detailed tables at the end of this section. These describe common unhealthy and healthy coping skills, and the scenarios where they are often present. Table 11-1 includes "unhealthy" skills, examples, and tools you can use to develop healthier coping. Table 11-2 includes "healthy" skills, examples, and ways to help the patient to utilize these skills. These tables will be useful for reference throughout your visits with patients.

TABLE 11-1 Unhealthy Coping Skills and Defense Mechanisms

PROBLEM	UNHEALTHY COPING SKILL/DEFENSE	EXAMPLE OF PATIENT RESPONSE	EXAMPLES OF PROVIDER RESPONSE	SUPPORTIVE TOOL USED	HEALTHIER COPING
Frequent readmissions	Denial	"It's not my fault my blood sugar is so high—I'm doing everything I can. If the pharmacy could remember to fill my insulin, I'd basically be healthy!"	I know it has been tough to manage your diabetes. It is a difficult disease but I think we can do this. What would you like to focus on? How are you managing the stress? Tell me about how you are feeling through this?	Validation Instill hope Problem focus Identifying emotions	Identify a specific goal Identify positives and rewards associated with achieving the goal
Housing issues	Projecting *Uncomfortable feeling is believed to come from someone else rather than oneself.* (here: anger)	"My sister threw me out onto the streets. She's just an angry and hateful person. I don't need her."	I can see why you might be angry with your sister as well. Do you think that has anything to do with your housing problems? How would you express that feeling to your sister?	Normalizing Problem focus Identifying emotion Role play	Express problems to a friend, a provider hotline, and sister when ready Channel anger: music, art, and activity
Substance abuse	Rationalization	"My wife is so annoying; I have to drink just so I can deal with her!"	It sounds like you and your wife are having some problems, and that you are looking for a way to deal with that. But your drinking is also causing problems, and maybe we can address that first? What else could you do when you feel annoyed with your wife?	Problem focus Summarizing Confrontation Socratic questioning	Support groups (alcoholic anonymous) Alternative hobbies for stress reduction Reducing triggers to drink
Pain	Externalization *Problems attributed to others or external factors*	"I gained 30 pounds since you stopped my opiates. I can't move with all this pain. It's impossible to be healthy now!"	I see your point, but what do you think your role is in all these? What sorts of things have you done to be healthy in the past?	Validation Socratic questioning Identifying coping skills already present	Meditation Deep breathing Exercise/physical therapy

Normalize

Patients who are struggling with the "common conditions" listed at the beginning of this chapter often share similar cognitive distortions or, fixed, false beliefs. Two of the most common distortions you will be working to adjust are patient's beliefs that their problems are unique and that their problems cannot be fixed. In dealing with difficult issues, patients feel alone and hopeless, which leads to additional suffering and interferes with coping.

Here, the task is to correct these false beliefs by normalizing. Reassure patients that their problems and feelings are not atypical or abnormal. Let them know there are others who share their difficulties and that people often get better. Your optimism will help patients to feel more hopeful and confident about reaching their goals.

Tools to Use:

Validate
• Give "permission" to have feelings.

Example of provider response: "Your mother was really hard on you, so it's ok to be angry with her."

Cheerlead
• Encourage patients to keep trying, even when they encounter set backs in their progress.
• Cheerlead toward a different goal if they cannot meet the original.

Example of provider response: "It's not uncommon for people to feel guilty after the loss of a loved one. You're a strong woman, and I know you will get through this."

Acceptance
• Use for emotions that cannot be resolved.
• Explain: understanding is helpful, even if "fixing" is not possible.

Teach

In supportive therapy, various tools can be used to teach patients and can be a fast way for them to gain insight and coping skills. Teaching can be done during the visit or by "assigning" patients to read, complete, or practice something before the next visit.

TABLE 11-2 Healthy Coping Skills and Defense Mechanisms

PROBLEM	HEALTHY COPING SKILL/DEFENSE	EXAMPLE OF PATIENT RESPONSE	EXAMPLE OF PROVIDER RESPONSE	SUPPORTIVE TOOL USED	NEXT STEP
Depression	Humor	"It's like I'm writing a book on 'how to ruin your life by 30.'"	You have a gift for making people laugh. Even you cheered up a bit with that joke.	Praise Naming emotions Identifying strengths	Set goals Increase frequency of coping skill use Teach how coping skill helps in meeting goals
Grief	Emotional reflection	"I'm not sure that I can handle this. I know it's silly, but sometimes I write my mom post-it notes and then rip them up. Then I will cry for hours."	You are sad and you cry. How do you feel after you cry? Oftentimes people feel a huge sense of relief after they let themselves cry. It is ok for everyone to feel sad from time to time.	Naming emotion Acceptance Normalizing	Listen empathically Suggest journaling, letter writing Identify "good" ways to experience grief
Family discord	Distraction	"Things are so bad at home; I've just been trying to stay busy with other things. I'm pretty sick of homework, but at least my grades are better."	It is great you can use your school work as an outlet. Are there other positive ways you can distract yourself? A lot of people feel better when they can take a break. Sometimes, just visualizing a calm, pleasant place can feel like getting away. Can you visualize a place like that?	Praise Teach new coping skill—visualization	Educate how healthy coping skills can be used to lessen distress and improve sense of control Practice visualization Identify other distractions to be used for coping, such as exercise, music, and hobbies
Anxiety	Channeling	"Sometimes I get so anxious; I feel like I'm going to explode. There's nothing I can do to make it go away."	Anxiety can feel that way! I know that when I feel nervous, channeling some of those feelings into exercise can really help. Can I give you some at-home workouts, or prices on gyms in your area?	Ally with patient Personal advice Role model Educate	Create concrete goals and educate about ability to control symptoms Identify other channeling activities
Recurrent hospitalization	Altruism and commitment to others	"I want to be a better parent. I know I should be healthy for my kids but it's so hard."	I have noticed how committed you are to your family. I am confident there are ways we can get you healthier. Do you have any specific goals you 'would like to work on to start?	Praise Empathy Problem focus	Create specific goals and how you will measure these goals Assign small tasks between visits

Giving advice and sharing personal examples can also be valuable teaching tools, and guide learning and show empathy.[4] Similarly role modeling healthy ways of dealing with emotions, such as anger and failure, can be very informative. Being relatable improves the alliance and offers the patient a chance to learn from your experience.[5]

Tools to Use:

Educate
- Share expertise.
- Use handouts to teach about symptoms (anxiety vs. cardiac-related pain, for example) and new coping techniques (guide to meditation).

Advice
- Can be personal or professional.
- Offer before giving.
- Use this sparingly, as it is best for patients to work with you and self-discover a healthy solution.

Example of provider response: "Would you like my medical opinion? I know a few things that helped people in similar scenarios."

Role play
- Ask patients what they would say/do if they were back in the scenario right now.

Self-esteem

Many patients suffer from low self-esteem, especially those with mood disorders, stress, pain, or loss of functioning.[6] In time, patients with healthier coping strategies experience higher self-esteem, but early in the process, support patients with genuine affirmation and reassurance. Sharing your expertise in treating similar patients will instill confidence and convey optimism.

Tools to Use:

Praise

- Point out *any* success.
- Point out use of healthy coping skills.

Example of provider response: "You were worried about using alcohol to cope with arguments with your wife. Instead, I noticed you took a healthier approach to deal with the anger by going to the gym. Good job!"

Instill hope

- Remain optimistic when they might not be able to do so.

Example of provider response: "You might be surprised how many people have trouble with finances, and most people can learn skills to help them get out of this problem. I know you can as well."

Confrontation

- It is ok to disagree with patient's choices and behaviors.
- Reinforce your role to support and help, while expressing concern in a nonjudgmental manner.
- Use this when patients are engaging in harmful behaviors (such as drugs or alcohol).

Example of provider response: "It sounds like the insomnia could be related to anxiety, but I'm more concerned about the amount you've been drinking, and how that's affecting your sleep."

STRUCTURING THE CLINIC VISITS

Clinic visit 1—use the entire visit (even if it is only 15 min) to do the following:

1. Problem focus—*find a specific problem to address and learn details.*
2. Identify emotions.
3. Identify coping skills used in the past.
4. Determine goals—*specific, realistic, and measurable.*
5. Teach—*in appointment, or with handout or homework that emphasizes steps 2, 3, or 4.*

Clinic visit 2—things to do:

1. Provider summarizes the problem.
2. Ask about emotions—*do not ask about new problems/concerns. Ask about feelings now or from the last visit; summarize if different from the last visit.*
3. Define coping skills—*explain that together you'll be coming up with coping skills—ways to manage the problem, lessen symptoms, and meet goal.*

4. Identify, educate, and build healthy coping skills (see Tables 11-1 and 11-2).
5. Assign coping skills between visits—*specify when, how often.*
6. Teach—*if time permits.*

Clinic visit 3 and additional visits:
   Goals and symptoms can be addressed with as few as 3 appointments. Additional appointments are structured similar to visit 3.

Things to do:

1. Review progress toward goal.
2. Identify coping skills used.
3. Connect how coping skills have helped reach goal, or improve function and symptom control.
4. Teach.
5. Plan—*define how patients will continue to work on problem and how often they will use coping skills.*
6. Offer additional resources—*yourself, books, support groups, etc.*

Case Vignette

Ms. Olive is a 26-year-old woman who comes to your clinic complaining of 1 month of poor sleep and daytime fatigue. Despite ideal weather, she has not been hiking, kayaking, or rock climbing with friends as she typically loves to do. She has gained 10 lbs, rarely leaves the house, and her blood sugars are significantly higher than before. She tearfully tells you, "I'm a wreck and no one seems to care. I don't want to do anything. I just hate my life right now."

Provider: "I can tell you're really upset. Can you tell me more about what's bothering you?" *Naming emotions and identifying a specific problem*

Patient: "I'm not myself. I don't want to get out of bed in the morning, but things are so busy at work, and I have to stay late every night. It's not like my friends want to hang out anymore, so I guess it doesn't matter that I'm at work all the time."

Provider: "Hmm. Can you tell me more about what's going on?" *Listens empathically, asks for details about problem*

Patient: "People used to call and invite me out to do things, but now I guess I'm not a very fun person. I'm too tired to talk anyway, so I rarely answer when friends call."

Provider: "And how does that make you feel?" *Identifying emotions*

Patient: "I feel like they don't care. It makes me sad and angry."

Provider: "That's understandable." *Normalizing, empathy*

Patient: "I wish they cared."

Provider: "It sounds like your friends have reached out and called you, but you've felt pretty down, and your sleep and energy are lousy. Is there anything that's been making you feel more down lately?"

continued

Summarizing, objective interpretation, connecting problems and symptoms

Patient: "I've been feeling really stressed at work and at home. And I'm so tired, and I don't want to exercise or be active like I used to. I guess that used to help relieve a lot of stress."

Provider: "You know, oftentimes when people feel depressed, they lose interest in doing things they once enjoyed, and everyday tasks become more difficult. It sounds like depression could be interfering with your ability to keep up your hobbies and friendships. I know that they've always been important to you. *Education, normalizing*

Patient: "Yes. that's true."

Provider: "What sorts of things do you do when you're feeling down or stressed?" *Identifying coping skills*

Patient: "Going outside has always helped me clear my head. But I'm so tired—I can't exercise like I used to."

Provider: "Sometimes, even a small amount of a good thing can really help our mood and sleep. What could you do to get outside more, and how often do you think you could do it in the next two weeks? Do you think this would help? *More education, surveying for coping*

Patient: "It probably would help. I could walk around the park twice a week. Maybe I could do it with friends, and that would help me feel better too. I guess my friends are pretty important to me."

Provider: "I think it's a great start and a good goal. Maybe we can check in again in 2 weeks and talk more about how you're dealing with stress. Everyone deals with challenges differently, and we could come up with some different strategies to help you feel like your old self and get your diabetes under control." *Instilling hope, defining coping skills, and aim of future visits*

Patient: "That sounds good. I feel better now that we have a plan. I'm glad I brought this up."

Provider: "Before our next visit, can you write down any other emotions you're struggling with? I can give you a handout on some common emotions. It sounds silly, but a lot of people find it helpful as they try to identify their feelings." *Setting goals, expectations, and education*

Patient: "Sure, if you think it will help. I'll write some things down before our next visit."

CONCLUSION

Supportive therapy techniques can be used in primary care to address common and complex issues. The acronym "PARENTS" will help providers remember core principles and skills, which can be learned quickly and applied effectively in just 3 visits. This type of treatment can offer substantial relief to many complex patients, particularly those with limited access to care, and those who cannot tolerate medications. By learning these skills, providers will be more equipped and more comfortable addressing the needs of their patients.

CME QUESTIONS

1. A 36-year-old female comes into your office to follow up on her hypertension. Upon walking in the room, she bursts into tears telling you her brother just passed away, and she has felt "hopeless" and "lost." She admits that she has completely neglected her own health, and when you check her blood pressure, it is 166/90. She does not think there is any reason to continue medications, when "I'll probably die soon anyway."

   WHICH OF THE FOLLOWING SUPPORTIVE THERAPY TECHNIQUES WOULD BE MOST APPROPRIATE?

   A. Ask her to list the evidence for and against the belief "I might die at any minute."
   B. Provide her with the phone number of a grief support group.
   C. Validate her feelings about being lost.
   D. Educate her about the importance of blood pressure management and the sequelae of uncontrolled hypertension.

   C is the correct answer. Supportive therapy techniques can be helpful for patients experiencing and processing acute grief. In this setting, it is important to listen empathically, convey concern, and give the patient permission to feel whatever she feels. This can be done by validating an emotion, which conveys understanding and acceptance without trying to change it.

   Asking a patient to list the evidence for and against her cognitive distortion "I'll probably die soon anyway" is a technique used in cognitive behavioral therapy (CBT) and does not address the emotions that she is experiencing in the here and now. While you may give the patient the phone number of a grief support group, this would not be appropriate to do before you validated and explored her grief. Given her degree of distress, she is unlikely to process or benefit from education on better blood pressure management. This also dismisses the problem she is attempting to address, and supportive therapy should be focused on problems identified by the patient. The patient's more pressing concern is her grief and should be the focus of the visit.

2. You are seeing a patient for follow-up on chronic pain. You have successfully tapered her hydrocodone dose by 50%, but she is resistant to further lowering the dose. You suggest that she stops her nighttime PRN Norco; however, she is worried that her pain will be so severe, she would not be able to function. Which of the following is a healthy coping skill the patient could use to manage pain?

A. Snapping a rubber band against her wrist to distract from pain
B. Engaging in one of her hobbies every evening around the time she would normally take her PRN Norco
C. Repeating "my pain does not exist" 5 to 10 times every night
D. Channeling her pain by inflicting pain on something else

B is the correct answer. Distraction can be a valuable coping skill, especially when the patient is worried about becoming fixated on something. Although distractions themselves can be both healthy and unhealthy, most people can identify and commit to use of some sort of positive distraction. Hobbies, leisure activity, and calling friends are all forms of healthy distraction that can help people cope.

Snapping a rubber band against one's wrist is a type of harm reduction technique often used in dialectical behavior therapy (DBT), but not supportive therapy. Repeating positive endorsements about oneself is sometimes used to address cognitive distortions in CBT, but this technique will likely make the patient more fixated on her pain and less able to cope. And while channeling can be used as a positive coping skill, it does not involve transferring one's own negative experience into something else. Rather, an unpleasant experience is channeled into something benign or healthy (like anger being channeled and released through exercise).

3. You are establishing care with a new patient who was discharged from the hospital last week with a new diagnosis of heart failure. As he begins to tell you how scary it was when he developed difficulty breathing, you look up from your computer screen and ask, "Any paroxysmal dyspnea, orthopnea, peripheral edema, or angina?" Not knowing what those terms mean, the patient shakes his head, "No." Sensing his anxiety, you tell him that with the right diet, limited fluid intake, and medication, he can prevent heart failure from getting worse. You tell him that your father-in-law has gained control over heart failure with some hard work.

WHAT DID THE PROVIDER DO TO HELP BUILD A THERAPEUTIC ALLIANCE?

A. Allow the patient to vent his feelings.
B. Speak to the patient in a conversational manner and avoiding medical jargon.
C. Ask clarifying questions and summarizing statements.
D. Self-disclose a personal example where appropriate.

D is the correct answer. The provider in the scenario appropriately utilizes self-disclosure through the example of his father-in-law to help reassure the patient that his disease is manageable. This tiny gesture shows the patient that the provider is willing to share part of themselves for the overall benefit of the patient. Unfortunately, the visit is off to a rough start. The provider interrupts the patient with a review of symptoms as he is trying to share his emotions and prevents the patient from venting his fears about losing his breath. The provider also uses a review of systems for heart failure symptoms with medical jargon that the patient may find unfamiliar and intimidating. Without clarification or summary statements about what the patient has stated, the patient does not feel like he is being heard by the provider.

RESOURCES

Psychology Today: https://www.psychologytoday.com/blog/fighting-fear/201306/supportive-psychotherapy.
Addiction.com: https://www.addiction.com/a-z/supportive-psychotherapy/.
NAMI: https://www.nami.org/Learn-More/Treatment/Psychotherapy.

REFERENCES

1. Cuijpers, P, Driessen, E, Hollon, SD, van Oppen, P, Barth, J, Andersson, G. The efficacy of non-directive supportive therapy for adult depression: a meta-analysis. *Clin Psychol Rev.* 2012;32(4):280-291.
2. Wolf, NJ, Hopko, DR. Psychosocial and pharmacological interventions for depressed adults in primary care: a critical review. *Clin Psychol Rev.* 2008;28(1):131-161.
3. Nieuwsma, JA, Trivedi, RB, McDuffie, J, Kronish, I, Benjamin, D, Williams, JW. Brief psychotherapy for depression: a systematic review and meta-analysis. *Int J Psychiatry Med.* 2012;43(2):129-151.
4. Misch, DA. Basic strategies of dynamic supportive therapy. *J Psychother Pract Res.* 2000;9(4):173-189.
5. Brenner, AM. Teaching supportive psychotherapy in the twenty-first century. *Harvard Rev Psychiatry.* 2012;20(5):259-267.
6. Battaglia, J. 5 keys to good results with supportive psychotherapy. *Curr Psychiatry.* 2007;6(6).

12

ADDICTION

Paul G. Kreis, MD and Charles De Mesa, DO, MPH

FAST FACTS

- Addiction is a primary, chronic disease of brain reward, motivation, memory, and related circuitry.
- Addiction is manifested through a series of neuroadaptations in different circuits in the brain.

NEUROBIOLOGY OF ADDICTION AND PAIN

"Addiction is a primary, chronic disease of brain reward, motivation, memory and related circuitry. Dysfunction in these circuits leads to characteristic biological, psychological, social and spiritual manifestations. This is reflected in an individual pathologically pursuing reward and/or relief by substance use and other behaviors."[1] Drug addiction as a brain disease is a concept that has emerged over the past 25 years owing to advances in the understanding of the brain reward circuitry. Use of euphorigenic substances such as alcohol, cocaine, heroin, methamphetamine, nicotine, and opioids can escalate to compulsive use that can result in progressive dysfunction in all areas of the individual's life. The American Medical Association has defined several International Classification of Diseases, Revision 10 categories associated with substance use disorder. Once a substance use disorder is identified in an individual, formal treatment is indicated. With respect to the neurobiology of addiction, much of the neural circuitry involving memory, mood, perception, and emotional states that is modified by addictive substances has been elucidated.[2,3] Repeated exposure to drugs of abuse can result in chronic long-term changes to these neural circuits that can affect the individual long after the individual discontinues use of the drug.[4,5] Addiction is manifested through a series of neuroadaptations in different circuits in the brain.[6-9] The reward and reinforcement centers in the ventral tegmental region associated with survival behavior are significantly affected. For instance, the inability to discontinue behavior that is clearly harmful inevitably affects the individual's marriage, children, family, career, health, and well-being of himself/herself or others. Distortions of cognitive and emotional functioning, which characterizes addiction, such as compulsion to use drugs, are the hallmarks of addiction. The drugs have usurped the brain's natural motivational control circuits, and consequently, drug *use* becomes the exclusive motivational priority. Higher inhibitory centers of the brain that modulate impulsive behavior, including the prefrontal cortex, are suppressed, leading to progressive loss of behavioral self-control.

In the clinical setting, primary care physicians may decide to discontinue chronic opioid therapy for chronic nonmalignant pain because of limited therapeutic benefit. If the physician were to offer the following dialogue to the patient: "*I'm concerned about the risk of the opioid medication. I think tapering off is the best thing for you at this time. What are your thoughts?*" The patient may exhibit signs of fear, anxiety, and opposition. As a physician who has the understanding that addiction has "changed his or her brain" and that the patient is no longer thinking rationally, he or she should be able to provide compassionate care and appropriate treatment resources.

REWARD REINFORCEMENT

The limbic system contains the brain's reward reinforcement circuitry. It links the structures of the brain that control and regulate the ability to feel pleasure. Feeling pleasure motivates individuals to repeat behaviors that are necessary for existence and survival. Therefore, the limbic system can be activated by healthy, life-sustaining activities such as eating and socializing. It can also be activated by drugs of abuse, such as cocaine, heroin, or opioids. Because the limbic system allows an individual to perceive other emotions that can be either positive or negative, it may account for the perception of the full range of the mood-altering properties of many drugs.[10]

There are 2 components involved in the reward reinforcement system.[8,9,11,12] First, the ventral tegmental dopaminergic brain circuitry (reward-reinforcement) mediates survival behavior, such as feeding, reproduction, and social behaviors. As this circuitry is usurped by drugs of abuse, discontinuation of the drug is interpreted by the individual as a limbic threat to survival. This unconscious reaction leads to great resistance to any discussion of tapering the addictive drug (i.e., opioids). The second is the physical withdrawal component and the impact on the reward reinforcement system. Negative reinforcement can be more powerful than the positive reinforcement of euphoria, and some data suggest that the negative (and not positive) reinforcement of physical withdrawal predicts increased difficulties associated with substance abuse over a person's lifetime. The strong negative reinforcement of physical withdrawal drives the individuals to attempt to avoid gaps in drug use. Given the patient's fear of physical withdrawal, therapists may apply strategies such as response prevention, generating alternative activities, environmental interventions within the family and community, and emotion regulation and distress tolerance skills. The intensification of the withdrawal syndrome, which is the hypo-dopaminergic state in the reward and reinforcement center, is the limbic survival call to action. By its very nature, any threat to survival has evolved to be noxious to get our attention. The more quickly the concentration of a drug falls to its nadir in the person's circulatory system, the more intense the withdrawal, the more miserable the person feels, and the greater this limbic call to action. From a societal standpoint, this manifests in many well-known behaviors such as stealing, armed robbery, and the taking of life, all of which are examples of the length individuals will go to escape withdrawal. The roller coaster rides of positive reinforcement (taking the drug for the euphoria) and negative reinforcement (taking the drug to avoid withdrawal) leads to behavior that appears to defy logic.[13] Because addiction is primarily a limbic disorder, attempts at a rational discussion with the substance-abusing individual are frequently unsuccessful.

OPIOIDS AND ADDICTION

Recently, there has been debate about the addictiveness of opioids.[14,15] The literature that emerged in the late 1990s downplayed the risk of addiction. In the setting of pain, addiction was estimated to be less than 1% in small studies advocating for use of opioids given this low risk in the pain, which were clearly not substantiated. At the same time, empirical evidence suggests that not everyone who drinks alcohol becomes an alcoholic. The genetic contribution to alcoholism risk is 40% to 50%.[16] Studies have assessed individuals who have experimented with a particular substance and examined the percentage of those individuals who eventually became users or addicts. Dependence among any time users for tobacco, heroin, alcohol, and illicit drugs are 31.9%, 23%, 15.4%, and 14.7%, respectively.[17] Dependence on opioid medications may fall within the range of these other addictive substances.

The fact that not every individual who uses a substance will become addicted highlights the genetic contribution to substance abuse risk. Animal models support the lack of complete penetrance and have demonstrated variations and differences in the amount of dopamine release when exposed to dopamine substances.[18,19] These may explain the varied responses that humans have to different substances. Advances in addiction treatment will complement new understanding of the disease process. Rather than incarcerating nonviolent offenders with drug addiction, alternatives such as in halfway houses, long-term substance abuse treatment centers with focus on family and communal support, are increasingly being considered.

OPIOID MISUSE

As physicians, we may encounter patients who require an opioid taper and/or discontinuation of conventional opioid therapy. Use of assessment tools such as the opioid risk tool (ORT) or the Screener and Opioid Assessment for Patients with Pain (SOAAP) helps identify patients at risk for opioid misuse. When aberrant behaviors surface, they may signal evidence of potential drug abuse and addiction. Some examples of aberrant behaviors include selling medications, forging prescriptions, using alternative routes of administration not prescribed, obtaining illicit prescriptions, and early refill trends. Abuse of prescription opioids, such as injecting, snorting, or smoking, is an attempt to modify the delivery system to achieve euphoria through rapid transmission of the medication into the blood stream. Aberrant behavior such as requesting early refills (on Friday afternoon), misplacing, or losing medication (i.e., my dog ate the medication), are warning signs of potential aberrancy that should result in an increased level of vigilance and oversight by the prescribing practitioner.

Signs of opioid misuse may also include taking pain medications for anxiety, sadness, or insomnia. In addition, borrowing pain medication from family members, getting prescribed controlled substances from more than one doctor, and having other family members obtain medication for them are red flags. Finally, taking more pain medication than prescribed and requesting additional prescriptions from other physicians in violation of the opioid agreement constitutes aberrant behavior.

A good physician-patient relationship is important in identifying individuals who are beginning to show signs of aberrant behavior associated with prescribed controlled substances. For early refills, a distinction must be made with regard to pseudoaddiction. **Pseudoaddiction** is a syndrome, not a diagnosis, and an individual with **pseudoaddiction** typically has pain that is partially but not adequately relieved by current pain management regimen.[10] This can be responsibly assessed by educating on initiation of chronic opioid therapy a trial of the medication, monitoring, and changes that will be made based on therapeutic effect. The monitoring of early refills will be an important consideration.

It is important that the patient understand that chronic prescription opioid therapy can result in **tolerance** to the medication, which is characterized as decreased pain relief to a given dose over time.[10] In addition, the patient can also develop **withdrawal**, which is manifested as the experience of more pain than he or she would have if he or she had not taken the medication in the first place. Tolerance and withdrawal are essential for the physician to recognize in any patient, whether or not they are addicted to opioids.

It is beneficial to distinguish among the different phases of opioid withdrawal highlighted in Table 12-1. For individuals suffering from opioid addiction, experiencing the negative physical effects of withdrawal can be rather worse than the positive physical effects of euphoria.

Significantly, the syndrome of protracted abstinence can last up to 6 months. This may explain why 30-day rehabilitation programs without a robust aftercare

program are often associated with high relapse rates.[21] The anhedonia and amotivational state of chronic withdrawal resulting from limbic and hypothalamic-pituitary-adrenal (HPA) axis alterations seen with chronic opioid use can take many months to recover.[2] Reduction in the rates of relapse may be seen in longer-term rehabilitation programs that emphasize family support.

For all the reasons mentioned, it is important for the practitioner to abide by accepted guidelines for the safe prescribing of controlled substances in all individuals, including the at-risk population. Similarly, one must emphasize pharmacovigilance, including the routine querying of state-run prescription drug monitoring programs and random urine drug screening. These topics are discussed in detail in Chapter 29 *Medicolegal Essentials and Best Practices in Opioid Prescribing*.

BUPRENORPHINE

Buprenorphine is associated with a lower risk of fatal respiratory depression than conventional opioids, including methadone.[22–25] Buprenorphine replacement therapy can be a useful adjunct in the treatment of prescription opioid and/or heroin addiction.[23] It is important to understand that, although buprenorphine is known to be safer than conventional opioids owing to the ceiling affect for respiratory depression, it can still theoretically cause fatal respiratory depression when combined with other respiratory depressants such as benzodiazepines. The following are some key characteristics of buprenorphine[26,27]:

- Partial mu receptor agonist
- Much lower incidence of QTc prolongation
- Reduced effect on HPA-reduced hypogonadism
- Does not cause spasm of the sphincter of oddi
- Anti-hyperalgesia
- Nonimmunosuppressive in animal models

Guidelines for the use of buprenorphine induction are provided by the American Society of Addiction Medicine (ASAM) and may be obtained from ASAM website resources.[28] The role of buprenorphine use in the primary care setting is further discussed in Chapter 30.

TABLE 12-1 The Different Phases of Opioid Withdrawal

1. Anticipatory withdrawal (3-4 h)
   a. Fear of withdrawal
   b. Anxiety
   c. Drug seeking
2. Early withdrawal (8-10 h)
   a. Anxiety
   b. Restlessness
   c. Nausea
   d. Nasal stuffiness
   e. Hypertension
   f. Tachycardia
   g. Yawning
   h. Sweating
   i. Abdominal cramps
   j. Drug seeking
   k. Rhinorrhea
   l. Lacrimation
3. Fully developed withdrawal (1-3 d)
   a. Severe anxiety
   b. Restlessness
   c. Muscle spasm
   d. Elevated blood pressure
   e. Fever/chills
   f. Dilated pupils
   g. Tremor
   h. Piloerection
   i. Vomiting/diarrhea
   j. Tachycardia
4. Protracted abstinence (up to 6 mo)
   a. Hypotension
   b. Bradycardia/insomina
   c. Loss of appetite
   d. Loss of energy
   e. Cue-induced craving[20]

REFERENCES

1. American Society of Addiction Medicine. *Public Policy Statement: Definition of Addiction*; 2011. Available from: https://www.asam.org/resources/definition-of-addiction. Accessed 21 February 2018.
2. Olds J. Hypothalamic substrates of reward. *Physiol Rev.* 1962;42:554-604.
3. Pulvirenti L, Koob GF. The neural substrates of drug addiction and dependence. *Funct Neurol.* 1990;5(2):109-119.
4. Koob GF, Nestler EJ. The neurobiology of drug addiction. *J Neuropsychiatry Clin Neurosci.* 1997;9(3):482-497.
5. Leshner AI. Addiction is a brain disease, and it matters. *Science.* 1997;278(5335):45-47.

6. Nestler EJ, Hope BT, Widnell KL. Drug addiction: a model for the molecular basis of neural plasticity. *Neuron.* 1993;11(6):995-1006.

7. Nestler EJ. Molecular neurobiology of drug addiction. *Neuropsychopharmacology.* 1994;11(2):77-87.

8. Pulvirenti L, Koob GF. Dopamine receptor agonists, partial agonists and psychostimulant addiction. *Trends Pharmacol Sci.* 1994;15(10):374-379.

9. Self DW, Nestler EJ. Molecular mechanisms of drug reinforcement and addiction. *Annu Rev Neurosci.* 1995;18:463-495.

10. Ries RK, Fiellin DA, Miller SC, Saitz R. *The ASAM Principles of Addiction Medicine.* 5th ed. Wolters Kluwer Lippincott Williams & Wilkins; 1796.

11. Leshner AI. Science-based views of drug abuse and addiction. *Isr J Psychiatry Relat Sci.* 2002;39(2):83-85.

12. Vorel SR, Ashby CR, Paul M, et al. Dopamine D3 receptor antagonism inhibits cocaine-seeking and cocaine-enhanced brain reward in rats. *J Neurosci.* 2002;22(21):9595-9603.

13. Olds J, Milner P. Positive reinforcement produced by electrical stimulation of septal area and other regions of rat brain. *J Comp Physiol Psychol.* 1954;47(6):419-427.

14. Porter J, Jick H. Addiction rare in patients treated with narcotics. *N Engl J Med.* 1980;302(2):123.

15. Leung PTM, Macdonald EM, Stanbrook MB, Dhalla IA, Juurlink DN. A 1980 letter on the risk of opioid addiction. *N Engl J Med.* 2017;376(22):2194-2195.

16. Knopik VS, Heath AC, Madden PA, et al. Genetic effects on alcohol dependence risk: re-evaluating the importance of psychiatric and other heritable risk factors. *Psychol Med.* 2004;34(8):1519-1530.

17. Anthony JC, Warner LY, Kessler RC. Comparative epidemiology of dependence on tobacco, alcohol, controlled substances, and inhalants: basic findings from the National Comorbidity Survey. *Exp Clin Psychopharmacol.* 1994;2:244-268.

18. Cadoni C. Fischer 344 and Lewis rat strains as a model of genetic vulnerability to drug addiction. *Front. Neurosci.* 2016;10.

19. Gardner EL. Endocannabinoid signaling system and brain reward: emphasis on dopamine. *Pharmacol Biochem Behav.* 2005;81(2):263-284.

20. Deborah M, Stephenson K, eds. *Guideline for Physicians Working in California Opioid Treatment Programs.* San Francisco, CA: California Society of Addiction Medicine; 2008:152.

21. National Institute on Drug Abuse. *Principles of Drug Addiction Treatment: A Research-Based Guide;* 2018.

22. Dahan A, Yassen A, Romberg R, et al. Buprenorphine induces ceiling in respiratory depression but not in analgesia. *Br J Anaesth.* 2006;96(5):627-632.

23. Campbell ND, Lovell AM. The history of the development of buprenorphine as an addiction therapeutic. *Ann N Y Acad Sci.* 2012;1248:124-139.

24. Davis MP. Twelve reasons for considering buprenorphine as a frontline analgesic in the management of pain. *J Support Oncol.* 2012;10(6):209-219.

25. Dahan A. Opioid-induced respiratory effects: new data on buprenorphine. *Palliat Med.* 2006;20(suppl 1):s3-s8.

26. Ding Z, Raffa RB. Identification of an additional supraspinal component to the analgesic mechanism of action of buprenorphine. *Br J Pharmacol.* 2009;157(5):831-843.

27. Pergolizzi J, Aloisi AM, Dahan A, et al. Current knowledge of buprenorphine and its unique pharmacological profile. *Pain Pract.* 2010;10(5):428-450.

28. Kraus ML, Alford DP, Kotz MM, et al. Statement of the American Society of Addiction Medicine Consensus Panel on the use of buprenorphine in office-based treatment of opioid addiction. *J Addict Med.* 2011;5(4):254-263.

III

FUNDAMENTALS OF PAIN HISTORY, PHYSICAL EXAM AND ASSESSMENT

13

NEUROPATHIC PAIN

Naileshni Singh, MD, Jon Zhou, MD and Samir J. Sheth, MD

FAST FACTS

- Neuropathic pain (NP) has a significant impact on function and quality of life.
- Due to the multiple etiologies of NP, it often is not straightforward to diagnose and can be difficult to treat.
- NP is best treated in a careful, stepwise fashion that utilizes a biopsychosocial model.

INTRODUCTION

Neuropathic pain (NP) is a difficult to diagnose and treat medical condition that affects millions of people worldwide. Adequately caring for those suffering from NP can be challenging due to its complex pathophysiology and multidimensional nature. This chapter reviews the mechanisms, assessment, and treatment of a variety of NP pain conditions.

DEFINITIONS AND MECHANISMS

Neuropathic pain is defined by the International Association for the Study of Pain (IASP) as "pain caused by a lesion or disease of the somatosensory nervous system." In contrast, nociceptive pain is defined as "pain that arrives from actual or threatened damage to non-neural tissue and is due to activation of nociceptors." The need for a "lesion" in the nervous system in the definition of NP may be difficult to assess for, even with diagnostic studies. Many NP conditions may not have demonstrable lesions or a known "disease" which makes the diagnosis largely determined by clinical information. The presence and level of severity of NP has significant levels of morbidity, higher depression, higher anxiety, compromised sleep, higher health care utilization, poorer quality of life, lost productivity, and increased health care costs as compared with the general population.[1-4]

NP can present in a variety of different ways, and the prevalence and incidence of NP conditions vary with each syndrome. For conditions such as diabetes, painful diabetic peripheral neuropathy (DPN) can occur in up to 30% of diabetics. The prevalence of phantom limb pain ranges from 40% to 80% of amputations but is based on patient-related factors and the site of the amputation.[5] Postsurgical pain is common after surgeries such as mastectomies and thoracotomies due to either direct or indirect nerve injury. See Table 13-1 for a description of the prevalence and incidence of common NP conditions.[6]

The research literature describes a variety of mechanisms which can lead to the experience of NP. The theories regarding causes of NP start peripherally and spread centrally in the nervous system. Specifically, mechanisms focus on abnormal firing of nerves, abnormal amplification or propagation of nerve signals, or altered inhibition of pain pathways.[6] Spontaneous neuronal activity from an injured primary afferent neuron such as a neuroma

TABLE 13-1 Prevalence and Incidence of Neuropathic Pain Conditions

NEUROPATHIC PAIN CONDITION	PREVALENCE (BEST ESTIMATE)	INCIDENCE
Painful diabetic neuropathy (DPN)	15%	15.3/100 000
Postherpetic neuralgia (PHN)	7%-27%	11-40/100 000
Human immunodeficiency virus (HIV) neuropathy	35%	Unknown
Acquired immunodeficiency syndrome (AIDS) neuropathy	50%	Unknown
Central poststroke pain	8%-11%	Unknown
Multiple sclerosis (MS) pain	23%	Unknown
Spinal cord injury (SCI) pain	40%-70%	Unknown
Phantom limb pain	53%-85%	Unknown
Trigeminal neuralgia	Unknown	5-8/100 000

Adapted from Sadosky A, McDermott A, Brandenberg N, et al. A review of the epidemiology of painful diabetic peripheral neuropathy, postherpetic neuralgia, and less commonly studied neuropathic pain conditions. Pain Pract. 2008;8(1):45-56. Copyright © 2008 Pain Practice. Reprinted by permission of John Wiley & Sons, Inc.

or lesion in the dorsal horn of the spinal cord, thalamus, or other supraspinal structures may cause pain. Upregulation of receptors such as voltage-gated sodium channels (Nav. 1.8) and transient receptor potential vanilloid (TRPV1) on nerves known to modulate NP has been demonstrated. Demyelination of nerves may cause abnormal signaling between pain fibers and other nonpain fibers. For example, ectopic discharges from damaged and demyelinated nerves may cause ephaptic crosstalk (i.e., communication) between nerves that typically propagate pain and ones that typically do not such as sympathetic fibers. Nonephaptic crosstalk through repetitive firing that releases neurotransmitters that activate nearby nonnoxious fibers may also occur.[6] Furthermore, functional reorganization of receptive fields, known as sprouting, occurs in spinal cord dorsal horn neurons such that sensory input from surrounding intact nerves emphasizes or aggravates input from the initial area of injury. Sprouting into the dorsal horn or dorsal root ganglion (DRG) causes increased activity to both noxious and nonnoxious stimuli. Additionally, loss of segmental inhibition or descending inhibition in the spinal cord may contribute to NP.[7] For instance, pain can occur if A beta fibers (touch, pressure, and vibration) fail to modulate input from unmyelinated C fibers and myelinated A delta fibers.

Neurotransmitters and neuropeptides have action on specific receptors that are involved in pain pathways. Understanding the interactions of these molecules in the propagation or attenuation of pain signals is important in choosing medications. Many NP medications and treatments will alter or enhance one or more neurotransmitters. For example, glutamate and aspartate along with the neuropeptide substance P are known to transmit pain. Substance P, along with other local mediators released by primary afferent neurons, may interact with C fibers to cause the perpetuation of pain chronically.[7] Endorphins and opioids are known to target both the ascending and descending pain pathways to inhibit pain. GABA and glycine are the main inhibitory neurotransmitters in the nervous system that modulate pain while serotonin is an inhibitory neurotransmitter involved in mood and emotion. Norepinephrine is involved in the descending inhibitory pain pathways.[7] Due to neurotransmitter and neuropeptide profiles, relevant drug targets may include the GABA pathways or agents that release norepinephrine and serotonin such as duloxetine. See Figure 13-1 for a diagram of the pain pathways and potential receptor and molecular targets of specific medication-based therapies.

The phenomenon of central and peripheral sensitization, as it relates to NP is of interest when considering the chronicity of many pain conditions which often exceeds the initial injury. Neuroinflammatory mediators such as substance P, cytokines, prostaglandins, and histamine can stimulate or sensitize pain fibers to cause peripheral sensitization of the nervous system. Through repetitive stimulation of pain fibers, molecular and anatomical changes occur in the central nervous system called central sensitization. Central sensitization occurs through multiple mechanisms that include abnormal signaling or altered inhibition from the peripheral nervous system.[6]

NP conditions such as postherpetic neuralgia (PHN) or painful. DPN have mechanisms that are complicated and specific to the condition. PHN is caused by reactivation of the Varicella zoster virus latent in the dorsal columns of spinal cord sensory neurons after an initial infection. The virus causes focal necrosis of neuronal cell bodies, decrease in epidermal nerve fiber density, neurogenic inflammation, and demyelination of neurons in the DRG and peripheral nervous system.[8] The virus may be reactivated in the elderly or immunocompromised leading to a severe pain condition. DPN has a mechanism of pain related to hyperglycemia causing nerve damage, sprouting and hyperexcitability of nerves, and the release of inflammatory mediators. Neurovascular changes causing hypoxia or sympathetic nervous system sprouting in the DRG are also thought to contribute to the pain experience in diabetics.[9] Mechanical pain associated with chronic nerve compression such as in trigeminal neuralgia (TN) or carpal tunnel syndrome may be relieved by decompression. Direct nerve injury and sensitization may occur during common surgical procedures such as mastectomy, inguinal herniorrhaphy, or thoracotomy.[10] Patients who undergo chemotherapy may experience pain due to neurotoxic therapeutic agents,

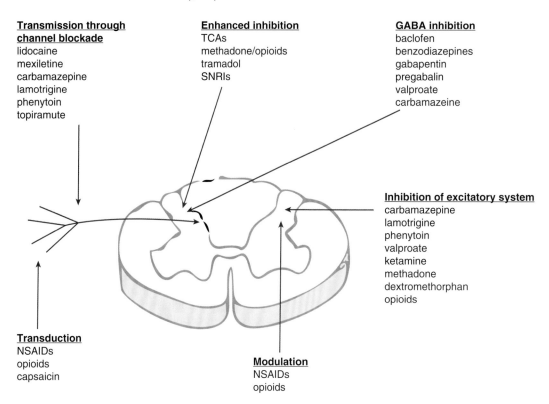

Transmission through
channel blockade
lidocaine
mexiletine
carbamazepine
lamotrigine
phenytoin
topiramute

Enhanced inhibition
TCAs
methadone/opioids
tramadol
SNRIs

GABA inhibition
baclofen
benzodiazepines
gabapentin
pregabalin
valproate
carbamazeine

Inhibition of excitatory system
carbamazepine
lamotrigine
phenytoin
valproate
ketamine
methadone
dextromethorphan
opioids

Transduction
NSAIDs
opioids
capsaicin

Modulation
NSAIDs
opioids

FIGURE 13-1 Pain pathways and potential receptor and molecular targets of specific medication-based therapies. NSAIDs, nonsteroidal anti-inflammatory drugs; SNRIs, serotonin–norepinephrine reuptake inhibitor; TCAs, tricyclic antidepressants.

such as platinum agents, vinca alkaloids, and taxanes. Radiation induced nerve injury is believed to be related to fibrotic compression of nerves, injury to the vascular supply, and direct axonal injury and demyelination from X-rays.[11] Sympathetically maintained pain in causalgia or complex regional pain syndrome (CRPS) is hypothesized to be related to dysfunction of the sympathetic nervous system along with neurogenic inflammation and sensitization of nociceptors; however, neuroplastic changes and autoimmune mechanisms have not been ruled out.[12] The myriad of conditions along with the differing pain mechanisms makes the treatment and diagnosis of NP challenging for clinicians and frustrating to patients.

CLINICAL PRESENTATION

The presentation of NP may be variable and specific to the underlying clinical condition. Patients who experience NP may describe the pain as "burning," "numbness," "itchy," "sharp," and "shooting" or "electric." The pain may be evoked or spontaneous. In DPN, the pain occurs in a "stocking glove pattern" sensitive to touch and typically in the lower extremities. Patients with radiculitis may report pain radiating to the extremities from the lumbar or cervical spine in a dermatomal pattern. Patients who suffer from TN may experience pain along any of the three dermatomal regions innervated by cranial nerve V, which is the trigeminal nerve. A thorough history may reveal a recent surgery, procedure, stroke,

injury, worsening diabetes or other metabolic disorder, new medications, or use of chemotherapy agents. However, in many cases, it may be idiopathic.

Physical examination and diagnostic testing may assist with the diagnosis of NP. Table 13-2 details physical examination maneuvers and diagnostic testing that may provide evidence for many common and uncommon NP conditions. Responses to physical examination may be illustrated through pain descriptors such as allodynia, hyperalgesia, or paresthesia, which are common in NP disorders. Additionally, NP screening and assessment tools may assist with describing the experience of pain and tracking response to treatments. See Table 13-3 for a list of NP clinical screening and assessment tools.[13] Validated tool and surveys can assess the quality of pain, severity of symptoms, exacerbating and alleviating factors, affective manifestations, and physical examination signs and other factors that may assist patients and clinicians in recognizing and treating NP (Table 13-4).

INTRODUCTION TO TREATMENTS

The treatment of NP conditions can be generally described as conservative or nonconservative. Conservative measures typically include physical therapy modalities, integrative therapies, and medications. Nonconservative measures may include interventional procedures, implanted devices, and surgery. Generally, the evidence for medication treatments includes first-line, second-line,

TABLE 13-2 Physical Examination and Diagnostic Testing for Neuropathic Pain

PHYSICAL EXAMINATION	DIAGNOSTIC TESTING
Touch	Comprehensive metabolic panel
Pinprick	Complete blood count
Pressure	Sedimentation rate
Cold	Folic Acid
Heat	Thyroid function test
Vibration	Hgb A1c and fasting glucose
Temporal summation	Infectious disease panel including
Measure affected areas	HIV, Hepatitis, and Lyme disease
Motor Strength	titer
Cranial nerves	MRI
Gait	CT
Reflexes	EMG/NCS
Skin changes	Skin biopsy
Atrophy	Vitamin B12 level
Rash	Heavy metal serum
Temperature	Serum electrophoresis and
Upper motor neuron signs	immunofixation
Palpation of masses or lymph	Antinuclear antibody
nodes	Rheumatoid factor
	Sjogren titers
	Cryoglobulins
	CSF study
	Orthostatic vital signs
	Urine or serum toxicology

Adapted from Kerstman E, Ahn S, Battu S, Tariq S, Grabois M. Neuropathic pain. Handb Clin Neurol. 2013;110:175-187. Copyright © 2013 Elsevier. With permission.

TABLE 13-3 Screening and Assessment Tools for Neuropathic Pain

SCREENING TOOLS	ASSESSMENT TOOLS
Leeds Assessment of Neuropathic Symptoms and Signs (LANSS)	Neuropathic Pain Scale (NPS)
Neuropathic Pain Questionnaire (NPQ)	Neuropathic Pain Symptom Inventory
Douleur Neuropathique 4 Questions (DN4) painDETECT	Short Form McGill Pain Questionnaire 2 (SF-MPQ-2)
ID Pain	
Standardized Evaluation of Pain	

Adapted by permission from Springer: Jones RC 3rd, Backonja MM. Review of neuropathic pain screening and assessment tools. Curr Pain Headache Rep. 2013;17(9):363. Copyright © 2013 Springer Science+Business Media New York.

TABLE 13-4 Pain Nomenclature and Definitions

PAIN NOMENCLATURE	DEFINITION
Allodynia	Pain due to a stimulus that does not normally provoke pain, lowered threshold stimulus, and response differ
Anesthesia dolorosa	Pain in an area or region which is anesthetic
Dysesthesia	An unpleasant abnormal sensation, whether spontaneous or evoked
Hyperalgesia	Increased pain to a normally painful stimulus
Hyperesthesia	Increased sensitivity to stimulation, excluding the special senses
Hyperpathia	Abnormally painful reaction to a stimulus, especially a repetitive stimulus
Hypoalgesia	Decreased pain in response to a normally painful stimulus
Neuralgia	Pain in the distribution of a nerve or nerves
Neuritis	Inflammation of a nerve or nerves
Neuropathy	A disturbance of function or pathological change in a nerve(s)
Paresthesia	An abnormal sensation, whether spontaneous or evoked

Adapted from the International Association for the Study of Pain's website: http://www.iasp-pain.org/Taxonomy.

and third-line recommendations. The research- and evidence-based guidelines on treatments options are usually divided by the specific pain condition.

Conservative, Integrative, and Alternative Modalities

Physical therapy (PT) modalities are often the first-line conservative treatment for most painful conditions. Exercise reduces NP symptoms in both experimental studies and clinical studies of DPN. Balance, mobility, strength, decreased inflammation, decreased allodynia, and increased hypoalgesia are some of the improvements seen with exercise therapy in peripheral neuropathic conditions such as DPN.[14] In CRPS, range of motion exercises are thought be a cornerstone of treatment that prevents loss in bone density and muscle atrophy and can reduce the symptoms of chronic pain. If PT and other movement-based or active therapies fail, other modalities can be considered.

Passive modalities for patients with NP may include transcutaneous electrical nerve stimulation (TENS), devices that are applied externally to painful areas which reduce action potentials and increase pain thresholds in the peripheral nervous system. TENS can be used for NP including DPN, TN, stump pain, phantom limb pain, radiculopathy, HIV (human immunodeficiency virus) neuropathy, CRPS, entrapment neuropathy, spinal cord injury, postlaminectomy, cancer-related NP, poststoke, and central pain where efficacy has been demonstrated.[15] Along with TENS, ultrasound and manual therapy may also be prescribed.

Acupuncture has a basis in Eastern Medicine and relies on carefully placed aseptic needles on points that elicit *deqi*, which is the sensation responsible for the therapeutic results. Acupuncture has been studied in clinical situations and is effective in back and neck pain and postoperative nausea and vomiting.[16] Acupuncture can decrease pain in PDH, Bell palsy, HIV neuropathy, spinal cord injury, and carpal tunnel syndrome.[17] As the risk of acupuncture intervention is low and the possible benefit high, acupuncture can be a useful first line treatment option.

Psychological Modalities

A multitude of psychological modalities and therapies can offer pain reduction and improved functioning in patients with NP. Cognitive behavioral therapy (CBT) addresses the negative thinking that causes distress and increased levels of pain in patients. CBT addresses pain catastrophizing, which is defined as an exaggerated response to pain or "overappraisal" of the sensation of pain.[18] CBT assists patients by teaching tools to counter negative and irrational thinking. Patients are asked to consciously address behaviors and thoughts that are counterproductive to the management of pain. To date, evidence suggest efficacy for the use of CBT in HIV neuropathy and spinal cord injury.[19]

Mindfulness-based strategies including mindfulness-based stress reduction (MBSR), mindfulness meditation, and mindfulness-based cognitive therapy are meditative schools of thought centered on awareness and attention in the moment without judgment. MBSR is typically a process that is taught in an 8- to 12-week session, but shorter mindfulness interventions have been described in the literature. Mindfulness has been used for decades to treat varied pain conditions such as PHN and chronic low-back pain resulting in improved functioning and decreased disability. Lifestyle issues that exacerbate pain such as stress, poor sleep, poor interpersonal interactions, and lack of exercise may be addressed through meditative modalities centered on mindfulness.[20-22] There is also some evidence that reduction in the depression and anxiety can be achieved with mindfulness.[22]

Medication-Based Modalities

"See chapter 34 *Neuropathic pain Medications*"!

Neuromodulation

Neuromodulation refers to the broad array of technologies that may alter the nervous system to decrease and improve the experience of pain for patients with NP conditions. This relies on the use of electrical energy that is applied near the spinal cord and dorsal horn that alters the pain pathways through multiple central and peripheral mechanisms. Neuromodulation is typically an invasive modality and used when other conservative therapies, including medications, fail.

The field of neuromodulation includes the technologies of spinal cord stimulation (SCS), peripheral field stimulation or peripheral nerve stimulation, deep brain stimulation (DBS), and motor cortex stimulation (MCS). These advanced therapies are used when conservative measures have been exhausted and patients have passed a thorough psychological evaluation to assess their appropriateness and preparedness for neuromodulation therapies. Patients with uncontrolled depression, anxiety, substance abuse, psychosis, pain catastrophizing, and inability to cope have poorer outcomes with spinal cord stimulation.[23,24] As an advanced technique, pain interventionalists and surgeons may offer this technology using fluoroscopic guidance. Wireless and injectable SCS systems are on the horizon which may make neuromodulation more readily available to other types of providers.

Spinal cord stimulation is the most common of the neuromodulation therapies and uses electrodes placed in the epidural space to cause paresthesias that are experienced by the patient. The proposed mechanism of SCS includes spinal modulation, attenuation of dorsal horn neurons, action on A beta fibers, and alteration of neurochemistry of the dorsal columns.[25] SCS is FDA approved for CRPS and failed back surgery syndrome (FBSS) but has been successfully used for many types of neuropathic and vascular pain conditions including peripheral neuropathy, DPN, peripheral vascular disease, and angina.[26] Typically, patients undergo percutaneous placement of leads with multiple electrodes into the epidural space using fluoroscopy. The dorsal columns of the spinal cord are stimulated and mapped during the one week trial to cover all the patient's pain locations. Patients may use a variety of preprogrammed options that offer combinations of amplitudes and frequencies of stimulation to see which experience provides the most pain relief and increased functioning. Some patients may be good candidates for high-frequency SCS which is a paresthesia-free option using high-frequency parameters to modulate pain.[27] Patients are also asked to monitor activity levels and functional goals to assess whether to proceed to the implantation of the SCS system and pulse generator. If SCS trial is difficult due to inability to place the percutaneous leads, then paddle leads, which have multiple imbedded leads in a "paddle" shape, may be placed by a surgeon through a laminotomy. SCS implantation is typically a minimally invasive outpatient procedure done in a surgical setting.

Other variations of neuromodulation have been found to be successful in pain conditions. High cervical SCS has been shown to be effective for intractable migraines or facial pain and stimulation of the DRG is as beneficial as traditional SCS.[28,29] Stimulation of the DRG, which is at the junction of the central and peripheral nervous system, has been successful for FBSS and other NP conditions.[29] Peripheral nerve field stimulation, where leads are placed over the area of a nerve subcutaneously, has been showed to be effective for illioinguinal neuritis and greater occipital neuritis through an A beta fiber pathway.[30] Peripheral nerve field stimulation uses leads typically placed in a nerve distribution and can be helpful for TN, head pain, face pain, and thoracic NP.[31,32] Peripheral neuromodulation has highlighted some initial efficacy in phantom limb pain and stump pain.[33] The type of neuromodulation system will largely depend on the patient's pain area and symptoms. Risks of neuromodulation include failure to manage pain, bleeding, infection, spinal cord injury, migration of the leads, equipment failure, urinary retention, and tolerance.

Deep brain stimulation is FDA approved for movement disorders intractable to conservative measures such as Parkinson disease and essential tremor. DBS has been used successfully for pain control in NP conditions such as CRPS, poststroke pain, spinal cord injury, facial pain, FBSS, and peripheral nerve plexus injury. DBS delivers constant electrical stimulation to areas of the brain, typically the thalamus and/or periventricular areas; however, this technology can be offered in many locations.[34] Similarly, motor cortex stimulation appears to be beneficial for phantom limb pain, TN or facial pain, and poststroke pain.[34] The invasiveness of these treatment modalities needs to be considered when assessing for patient appropriateness. Noninvasive transcranial magnetic stimulation over the primary somatosensory area or the premotor cortex using a high frequency that activates neurons has been used successfully for short-term pain management.[35]

Lastly, intrathecal therapies that deliver low-dose medications into the CSF may be a last resort modality for NP conditions. Opioids, baclofen, and ziconitide are FDA-approved medications for intrathecal therapy. Ziconitide is a calcium channel blocker which has been used for refractory NP.[36] The side effect profile of mood changes, ataxia, nausea, dizziness, sedation, altered mentation, and urinary retention may make this medication challenging to tolerate. However, lower doses of ziconitide can be combined with other intrathecal medications such as opioids or local anesthetics to be used for NP conditions.

Nerve and Spinal Cord Ligation

Stump pain due to a neuroma is often a consequence of amputations and is a separate entity from phantom limb pain or phantom limb sensations. Patients may present with point tenderness at the stump and NP qualities such as numbness. Surgical neuroma excision and steroid injections performed perineurally (surrounding the neuroma) are effective in treating stump pain.[37,38]

Dorsal root entry zone (DREZ) lesioning of the spinal cord causes deafferentation of pain fibers and has had successes in facial pain, refractory TN, spinal cord injury, phantom limb pain, and brachial plexus avulsion.[39,40] This involves surgically placed lesions in the spinal cord that disrupt the dorsal columns. A more targeted approach for central pain management may also be accomplished by gamma knife surgical techniques that use focused doses of radiation in conditions such as TN.[41] Gamma knife may be performed before microvascular decompression as a less invasive modality for TN and can be repeated if the pain reoccurs.

Nerve Blocks and Ablation

A variety of nerves can be "blocked" temporarily or permanently by local anesthetic, local anesthetics plus steroids, nerve degenerative solutions such as phenol or glycerol, or ablated using high-level thermal energy (80°C) or low-level pulsing energy (pulse dose radiofrequency at lower temperature but longer treatment time). There is evidence for steroid and local anesthetic blocks of the greater and lesser occipital nerve for occipital neuralgia and other headache disorders.[42] Headache and facial pain can also be treated by blocks of the third occipital, supraorbital, auriculotemporal, supratrochlear nerves and the sphenopalatine ganglion.[43,44] Gasserian ganglion radiofrequency (RF) thermal lesioning and neurolytic lesioning has been shown to be effective for facial pain due to TN.[45] Pulsed RF is efficacious in TN, facial pain, postthoracotomy pain, radicular pain, joint pain, peripheral neuropathy, and myofascial pain.[46] The intercostal nerves (or the corresponding DRG) may undergo cryoablation, pulsed or thermal radiofrequency ablation, or even surgical neurectomy to relieve postthoracotomy pain.[47] Sympathetically maintained pain conditions such as causalgia and CRPS types I and II can be diagnosed and treated with blockade of the sympathetic nervous system.[48-50] Chronic pelvic pain, coccydynia, or perineal pain may be relieved by an impar ganglion, which is the most distal aspect of the sympathetic chain.[50] Lastly, patients with intractable abdominal pain from malignancy may benefit from a neurolytic celiac plexus block or hypogastric block with alcohol, phenol, or glycerol.[51]

Botulinum Toxin

Botulinum toxin A has been used for dystonia, spasticity, and migraines as well as peripheral NP. However, the evidence behind its efficacy for decreasing NP is equivocal with botulinum being recommended as a third-line medication for peripheral NP.[52] The antinociceptive effects of Botulinum Toxin A are attributed to the inhibition of inflammatory mediators from peripheral sensory nerves, including substance P, glutamate, and calcitonin gene-related peptide (CGRP). There are no guidelines for the ideal dosage of Botulinum Toxin A for NP, but most studies evaluated used 50 to 200 units at the site of pain.[53] Smaller trials have shown efficacy in decreasing DPN pain with injections directly into the patient's feet when compared with placebo.[54] Botulinum toxin A has a low side effect profile with the most common side effect listed as neck pain, injection site pain, and muscular weakness. Overall, smaller trials show efficacy with use of botulinum toxin A for TN, DPN, but others show no improvement in occipital neural pain or CRPS. The true potential of this medication for peripheral neuropathy requires more research as most studies have small enrollment numbers and have varying doses of toxin given.

Neuropathic Pain Conditions

A few of the most common NP conditions will be described in detail below. A more complete list of conditions is shown in Table 13-5.

TABLE 13-5 Neuropathic Pain Conditions and Diagnoses

TYPE OF NEUROPATHY	CLINICAL CONDITIONS
Peripheral neuropathy	Phantom pain, stump pain, nerve injury, nerve root avulsion, neuroma, posttraumatic neuralgia, entrapment syndrome, Morton neuralgia, painful scar, herpes zoster (acute and chronic), diabetic neuropathy, diabetic amyotrophy, ischemic neuropathy, borreliosis, vasculitis or connective tissue disease, neuralgic amyotrophy, peripheral nerve tumor, radiation-induced neuropathy, plexus neuritis, trigeminal neuralgia, glossopharyngeal neuralgia, vagus neuralgia, pudendal neuralgia, vascular compression syndrome, postsurgical pain (postmastectomy or postthoracotomy)
Generalized neuropathy	Metabolic or nutritional: diabetes, alcoholism, amyloidosis, hypothyroidism, beri beri, pellagra
	Drug related: examples are chemotherapy agents and antiretrovirals
	Toxin-related: examples are arsenic and thallium
	Hereditary: amyloid neuropathy, Fabry disease, Charcot–Marie–Tooth disease, hereditary autonomic and sensory neuropathy
	Malignant: paraneoplastic neuropathy, myeloma
	Infectious or immune related: acute or inflammatory polyradiculoneuropathy (Guillain–Barre syndrome), borreliosis, HIV (human immunodeficiency virus) neuropathy, syphilis
	Other or unknown: idiopathic small-fiber neuropathy, trench foot, erythromelalgia
Central pain syndromes	Vascular lesions in the brain and spinal cord, multiple sclerosis, traumatic spinal cord injury, traumatic brain injury, atypical facial pain, syringomyelia and syringobulbia, tumor and abscess (depends on location), myelitis, epilepsy, Parkinson disease
Sympathetically maintained pain	Chronic regional pain syndrome (types I and II)
Mixed pain syndromes or unknown	Low-back or neck pain with radiculitis or radiculopathy, malignant plexus invasion, functional abdominal pain, coccydynia, orofacial dystonia, burning mouth syndrome

Adapted from Baron R, et al. Neuropathic pain: diagnosis, pathophysiological mechanisms, and treatment. Lancet Neurol. 2010;9(8):807-819. Copyright © 2010 Elsevier. With permission.

Trigeminal Neuralgia

TN, which is also called *tic douloureux*, is a chronic NP status that primarily affects the 5th cranial nerve, the trigeminal nerve. The disease typically presents in patients over the age of 50 years and is more common in females. The presentation of TN is an evoked, severe, and burning pain that may last from several seconds to a few minutes located in the dermatomes of the trigeminal nerve. Patients may have dozens of these episodes in a day. An atypical presentation is a lower intensity NP state that lasts longer than the time frame of the typical presentation.[55] The diagnosis of TN is mainly through the physical examination and patient history, but most patients require MRI (magnetic resonance imaging) to rule out tumor, vascular impingement, or multiple sclerosis as the primary cause. A fine cut high-resolution MRI will follow the course of the trigeminal nerve to see if there is mechanical impingement as the nerve exits the neural foramen and enters the face.

There are various causes of TN, one of which may be vascular in origin where an aberrant branch of the superior cerebellar artery applies pressure onto the trigeminal nerve causing myelin sheath irritation and injury. Central nervous system disorders such as multiple sclerosis may also cause degradation of the myelin that causes TN pain. Other less common causes may include tumors, facial trauma, jaw pain, dental-related pain, Bell palsy, stroke, and ear, nose, or throat diseases or malignancies that may produce TN pain.

Treatment options are primarily pharmacological, with microvascular surgery reserved for intractable TN pain from a vascular impingement. Medications used first line include sodium channel blockers and calcium channel blockers such as gabapentin and carbamazepine and tricyclic antidepressants (TCAs) such as amitriptyline. Due to the neuropathic nature of TN, μ agonists such as opioids are not reliably effective and thus not recommended as the first-line pharmacological agent. If the patient suffers relapse despite medications, other neurosurgical procedures such as gamma knife stereotactic radiotherapy or ablation are available to treat the symptoms from trigeminal nerve injury. The risks involved in surgery include damage to other nerves and cerebrospinal fluid leak.

Diabetic Neuropathy

DPN is a neuropathic condition associated with diabetes mellitus and is often the result of microvascular injury due to the chronic hyperglycemic state. DPN affects all the peripheral nerves including the small pain fibers, the autonomic system, and even motor neurons. DPN presents as a symmetrical, length-dependent sensorimotor polyneuropathy. The pathophysiology of the diabetic neuropathy is multifactorial, with microvascular narrowing of vessels that supply the peripheral nerves as one of the main causes. Elevated levels of glucose may cause increased inflammatory states thus worsening of DPN. EMG/nerve conduction testing will typically show reduced functioning of peripheral nerves by demonstrating positive sharp waves, decreased amplitudes, slower conduction velocity, and spontaneous discharges.[56]

Patients with severe DPN may have decreased sensation in their extremities, often described as a glove-stock distribution with numbness and dysesthesia. Diagnosis is primarily based on physical examination of the patient showing decreased sensation and/or pain in the extremities and impaired or lost reflexes. Small fiber neuropathy can be assessed with pinprick and temperature sensation while large fiber neuropathy can be assessed with proprioception maneuvers and the use of a 128 Hz tuning fork for vibration sense.[57] Autonomic manifestations of DPH should also be evaluated such as heart rate abnormalities with Valsalva maneuver and standing, R-R interval variation, orthostatic hypotension, gastroparesis, tachycardia, sudomotor dysfunction, and erectile dysfuction.[58] Patients are at an elevated risk of injuring themselves when ambulating and developing ulcers and infections in the lower extremity which may lead to amputation, falls, and fractures. Other disorders should be considered in the differential such as prediabetes, thyroid disease, vasculitis, vitamin deficiency, alcohol abuse, heavy metal poisoning, chronic inflammatory demyelinating polyradiculoneuropathy, or HIV neuropathy when making the diagnosis of DPN.[57]

Treatment for DPN includes pharmacological agents that are used to treat many other neuropathic conditions including anticonvulsants, tricyclic antidepressants, and topical agents. The three FDA-approved medications for DPN are the calcium channel blocker, pregabalin, the serotonin–norepinephrine reuptake inhibitor duloxetine, and tapentadol extended release. Tapentadol is a centrally acting mu opioid agonist and a norepinephrine reuptake inhibitor, with a similar mechanism of action to tramadol. The use of pure mu agonist opioids for DPN is controversial due to long-term side effects of opioids including dependence, constipation, and opioid-induced hyperalgesia. Other nonpharmacological agents include acupuncture and capsaicin for DPN, although further research needs to be conducted to establish efficacy. Long-term treatment of DPN depends on improved glucose control through lifestyle management.

Postherpetic Neuralgia

PHN is a pain condition stemming from the reactivation of herpes zoster virus that may result in a chronic condition with a significant amount of morbidity. The course of the disease starts with an initial contagious infection (chickenpox) with varicella zoster virus, often in childhood. The virus then becomes latent in the dorsal column sensory ganglia and reactivates decades later to produce NP and a rash in a dermatomal pattern. In contrast, zoster sine herpete is another version of the disease manifestation but without a rash. Studies vary but as many as half of individuals who present with herpes zoster (HZ) may develop the chronic painful condition. The skin manifestation presents as a maculopapular rash in a unilateral dermatomal pattern typically in the thoracic spine, high lumbar spine, and rarely in the distribution of cranial nerve V. Patients present with allodynia, dysesthesia, sensitivity to thermal stimuli, and hyperalgesia.[59] Those with facial symptoms (HZ ophthalmicus) in the ophthalmic branch of the facial nerve are at risk of blindness due to retinal damage and should be treated right away.

The shingles vaccine with live attenuated varicella zoster virus may prevent the development of HZ and PHN for individuals aged 60 years or older.[60] Those with the acute phase of the infection should be treated with opioid therapy, oral or ophthalmic steroids, and a 7 to 10-day course of antiviral agents such as acyclovir, famciclovir, or valacyclovir which can decrease the viral load and the severity of HZ.[61] Those who are immunocompromised and elderly are at higher risk of developing HZ. The chronic disease of pain that persists longer than 30 days after the disease onset is termed PHN. PHN can be treated with a multiple of options including calcium channel agents, lidocaine patches or topical agents, capsaicin, and TCAs.

Treating Neuropathic Pain in Patients With Comorbid Conditions

Individuals with NP may also have multiple medical comorbidities which can complicate treatment. An awareness of pharmacokinetics and pharmacodynamics along with drug–drug interactions should be considered when offering polypharmacy. Adverse drug reactions from neuropathic agents can be life-threatening such as in cases with increased suicidal thoughts, prolonged QTc, Steven–Johnson syndrome with AEDs, and serotonin syndrome. Anticholinergic medications, such as TCAs, should be avoided in those being treated with anticholinesterase drugs such as in Alzheimer disease or have acute angle glaucoma. Many interactions are due to isoenzymes of the hepatic cytochrome P450 (CYP) system. Some medications may induce or mitigate the effect of other medications through the CYP system. For example, carbamazepine may reduce the serum levels of TCAs or the anticoagulation effects of warfarin.[62] Codeine and tramadol are those medications whose actions depend on the CYP system, and therefore effects can be variable depending on whether the patient is a rapid metabolizer or does not biotransform the medication.[62]

Patients with liver or kidney disease will need their medications carefully monitored and dosed appropriately. Gabapentin is excreted unchanged in the urine but will need to be renally dosed in the setting of kidney disease. Nonsteroidal anti-inflammatory drugs (NSAIDs) will also need to be used sparingly in those with renal disease but topical NSAIDs may be a better option in this setting. Neurotoxic metabolites of morphine may accumulate in those with renal failure. Liver cirrhosis may cause alterations in drug metabolism, plasma protein binding, elimination, and distribution. TCAs, duloxetine, carbamazepine, and opioids should be used with extreme caution in those with liver disease.[62] MAO inhibitors are contraindicated in patients on norepinephrine modulating medications such as venlafaxine or duloxetine. Furthermore, hypertension can be a side effect of venlafaxine and duloxetine or NSAIDs. EKG changes such as prolonged QTc can be seen with methadone and TCAs. Weight gain and congestive heart failure have been described with pregabalin, especially in the elderly. Opioids may also affect the cardiovascular system by causing hypotension or hypertension, bradycardia, sleep apnea, and respiratory depression. Respiratory depression occurs more frequently at higher opioid doses and when combined with benzodiazepines or alcohol. AEDs, which are often teratogenic, should be avoided in those planning on getting pregnant. The first trimester is crucial in avoiding medications that may cause complications for the mother and fetus. The lowest effective dose should be recommended along with supplementation with folic acid.[62] Most neuropathic agents, except gabapentin and high-dose opioids, pass into breast milk sparingly or without clinical effect.

The elderly is a group susceptible to NP due to progression of comorbid conditions, overwhelming polypharmacy, or risk of developing PHN and other illnesses. NP is overrepresented in those who are elderly with high levels of morbidity.[4,63] There are challenges in treating this group of individuals which includes their ability to communicate pain or show signs of classical clinical presentations. Additionally, fall risk and subsequent injury makes the use of medications or other aggressive treatments challenging. Aging itself alters pharmacokinetics and pharmacodynamics of water soluble and fat soluble medications along with changes in the metabolic liver pathways. A practical approach where adverse drug effects are screened for frequently and the lowest effective doses are used is likely the best treatment plan for elderly patients in preserving independence and functionality.

CONCLUSIONS

The assessment and treatment of patients with NP remains a challenge for providers, but the high levels of morbidity and suffering cannot be discounted. The multitude of pharmacological, nonpharmacological, and intervention-based treatments for NP offers clinicians and patients treatment options that fit personal goals.

REFERENCES

1. Doth AH, Hansson PT, Jensen MP, Taylor RS. The burden of neuropathic pain: a systematic review and meta-analysis of health utilities. *Pain*. 2010;149(2):338-344.
2. Schaefer C, Sadosky A, Mann R, et al. Pain severity and the economic burden of neuropathic pain in the United States: BEAT Neuropathic Pain Observational Study. *Clinicoecon Outcomes Res*. 2014;6:483-496.
3. Schaefer C, Mann R, Sadosky A, et al. Burden of illness associated with peripheral and central neuropathic pain among adults seeking treatment in the United States: a patient-centered evaluation. *Pain Med*. 2014;15(12):2105-2119.
4. McDermott AM, Toelle TR, Rowbotham DJ, Schaefer CP, Dukes EM. The burden of neuropathic pain: results from a cross-sectional survey. *Eur J Pain*. 2006;10(2):127-135.
5. Luo Y, Anderson TA. Phantom limb pain: a review. *Int Anesthesiol Clin*. 2016;54(2):121-139.
6. Kerstman E, Ahn S, Battu S, Tariq S, Grabois M. Neuropathic pain. *Handb Clin Neurol*. 2013;110:175-187.
7. Benzon HT, Raja SN, Liu SS, Fishman SM, Cohen SP. *Essentials of Pain Medicine*. 3rd ed. Philadelphia, PA: Elsevier; 2011.
8. Opstelten W, McElhaney J, Weinberger B, Oaklander AL, Johnson RW. The impact of varicella zoster virus: chronic pain. *J Clin Virol*. 2010;48(suppl 1):S8-S13.
9. Aslam A, Singh J, Rajbhandari S. Pathogenesis of painful diabetic neuropathy. *Pain Res Treat*. 2014;2014:412041.
10. Rashiq S, Dick BD. Post-surgical pain syndromes: a review for the non-pain specialist. *Can J Anaesth*. 2014;61(2):123-130.
11. Delanian S, Lefaix JL, Pradat PF. Radiation-induced neuropathy in cancer survivors. *Radiother Oncol*. 2012;105(3):273-282.
12. Tajerian M, Clark JD. New concepts in complex regional pain syndrome. *Hand Clin*. 2016;32(1):41-49.
13. Jones RC, Backonja MM. Review of neuropathic pain screening and assessment tools. *Curr Pain Headache Rep*. 2013;17(9):363.
14. Cooper MA, Kluding PM, Wright DE. Emerging relationships between exercise, sensory nerves, and neuropathic pain. *Front Neurosci*. 2016;10:372.
15. Johnson MI, Bjordal JM. Transcutaneous electrical nerve stimulation for the management of painful conditions: focus on neuropathic pain. *Expert Rev Neurother*. 2011;11(5):735-753.
16. Tang Y, Yin HY, Rubini P, Illes P. Acupuncture-induced analgesia: a neurobiological basis in purinergic signaling. *Neuroscientist*. 2016;22(6):563-578.
17. Dimitrova A, Murchison C, Oken B. Acupuncture for the treatment of peripheral neuropathy: a systematic review and meta-analysis. *J Altern Complement Med*. 2017;23(3):164-179.
18. Severeijns R, Vlaeyen JW, van den Hout MA, Weber WE. Pain catastrophizing predicts pain intensity, disability, and psychological distress independent of the level of physical impairment. *Clin J Pain*. 2001;17(2):165-172.
19. Jones RC, Lawson E, Backonja M. Managing neuropathic pain. *Med Clin North Am*. 2016;100(1):151-167.
20. Meize-Grochowski R, Shuster G, Boursaw B, et al. Mindfulness meditation in older adults with postherpetic neuralgia: a randomized controlled pilot study. *Geriatr Nurs*. 2015;36(2):154-160.
21. Poulin PA, Romanow HC, Rahbari N, et al. The relationship between mindfulness, pain intensity, pain catastrophizing, depression, and quality of life among cancer survivors living with chronic neuropathic pain. *Support Care Cancer*. 2016;24(10):4167-4175.
22. Creswell JD. Mindfulness interventions. *Ann Rev Psychol*. 2017;68:491-516.
23. Sparkes E, Duarte RV, Mann S, Lawrence TR, Raphael JH. Analysis of psychological characteristics impacting spinal cord stimulation treatment outcomes: a prospective assessment. *Pain Phys*. 2015;18(3):E369-E377.
24. Fama CA, Chen N, Prusik J, et al. The use of preoperative psychological evaluations to predict spinal cord stimulation success: our experience and a review of the literature. *Neuromodulation*. 2016;19(4):429-436.
25. Meyerson BA, Linderoth B. Mechanisms of spinal cord stimulation in neuropathic pain. *Neurol Res*. 2000;22(3):285-292.
26. Verrills P, Sinclair C, Barnard A. A review of spinal cord stimulation systems for chronic pain. *J Pain Res*. 2016;9:481-492.
27. Bicket MC, Dunn RY, Ahmed SU. High-frequency spinal cord stimulation for chronic pain: pre-clinical overview and systematic review of controlled trials. *Pain Med*. 2016;17(12):2326-2336.

28. Lambru G, Trimboli M, Palmisani S, Smith T, Al-Kaisy A. Safety and efficacy of cervical 10 kHz spinal cord stimulation in chronic refractory primary headaches: a retrospective case series. *J Headache Pain.* 2016;17(1):66.

29. Liem L. Stimulation of the dorsal root ganglion. *Prog Neurol Surg.* 2015;29:213-224.

30. Chakravarthy K, Nava A, Christo PJ, Williams K. Review of recent advances in peripheral nerve stimulation (PNS). *Curr Pain Headache Rep.* 2016;20(11):60.

31. Mitchell B, Verrills P, Vivian D, DuToit N, Barnard A, Sinclair C. Peripheral nerve field stimulation therapy for patients with thoracic pain: a prospective study. *Neuromodulation.* 2016;19(7):752-759.

32. Verrills P, Rose R, Mitchell B, Vivian D, Barnard A. Peripheral nerve field stimulation for chronic headache: 60 cases and long-term follow-up. *Neuromodulation.* 2014;17(1):54-59.

33. Soin A, Fang ZP, Velasco J. Peripheral neuromodulation to treat postamputation pain. *Prog Neurol Surg.* 2015;29:158-167.

34. Honey CM, Tronnier VM, Honey CR. Deep brain stimulation versus motor cortex stimulation for neuropathic pain: a minireview of the literature and proposal for future research. *Computat Struct Biotechnol J.* 2016;14:234-237.

35. O'Connell NE, Wand BM, Marston L, Spencer S, Desouza LH. Non-invasive brain stimulation techniques for chronic pain. *Cochrane Database Syst Rev.* 2014(4):Cd008208.

36. Rauck RL, Wallace MS, Burton AW, Kapural L, North JM. Intrathecal ziconotide for neuropathic pain: a review. *Pain Pract.* 2009;9(5):327-337.

37. Domeshek LF, Krauss EM, Snyder-Warwick AK, et al. Surgical treatment of neuromas improves patient-reported pain, depression, and quality of life. *Plast Reconstr Surg.* 2017;139(2):407-418.

38. Hung YH, Wu CH, Ozcakar L, Wang TG. Ultrasound-guided steroid injections for two painful neuromas in the stump of a below-elbow amputee. *Am J Phys Med Rehabil.* 2016;95(5):e73-e74.

39. Haninec P, Kaiser R, Mencl L, Waldauf P. Usefulness of screening tools in the evaluation of long-term effectiveness of DREZ lesioning in the treatment of neuropathic pain after brachial plexus injury. *BMC Neurol.* 2014; 14:225.

40. Chivukula S, Tempel ZJ, Chen CJ, Shin SS, Gande AV, Moossy JJ. Spinal and nucleus caudalis dorsal root entry zone lesioning for chronic pain: efficacy and outcomes. *World Neurosurg.* 2015;84(2):494-504.

41. Regis J, Tuleasca C, Resseguier N, et al. Long-term safety and efficacy of Gamma Knife surgery in classical trigeminal neuralgia: a 497-patient historical cohort study. *J Neurosurg.* 2016;124(4):1079-1087.

42. Choi I, Jeon SR. Neuralgias of the head: occipital neuralgia. *J Korean Med Sci.* 2016;31(4):479-488.

43. Blumenfeld A, Ashkenazi A, Napchan U, et al. Expert consensus recommendations for the performance of peripheral nerve blocks for headaches–a narrative review. *Headache.* 2013;53(3):437-446.

44. Robbins MS, Robertson CE, Kaplan E, et al. The sphenopalatine ganglion: anatomy, pathophysiology, and therapeutic targeting in headache. *Headache.* 2016;56(2):240-258.

45. Peters G, Nurmikko TJ. Peripheral and gasserian ganglion-level procedures for the treatment of trigeminal neuralgia. *Clin J Pain.* 2002;18(1):28-34.

46. Chua NH, Vissers KC, Sluijter ME. Pulsed radiofrequency treatment in interventional pain management: mechanisms and potential indications-a review. *Acta Neurochir.* 2011;153(4):763-771.

47. Cohen SP, Sireci A, Wu CL, Larkin TM, Williams KA, Hurley RW. Pulsed radiofrequency of the dorsal root ganglia is superior to pharmacotherapy or pulsed radiofrequency of the intercostal nerves in the treatment of chronic postsurgical thoracic pain. *Pain Phys.* 2006;9(3):227-235.

48. Imani F, Hemati K, Rahimzadeh P, Kazemi MR, Hejazian K. Effectiveness of Stellate Ganglion Block under fuoroscopy or ultrasound guidance in upper extremity CRPS. *J Clin Diagn Res.* 2016;10(1):Uc09-12.

49. van Eijs F, Stanton-Hicks M, Van Zundert J, et al. Evidence-based interventional pain medicine according to clinical diagnoses. 16. Complex regional pain syndrome. *Pain Pract.* 2011;11(1):70-87.

50. Walters A, Muhleman M, Osiro S, et al. One is the loneliest number: a review of the ganglion impar and its relation to pelvic pain syndromes. *Clin Anat.* 2013;26(7):855-861.

51. Mercadante S, Klepstad P, Kurita GP, Sjogren P, Giarratano A. Sympathetic blocks for visceral cancer pain management: a systematic review and EAPC recommendations. *Crit Rev Oncol Hematol.* 2015;96(3):577-583.

52. Finnerup NB, Attal N, Haroutounian S, et al. Pharmacotherapy for neuropathic pain in adults: a systematic review and meta-analysis. *Lancet Neurol.* 2015; 14(2):162-173.

53. Oh HM, Chung ME. Botulinum toxin for neuropathic pain: a review of the literature. *Toxins.* 2015;7(8):3127-3154.

54. Chen WT, Yuan RY, Chiang SC, et al. OnabotulinumtoxinA improves tactile and mechanical pain perception in painful diabetic polyneuropathy. *Clin J Pain.* 2013;29(4):305-310.

55. Cruccu G, Finnerup NB, Jensen TS, et al. Trigeminal neuralgia: new classification and diagnostic grading for practice and research. *Neurology.* 2016;87(2):220-228.

56. Bagai K, Wilson JR, Khanna M, Song Y, Wang L, Fisher MA. Electrophysiological patterns of diabetic polyneuropathy. *Electromyogr Clin Neurophysiol.* 2008;48(3-4):139-145.

57. Pop-Busui R, Boulton AJ, Feldman EL, et al. Diabetic neuropathy: a position statement by the American Diabetes Association. *Diab Care.* 2017;40(1):136-154.

58. Vinik AI, Maser RE, Mitchell BD, Freeman R. Diabetic autonomic neuropathy. *Diab Care.* 2003;26(5):1553-1579.

59. Mallick-Searle T, Snodgrass B, Brant JM. Postherpetic neuralgia: epidemiology, pathophysiology, and pain management pharmacology. *J Multidiscip Healthc.* 2016;9:447-454.

60. Gagliardi AM, Andriolo BN, Torloni MR, Soares BG. Vaccines for preventing herpes zoster in older adults. *Cochrane Database Syst Rev.* 2016;3:Cd008858.

61. Whitley RJ, Volpi A, McKendrick M, Wijck A, Oaklander AL. Management of herpes zoster and post-herpetic neuralgia now and in the future. *J Clin Virol.* 2010;48(suppl 1):S20-S28.

62. Haanpaa ML, Gourlay GK, Kent JL, et al. Treatment considerations for patients with neuropathic pain and other medical comorbidities. *Mayo Clin Proc.* 2010;85(3 suppl):S15-S25.

63. Schmader KE, Baron R, Haanpaa ML, et al. Treatment considerations for elderly and frail patients with neuropathic pain. *Mayo Clin Proc.* 2010;85(3 suppl):S26-S32.

64. http://www.iasp-pain.org/Taxonomy. Accessed March 22, 2017.

14

HEADACHES AND OTHER FACIAL PAIN SYNDROMES

Shweta Teckchandani, DO, Marc Lenaerts, MD, FAHS and Charles De Mesa, DO, MPH

INTRODUCTION

Headaches are a worldwide problem affecting people of all ages, socioeconomic backgrounds, and races. According to the World Health Organization,[1] 50% of the general population have headaches during any given year. Headache disorders are a public health concern, given the socioeconomic burden directly due to health care costs and indirectly due to missed workdays or reduced competence.[2] Given that most patients with headache initially present in a primary care setting, it is highly important to obtain the correct diagnosis with an appropriate plan of care. Headaches fall under two

categories namely, "primary" and "secondary." By definition, a primary headache is due to the headache itself, whereas a secondary headache is due to a demonstrable organic disease or an underlying structural abnormality. Ninety percent of headaches seen in practice are primary headaches, and less than ten percent are secondary headaches.[3] Because secondary headaches are rare and pose significant risks, they must be effectively ruled out.

PRIMARY HEADACHE DISORDERS

The 3 types of primary headaches are migraine, tension type, and trigeminal autonomic cephalgias (TACs).[4,5] Tension-type headache (TTH) is the most prevalent affecting 60% to 80% of the population.[6] However, in the outpatient setting, migraine is far more common than tension type and cluster because it is disabling enough for an individual to seek medical attention.[7]

MIGRAINE

The estimated global prevalence of migraine is 14.7% (1 in 7 people).[8] It is more prevalent than diabetes, epilepsy, and asthma combined.[9] Clinical features of migraine include localized unilateral headaches but may present as bilateral, retro-orbital, occipital/suboccipital, parietal, or central facial. It is throbbing in quality, and the intensity is variable from mild to extremely severe and disabling. The patient may be irritable and complain of symptoms of photophobia, phonophobia, osmophobia, and kinesiophobia (fear of physical movement). There may be accompanying gastrointestinal symptoms of anorexia, nausea, vomiting, or diarrhea. Occasionally, patients will present with migraine with an aura which may include cortical symptoms such as visual spots and flashes of lights. Other less common aura symptoms include hemiparesis, hemisensory loss, aphasia, confusion, and amnesia, which are fully reversible.

DIAGNOSTIC CRITERIA[4]

A. At least 5 attacks fulfilling criteria B-D

B. Headache attacks lasting 4 to 72 hour (untreated or unsuccessfully treated)[2,3]

C. Headaches have at least 2 of the following 4 characteristics:
1. unilateral location
2. pulsating quality
3. moderate or severe pain intensity
4. aggravation by or causing avoidance of routine physical activity (e.g., walking or climbing stairs)

D. During headache at least 1 of the following accompanies:
1. nausea and/or vomiting
2. photophobia and phonophobia

E. Not better accounted for by another *International Classification of Headache Disorders*-3 (ICHD-3) diagnosis.

TREATMENT

Treatment strategies should focus on improvement in functionality and reduction in the number of headache days. The best approach to manage migraine is to individualize the treatment based on the patient's unique symptoms and should include medication management and other nonpharmaceutical treatment strategies.

Have a low threshold for treatment and be an advocate for prevention because it will help prevent transformation into chronic migraine. Prophylaxis is indicated for greater or equal to 3 attacks a month. Monitoring side effects and reassessing efficacy are important. Consider comorbid conditions in treatment such as hypertension, depression, and seizures because they may help guide medication selection. Attempt therapy long enough to determine effects. For example, provide greater and equal to a 6-week trial with greater than or equal to 6-month maintenance. Do not stop too quickly as these regress the benefit of treatment strategies.

If the individual experiences one headache a month but nothing else helps, then prevention or prophylaxis is still reasonable. The goal in prevention is fewer headaches (e.g., decrease frequency by 50%), decrease in intensity and duration of pain, reduced need for rescue medication, and improved efficacy of abortive therapy. Understand and explain to the patient that this may take 2 months for full benefit.

An important consideration before prophylaxis is initiated is to assess for medication-overuse headaches. If the patient is using abortive therapy more than 10 days a month, he or she may be experiencing rebound headaches. In such cases, the abortive medication should be withdrawn before starting prophylactic therapy.[9]

Migraine Abortive Treatment

Early abortive treatment is essential in migraine management for maximum benefit. A study using almotriptan (Axert) showed that abortive therapy when initiated within 1 hour of headache onset has greater relief and lower recurrence rates of pain than nonearly users.[10] When deciding for treatment, aggressive and larger dose of the variety of choices may be selected, and this may vary over time. It may be necessary to change medication that is a therapeutic failure. The goal of aborting a headache is to stop it as early and aggressively as possible with the least side effects to improve quality of life and function.

Categories can be nonspecific or specific. Nonspecific medications include acetylsalicylic acid (ASA), N-acetyl-p-amino-phenol (APAP), and nonsteroidal anti-inflammatory drugs (NSAIDs) (although some specificity is present because these act on inflammation not just pain). Triptans are first-line therapies for moderate to severe migraine, or mild to moderate migraine, that has not responded to adequate doses of simple analgesics.[11] They can be effective by activating serotonin receptor type 1 subtypes b, d, and f. They are more targeted because they do not act on the dopamine receptor and therefore do not cause nausea, whereas dihydroergotamine (DHE) and older ergotamines can cause nausea. Other potential options with good evidence of efficacy for migraine abortive therapy include antiemetic agents such as promethazine, prochlorperazine, and metoclopramide.[12]

Adverse effects should be explained including chest, neck, and head pressure; tingling; paresthesia; and flushing, as well as central effects of dizziness and sedation. These are transient though and are not indicative of absence of relief. Such counseling can be effective for the patient. Contraindications are coronary artery and cardiovascular diseases. Relative contraindications are in hemiplegia, brainstem, and aura migraines.

MIGRAINE PROPHYLAXIS

Pharmacologic treatment typically involves daily preventive medication. It should be noted that only 2 agents (onabotulinumtoxinA and topiramate) have strong evidence in chronic migraine,[13] although there are other medications for episodic migraine. First-line agents typically used with evidence of efficacy belong to 3 broad classes namely antihypertensives, antiepileptics, and antidepressants (see Table 14-1).[14] The doses vary highly, the medication must be titrated slowly, and the patient must be informed that titration may take weeks for the individual to tolerate it.

Calcium channel blockers are not as effective as beta-blockers but well tolerated in some patients. Several studies have also shown efficacy of nutraceuticals such as riboflavin, magnesium, and coenzyme Q10 for prophylaxis.[15] If the individual has high blood pressure, medications used such as lisinopril and candesartan demonstrate randomized control trials with data to support their use, but these are generally of shorter duration. Nevertheless, they are good choices for those unable to use the other medications. Smaller study on tizanidine appears supportive as well.

OnabotulinumtoxinA injection therapy is FDA approved only for chronic migraine, and emerging

TABLE 14-1 Migraine Prophylaxis

MEDICATION	DAILY DOSE RANGE	POSSIBLE ADVERSE EFFECTS	CONTRAINDICATIONS
Antiepileptic Drugs			
Valproate	250-500 mg bid	Alopecia, weight gain, tremors	Pregnancy Liver disease
Topiramate	50 mg bid	Paresthesias, word-finding difficulty, cognitive slowing	Pregnancy history of nephrolithiasis Glaucoma
Beta-Blockers			
Propranolol	80-240 mg divided bid or tid	Hypotension, fatigue	Asthma Diabetes
Tricyclic Antidepressants			
Nortriptyline	10-150 mg daily	Weight gain, dry mouth, drowsiness	Cardiac conduction abnormalities
Amitriptyline	30-150 mg daily		
Venlafaxine	75-150 mg daily	Nausea vomiting	Do not use with MAOIs—increases risk of serotonin syndrome
Calcium Channel Blockers			
Verapamil	80-480 mg divided tid	Constipation, atrioventricular conduction disturbances	Cardiac conduction abnormalities
Angiotensin-Converting Enzyme Indicator			
Lisinopril, generic	5-40 mg daily	Hypotension	History of angioedema
Angiotensin-Receptor Blocker			
Candesartan	8-21 mg daily	Hypotension	Allergic to sulfonamide drugs

Republished with permission of Dove Medical Press Ltd from Garza I, Swanson JW. Prophylaxis of migraine. Neuropsychiatr Dis Treat. 2006;2(3):281-291; permission conveyed through Copyright Clearance Center, Inc.

data suggest this treatment modulates central sensitization rather than a muscle effect. Injections are repeated every 12 weeks and are based on the PREEMPT protocol (Figure 14-1). This treatment does not work in episodic migraine or TTH contrary to one would presume.

In addition to medication management, treatment with nonpharmaceutical strategies should be considered as well. Cognitive behavioral therapy, physical therapy, biofeedback, and mindfulness training as a form of relaxation therapy may be useful.[16] Other potential options include neurostimulation devices such as Cefaly and Spring transcranial magnetic stimulation (TMS) device.

TENSION-TYPE HEADACHES

TTHs are recurrent episodes of bilateral headaches lasting minutes to weeks. Pain is mild to moderate in intensity with a pressing or tightening in quality. TTH may be distinguished from migraines by location (generally bilateral), absence of associated nausea/vomiting, and symptoms that typically *do not* worsen with physical activity.

TRIGEMINAL AUTONOMIC CEPHALGIAS

Trigeminal autonomic cephalgias or TACs are a group of primary headache disorders characterized by unilateral trigeminal distribution pain that is associated with ipsilateral cranial autonomic features. These include cluster headaches, paroxysmal hemicrania, hemicrania continua, and short-lasting unilateral neuralgiform headache with conjunctival injection and tearing (SUNCT) or with cranial autonomic features (SUNA). Cluster headache is characterized by attacks of severe orbital, supraorbital, or temporal pain, accompanied by autonomic phenomena and/or restless or agitation.[17] These occur in cyclical patterns or clusters and are one of the most painful types of headache. Individuals with cluster headaches may commonly experience nighttime awakening by an intense pain in or around one eye on one side of the head.[18] Ipsilateral autonomic symptoms including conjunctival injection, eyelid closure, lacrimation, and rhinorrhea may be present.[19]

A summary of available treatments for TTH, cluster, and other selected headaches are listed in the rapid reference table (Table 14-2).

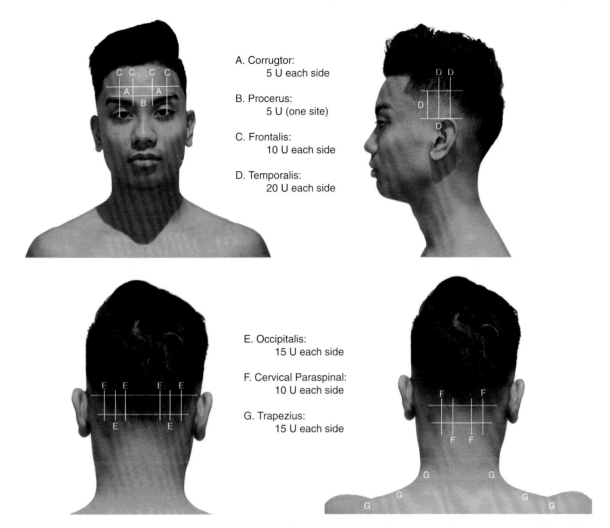

A. Corrugtor:
5 U each side

B. Procerus:
5 U (one site)

C. Frontalis:
10 U each side

D. Temporalis:
20 U each side

E. Occipitalis:
15 U each side

F. Cervical Paraspinal:
10 U each side

G. Trapezius:
15 U each side

FIGURE 14-1 Botulinum toxin injection sites and doses for chronic migraine prophylactic treatment. Read the package insert for full details of this treatment option.

MEDICATION-OVERUSE HEADACHES

Patients should be educated on medication-overuse headaches. As a general rule, abortive medications may not be used for more than 10 days a month (may use more than once a day up to the maximum recommended dose). Another important point of discussion includes opioids in management of headaches. Every physician regardless of his or her practice will encounter patients using opioids. Recent evidence suggests that opioids are not an effective treatment for headaches and, in fact, lead to development of chronic daily headaches[20] in addition to other potential risks. Opioids may also render use of other prophylactic and abortive medications ineffective[4] and therefore should be avoided in headache management.

PRIMARY VERSUS SECONDARY HEADACHES

Carefully obtain a history to distinguish between primary and secondary headaches because they may share similar features (e.g., visual or sensory auras may mimic sudden neurologic symptoms of transient ischemic attacks [TIAs] or seizures). The physical examination for primary headaches will be essentially normal in comparison with secondary headaches. Identifying "red flags" are essential for appropriately working up, managing, and treating secondary headaches in a time-sensitive fashion.[21]

RED FLAGS

First or worst headache ever
New-onset headache
Onset after age 50 years
Change in the pattern of headache
Worsening headache
Acute or sudden onset
Sudden onset during exertion, coughing, sneezing, and
    sex-related
Headache with postural link
Headache in setting of malignancy or HIV
Systemic symptoms (fever, weight loss, coughing)
Neurologic symptoms or signs
    A rapid approach to effectively identify and exclude secondary headaches based on history, and an

TABLE 14-2 Treatment for Tension-type Cluster and Other Headaches

Tension-Type Headache*

Medication	Daily Dose Range
Naproxen sodium	500 mg PO qd or bid
Acetaminophen	500-1000 PO bid or tid
Amitriptyline	25-100 mg PO qd

Cluster Headache

Medication	Daily Dose Range
Prophylactic	
Prednisone	100 mg PO qd tapered over a week; low dose may need to be maintained for a longer time
Verapamil	240-720 mg PO qd
Lithium	300-900 mg PO qd
Valproate sodium	500 mg PO bid or tid up to 2000 mg/day in equally divided doses
Ergotamine tartrate	1 mg PO qd or bid
Symptomatic	
Oxygen	10 L per minute by nasal cannula for 10 to 15 min
Sumatriptan	6 mg subcutaneously bid
Dihydroergotamine	1 mg IV with or without pretreatment with a dopamine antagonist to counteract adverse effects of DHE

Chronic Paroxysmal Hemicrania and Hemicrania Continua

Medication	Daily Dose Range
Indomethacin	25 mg PO bid or tid up to 225 mg per day in equally divided dose

*Nonpharmacologic treatments should be considered with referral to a psychologist or a physical therapist with proficiency in the field.
bid, twice a day; PO, by mouth; IV, Intravenously; qd, each day; tid, 3 times a day.

examination is achieved by applying the mnemonic SNOOP.[22] This stands for:

- **S**ystemic symptoms: constitutional symptoms, presence of secondary risk factors that predispose one to secondary headaches, such as immunocompromised status (HIV or cancer)
- **N**eurologic signs or symptoms: finding papilledema on funduscopic examination, which suggests increased intracranial pressure
- **O**ld age: first-onset headache after age 50 years
- **O**nset: quick- or sudden-onset headache (e.g., "thunderclap" headache)
- **P**attern: remarkable change in the frequency, severity, or type of headache

History and a complete physical examination including a neurologic and ophthalmologic examination are paramount to establishing the kind of symptoms and quantitative assessment. For example, the physician may ask the following:

Onset: Old versus new? Sudden versus gradual onset?

Family history: Is there a history of migraine? Aneurysm?

Duration: How often do you have headaches and how long do they last?

Associated symptoms: GI symptoms? Neurologic symptoms?

Characterizing the headache symptoms enables one to reach an appropriate diagnosis, obtain further diagnostic studies if necessary, and implement an individualized treatment.

A physician may also use available tools to determine the disability or limitation of activities during the headache specifically for migraine. One example is the Migraine Disability Assessment Test (MIDAS) instrument.[7,23,24]

The MIDAS Questions

1. *On how many days in the last 3 months did you miss work or school because of your headaches?*
2. *How many days in the last 3 months was your productivity at work or school reduced by half or more because of your headaches? (Do not include days you counted in question 1 where you missed work or school.)*
3. *On how many days in the last 3 months did you not do household work because of your headaches?*
4. *.How many days in the last 3 months was your productivity in household work reduced by half of more because of your headaches? (Do not include days you counted in question 3 where you did not do household work.)*
5. *On how many days in the last 3 months did you miss family, social, or leisure activities because of your headaches?*

The patient's score consists of the total of these 5 questions. Moreover, there is a section for patients to share with their doctors:
What your physician needs to know:

A. *How many days in the last 3 months did you have a headache? (If a headache lasted more than 1 d, count each day.)*
B. *On a scale of 0 to 10, on average how painful were these headaches? (where 0 = no pain at all and 10 = pain as bad as it can be.)*

Scoring:
Once scored, the test gives the patient an idea of how debilitating his or her migraines are based on this scale:
0 to 5, MIDAS Grade I, little or no disability
6 to 10, MIDAS Grade II, mild disability
11 to 20, MIDAS Grade III, moderate disability
21+, MIDAS Grade IV, severe disability

LOCATION

Location of the headache/radiation: Certain headaches have characteristic patterns of location and radiation. For instance, occipital neuralgia typically begins in the occipital region (near the occipital notch) and can radiate forward, sometimes becoming retro-orbital.[25] Laterality can be a distinguishing feature as some individuals may experience a headache that changes sides or stays strictly unilateral from day to day. Hemicrania continua, a "side-locked" headache, is one example of a headache that always stays on one side of the head. How the pain radiates helps determine the type of headache. For instance, a headache that originates in the neck and travels to the occipital region may be indicative of cervicogenic headache, whereas migraine headaches usually occur relatively unilaterally along the temporal, parietal, occipital/suboccipital, and/or retro-orbital regions. Approximately 75% of migraine patients have neck pain, so careful assessment is needed to differentiate migraine from cervicogenic headache.[26] Because of overlapping nerve supply and convergent projection, pain is referred to a larger area distally.

ALLEVIATING AND EXACERBATING FACTORS

This is helpful in assessing headaches related to intracranial pressure. For example, when sitting up, high-pressure headaches such as idiopathic intracranial hypertension are relieved, whereas low-pressure headaches such as postdural puncture headaches may become worse.

Environmental, dietary, and hormonal triggers may influence migraine attacks. Determining a link with menstrual cycle or with eating certain foods such as chocolate suggests the possibility of migraine. On the other hand, a cyclical or aggregate pattern is suggestive of cluster headaches. If increased activity levels or changes in environmental altitude do not change the headache, then TTH may be the likely diagnosis.

NEUROLOGIC SYMPTOMS

Carefully assess neurologic complaints such as seizures, syncope, visual changes, slurring of speech, and weakness. Behavioral changes during an attack may point to certain diagnoses. For instance, irritability and absent mindedness with the headache suggest migraine that is explained by hypothalamic dysfunction. Restlessness and lack of sleep are more likely to accompany cluster headaches.[4,27] Auras may precede or accompany migraine headaches. Visual auras are most common and are followed by paresthesia or speech difficulty. An aura is a benign abnormal neurologic phenomenon. Any brain can experience an aura although migraine makes an individual genetically more prone to it. Auras occur in succession, and the same patient may have a visual aura followed by sensory paresthesia or speech difficulty suspected from cortical spreading depression (CSD). In CSD, there is abnormal neuronal activation involving interstitial fluid and astrocytes with waves of electrophysiological hyperactivity followed by a wave of inhibition. This flow is a 3 mm per minute wave at the time when the

area of the brain is hyperactive. There is a bright shiny image of light in the corresponding visual field, and once the wave has swept that area, the neurons are in an inhibition state (ineffective). An individual may experience a blinded or blurred area that eventually recovers. If there is sensory involvement, then one experiences an area of numbness and tingling. If it affects a motor region, one experiences weakness, and if the wave affects the temporal lobe, one experiences dizziness. The propensity overall is far greater in the occipital because it is more of a receptive part of the cortex. In summary, neuronal activation is followed by inhibition then recovery, and the slow sweeping pattern clearly explains the symptoms. The benign electric wave in the brain responsible for such symptoms can in turn trigger inflammation in the dura from the metabolic alterations explaining why pain follows.

DIAGNOSTIC STUDIES AND THERAPEUTIC INTERVENTIONS

Performing a funduscopic examination to assess intracranial hypertension along with ear, nose, throat (ENT) evaluation is important in assessing sinus disease in headaches although frankly a sinus headache is often overdiagnosed. Full neurologic examination will complete the critical components of the physical examination. Generally, it is essential to assess ENT evaluation specifically to exclude giant cell arteritis (GCA), peri-cranial muscle tenderness, and temporomandibular joint disease as these conditions may mimic partial symptomatology or will need to be treated if diagnosed based on history and examination. Erythrocyte sedimentation rate (ESR) and C-reactive protein (CRP) may be useful if suspecting temporal arteritis and both values will be elevated. Biopsy of the superficial temporal artery confirms the diagnosis. CT scan is indicated for expeditious examination of an individual suspected to have an intracranial disorder such as increased CSF pressure, subarachnoid hemorrhage, epidural or subdural hematoma, brain parenchymal bleeding, infarct, or mass effect from tumor. Magnetic resonance angiogram (MRA) and magnetic resonance imaging (MRI) with and without contrast can further assess vascular and structural abnormalities to exclude secondary causes of headaches. MRI may also be indicated if headache pain intensity increases, if it is the first time the person has a headache requiring urgent medical attention, or the headache now lasts several weeks.

Always ask accompanying autonomic signs and symptoms in patients with headaches. Ipsilateral headaches associated with lacrimation, nasal stuffiness, conjunctival injection, facial swelling, or Horner syndrome should alert you to possible cluster headaches or one of the TACs. It is essential to exclude other possible causes of Horner syndrome. For instance, a chest X-ray may be useful to rule out Pancoast tumor in a patient with a history of smoking. Cervical MRA or MRI may be indicated in a patient with neck trauma.

With headache present on awakening in the morning, one has to suspect obstructive sleep apnea, poorly controlled hypertension, elevated intracranial pressure, or migraine. Sleep study will be helpful particularly in a patient with chronic pain who may be using opioid therapy in combination with a benzodiazepine. This combination therapy is not recommended for treatment of headaches because it exacerbates symptoms and poses significant health risks. If seizures are in the differential diagnosis for a headache assessment, then electroencephalogram (EEG) and MRI are important diagnostic studies.

SECONDARY HEADACHES

Traumatic injuries leading to headaches are commonly encountered in the primary care setting. One may suffer from posttraumatic headache (PTH), which is defined as a headache which develops within 7 days of the injury or after regaining consciousness.[4]

Trauma can also significantly change the course of a pre-existing headache as in migraine condition. For instance, an individual with migraine may now have daily headaches after trauma. Although the trauma is an exacerbating factor, the individual still has a migraine condition and requires migraine treatment. The effect of trauma needs to be carefully reviewed in history. Critical appraisal of prior workup, current management, and adherence to medical therapy is essential.

Other secondary headache disorders include headaches attributed to brain tumors, intracranial hypertension or hypotension, temporal arteritis, subarachnoid hemorrhage, and substance use or withdrawal and due to underlying systemic disease.

MIGRAINE MIMICS AND OTHER CONSIDERATIONS

Conditions that can mimic a migraine aura include strokes, TIAs, seizure disorders, tumors, venous thrombosis, arteriovenous malformations, and carotid dissections. The onset, progression, and duration of the symptoms help differentiate between a migraine aura and a TIA or a seizure. Difficulty in making a distinction between these entities occurs when the aura is not followed by a headache. A gradual onset and progression over a few minutes is a characteristic of a migraine aura compared with a sudden onset in a TIA or a seizure. The classical duration of a migraine aura is 20 to 30 minutes as compared with a significantly shorter duration for a seizure and a longer one for a TIA.

Headaches may share associated symptoms (see Figure 14-2). For instance, autonomic features such as conjunctival injection, lacrimation, and rhinorrhea may occur in migraine or cluster headaches. Autonomic symptoms are triggered by food or stress that alters the trigeminovascular system. A key region within this system is the trigeminal nucleus caudalis of the brainstem that drives this

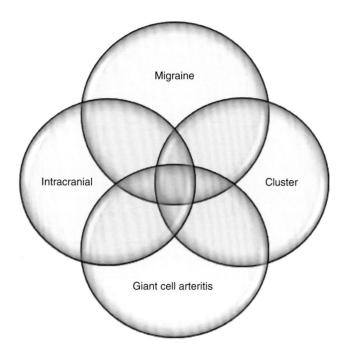

FIGURE 14-2 Shared associated symptoms in selected headaches.

phenomenon. In the case of migraine, the superior salivatory nucleus of the brain stem is responsible for gastrointestinal symptoms (appetite changes, nausea, vomiting).

Cluster headaches and headaches from GCA, also known as temporal arteritis, share painful symptoms around the eye. Cluster headache involves periorbital pain, whereas GCA involves pain localized to the superficial temporal artery along the "temple" (i.e., above the zygomatic arch of the temporal bone). Fever is an associated symptom of both GCA and intracranial disorders such as a brain tumor, high or low cerebrospinal fluid pressures, hypothalamic dysfunction, or infections (meningitis). Vomiting is a common feature of migraines or intracranial disorders.

Unique features of the selected headaches help distinguish them. For migraine, hypersensitivity symptoms of photophobia, phonopobia, osmophobia, and kinesiophobia are distinctive. Cluster headaches have an aggregate periodicity as the name suggests. GCA will have tenderness to palpation of the superficial temporal arteries, jaw pain when chewing, and vision problems. Intracranial disorders will have changes in cognition that may include memory impairment.

CONCLUSION

Diagnosing a headache requires careful attention to history, examination, and prior treatments. Diagnostically excluding secondary headaches is imperative, and treatment strategies should be adequately attempted before considering failure. A multimodal approach is beneficial, and the emphasis is to decrease pain intensity and improve functional quality of life.

REFERENCES

1. WHO. *Headache Disorders.* 2016. Available from: http://www.who.int/mediacentre/factsheets/fs277/en/.

2. Rasmussen BK. Epidemiology and socio-economic impact of headache. *Cephalalgia.* 1999;19(suppl 25):20-23.

3. Rasmussen BK, Jensen R, Schroll M, Olesen J. Epidemiology of headache in a general population–a prevalence study. *J Clin Epidemiol.* 1991;44(11):1147-1157.

4. Headache Classification Committee of the International Headache Society. The international classification of headache disorders. *Cephalalgia.* 2013;33(9):629-808.

5. Headache Classification Committee of the International Headache Society. The international classification of headache disorders, 2nd ed. *Cephalalgia.* 2004;24(suppl 1):9-160.

6. Ahmed F. Headache disorders: differentiating and managing the common subtypes. *Br J Pain.* 2012;6(3):124-132.

7. Lipton RB, Dodick D, Sadovsky R, et al. A self-administered screener for migraine in primary care: The ID Migraine validation study. *Neurology.* 2003;61(3):375-382.

8. Steiner TJ, Stovner LJ, Birbeck GL. Migraine: the seventh disabler. *Headache.* 2013;53(2):227-229.

9. Dikran P. Migraine prophylaxis in adult patients. *West J Med.* 2000;173(5):341-345.

10. Goadsby PJ, Zanchin G, Geraud G, et al. Early vs. non-early intervention in acute migraine-'Act when Mild (AwM)'. A double-blind, placebo-controlled trial of almotriptan. *Cephalalgia.* 2008;28(4):383-391.

11. Gilmore B, Michael M. Treatment of acute migraine headache. *Am Fam Physician.* 2011;83(3):271-280.

12. Kelley NE, Tepper DE. Rescue therapy for acute migraine, part 3: opioids, NSAIDs, steroids, and post-discharge medications. *Headache.* 2012;52(3):467-482.

13. Chiang CC, Schwedt TJ, Wang SJ, Dodick DW. Treatment of medication-overuse headache: A systematic review. *Cephalalgia.* 2016;36(4):371-386.

14. Garza I, Schwedt TJ. Diagnosis and management of chronic daily headache. *Semin Neurol.* 2010;30(2):154-166.

15. D'Onofrio F, Raimo S, Spitaleri D, Casucci G, Bussone G. Usefulness of nutraceuticals in migraine prophylaxis. *Neurol Sci.* 2017;38(suppl 1):117-120.

16. Saper JR, Dodick D, Gladstone JP, Management of chronic daily headache: challenges in clinical practice. *Headache.* 2005;45 (suppl 1):S74-S85.

17. Teckchandani S, Barad M. Treatment strategies for the opioid-dependent patient. *Curr Pain Headache Rep.* 2017;21(11):45.

18. Lenaerts ME. Headache. In: Rosenberg RN, ed. *Atlas of Clinical Neurology.* Current Medicine Group; 2009.

19. May A. Headaches with (ipsilateral) autonomic symptoms. *J Neurol.* 2003;250(11):1273-1278.

20. Gelfand AA, Goadsby PJ. A neurologist's guide to acute migraine therapy in the emergency room. *Neurohospitalist.* 2012;2(2):51-59.

21. Evans RW. Diagnostic testing for headache. *Med Clin North Am.* 2001;85(4):865-885.

22. Dodick DW. Diagnosing headache: clinical clues and clinical rules. *Adv Stud Med.* 2003;2:87-92.

23. Stewart WF, Lipton RB, Kolodner K, Liberman J, Sawyer J. Reliability of the migraine disability assessment score in a population-based sample of headache sufferers. *Cephalalgia.* 1999;19(2):107-114. discussion 74.

24. Stewart WF, Lipton RB, Kolodner KB, Sawyer J, Lee C, Liberman JN. Validity of the Migraine Disability Assessment (MIDAS) score in comparison to a diary-based measure in a population sample of migraine sufferers. *Pain.* 2000;88(1):41-52.

25. Sheikh HU. Approach to chronic daily headache. *Curr Neurol Neurosci Rep.* 2015;15(3):4.

26. Ravishankar K. The art of history-taking in a headache patient. *Ann Indian Acad Neurol.* 2012;15(suppl 1):S7-S14.

27. Cohen AS, Burns B, Goadsby PJ, High-flow oxygen for treatment of cluster headache: a randomized trial. *JAMA.* 2009;302(22):2451-2457.

28. Garza I, Swanson JW. Prophylaxis of migraine. *Neuropsychiatr Dis Treat.* 2006;2(3):281-291.

15

CERVICAL SPINE

Charles De Mesa, DO, MPH and Omar Dyara, DO

FAST FACTS

- Neck pain is the third most common pain condition reported nationally and a frequent reason for seeking medical attention.
- Most episodes of acute neck pain are self-limited, but nearly 50% of individuals will continue to experience some level of pain or frequent occurrences.
- Excluding red flags is essential for early identification and management of more serious diagnoses of neck pain.
- Success of therapeutic procedures and surgeries relies heavily on appropriate patient identification/selection.

INTRODUCTION

Neck pain is the third most common pain condition reported nationally and a frequent reason patients visit their primary care physician.[1] Pathology in the cervical spine can radiate to the head, shoulder, arm, or hand. When a severe injury to the neck occurs, the spinal cord can be affected, which may lead to impaired function of all extremities. For this reason, identifying the specific pain generator and accompanying symptoms is essential in creating a differential diagnosis of neck pain.

Significant uncertainty surrounds the pathophysiology of *chronic* neck pain, and in many cases, the chance of accurately identifying a specific cause is low.[2] The most critical task is to evaluate patients with neck pain for myelopathy, radiculopathy, and dangerous underlying causes such as cancer, fractures, and osteomyelitis.

To be more specific when referring to cervical pain, it is described as the region bounded superiorly by the superior nuchal line and inferiorly by an imaginary transverse line through the T1 spinous process. Few diagnoses cause neck pain alone and referred pain is common. A clinician's role is to determine the most likely pain generator that can be difficult but not impossible (Table 15-1).

HISTORY

In addition to determining pain onset, location, duration, character, aggravating/alleviating factors, radiating features, and timing, a careful determination of recent trauma and mechanism of injury is imperative. Although the majority of patients presenting to primary care physicians with a chief complaint of neck pain will not have a serious condition, it is important to exclude serious causes. Symptoms that may suggest significant pathology include fever, chills, extremity weakness or clumsiness, gait disturbance, and bowel or bladder dysfunction.

A pertinent history of past cancer, unexplained weight loss, and pain lasting more than 1 month are key features suggesting cancer-related cervical spine pain.[3] Immunosuppression, chronic steroid use, and IV drug use are antecedent factors that may predispose a patient to conditions such as osteomyelitis or fractures with associated myelopathy.[4] A diagnosis of vertebral artery dissection should always be considered in a patient with neck pain following relatively minor trauma because it can be life-threatening.[5] In elderly individuals with severe osteoarthritis of the neck, the development of neurologic injury may occur from minor trauma or strenuous lifting—a condition known as cervical spondylotic myelopathy.[6]

TABLE 15-1 Differential Diagnosis of Neck Pain

DIAGNOSIS	PHYSICAL EXAMINATION	WORKUP	TREATMENT	WHEN TO REFER
Cervical strain/ sprain	Decreased cervical range of motion (ROM) Tender to palpation of neck, upper trapezius, and sternocleidomastoid muscles Neurologic examination normal	Imaging or electrodiagnostic examination not indicated unless neurologic impairment If considering X-rays, assess for alignment and fractures	Physical therapy (PT) functional restoration Nonsteroidal anti-inflammatory drugs (NSAIDs) acetaminophen Osteopathic manipulative treatment (OMT) Massage Heat Transcutaneous electrical nerve stimulation (TENS) Soft collar (kinesthetic reminder, limit use to 3 d)	If no improvement after 1-2 mo, consider additional imaging (X-ray, MRI) and referral to pain medicine or physical medicine and rehabilitation
Cervical radicular pain (cervical radiculitis)	Upper limb pain Neurologic examination normal. Special tests: Spurling examination Perform shoulder examination to rule out rotator cuff pathology	X-rays (anterior-posterior and lateral) Flexion and extension X-rays if concern for instability or before prescribing PT rehabilitation MRI-C spine	PT—cervicothoracic stabilization Scapulothoracic kinetic efficiency NSAIDs, acetaminophen Neuropathic drugs (Neurontin, TCA) Muscle relaxants (tizanidine)	If no clinical improvement after conservative management, referral to pain medicine
Cervical radiculopathy	Any combination of neurologic deficits: ↓ sensory, ↓ motor, and/or ↓ reflex	MRI EMG	Activity modification, PT (as above in radiculitis), analgesics	If no improvement or if concern of neurologic compromise, referral to orthopedic or neurosurgery
Cervical zygapophyseal (facet) joint disease (e.g., arthritis)	Pain in distinct pain referral distribution (Dwyer et al.) ↓ ROM	X-ray AP and lateral CT if still concern for fracture or to delineate joint fracture (note: ↑ radiation exposure with this examination, so weigh risks/benefits in pursuing this study)	PT (cervicothoracic stabilization exercises, analgesics, cervical collar)	If no improvement with conservative therapy, refer to pain medicine for diagnostic facet joint blocks (medial branch blocks) Referral to orthopedic or neurosurgery for fractures or concern for neurologic compromise
Cervical spondylolisthesis		X-ray cervical A/P, lateral, flexion, and extension films (assess for instability)		Neurosurgical referral when signs of myelopathy and/or instability
Cervical intervertebral disk disruption	Tenderness to palpation affected cervical region, head, neck, trapezius, and interscapular pain, which is nonradicular Trauma worse with sitting and Valsalva (coughing, sneezing)	X-ray A/P and lateral concomitant spondylosis likely to be present MRI shows ↓ signal on T2-weighted sequence	PT (functional restoration), analgesics	Failure of conservative treatment, then refer to pain medicine for consideration of injection therapies Refer to orthopedic or neurosurgery surgery for severe axial pain discogenic in origin which has failed injection therapy, such as epidural steroid injection Surgeries may include anterior cervical discectomy and fusion or posterior fusion

(Continued)

TABLE 15-1 Differential Diagnosis of Neck Pain (Continued)

DIAGNOSIS	PHYSICAL EXAMINATION	WORKUP	TREATMENT	WHEN TO REFER
Cervical myelopathy (also myeloradiculopathy)	(males > females) Numbness and paresthesia of the distal limbs and extremities Δ in pain/temp sensory testing Lower limb > upper limb involvement Atrophy hand intrinsics +Hoffman and/or Babinski signs	X-ray A/P and lateral (central canal diameter less than 10 mm indicates myelopathy if patient has + physical exam findings) MRI may demonstrate cervical spondylosis, myelomalacia, ↓ CSF flow EMG to establish nerve root injury	PT, occupational therapy (OT) for manual dexterity and activities of daily living (ADLs); cervical orthosis for mild or static symptoms without evidence of gait disturbance	Refer to orthopedic or neurosurgery for severe and progressive symptoms
Cervical stenosis	Spurling may be positive for cervical radicular pain to shoulder and relieved by holding hand overhead. Assess for upper motor signs including Hoffman sign and wrist clonus (which indicate myelopathy). Assess for sensory ataxia due to posterior column dysfunction via Romberg test. Wide-based gait and loss of dexterity may be observed all point to progression due to cervical spondylotic myelopathy	X-ray cervical A/P, lateral, flexion, and extension films Torg-Pavlov ratio (i.e., sagittal diameter of the cervical canal: width of a mid-cervical vertebral body Cervical MRI EMG (in some cases)	Early cervical stenosis with mild-to-moderate cord compression without edema is usually treated nonoperatively • Physical therapy • Serial neurologic examinations every 6 mo to ensure early myelopathic symptoms are not missed	Neurosurgic referral when signs of myelopathy are present, cord compression is severe, or edema is seen on MRI

Assessing demographic information and past diagnoses will aid the management plan. For instance, an elderly, osteoporotic individual with a recent fall may be more likely to suffer a fracture and/or develop cervical myelopathy. A 45-year-old nurse who lifts patients and engages in repetitive computer charting for employment may have a postural disorder leading to cervical strain. This may be accompanied by symptoms of neck pain, soreness, triggered by neck movement in a nondermatomal radiation pattern. If she experiences focal point tenderness and reproduction of pain upon palpation, it may be consistent with myofascial trigger points.[7] These have a fairly consistent distribution (Figure 15-1).

MECHANISM OF INJURY

The mechanism of injury for neck pain can help discern a diagnostic hypothesis. For example, did the painful symptoms appear over time and as a result of poor posture while performing computer work or use of heavy attire? Or did the pain develop after a motor vehicle collision?

These would suggest distinct etiologies including neck strain and cervical zygapophyseal joint (Z-joint)–mediated pain, respectively.

Establishing the sequence and time course of each of the symptoms will lead to more accurate assessment. For

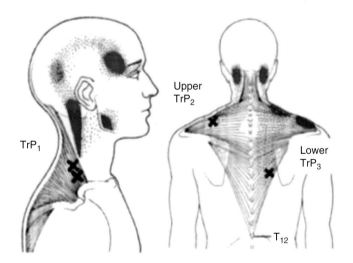

FIGURE 15-1 Example of a trigger point referral pattern of the upper trapezius muscles.[8]

example, acute pain from sharply turning one's head may result in an acute cervical strain. This is common because cervical muscles attach to bone through myofascial tissue. On the other hand, a rear-end collision with resulting whiplash injury may lead to chronic, painful symptoms from biomechanical stress on cervical Z-joints. This is a leading source of chronic neck pain with a consistent distribution (Figure 15-2). Z-joints are also known as facet joints.

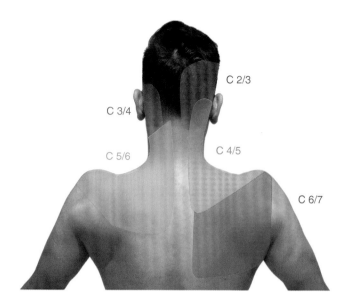

FIGURE 15-2 Cervical facet joint—pain referral patterns.

LOCATION

Pain that originates from the upper cervical spine may travel into regions of the head resulting in cervicogenic headache. An explanation for the considerable overlap between the head and neck is a result of convergence. In this process, pain afferent (A-delta and C) nerve fibers from tissues converge onto the same spinal neuron, thereby referring pain in a segmentally shared distribution. For instance, cervical afferents and trigeminal afferents may converge in the dorsal horn of C1-C3 segments of the spinal cord leading to symptoms of pain around the temples or the eyes, which originate from the upper cervical spine. The convergence of cervical afferents and the C2 spinal segment may cause episodes of lancinating pain in the occipital region radiating to the frontal and temporal areas.[2]

Characteristic features of myofascial pain due to trigger points of the cervical and periscapular region are relatively distinct. The key features that distinguish this from Z-joint–mediated pain include focal point tenderness, reproduction of pain upon palpation, hardening of the muscle upon palpation, pseudoweakness of involved muscle, and referred pain. Cervical discogenic pain may cause referral of pain into the neck, occiput, face, shoulder, interscapular region, and upper limb.[9] Three types of disk disease include (1) disk degeneration, (2) internal disk disruption, and (3) disk herniation.

In disk degeneration, there may be a disk bulge present where 50% of the disk is exposed over the surface of the vertebral body. The disk is thinner with less water content, and it is usually accompanied by degenerative zygapophyseal (facet) and Luschka joints. Disk degeneration is commonly seen in asymptomatic individuals.

In cervical internal disk disruption the internal architecture of the disk is disrupted although exterior surface is normal without bulge or herniation. A degrading nucleus with radial fissures may extend to the outer

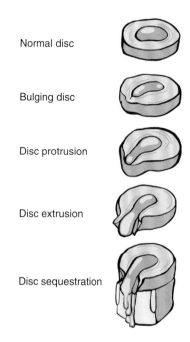

FIGURE 15-3 Cervical disc pathology.

third of the annulus, which can be painful.[2,4] This too is accompanied by arthritis of zygapophyseal (facet) and Luschka joints.

Disk herniation occurs when less than 50% of the disk is exposed beyond the surface of the vertebrae. The narrower diameter of the portion of the disk jutting past the vertebrae may be contained (extruded) or uncontained (sequestered) by annular fibers (see herniation types Figure 15-3). Herniation may lead to ipsilateral pain, whereas disk degeneration may not. Interestingly, these conditions do not follow a dermatomal distribution.

Similarly, cervical radicular pain is not necessarily dermatomal. Radicular pain is perceived deeply through the shoulder girdle and into the upper limb. Cervical radicular pain from the C5 nerve root tends to remain in the arm, but pain from C6, C7, and C8 nerve roots extends into the forearm and hand.[2]

Cervical radicular pain (cervical radiculitis) occurs when compression or compromise of the dorsal root ganglion with a shooting, stabbing electrical quality traveling distally into the affected limb is experienced. This occurs because afferent (sensory) fibers including Ab fibers and C fibers are disturbed. Ab fiber discharge is consistent with numbness and tingling pain. C fibers pain may be characterized as dull, deeper, second pain.[2,9]

In contrast, cervical radiculopathy is characterized by objective signs of loss of neurologic function with some combination of sensory or motor loss or depressed reflexes. *Cervical radiculopathy occurs in a dermatomal or myotomal distribution* (see Figure 15-4). The reason for this is compression or compromise to a cervical spine nerve or its roots. These structures do not elicit pain.

In cervical radiculopathy, symptoms are mainly sensory with neck or radicular pain (98%), paresthesias (90%), radicular pain (66%), and weakness (15%).[9] In the cervical spine, confirmed disk protrusion was responsible

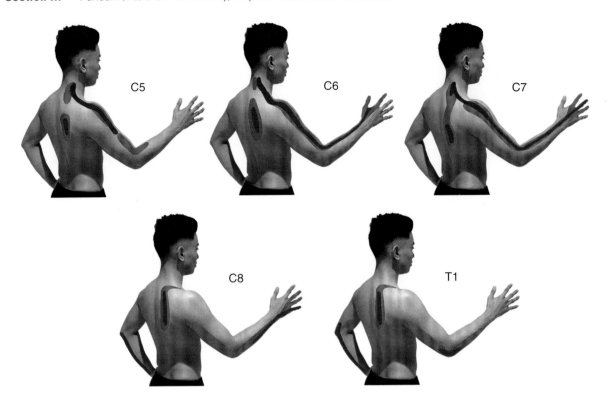

FIGURE 15-4 Cervical radicular pain distribution based on cervical root level.

for cervical radiculopathy in 22 % of patients, whereas 68% were related to spondylosis, disk, or both.[3,4,9,10] One should consider the cause of radiculopathy as disk herniation for patients 50 years or younger or osteophyte spurring for those 50 years or older.[3,4,9]

ALLEVIATING AND EXACERBATING FACTORS

When considering disorders of the cervical spine that result in shoulder pain, certain activities can make pain better or worse. In the case of cervical spondylosis (also known as zygapophyseal or facet joint arthritis), axial neck and posterior shoulder pain is exacerbated with cervical extension. In contrast, cervical radicular pain may worsen with cervical rotation and lateral bending toward the symptomatic side owing to narrowing of the intervertebral foramen where the affected nerve root exits. Cervical radicular pain may improve with lifting the affected limb overhead and placing the ipsilateral hand behind the head.

Dull, head and neck pain alleviated by exercise yet not fully improved with physical therapy or analgesics may suggest cervicogenic headache. Key exacerbating factors include rotation of the head and use of heavy clothing/equipment at work such as a utility vest or backpack. In contrast, dull, neck and *shoulder* pain relieved only temporarily with analgesics and made worse with neck extension and rotation suggests cervical Z-joint–mediated pain.

Ipsilateral shoulder or arm pain alleviated by lifting over the head yet worsening when dropped alongside of the body gives clues to a diagnosis of cervical radicular pain. Reproduction of shoulder or arm pain with turning the head toward the affected side while extending the neck also provokes cervical radicular pain on physical examination (this is known as Spurling manuever).

NEUROLOGIC SYMPTOMS

C5-8 cervical nerve roots are most commonly involved in compressive radiculopathies. C7 is involved around 50% of the time, and C6 is involved about 25% of the time.[10] Only a few patients describe trauma or physical exertion preceding their pain.

Localizing the lesion is important, and reflex testing will help distinguish between an upper motor neuron (UMN) lesion versus a lower motor neuron (LMN) lesion. Reflexes are decreased with LMN lesions such as cervical radiculopathy and increased with UMN lesions such as stroke (a brain lesion) or cervical myelopathy (a spinal cord lesion). Other pathological signs in *upper motor neuron* lesions include Hoffman sign, wrist clonus, and Lhermitte sign (an electric shock–like sensation that radiates down the spine and occurs with neck flexion). Reflexes may not change in the face of a lesion because of multiple root innervations for each reflex. They can also be influenced by metabolic changes, electrolyte abnormalities, and anxiety level. It is important therefore to check multiple reflexes and compare both sides.

This can be accomplished efficiently and thoroughly with an understanding of cervicothoracic dermatomes, myotomes, and reflexes. A sufficient examination for screening strength would include an assessment of elbow flexion (C5), wrist extension (C6), elbow extension (C7), finger flexion (C8), and finger abductors (T1). A screening sensory examination should include the C5-T1 dermatomes (Figure 15-4). Reflex examination should include biceps (primarily C5), brachioradialis (C6), and triceps (C7) with particular attention to asymmetry from side to side. Additionally, an assessment for UMN signs is imperative.

ASSOCIATED SYMPTOMS

Onset of symptoms of cervical myelopathy is often insidious and gradual with years going by before the patient seeks medical attention.[11] However, patients can present with sudden or episodic worsening usually associated with abrupt hyperextension trauma. Cervical spinal stenosis may result from degenerative osteoarthritis of the spine. If symptoms are mild at onset, the clinical course most commonly remains dormant. Occasionally, a steady progression of symptoms occurs.[12,13]

Symptoms are variable and may include[4,14]:

- Significant pain in the neck, shoulders, or arms (although not present in most patients)
- Gait spasticity
- Upper extremity numbness

Many spinal cord tumors present with pain. Extramedullary and extradural spinal cord tumors can cause severe local pain and tenderness. Pain and muscle weakness follow patterns according to root distribution. Horner syndrome may occur with lesions at the cervicothoracic junction (C8) as a result of automatic nervous system dysfunction. Horner syndrome includes ptosis of the eyelid with pupillary constriction (miosis) and anhydrosis on the affected side. This can occur unilaterally or bilaterally. Pancoast tumors affecting the apex of the lung may present with Horner syndrome.

Intramedullary tumors include intradural lesions, which arise within the substance of the tracts and central gray matter. These may affect the spinothalamic tract affecting the ascending pain and temperature pathway. Syringomyelia may involve the enlargement of a fluid-filled cyst (syrinx) within the spinal cord over time, which may damage the spinal cord causing pain originating at the site of injury, weakness, and stiffness. Early signs and symptoms of syringomyelia may affect the back of the neck, shoulders, arms, and hands first (sensory impairment in a "cape distribution"). Key findings include muscle weakness, atrophy, loss of reflexes, and decreased pain and temperature below the extent of the lesion (Table 15-2).

DIAGNOSTIC STUDIES AND THERAPEUTIC INTERVENTIONS

Whenever possible, it is helpful to evaluate a patient's prior diagnostic and therapeutic interventions. Such information provides you with past diagnoses and therapeutic failures to guide future approaches to treatment. For instance, prior X-ray, magnetic resonance imaging (MRI), and electrodiagnostic studies may help narrow your working diagnosis and restructure your treatment plan. It is important to note that the incidental abnormalities on imaging may be asymptomatic.[15] Therefore, it is important to correlate the history and physical examination with the imaging findings to provide appropriate individualized treatment.

Prior treatments may include medications (oral and topical), physical therapy, procedures, surgeries, and other treatments such as manipulation, massage therapy, and acupuncture. If a particular treatment was not effective, it is essential to know what the treatment consisted of, its frequency, course, and duration before determining whether it was a failure. For instance, a topical anti-inflammatory medication may have been deemed a "failure" when it was only used once.

TABLE 15-2 Cervical Root Level Pathology, Accompanying Pain Referral Pattern, and Neurologic Impairment

ROOT	PAIN	NUMBNESS	WEAKNESS	REFLEX AFFECTED
C5	Neck, shoulder, scapula	Lateral arm (in distribution of axillary nerve)	Shoulder abduction, external rotation, elbow flexion, forearm supination	Biceps, brachioradialis
C6	Neck, shoulder, scapula, lateral arm, lateral forearm, lateral hand	Lateral forearm, thumb, and index finger	Shoulder abduction, external rotation, elbow flexion, forearm supination, and pronation	Biceps, brachioradialis
C7	Neck, shoulder, middle finger, hand	Index and middle finger, palm	Elbow and wrist extension (radial), forearm pronation, wrist flexion	Triceps
C8	Neck, shoulder, medial forearm, fourth and fifth digits, medial hand	Medial forearm, medial hand, fourth and fifth digits	Finger extension, wrist extension (ulnar), distal finger flexion, extension, abduction and adduction, distal thumb flexion	None
T1	Neck, medial arm, and forearm	Anterior arm and medial forearm	Thumb abduction, distal thumb flexion, finger abduction and adduction	None

TABLE 15-3 Indications for Cervical X-Ray

- Trauma
- Presence of any red flags indicating possible fracture, infection, or malignancy
- Clinical suspicion of ankylosing spondylitis, rheumatoid arthritis
- Suspicion of spinal deformity
- Suspicion of instability (include flexion/extension views)
- Unusual presentation

TABLE 15-4 These are Common Clinical Indications for Obtaining a Cervical MRI

- Suspected metastasis, tumor, osteomyelitis, discitis, or paraspinal abscess
- Congenital/traumatic spinal deformities
- Severe pain
- Progressively severe symptoms or neurologic dysfunction
- Myelopathy
- Radicular pain >7 wk
- Suspected vascular malformation
- Compression fracture in the elderly

Because most neck pain will resolve with time, it is not always recommended to obtain imaging in the first 6 weeks unless clinical suspicion is high, and red flags are evident for signs and symptoms of infection, malignancy, or progressive neurologic deficits.

Plain X-ray films are used to assess degenerative changes, alignment, compression, and other fractures (Table 15-3). Dynamic flexion and extension X-ray assessments help evaluate spinal instability.

In diagnostic myelography, a contrast dye is injected into the spinal canal, and X-ray films are then obtained. A "silhouette" of the spinal cord as well as nerve roots is observed because the dye spreads into the cervical spinal fluid (CSF) and subarachnoid space surrounding spinal cord and nerve roots. This provides the ability to assess central canal narrowing, foraminal narrowing, and/or nerve root pathology due to masses (e.g., nerve root–associated tumors or arachnoiditis). Such conditions are seen better with myelography in comparison with plain X-ray films alone. However, abnormalities *within* the spinal cord as well as *within* the nerve roots *cannot* be seen.

Computed tomography (CT) is the same basic technology as plain X-ray films except that a rotating X-ray source is present with a rotating detector "array." It has multiple detectors as opposed to a single detector, which is utilized in plain X-ray films. This diagnostic procedure exposes patients to more ionizing radiation. In spine imaging, CT scan allows you to see the bony structures including the neural foramen and central canal. Additionally, one can see soft tissues better than when using plain films but not as good as MRI. CT scans are used to assess degenerative changes such as osteophytes, fracture, and malalignment. However, CT cannot effectively evaluate the spinal cord or the nerve roots.

CT myelography is essentially very similar to plain film with myelography in the sense that one can see the outline of the spinal cord and the nerve roots after injection of contrast dye in the subarachnoid space. One can examine more with CT than with plain film because the anatomic details are better with 2-dimensional (2-D) and 3-dimensional (3-D) imaging. However, when a contrast dye is injected into the subarachnoid space, it surrounds the spinal cord and nerve roots, thereby illustrating the contour of the structures and allowing for evaluation of compression or mass lesions with one of the nerve roots in multiple dimensions. Therefore, CT myelography is used to assess spinal cord compression or nerve root pathology due to masses and arachnoiditis and is an alternative or an adjunct to MRI.

MRI is completely different from plain film and CT. It does not involve ionizing radiation. One can visualize soft tissues extremely well in MRI including the spinal cord, nerve roots, paraspinal soft tissues, and intervertebral disks and joints. However, bone is poorly visualized in MRI compared to CT, although it is still possible to identify marrow abnormalities. MRI is best used to assess degenerative pathology including spinal cord or nerve root compression and for the assessment of patients who experience trauma or soft tissue injuries, infection, and neoplasm.

MRI can be limited by hardware, for example, in a spinal fusion containing plates, rods, and screws. These can cause artifacts that impair the ability to detect pathology. To reduce the artifacts, request the radiologist to complete nongradient sequences. This change will improve visualization of structures in the MRI study. It is important to appreciate that while not perfect, it will enhance the study when hardware is present (Table 15-4).

Electromyography (EMG) and nerve conduction studies (NCS) help to identify abnormalities of peripheral nerve, muscle, and neuromuscular junction (NMJ) function. They can provide information on location of pathology, chronicity, and severity. EMG and NCS also help determine the progression of abnormalities or recovery from abnormal function. Note that contraindication to this examination includes INR >3 or pacemakers (relative). The test is also operator dependent and may be limited by patient tolerance of the examination.

CONCLUSION

The cervical spine is slender and flexible but strong enough to support the weight of the head. It is vulnerable to injury because it must secure the mass of the head at its apex.[15] Neck pain may be associated with neurologic injury and therefore a careful review of history and physical examination assessment must exclude this and other red flags. Neck pain can usually be alleviated with rest and ice and physical therapy. Sometimes, medications or injection therapies may be needed. Some cases may require surgical intervention particularly if there are signs and symptoms of neurologic deterioration.

REFERENCES

1. Statistics, N.C.f.H. *Special Feature: Pain. Chartbook on Trends in the Health of Americans*; 2006.

2. Bogduk N. The anatomy and pathophysiology of neck pain. *Phys Med Rehabil Clin N Am.* 2003;14(3):455-472.

3. Magee DJ. *Orthopedic Physical Assessment.* 4th ed. Philadelphia, PA: W.B. Saunders; 2002.

4. Braddom RL. *Physical Medicine & Rehabilitation.* Philadelphia: Saunders; 1996.1301 p.

5. Dziewas R, Konrad C, Dräger B, et al. Cervical artery dissection–clinical features, risk factors, therapy and outcome in 126 patients. *J Neurol.* 2003;250(10):1179-1184.

6. Klineberg E. Cervical spondylotic myelopathy: a review of the evidence. *Orthop Clin North Am.* 2010;41(2):193-202.

7. Bennett R. Myofascial pain syndromes and their evaluation. *Best Pract Res Clin Rheumatol.* 2007;21(3):427-445.

8. David G, Simons DG, Travell JG, Simons LS, Cummings BD. *Myofascial Pain and Dysfunction: The Trigger Point Manual, Vol. 1-Upper Half of Body.* 2nd ed. Lippincott Williams & Wilkins; November 1, 1998.

9. Radhakrishnan K, Litchy WJ, O'Fallon WM, Kurland LT. Epidemiology of cervical radiculopathy. A population-based study from Rochester, Minnesota, 1976 through 1990. *Brain.* 1994;117(Pt 2):325-335.

10. Levin KH, Covington EC, Devereaux MW. Neck and low back pain. *Continuum.* 2001;7:7-43.

11. McCormick WE, Steinmetz MP, Benzel EC. Cervical spondylotic myelopathy: make the difficult diagnosis, then refer for surgery. *Cleve Clin J Med.* 2003;70(10):899-904.

12. Kadanka Z, Mares M, Bednarík J, et al. Predictive factors for spondylotic cervical myelopathy treated conservatively or surgically. *Eur J Neurol.* 2005;12(1):55-63.

13. Kadanka Z, Mares M, Bednarík J, et al. Predictive factors for mild forms of spondylotic cervical myelopathy treated conservatively or surgically. *Eur J Neurol.* 2005;12(1):16-24.

14. Lunsford LD, Bissonette DJ, Zorub DS. Anterior surgery for cervical disc disease. Part 2: treatment of cervical spondylotic myelopathy in 32 cases. *J Neurosurg.* 1980;53(1):12-19.

15. Bogduk N. Functional anatomy of the spine. *Handb Clin Neurol.* 2016;136:675-688.

16. Hooten WM, Cohen SP, Rathmell JP. Introduction to the symposium on pain medicine. *Mayo Clin Proc.* 2015;90(1):4-5.

16

SHOULDER PAIN

Charles De Mesa, DO, MPH, Brian A. Davis, MD, FACSM
and Misty Humphries, MD, MAS, RPVI, FACS

FAST FACTS

- Shoulder pain usually arises from the shoulder joint itself and can be due to bursitis, tendinopathy or tear, instability arthritis, or fractures.
- It can be due to referred pain from the neck, thorax, or abdomen.
- Shoulder pain may be divided into four categories: musculoskeletal, neurologic, vascular, and referred visceral-somatic pain.
- A systematic approach is essential for effective management of shoulder pain.

INTRODUCTION

Shoulder pain is the third most common pain complaint in the primary care setting and accounts for approximately 16% of all musculoskeletal complaints.[1] The shoulder is a complex structure. Therefore, it is important to define the shoulder by region to better identify the location of perceived pain, as it may originate from somewhere else. This chapter will identify shoulder girdle pain as the perception of pain located within the bones which connects the arm to the axial skeleton on each side, namely, the clavicle, scapula, humerus and the joints, tendons ligaments, muscles, subcutaneous tissue, and skin subserving this location. Shoulder pain may be divided into four categories: musculoskeletal, neurologic, vascular, and referred visceral–somatic pain (see Tables 16-1 to 16-4).[2]

In contrast, the "neck pain chapter" will identify neck pain as the region bounded superiorly by the superior nuchal line, laterally by the lateral margins of the neck, and inferiorly by an imaginary transverse line through the T1 spinous process.[3]

HISTORY

Physicians make a correct diagnosis about 80% of the time based on history and physical examination alone.[4] The pain history requires a detailed interview which includes the chief complaint, mechanism of injury, accompanying symptoms, prior treatments, and impact on function and quality of life. The character, quality, and location of the pain including perceived level of pain are also important. Ways of conveying this information may include a numeric rating pain score with 0 being no pain and 10 being the worst possible pain. Ascertaining the pain score for current pain, average pain for the last week, lowest and worst pain in the last 24 hours allow for characterization of the pain leading up to the office visit. A pain diagram illustrating the location is useful in communicating the pattern of pain and for interval assessment following treatment.

MECHANISM OF INJURY

Acute versus chronic injuries are important considerations in the assessment of shoulder pain (Table 16-5). Trauma from a motor vehicle collision or accidental fall may imply acute pain while overuse or repetitive activities are indicative of chronic microtrauma leading to pain. It is important to identify the acute presentation of neuropathic pain as a result of trauma. For example, falls in the elderly may result in cervical extension injury leading to shoulder pain referred from the neck.

TABLE 16-1 Musculoskeletal Shoulder Pain[1-22]

DIAGNOSIS	PHYSICAL EXAMINATION	WORK-UP	TREATMENT	WHEN TO REFER
Rotator cuff tendinitis (RCT) with or without calcification	Shoulder external rotation (ER) usually weaker than internal rotation (IR) Hawkins–Kennedy test, the infraspinatus muscle test, and the painful arc sign Cervical spine examination to rule out spine pathology	X-rays (anterior–posterior [AP], axillary, and supraspinatus outlet) assess for alignment and degenerative changes Ultrasound (dynamic study to assess injury although operator dependent) MRI (magnetic resonance image) shoulder MR (magnetic resonance) arthrogram for clinical suspicion of a full thickness rotator cuff and/or a labral tear or postoperative complications	Activity modification, physical therapy (PT), analgesics, subacromial corticosteroid injection For calcifications: • ultrasound-guided percutaneous lavage (UGPL) • extracorporeal shock wave therapy	If refractory rotator cuff tendinitis with calcification, refer to physical medicine and rehabiliation, sports, or pain medicine for UGPL
RCT, partial	Shoulder ER usually weaker than IR Special tests: External rotation lag sign (ERLS), the dropping sign, the hornblower's sign, and the internal rotation lag sign (IRLS) Cervical spine examination to rule out spine pathology	X-rays (AP, axillary, and supraspinatus outlet) assess for alignment and degenerative changes Ultrasound (dynamic although operator dependent) MRI shoulder MR arthrogram for clinical suspicion of a full thickness RCT and/or a labral tear or postoperative complications.	Activity modification, PT, analgesics, subacromial corticosteroid injection	No improvement after 3-6 mo of therapy, surgical consultation
RCT, complete	Shoulder ER usually weaker than IR Special tests: External rotation lag sign, the dropping sign, the hornblower's sign, and IRLS Cervical spine examination to rule out spine pathology	X-ray Ultrasound MR arthrogram for clinical suspicion of a full thickness RCT and/or a labral tear or postoperative complications	Activity modification, PT, analgesics, surgery, (subacromial corticosteroid injection)	Acute, full thickness, with minimal amount of fatty infiltration—orthopedic surgical referral
Acromioclavicular (AC) joint arthritis	Painful palpation at AC joint Special tests: Horizontal cross arm adduction test localizes pain over the AC joint	X-ray AP and lateral Note: acromion morphology: • Flat • Curved • Hooked AC joint morphology: • Flat • Curved • Horizontal Hooked acromion and horizontal AC joints may have risk of developing localized impingement symptoms requiring surgery	PT, analgesics, acromioclavicular joint corticosteroid injection	If no improvement after 3-6 mo of therapy, analgesics and corticosteroid injection, then referral to orthopedic surgery for excision of the isolated painful joint or localized impingement region affecting functional quality of life

(Continued)

TABLE 16-1 Musculoskeletal Shoulder Pain[1-22]   (Continued)

DIAGNOSIS	PHYSICAL EXAMINATION	WORK-UP	TREATMENT	WHEN TO REFER
Glenohumeral arthritis	• Local glenohumeral joint line tenderness and swelling anteriorly • Reduced range of motion (ROM), external rotation, and abduction • Atrophy of the rotator cuff muscles over the scapula • Crepitation	X-ray AP and lateral external rotation, Y-outlet, and axillary views	PT, nonsteroidal anti-inflammatory drugs (NSAIDs), and occasionally intra-articular injection	Failure of conservative treatment, continued impairment in shoulder function affecting daily activities and associated with intractable pain should be referred to orthopedic surgery for prosthetic replacement (except in patients younger than 50 y in whom arthroscopic debridement and removal of osteophytes might be attempted to delay the need for prosthetic replacement)
Adhesive capsulitis	Stiffness, decreased ROM ER and abduction	X-ray (rule out other diagnoses) Ultrasound evaluation to rule out rotator cuff pathology MR arthrogram axillary recess may show thickening ≥1.3 cm	PT, occupational therapy (OT), gentle ROM exercises (e.g., pendulum swings) provided they do not cause undue discomfort As pain allows, patients can add stretching and strengthening exercises Intra-articular corticosteroid injection Ultrasound-guided intra-articular dilation (distension)	Refer to sports or pain medicine for intra-articular dilation For refractory adhesive capsulitis affecting function and quality of life, referral for arthroscopic surgical release (e.g. bipolar radiofrequency controlled capsular release)
Bicipital tenosynovitis	Painful palpation to the proximal aspect of the long head of the biceps (LHB), pain with activities that require eccentric deceleration of the upper extremity (such as throwing or swinging an object), and pain with muscular loading of the biceps (especially during shoulder flexion and arm supination)	X-ray (rules out fractures/dislocations) Ultrasound (dynamic diagnostic evaluation can exclude subluxation) MRI evaluation of the superior labral complex and biceps tendon	Analgesia with NSAIDs, acetaminophen (to avoid side effects from NSAIDs), ice, rest from overhead activity, or physical therapy. Biceps tendon sheath corticosteroid injection and/or needle tenotomy	Physical Medicine and Rehabilitation, sports referral for ultrasound-guided injections Orthopedic referral if no improvement after conservative measures for consideration of surgical debridement, tenodesis, or tenotomy

Biceps tendon tear	Tenderness with palpation over biceps groove worse with arm internally rotated 10 degrees "Popeye" deformity indicates rupture	• Ultrasound: can show thickened tendon within bicipital groove
		• MRI: can demonstrate thickening and tenosynovitis of proximal biceps tendon increased T2 signal around biceps tendon
			• Nonoperative
			  • NSAIDS
			  • PT
			  • steroid tendon sheath injections
			• Operative
			  • arthroscopic tenodesis
			  • tenotomy
				Referral for orthopedic surgery if no improvement after conservative therapy for evaluation of surgical debridement, tenodesis, or tenotomy

External impingement (with accompanying subacromial bursitis)	Shoulder ER usually weaker than IR. Hawkins–Kennedy test, the infraspinatus muscle test, and the painful arc sign Cervical spine examination to rule out spine pathology.	X-ray orthogonal views Ultrasound MRI shoulder	Activity modification, PT, and analgesic medications. Subacromial corticosteroid injection	Orthopedic surgical referral if no improvement after 3-6 mo of nonsurgical management

TABLE 16-1 Musculoskeletal Shoulder Pain[1-22] (Continued)

DIAGNOSIS	PHYSICAL EXAMINATION	WORK-UP	TREATMENT	WHEN TO REFER
Internal impingement	Shoulder IR usually weaker than ER Muscular asymmetry with deep posterior pain with 90°-110° of abduction, slight extension, and maximal external rotation with scapula stabilized	X-ray orthogonal views Ultrasound MRI arthrogram to evaluate damage to the labrum or to assess capsular laxity and in those with prior surgery	Activity modification, PT and analgesic medications. Subacromial corticosteroid injection	Orthopedic surgical referral if no improvement after 3-6 mo of nonsurgical management
Proximal humerus fracture (PHF)	Inspection: ecchymosis of chest, arm, and forearm neurovascular examination: 45% incidence of nerve injury (axillary most common)	X-ray complete trauma series • true AP • scapular Y • axillary CT scan to characterize injury and for preoperative planning	Majority of nondisplaced fractures are Neer one-part fractures. PHFs are considered nondisplaced if no segment is displaced more than 1 cm or angulated more than 45°	For complex fractures with significant displacement and/or if nerve injury is suspected, a surgical referral is indicated
Glenohumeral instability or dislocation	Shoulder IR usually weaker than ER Special attention to muscle tone, symmetry, and deformity. Passive ROM no more than 90° in any direction (risks redislocating) Apprehension and anterior release tests	X-ray shoulder, AP (external rotation), and scapula, lateral (Y view) MRI shoulder (if weakness persists after 4 wk of PT)	Pre- and postreduction X-rays to assess for humeral head location. Pre and post neurovascular examination. Sling immobilization following reduction (avoid NSAIDS may impair bony healing) PT/OT first 1-2 wk after dislocation, gentle ROM to minimize capsular contraction Reevaluation at 2 and 4 wk. If weakness persists at 4-wk, consider advanced imaging Restrictions for the first 4-6 wk include no abduction and ER at 90° to prevent redislocation Scapular strengthening introduced at 6-wk; continue strengthening dynamic/static stabilizers	Refer to surgery under following circumstances: >50% rotator cuff tear, glenoid osseous defect >25%, humeral head articular surface osseous defect >25%, PHF requiring surgery, irreducible dislocation, failed trial of rehabilitation, inability to tolerate shoulder restrictions, and inability to perform sport-specific drills without instability
Acromioclavicular separation	AC joint "step-off" on observation	X-ray AP bilateral for comparison and lateral additional projections include zanca view	Sling, cold packs, and medications can often help manage the pain.	Orthopedic surgical referral indicated for grade 3 Rockwood classification (AC and coracoclavicular [CC] ligaments are torn) with the CC distance is 25%-100% of the other side

(Continued)

TABLE 16-1 Musculoskeletal Shoulder Pain[1-22]   (Continued)

DIAGNOSIS	PHYSICAL EXAMINATION	WORK-UP	TREATMENT	WHEN TO REFER
Rheumatoid arthritis	Local glenohumeral joint line tenderness and swelling, atrophy, accompanying Metacarpophalangeal and proximal interphalangeal joint arthritis	Laboratory tests: • erythrocyte sedimentation rate (ESR) • C-reactive protein (CRP) • rheumatoid factor (RF) • anti–cyclic citrullinated peptide (CCP) antibodies • antinuclear antibodies (ANA) Arthrocentesis: if there is diagnostic uncertainty	DMARD (e.g., methotrexate), NSAIDs, or glucocorticoids	Rheumatology referral to start DMARD therapy, prevent progressive joint injury and associated functional decline
Infectious (septic) arthritis	Monoarticular joint pain, swelling, warmth, and restricted movement	Synovial fluid aspiration performed (prior to administration of antibiotics); fluid should be sent for Gram stain and culture, leukocyte count with differential, and assessment for crystals.	Antimicrobial regimen based on coverage of the most likely organisms to cause infection More than 80% of septic arthritis cases are caused by *S. aureus* and other gram-positive organisms	Refer to infectious disease if poor response to therapy, coexistent renal or cardiac disease, and immunosuppression Surgical referral for refractory antibiotic treatment
Myofascial pain	Hyperirritable nodules within taut skeletal muscle bands when palpated produce a muscle twitch and reproduction of the patient's *referred* pain	Laboratory tests: • complete blood count (CBC), urinalysis • renal and liver function, serum calcium, albumin, phosphate, TSH, CK, 25-hydroxyvitamin D Not routinely ordered but maybe helpful for myalgia.	Trigger point injections or dry needling (dry needling uses an acupuncture needle without introducing an injectate).	Consider referral to rheumatology if suspected polymyalgia rheumatica Consider physical medicine and rehabilitation referral for ongoing management

TABLE 16-2 Neurologic Shoulder Pain[1-15,19]

DIAGNOSIS	PHYSICAL EXAMINATION	WORK-UP	TREATMENT	WHEN TO REFER
Neurogenic thoracic outlet syndrome (nTOS) Anterior scalene syndrome	Tenderness over the scalene muscles above the clavicle	Scalene muscle blocks; electromyography nerve conduction studies (EMG/NCS): measurement of sensory medial antebrachial cutaneous nerves, C8 nerve conduction velocity	Thoracic outlet—protocol-specific PT. First rib resection with or without scalenectomy	Refer to pain medicine for muscle block
Claviculocostal syndrome	Tenderness along the clavicle and first rib	EMG/NCS	Thoracic outlet—protocol-specific PT. First rib resection with or without scalenectomy	Refer to pain medicine for muscle block
Pectoralis minor syndrome	Tenderness PMMs and axilla below the clavicle.	Pectoralis minor block EMG/NCS	Thoracic outlet—protocol-specific PT. Pectoralis minor tenotomy in combination with thoracic outlet decompression	Refer to pain medicine for muscle block

TABLE 16-2 Neurologic Shoulder Pain[1-15,19]   (Continued)

DIAGNOSIS	PHYSICAL EXAMINATION	WORK-UP	TREATMENT	WHEN TO REFER
Traction injury	Muscle weakness and sensory changes of affected parts of the brachial plexus (upper trunk cannot lift arm vs. lower trunk cannot move hand) Muscle weakness predominates in neuropraxic lesions, obstetric and backpack palsies, posterior and anterior root avulsions Sensory symptoms predominate in neoplastic or radiation-induced plexopathies and neurogenic TOS	X-ray orthogonal views MRI brachial plexus EMG/NCS	Nonsurgical • Short duration immobilization at onset • Bracing/compression garment • Medications • Transcutaneous nerve stimulation (TENS) • Acupuncture • Nerve blocks • Therapy, ROM, home exercises Surgical • Neurolysis and grafting: usually performed for less than antigravity strength with plateau in recovery before age 12 mos. (avoids denervation atrophy) • Nerve transfers: staged intervention to add nerve supply • Muscle/tendon transfers: release IR/adductors at shoulder; augment ER by changing insertion • Capsulodesis for subluxation • Derotational osteotomy	Refer to neurology and/or physical medicine and rehabilitation and surgery
Penetrating injury	Muscle weakness and sensory changes of injured parts of the brachial plexus	X-ray MRI brachial plexus EMG/NCS	Nerve transfers • Muscle/tendon transfers Capsulodesis to address subluxation	Refer to surgery if limited recovery of functional strength and nerve injury

Brachial plexitis	Sudden, abrupt, unilateral shoulder pain, ↑ severity and intensity
	Acute pain replaced with weakness, reflex changes, and sensory abnormalities
	Antecedent influence
	
	• Surgical
	• Infectious
	• Traumatic
	• Therapeutic
	   • vaccinations
	   • antibiotic treatments
	   • postsurgical
		X-ray
		MRI brachial plexus
		EMG/NCS
			Opioid/nonsteroidal anti-inflammatory drug (NSAID)/steroids/neurontin
			OT for ROM and strengthening
				Functional recovery is usually good in most cases
				
				~80% by 2 y
				
				~90% by 3 y
				
				Refer to surgery if limited recovery of functional strength and/or EMG findings of no reinnervation

Pancoast tumor	Pain (in the distribution of the C8, T1, and T2 dermatomes), Horner syndrome, weakness and atrophy of the muscles of the hand	X-ray chest CT/MRI chest PET scanning is necessary for preoperative evaluation of mediastinal lymph nodes as well as distant metastases Core needle biopsy of superior sulcus tumor	Induction chemoradiotherapy plus surgery for tumors without distant or mediastinal metastases. Definitive chemoradiotherapy for medically inoperable or who have locally advanced, unresectable disease Thoracic radiotherapy for distant metastatic disease or a poor performance status Systemic chemotherapy for locally advanced or metastatic disease	Oncology and thoracic surgery

(Continued)

TABLE 16-2 Neurologic Shoulder Pain[1-15,19]   (Continued)

DIAGNOSIS	PHYSICAL EXAMINATION	WORK-UP	TREATMENT	WHEN TO REFER
Poststroke hemiplegic shoulder pain	Shoulder subluxation, limited active and passive ROM with atrophy of rotator cuff muscles and deltoid. Spasticity and hyperreflexia of affected shoulder	X-ray shoulder Ultrasound	Occupational therapy (OT) for preventative measures, restoration of ROM and degree of function, compensatory strategies. Oral medications or botulinum toxin injections to reduce arm spasticity. Nerve blocks and corticosteroid injections to relieve pain. Communication with the occupational therapist plays an important role in reporting efficacy, and alignment of treatment is imperative	Physical medicine and rehabilitation for spasticity management Pain medicine referral for refractory pain or short term peripheral nerve stimulation (PNS) therapy

TABLE 16-3 Vascular

DIAGNOSIS	PHYSICAL EXAMINATION	WORK-UP	TREATMENT	WHEN TO REFER
Arterial thoracic outlet syndrome	Cold, discolored painful hand with upper limb paresthesia and ischemic changes. Diminished pulses and reduced blood pressure	Radiography can be useful for identifying bony abnormalities (cervical ribs, elongated transverse process of C7), CT/MRI angiograms for arterial compression, MRI for brachial plexus analysis, and ultrasound as an adjunctive tool for detection of anatomic vessel abnormalities and pulse volume recording	First rib resection with or without scalenectomy	Vascular surgery based on work-up and clinical correlation
Venous thoracic outlet syndrome	Swelling, discoloration, pain, and paresthesia of the arm with venous engorgement	X-ray cervical spine CT/MRI angiogram Ultrasound as adjunctive to detect anatomic vessel abnormalities and vascular flow	Clot dissolution First rib resection and venolysis Venogram and balloon angioplasty (if necessary) Open angioplasty and venous reconstruction is rare	Vascular surgery based on work-up and clinical correlation.

From Sanders RJ, Annest SJ. Thoracic outlet and pectoralis minor syndromes. Semin Vasc Surg. 2014;27(2):86-117.

TABLE 16-4 Referred Visceral–Somatic Pain[1-20]

DIAGNOSIS	PHYSICAL EXAMINATION	WORK-UP	TREATMENT	WHEN TO REFER
Cardiac angina pain	Radiates to other parts of the body, including the upper abdomen (epigastric), shoulders, arms (upper and forearm), wrist, fingers, neck and throat, lower jaw, and teeth (but not upper jaw)	EKG (electrocardiogram) X-ray chest Troponins	Stable: beta blockers, calcium channel blockers, and nitrates Unstable: morphine, oxygen, sublingual nitroglycerin, aspirin	Unstable angina call 911 or go to nearest Emergency Department
Gallbladder	Sudden and rapidly intensifying pain in the right upper quadrant or center of the abdomen below the sternum Back pain between shoulder blades and **right** shoulder pain	CBC, LFTs CT scan Hepatobiliary iminodiacetic acid (HIDA) scan, MRI/MR endoscopic retrograde cholangiopancreatography (ERCP)	Ursodeoxycholic acid (UDCA) enhances gallstone dissolution Cholecystectomy	Surgical referral

TABLE 16-4 Referred Visceral-Somatic Pain[1-20]   (Continued)

DIAGNOSIS	PHYSICAL EXAMINATION	WORK-UP	TREATMENT	WHEN TO REFER
Diaphragmatic	Splenomegaly with associated **left** shoulder pain. Percussion of Traube space, a semilunar tympanitic area overlying the gas bubble in the stomach, is a valuable maneuver in this regard: obliteration of Traube space favors a pleural effusion	CBC, clotting factors Ultrasound of abdomen CT scan abdomen	Depending on degree of injury, may require surgical repair—partial or complete removal	Surgical evaluation and treatment
Complex regional pain syndrome (sympathetically mediated)	**Sensory:** Allodynia (to light touch and/or temperature sensation and/or deep somatic pressure and/or joint movement) and/or hyperalgesia (to pinprick) **Vasomotor:** Temperature asymmetry (more than 1 degree) and/or skin color changes and/or skin color asymmetry **Sudomotor/edema:** Edema and/or sweating changes and/or sweating asymmetry **Motor/trophic:** Decreased range of motion and/or motor dysfunction (weakness, tremor, dystonia) and/or trophic changes (hair/nail/skin)	Laboratory tests and imaging to exclude other conditions: vascular and rheumatologic studies EMG to exclude other neuropathies and may be useful in the diagnosis of CRPS type II to demonstrate nerve injury MRI to assess muscle, joint, or soft tissue etiologies of pain. Triple-phase bone scans to further narrow the differential, but these show no diagnostic utility in CRPS	PT/OT Tactile (or sensory) discrimination training—desensitization Mirror box therapy Graded motor imagery Transcutaneous nerve stimulation (TENS) Cognitive behavioral therapies Medications: • NSAIDs (nonsteroidal anti-inflammatory drugs) • Gabapentin, pregabalin, topiramate, carbamazepine • Bisphosphonates • Calcitonin • Corticosteroids • Tizanidine • Opioids • Ketamine • Topical lidocaine or compounded medications (e.g. including isosorbide dinitrate, clonidine, diclofenac) Interventions: • Sympathetic blocks • intravenous regional blocks • Spinal cord stimulation • Dorsal root ganglion stimulation • Radiofrequency sympathectomy Surgery: • Surgical sympathectomy • Motor cortex stimulation • Deep brain stimulation	Referral to pain medicine. If refractory to pain medicine interventions then consider referral to neurosurgery

Accompanying symptoms of abnormal gait or poor hand dexterity/fine motor skills point toward cervical myelopathy which requires urgent care and investigation. Similarly, even minor trauma that includes some degree of cervical alteration may lead to vertebral artery dissection (VAD), and this differential diagnosis must be entertained because it can be lethal[5]. Atraumatic acute shoulder pain accompanied by chest and jaw pain plus diaphoresis may be indicative of cardiac disease necessitating urgent treatment.

Musculoskeletal shoulder pain may be degenerative and related to overuse injuries. One of the most common injuries affecting individuals over the age of 40 years include tendinitis with or without calcific deposits

TABLE 16-5 Possible Diagnoses Based on Timing/Onset of Pain

ACUTE	INSIDIOUS	CHRONIC
Dislocation (glenohumeral instability—trauma)	Dislocation (glenohumeral instability—subluxation)	Rotator cuff injuries
• Fall on outstretched hand		
Acromioclavicular joint separation		Acromioclavicular joint arthritis
• Fall on adducted arm		
Fracture		
• Cervical		
• Clavicular		
• Humeral		
• Scapular		
	Thoracic outlet syndrome	Thoracic outlet syndrome
Brachial neuritis (traumatic)	Brachial neuritis (idiopathic, viral, or immunization antecedent factor)	
Glenohumeral arthritis	Spinal accessory neuropathy	Glenohumeral arthritis
Glenoid labral tears	Suprascapular neuropathy	
Subacromial bursitis	Long thoracic neuropathy	
Myofascial pain	Myofascial pain	Myofascial pain
	Polymyalgia rheumatica	Polymyalgia rheumatica

typically affecting the tendons of the supraspinatus and infraspinatus rotator cuff muscles. Partial or complete rotator cuff injuries may also occur. Key features that point toward a degenerative process are pain and weakness in lifting the arm overhead. The supraspinatus muscle and tendon are responsible for shoulder abduction. From a mechanical perspective, the tendon is placed at increased risk of rupture because its path from origination to insertion involves an approximate 90-degree sharp turn when abducted. The space through which it must traverse is narrow, and therefore any process that further restricts its motion such as arthritis, edema, or inflammation can result in fraying and further damage. Finally, traction upon the cuff from the dependent arm or pull from the contracting cuff muscle elongates the tendon and renders the critical zone relatively ischemic. The area that becomes compressed within the supraspinatus tendon is the critical zone which is the portion with

the greatest tensile strength and also the region accumulating calcium deposits thus commonly the site of cuff ruptures.[2,6,7]

Traumatic injuries are more common in younger age groups and may result in fractures or shoulder dislocations, acromioclavicular separation, or (long head) biceps tendon tear. Fractures along the clavicle will most commonly occur at the junction of the middle and distal thirds of the clavicle because the bone is thinnest at this location. Scapular fractures are rare and commonly occur following motor vehicle collision or other high-velocity impact occurrence. Humeral head fractures may result from a fall in elderly individuals leading to minimally displaced proximal humerus fractures in 85% of individuals.[8,9] Such fractures including greater tuberosity fractures, displaced <5 mm, or minimally displaced surgical neck fractures can be treated nonoperatively. Operative management is indicated for multiple part fractures or if the greater tuberosity is displaced >5 mm. Surgical interventions may include closed reduction percutaneous pinning and open reduction internal fixation for multiple part fractures.

Dislocation may be common with shoulder instability. Typically shoulder dislocations involve displacement of the humeral head anteriorly and inferiorly relative to the glenoid. Prior dislocation is a risk factor for recurrent dislocation.

Acromioclavicular separations may occur when the mechanism of injury involves falling on top of the shoulder which causes depression of the acromion with respect to the clavicle (see Figures 16-1 to 16-3). A classic example is a running-back holding a football who is tackled to the ground and consequently impacting his shoulder with ball in hand.

A biceps tendon tear may occur from excessive load from resisted elbow flexion and supination activities resulting in rupture. This may lead to pain swelling and deformity as the biceps balls up in the arm (Popeye sign). Such injuries are frequently accompanied by shoulder pain because the long head of the biceps tendon originates from the superior labrum within the glenohumeral joint (Figure 16-1).

Bacterial, viral, or fungal infections can lead to septic arthritis which may affect the shoulders. Septic arthritis may occur in younger or older adults or immunocompromised individuals. The most common bacterial species responsible for septic arthritis is *Staphylococcus aureus.*[10] It can occur as a result of skin or urinary infection which travels through the bloodstream to the shoulder joint.

Thoracic outlet syndrome (TOS) is a constellation of symptoms resulting from compression of the neurovascular bundle as it courses from its cervical origins to the upper extremity including the shoulder. Intermittent upper extremity paresthesia or pain, numbness, and occasionally weakness are the most common manifestations of TOS, although symptoms can become persistent and severely debilitating. TOS is an umbrella diagnosis because symptoms can occur due to arterial, venous, or neurogenic compromise, either above or below the clavicle (Figure 16-4).[11] Pathological compression above the clavicle

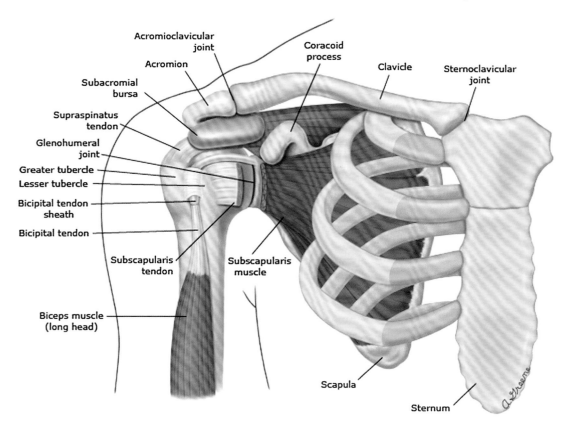

FIGURE 16-1 Anterior view of shoulder anatomy. Reproduced with permission from Simons SM, Roberts M. Patient education: rotator cuff tendinitis and tear (Beyond the Basics). In: Post TW, ed. *UpToDate*. Waltham, MA: UpToDate. Accessed October 30, 2018. Copyright © 2019 UpToDate, Inc. For more information visit www.uptodate.com.

is the most common form of TOS. Below the clavicle, impingement by the pectoralis minor muscle (PMM) leading to pectoralis minor syndrome (PMS) may be present independently or in conjunction with TOS. Isolated PMS is most frequently seen in teenagers or young adults, particularly ones that participate in sports requiring repetitive scapular retraction such as swimming, baseball, and weight lifting, which causes stretching of the PMM.[12]

Vascular causes of shoulder pain may be associated with either arterial or venous thoracic outlet syndrome (TOS) (Table 16-4). Shoulder pain may not necessarily be the primary pain complaint yet due to the distribution of the neurovascular bundle which originates along the neck traveling distally past the shoulder to the hand, such symptoms may arise. For instance, *arterial* TOS presents clinically with a cold, discolored painful hand. This may include paresthesia along the upper limb and ischemia or gangrene of the hand if severe. Physical examination will detect diminished pulses, reduced blood pressure, and ischemic fingers. This can be due to cervical or anomalous first rib causing subclavian artery thrombus, possible aneurysm formation, and emboli to the hand or fingers. In contrast, shoulder pain due to arterial pectoralis minor syndrome may be seen in competitive athletes who throw overhead who experience obstruction or aneurysm formation with thrombosis of the axillary artery or one of its branches with emboli traveling to the hand or fingers.

In contrast, *venous* TOS syndrome presents with swelling, discoloration, pain, and paresthesia of the arm. It is caused by obstruction of the subclavian or axillary vein with or without thrombosis. Physical examination demonstrates a swollen, discolored arm with venous engorgement. Venous TOS occurs from repetitive overhead upper limb activities with subclavian vein contacting the costoclavicular ligament or subclavius tendon. Like arterial TOS, this may result in propensity to form a clot. Venous pectoralis minor syndrome is less common and is the result of the pectoralis minor compressing the axillary vein.

LOCATION

Pain location and radiation patterns are helpful in making an accurate diagnosis. Patients with cervical spondylosis (zygapophysial or facet arthropathy) will classically report radiation of pain into the occiput, shoulder, scapula, and proximal upper arm.[13] Cervical discogenic pain may cause referral of pain into the neck, occiput, face, shoulder, interscapular region, and upper limb.[14] Interestingly, these conditions do not follow a dermatomal distribution. Similarly, cervical radicular pain is not necessarily dermatomal. Radicular pain is perceived deeply, through the shoulder girdle and into the upper limb. Cervical radicular pain from C5 tends to remain in the arm, but pain from C6, C7, and C8 extends into the forearm and hand (see Figure 16-5).[3] In contrast, cervical

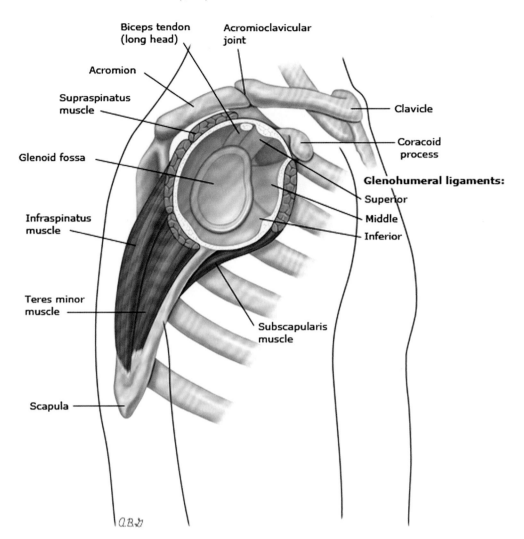

FIGURE 16-2 Lateral view of the shoulder anatomy. Reproduced with permission from Simons SM, Roberts M. Patient education: rotator cuff tendinitis and tear (Beyond the Basics). In: Post TW, ed. *UpToDate*. Waltham, MA: UpToDate. Accessed October 30, 2018. Copyright © 2019 UpToDate, Inc. For more information visit www.uptodate.com.

radiculopathy is characterized by objective signs of loss of neurologic function with some combination of sensory or motor loss or depressed reflexes. Cervical radiculopathy *does* occur in a dermatomal or myotomal distribution. The reason for this is because compression or compromise to a cervical spine nerve or its roots occurs. These diagnoses are further described in the neck pain chapter.

Pain can occur in different patterns based on underlying pain generator. For instance, individuals with glenohumeral arthritis or labral tears may complain of a deep, diffuse pain. Alternatively, one may describe a painful rotator cuff injury as originating along the anterolateral shoulder radiating to the distal deltoid muscle.[15] Similarly, acromioclavicular joint arthritis would be distinguished and localized to the skin area overlying the joint.

In contrast, pain that occurs in other joints without trauma may be related to infectious or immunologic or systemic connective tissue diseases.

Inflammatory causes of musculoskeletal shoulder pain may be related to rheumatic arthritis (RA). Typically, in RA onset is insidious, often beginning with fever,

malaise, arthralgias, and weakness before progressing to joint inflammation and swelling. It is characterized as a persistent symmetric polyarthritis (synovitis) of hands and feet (hallmark feature) that may affect other joints as well. If RA is to affect the shoulder, it may include the acromioclavicular joint and glenohumeral joint.

Polymyalgia rheumatica (PMR) is an inflammatory condition of unknown cause which is characterized by severe bilateral pain and morning stiffness of the shoulder, neck, and pelvic girdle. The most characteristic presenting feature of PMR is bilateral shoulder pain and stiffness of acute or subacute onset with bilateral upper arm tenderness.

ALLEVIATING AND EXACERBATING FACTORS

Identification of movements and positions that exacerbate or alleviate pain can be helpful in guiding diagnosis and treatment (Table 16-6).

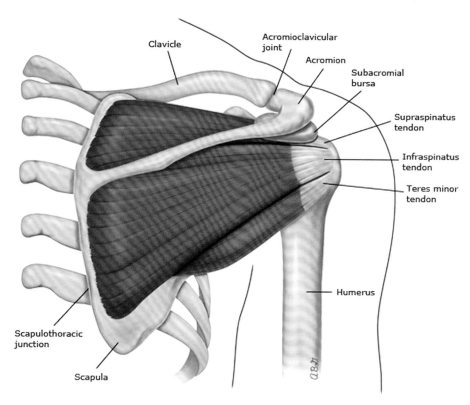

FIGURE 16-3 Posterior view of shoulder anatomy. Reproduced with permission from Simons SM, Roberts M. Patient education: rotator cuff tendinitis and tear (Beyond the Basics). In: Post TW, ed. *UpToDate*. Waltham, MA: UpToDate. Accessed October 30, 2018. Copyright © 2019 UpToDate, Inc. For more information visit www.uptodate.com.

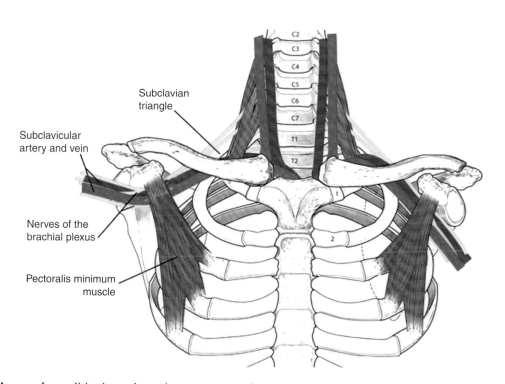

FIGURE 16-4 Areas of possible thoracic outlet entrapment between the scalene muscles, at the costoclavicular region (clavicle and first rib) and the level of the pectoralis minor muscle. Reprinted from Sanders RJ, Annest SJ. Thoracic outlet and pectoralis minor syndromes. *Semin Vasc Surg.* 2014;27(2):86-117. Copyright © 2014 Elsevier. With permission.

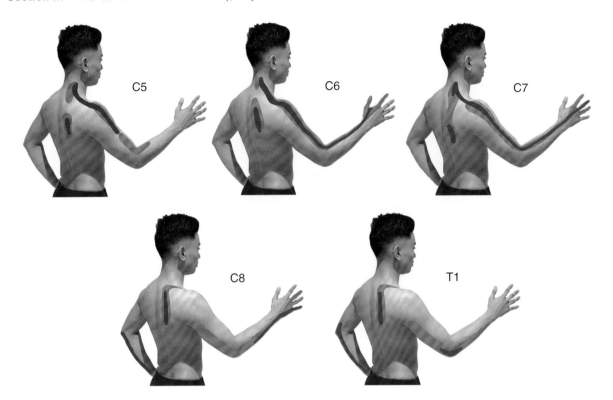

FIGURE 16-5 Cervical radicular pain referral pattern.

TABLE 16-6 Suspected Diagnoses Based on Alleviating Versus Exacerbating Factors

DIAGNOSIS	ALLEVIATING FACTORS	EXACERBATING FACTORS
Thoracic outlet syndrome, spinal accessory, suprascapular and long thoracic neuropathy	Rest with arm held in relaxed position	Overhead or shoulder abduction and rotating head away from symptomatic side
Rotator cuff injuries (tears/strains), subacromial bursitis	Rest	Overhead activities Sleeping or side-lying on affected shoulder
Acromioclavicular arthritis	Rest	Sleeping or side-lying on affected shoulder
Dislocation (Glenohumeral instability)	Supporting the upper limb	Upper limb in dependent position

Pain due to rotator cuff tears and/or subacromial bursitis will worsen with overhead activities. In contrast, pain from acromioclaviular joint arthritis usually worsens with arm adduction because a compressive force is applied to the joint. In both subacromial bursitis and acromioclavicular joint arthritis, sleeping on the affected shoulder will cause pain.

Bicepital tendonitis may be exacerbated by forearm supination and elbow flexion which are the muscle actions used to uncork a bottle of wine. The pain will be alleviated with ice, rest, and acetaminophen or nonsteroidal anti-inflammatory drugs (NSAIDs) as needed.

Labral tears are exacerbated by activities such as overhead pitching, throwing, or reaching for objects from a kitchen cabinet. Shoulder labral pathology may also get better with ice, relative rest, and acetaminophen or NSAIDs as needed.

Glenohumeral arthritis pain will be accompanied by stiffness and worsen with activities approaching the end range of motion. It may be relieved with rest, ice, gentle range of motion, and anti-inflammatory medications.

Adhesive capsulitis (frozen shoulder) is characterized with pain, stiffness, and decreased range of motion in external rotation and/or abduction.[16] There is a loss of both passive and active range of motion. Adhesive capsulitis can be divided into three stages: First is the painful stage which is progressive during which a vague pain may be present for approximately 8 months. Second is the stiffening stage where decreased range of motion occurs and lasts for 8 months. The third stage is the thawing stage which is discernable by increase in range of motion and decrease in pain. Adhesive capsulitis is a consequence of the synovial tissue of the capsule and bursa becoming adherent to one another. Older patients often with diabetes, stroke, or injury are typically affected.

Soft tissue injuries such as strains may occur with any of the muscles supporting and contributing to the movement of the shoulder. Exacerbating factors include motion, while relieving factors include rest or even stretch. Myofascial trigger points to the periscapular area result in pain that radiates following palpation of a trigger point. Trigger points are hyperirritable nodules within taut bands of skeletal muscle, the palpation of which can produce a muscle twitch and referred pain.[16,17] Active trigger points, which are associated with pain, are acutely tender to palpation and may contribute to motor dysfunction such as stiffness and restricted range of motion.

NEUROLOGIC SYMPTOMS

During a musculoskeletal examination, it is imperative to complete a neurological investigation including sensory, motor, and reflex testing. Neurological disease may be distinguished as upper motor neuron versus lower motor neuron process or injury. For example, weakness, spasticity, and brisk reflexes may point toward an upper motor neuron disorder such as stroke or cervical myelopathy. A lower motor neuron disorder may include segmental distribution of sensory or motor loss with depressed reflexes as in the case of a C6 right cervical radiculopathy.

Vision changes, vertigo, numbness, nausea, and vomiting are usually only associated with vertebrobasilar artery insufficiency secondary to atlantoaxial instability or even stroke. Facial numbness and dysesthesias are common symptoms of vertebral artery dissection.

Weakness associated with neck or shoulder pain can be categorized into proximal (shoulder girdle) or distal (intrinsic hand) weakness. Painless proximal weakness may be a sign of suprascapular, long thoracic, spinal accessory, or traction mononeuropathies.[18,19] Suprascapular neuropathy results in shoulder abduction and external rotation weakness. If there is isolated infraspinatus atrophy, it may indicate more distal entrapment possibly related to paralabral cyst. Long thoracic neuropathy may be recognized by winging of the scapula and limited overhead strength, while a spinal accessory neuropathy involves weakness with shoulder shrug, shoulder abduction, and head rotation. Proximal upper brachial plexus lesions result in the inability to lift the arm while lower plexus lesions result in hand weakness.

Distal upper limb weakness with neck and shoulder pain may indicate cervical radiculopathy, although other conditions such as cervical myelopathy, (Pancoast, extramedullary, intramedullary) tumors, and thoracic outlet syndromes must be excluded.

Inflammatory conditions such as brachial neuritis (plexitis or Parsonage Turner syndrome) present clinically with severe, burning, constant pain of the shoulder girdle with sudden onset and radicular symptoms extending to the trapezius, upper arm forearm, and hand.[20] The pain may last 2 weeks and is nonpositional and worse at night therefore impairing sleep. It is not accompanied by constitutional symptoms. Surgical procedures, trauma, viral infection, and recent immunization are known antecedent factors.

Central nervous system disorders such as stroke can lead to hemiplegic shoulder pain with features of joint subluxation, range of motion limitations, and muscle atrophy and weakness. Muscle spasticity and the development of contracture are also elements of poststroke hemiplegic shoulder pain which may be addressed to prevent complications leading to skin breakdown.

ASSOCIATED SYMPTOMS

If shoulder pain is accompanied by neck pain, then it is important to consider cervical facet arthropathy. There is referred pain that follows a common pattern as demonstrated by Dwyer et al. (see Figure 16-6).[21] Higher cervical levels are associated with head pain (usually the back of the head) whereas midcervical levels are associated with neck pain and lower cervical levels refer pain to the trapezius and posterior shoulder. Cervical facet-mediated pain is commonly experienced following whiplash injuries from motor vehicle collisions.

A clicking or popping noise associated with shoulder pain is indicative of shoulder instability. Most commonly, the instability is unidirectional (with dislocation in the anterior-inferiorly) and infrequently multidirectional. A prior shoulder dislocation or subluxation places an individual at risk for recurrence. Labral injuries, such as Bankhart lesions, are a common consequence of shoulder instability and associated damage to the humeral head (hill sacks deformities).

Diffuse soft tissue shoulder pain may occur in other systemic or inflammatory conditions or fibromyalgia.[22] These may be accompanied by pain affecting sleep and daytime fatigue.

PRIOR DIAGNOSTIC STUDIES AND THERAPEUTIC INTERVENTIONS

Assessment of prior diagnostic studies including X-rays and magnetic resonance images (MRIs) can be helpful. Available electromyography (EMG) nerve conduction studies would also facilitate treatment because these may narrow differential diagnosis (e.g., exclude cervical radiculopathy, suprascapular neuropathy, upper trunk plexopathy). Inquiring about prior treatments including physical therapy, oral and/or topical pain medications,

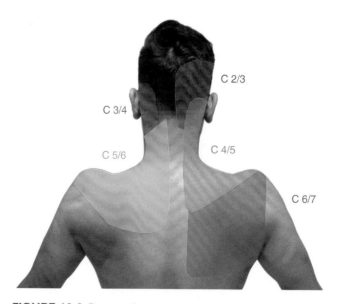

FIGURE 16-6 Dwyer diagram demonstrating the cervical zygapophysial (facet) joint pain referral pattern.

Anterior   Posterior

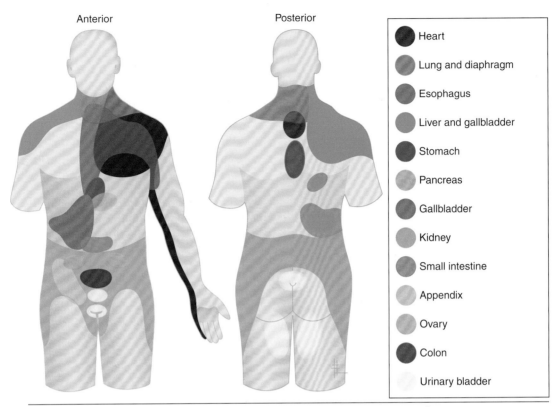

Heart

Lung and diaphragm

Esophagus

Liver and gallbladder

Stomach

Pancreas

Gallbladder

Kidney

Small intestine

Appendix

Ovary

Colon

Urinary bladder

Referred pain. The sites for referred pain from various organs are shown.

FIGURE 16-7 Areas of visceral referred pain.

previous injections, chiropractic treatment, osteopathic manipulation, acupuncture, use of a tens unit, or surgical interventions is helpful in determining an appropriate treatment plan.

Factors for therapeutic failure may be related to various reasons. In the case of physical therapy, perhaps the diagnosis was nonspecific and therefore the therapy prescribed and received may not have addressed the underlying issue. The quality of physical therapy instruction and patient adherence to treatments or home exercises may have been inconsistent. Determination of the type of physical therapy performed, duration, and modalities used for pain control are key elements of the history. It is beneficial to ask the patient to demonstrate the type of home exercise performed which will help to ascertain compliance and to assess both form and technique. Reasons for why physical therapy was discontinued should also be investigated. Similarly, when reviewing medications, the type, effectiveness, dosages, and side effects should be assessed and reasons for discontinuation considered. These are also important with regard to injection, procedures, or surgeries.

CONCLUSION

The shoulder is a complex structure with less stability and increased range of motion when compared with other joint complexes such as the hip. Shoulder pain usually arises from the shoulder joint itself and can be due to

bursitis, tendinopathy or tear, instability arthritis, or fractures. It can be due to referred pain from the neck, thorax, or abdomen. It is useful to divide shoulder pain into four categories in developing a differential diagnosis: musculoskeletal, neurologic, vascular, and referred visceral-somatic pain (see Figure 16-7 for visceral referred pain). A systematic approach is essential for effective management of shoulder pain.

REFERENCES

1. Burbank KM, Stevenson JH, Czarnecki GR, Dorfman J. Chronic shoulder pain: part I. Evaluation and diagnosis. *Am Fam Physician.* 2008;77(4):453-460.

2. Cailliet R. *Shoulder Pain.* Philadelphia, PA: FA Davis Publishers; 1991.

3. Bogduk N. The anatomy and pathophysiology of neck pain. *Phys Med Rehabil Clin N Am.* 2011;22(3):367-382, vii.

4. Paley L, Zornitzki T, Cohen J, Friedman J, Kozak N, Schattner A. Utility of clinical examination in the diagnosis of emergency department patients admitted to the department of medicine of an academic hospital. *Arch Intern Med.* 2011;171(15):1394-1396.

5. Inamasu J, Guiot BH. Vertebral artery injury after blunt cervical trauma: an update. *Surg Neurol.* 2006;65(3):238-245; discussion 245-6.

6. Codman EA. Rupture of the supraspinatus tendon. 1911. *Clin Orthop Relat Res.* 1990;(254):3-26.

7. Lohr JF, Uhthoff HK. The microvascular pattern of the supraspinatus tendon. *Clin Orthop Relat Res.* 1990;(254):35-38.

8. Lefevre-Colau MM, Babinet A, Fayad F, et al. Immediate mobilization compared with conventional immobilization for the impacted nonoperatively treated proximal humeral fracture. A randomized controlled trial. *J Bone Joint Surg Am.* 2007;89(12):2582-2590.

9. Platzer P, Thalhammer G, Oberleitner G, et al. Displaced fractures of the greater tuberosity: a comparison of operative and nonoperative treatment. *J Trauma.* 2008;65(4):843-848.

10. Dubost JJ, Soubrier M, De Champs C, Ristori JM, Bussiére JL, Sauvezie B. No changes in the distribution of organisms responsible for septic arthritis over a 20 year period. *Ann Rheum Dis.* 2002;61(3):267-269.

11. Sanders RJ, Hammond SL, Rao NM. Thoracic outlet syndrome: a review. *Neurologist.* 2008;14(6):365-373.

12. Sanders RJ, Annest SJ. Thoracic outlet and pectoralis minor syndromes. *Semin Vasc Surg.* 2014;27(2):86-117.

13. Aprill C, Dwyer A, Bogduk N. Cervical zygapophyseal joint pain patterns. II: A clinical evaluation. *Spine (Phila Pa 1976).* 1990;15(6):458-461.

14. Bogduk N. The anatomical basis for spinal pain syndromes. *J Manipulative Physiol Ther.* 1995;18(9):603-605.

15. Cohen RB, Williams GR. Impingement syndrome and rotator cuff disease as repetitive motion disorders. *Clin Orthop Relat Res.* 1998;(351):95-101.

16. Neviaser AS, Hannafin JA, Adhesive capsulitis: a review of current treatment. *Am J Sports Med.* 2010;38(11):2346-2356.

17. Shah JP, Thaker N, Heimur J, Aredo JV, Sikdar S, Gerber L. Myofascial trigger points then and now: a historical and scientific perspective. *PM R.* 2015;7(7):746-761.

18. Macaluso S., Ross DC, Doherty TJ, Doherty CD, Miller TA. Spinal accessory nerve injury: a potentially missed cause of a painful, droopy shoulder. *J Back Musculoskelet Rehabil.* 2016;29(4):899-904.

19. Srikumaran U, Wells JH, Freehill MT, Tan EW, Higgins LD, Warner JJ. Scapular winging: a great masquerader of shoulder disorders: AAOS exhibit selection. *J Bone Joint Surg Am.* 2014;96(14):e122.

20. Feinberg JH, Radecki J. Parsonage-turner syndrome. *HSS J.* 2010;6(2):199-205.

21. Dwyer A, Aprill C, Bogduk N. Cervical zygapophyseal joint pain patterns. I: A study in normal volunteers. *Spine (Phila Pa 1976).* 1990;15(6):453-457.

22. Bardal EM, Roeleveld K, Mork PJ. Aerobic and cardiovascular autonomic adaptations to moderate intensity endurance exercise in patients with fibromyalgia. *J Rehabil Med.* 2015;47(7):639-646.

17

CHEST WALL PAIN

Zar Baqai, MD and Jon Zhou, MD

OVERVIEW
INTRODUCTION
HISTORY
MECHANISM OF INJURY
LOCATION
DIAGNOSTIC STUDIES
THERAPEUTIC INTERVENTIONS
CONCLUSION
   References

FAST FACTS

- Chest pain is a common presenting symptom in primary care.
- There are noncardiac causes of chest pain.
- Accurate assessment is essential to ensure appropriate management.
- Assessment is largely based on history and physical examination.

INTRODUCTION

The chief complaint of "chest pain" is one of the most common, high-risk presentations encountered in the medical field.[1] Owing to the potential for a life-threatening condition, it is imperative to diagnose and treat patients with acute myocardial infarction, thoracic aortic dissection, or pulmonary embolism. However, in the primary care setting, studies show that more benign conditions such as musculoskeletal chest wall pain account for nearly half of all chest pain complaints.[2,3] The purpose of this chapter is to aid primary care physicians in both recognizing and managing various types of chest wall pain.

HISTORY

There are 3 general categories of musculoskeletal chest pain: isolated musculoskeletal pain syndromes, rheumatic disease–related pain, and systemic nonrheumatologic conditions. The history and physical examination are essential in making an accurate diagnosis, especially in isolated musculoskeletal pain syndromes such as costochondritis where no confirmatory laboratory test or imaging study currently exists. A large study by Bosner et al. found that 4 determinants were particularly useful in diagnosing musculoskeletal chest pain: localized muscle tension, stinging pain, pain reproducible by palpation, and absence of cough. The presence of 2 out of 4 determinants leads to a greater than 60% sensitivity and specificity for the diagnosis of musculoskeletal chest pain.[2]

A thorough history including pain location, quality, severity, onset, setting, aggravating/alleviating factors, and associated symptoms should be completed. Past medical history may disclose systemic conditions including osteoporosis, chronic renal disease, or cancer, which may be related to the pain complaint. The family history will aid in identifying individuals with genetic predisposition to diseases including rheumatologic conditions. The social history may indicate whether there has been a change in physical activity or if work or recreational activities that are frequent and repetitive are implicated. Travel history helps determine exposure to infections, for example, those caused by tick-borne diseases in endemic areas leading to the complaint of musculoskeletal chest wall and joint pain.

Inspection and palpation are essential physical examination elements in patients complaining of musculoskeletal chest pain. Visual inspection of the location of pain is essential to evaluate for obvious infection, trauma, scarring, tumor, erythema, and swelling. Examining areas that are tender to palpation helps narrow the diagnosis. Specifically, the costochondral junctions, clavicular articulations, manubrium, sternum, xiphoid, and ribs should be palpated. Positive findings on palpation of the costal margins and techniques such as the "hooking maneuver" can aid in the diagnosis of painful rib syndrome otherwise known as slipping rib syndrome[4] (see Figure 17-1). All patients should have an examination of the spine, hips, and pelvic girdle evaluating for tenderness, flexion and extension, stiffness, and rotation. Patients with restriction to flexion

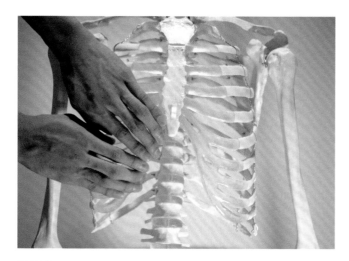

FIGURE 17-1 Hooking maneuver.

of the lumbar spine, tenderness in the sacroiliac joint, and morning stiffness may have ankylosing spondylitis, which is associated with tenderness in the sternum and sternoclavicular joints. The presence of uveitis or dactylitis would further support this diagnosis. A thorough examination of more distal joints should be performed as well to evaluate for other types of rheumatologic disease (Table 17-1).

MECHANISM OF INJURY

The mechanism of injury is important as it allows the physician to narrow the differential diagnosis and provides insight into the pathophysiology of the pain itself and guides treatment. It is essential to view the illness in the clinical context. For example, elderly women are prone to osteoporosis and insufficiency fractures. Patients who have a history of cancer may have pathologic fractures that are causing chest pain. Elderly patients with unilateral nerve pain and rashes may have zoster and postherpetic neuralgia, which have a predilection for the thoracic nerve dermatomes. Those with pain from repetitive activities may have stress fractures

TABLE 17-1 Musculoskeletal Chest Wall Pain

CAUSES	SYMPTOMS	PHYSICAL EXAM	LABS/IMAGING
Costochondritis	Pain at costochondral joint	Tender to palpation	NA
Lower rib pain syndrome/ slipping Rib syndrome	Pain at costal margin	Tender to palpation	NA
Post-thoracotomy pain	Incisional pain/neuropathy	Tender to palpation	NA
Sternalis syndrome	Pain over sternum	Tender to palpation	NA
Xiphoidalgia	Pain over xiphoid	Tender to palpation	NA
Fibromyalgia	Fatigue, diffuse pain, waking unrefreshed	Trigger points	NA
Rheumatoid arthritis	Joint pain, morning stiffness	Tender, swollen, deformed joints	RF, anti-CCP, ESR, CRP, and X-ray/ US showing inflammation and arthritis
Ankylosing spondylitis	Joint pain, back pain, stiffness	Joint tenderness, dactylitis	HLA-B27, pelvic X-ray, and MRI SI joint
Systemic lupus erythematosus	Can affect the kidneys, lungs, heart, brain, bone marrow, muscles, joints	Malar rash, joint involvement	ANA, ESR, CRP, anti-ds-DNA, anti-Sm, proteinuria, CBC, creatinine, anti-phospholipid ab, C3, C4
Insufficiency or stress fractures	Localized pain	Tender to palpation/ swelling	X-ray (inexpensive, higher propensity for false negative than MRI) MRI (expensive, more accurate than X-ray)
Malignancy	Systemic, vary based on types	Tumor, swelling	CT chest
Tietze syndrome	Pain and swelling at costosternal, costochondral, or sternoclavicular joints, younger patients, usually second or third ribs	Tenderness, swelling	NA

from microtrauma to the area. A history of thoracotomy raises concern for postthoracotomy pain experienced by roughly 50% of postthoracotomy patients chronically.[5] The presence of symptoms such as joint pain, morning stiffness, and fatigue indicates the possibility of a rheumatologic process, which has a different pathophysiologic profile compared with an isolated musculoskeletal chest syndrome.

LOCATION

Given a clinical context, the location of the chest wall pain may help pinpoint a diagnosis. Costochondritis often involves tenderness in the costosternal and costochondral junctions. Costochondritis typically affects the third, fourth, and fifth costosternal joints, whereas Tietze syndrome, another similar condition, usually affects the second or third costosternal joint. Pain in the lower ribs along the costal margins with a positive "hooking maneuver" suggests slipping rib syndrome, which is defined by reproducible pain in the lower costal margins. Pain directly over the sternum and sternalis muscle that radiates out when palpated may be a sign of sternalis syndrome. Another syndrome associated with midline sternal pain is poststernotomy pain in patients who have undergone coronary artery bypass graft surgery. Pain when palpating the xiphoid may indicate xiphoidalgia. A more diffuse complaint of pain along with fatigue and cognitive symptoms may point toward fibromyalgia. Those with rheumatologic disease often have pain in the small joints of the hands and feet. In terms of chest wall pain, this is more likely to present in the sternoclavicular, costovertebral, costosternal, and manubriosternal joints.[6]

DIAGNOSTIC STUDIES

Isolated musculoskeletal chest wall syndromes are not associated with specific laboratory tests or imaging studies. They are often thought to be a result of overuse, trauma, twisting, weight-bearing, or repetitive activity. The diagnosis is clinical and based on history and physical examination. In many ways, it is a diagnosis of exclusion, which means both rheumatic pain and systemic nonrheumatologic disease should be ruled out. The most common isolated musculoskeletal chest wall pains include costochondritis and lower rib pain syndromes. Costochondritis is usually characterized by pain in one or more costochondral or costosternal junctions, where pain is reproducible on palpation. Furthermore, there is lack of swelling and erythema in the region of pain. Lower rib pain syndromes involve pain in the lower ribs reproducible on palpation. The "hooking maneuver" is a diagnostic test performed by gently curling one's fingers under the suspected costal margin and pulling outward.

Rheumatologic disease–related chest wall pains have been linked to many conditions including rheumatoid arthritis, ankylosing spondylitis, psoriatic arthritis, fibromyalgia, and systemic lupus erythematosus. Laboratory and imaging tests can increase the accuracy of the diagnosis when used in conjunction with the clinical presentation. For ankylosing spondylitis, HLA-B27 has a high sensitivity. Anterior-posterior radiographs of the pelvis are cost-effective and allow grading of the degree of sacroiliitis. An MRI of the sacroiliac joints can sometimes show early changes and bone marrow edema, with the major limitation being high cost. For rheumatoid arthritis, there are 2 major laboratory tests: rheumatoid factor (RF) and anti-CCP. RF has a higher sensitivity, and anti-CCP has a much higher specificity at 96%.[7] For systemic lupus erythematosus, laboratory tests include antinuclear antibody (ANA), double-stranded DNA (ds-DNA) antibodies, and anti-Smith (anti-Sm) antibodies. ds-DNA and anti-Sm antibodies are more specific for lupus (99% for anti-Sm), although the sensitivity of anti-Sm is low at 40%.[8,9] The remaining rheumatologic diseases are not associated with specific tests. However, chest X-ray and ultrasound can reveal inflammation or bony changes consistent with the pattern of pain and may aid in the diagnosis. Erythrocyte sedimentation rate (ESR) and C-reactive protein (CRP) are acute phase reactants and are nonspecific tests.

Systemic nonrheumatologic conditions causing chest wall pain include stress fractures, insufficiency fractures, sickle cell disease, and malignancy involving the chest wall. Diagnostic studies will depend on the specific clinical scenario. Fractures can be seen with a chest radiograph. However, stress fractures may be missed with X-ray alone. MRI, though more expensive, is more accurate.[10,11] If neoplasm or metastasis is suspected, a CT scan of the chest may be warranted. In patients with sickle cell anemia, acute chest syndrome should be worked up in the emergency room before considering chronic pain or rib infarction.

THERAPEUTIC INTERVENTIONS

The initial approach for treatment of isolated musculoskeletal chest wall pain may include conservative measures such as rest and application of heat (muscle spasm) and ice (swelling). Formal physical therapy programs may help patient focus on stretching and strengthening the soft tissue region to decrease pain. Medications used for isolated musculoskeletal chest wall pain are similar to other muscular conditions including acetaminophen, NSAIDs, and topical analgesics such as a lidocaine patch. Interventional pain treatments include local anesthetic and steroid injections into the painful regions. However, they are not permanent solutions and require close monitoring. Anti-inflammatory medications and disease-modifying agents (DMARDs) should be used to treat the underlying condition of chest wall pain associated with rheumatologic conditions. Similarly, chest pain from systemic nonrheumatologic disease should be managed based on the underlying disease state.

CONCLUSION

Chest wall pain continues to be a common complaint in the primary care setting with a broad range of etiologies. By using a categorical approach, the differential diagnoses can be significantly narrowed into 3 categories: isolated musculoskeletal pain syndromes, rheumatic disease–related pain, and systemic nonrheumatologic conditions. This delineation not only helps in diagnosis but also separates conditions based on the treatment approach. This chapter aims to provide clinicians with enhanced, efficient utilization of the history, physical examination, laboratory tests, and imaging in order to both diagnose and treat patients with chest wall pain effectively.

QUESTION

1. A 23-year-old man presents with a 1-day history of pain and swelling in his right upper chest with no other associated symptoms. No history of trauma to the area. ECG is unremarkable, and troponin is negative. Physical examination reveals swelling and tenderness along the second rib. Which of the following is the most likely diagnosis?

   A. Myocardial infarction
   B. Costochondritis
   C. Tietze syndrome
   D. Fibromyalgia

   C is the correct answer. Tietze's syndrome is a rare syndrome that typically manifests with pain and nonsuppurative swelling over the second or third rib. A key distinction between Tietze syndrome and costochondritis is the presence of swelling. Likewise, fibromyalgia may be associated with chest pain but not a localized swelling. Myocardial infarction is unlikely in an otherwise healthy young woman with a normal ECG and negative troponin.

2. A 35-year-old woman presents with complaints of chest wall pain, joint pain, and morning stiffness. Physical examination reveals tenderness in the sternoclavicular joints as well as PIP joints in the hand. Laboratory testing reveals a positive rheumatoid factor and a positive anti-CCP antibody. You decide to start DMARD therapy. Which of the following tests should be performed before initiating treatment?

   A. Hepatitis panel
   B. HIV
   C. TB screen
   D. A and C

   D is the correct answer. Before initiating DMARD therapy, both hepatitis panel and TB screen should be performed to avoid reactivation of disease.

3. A 43-year-old woman presents with a 6-month history of fatigue, sleep disturbance, and diffuse pain. Physical examination reveals tenderness in the neck, shoulders, upper chest, and hips. CBC, BMP, TSH, T4, HLA-B27, ANA, ds-DNA, C3, C4, RF, anti-CCP, ESR, and CRP are all within normal limits. Which of the following is the most likely diagnosis?

   A. Lupus
   B. Hypothyroidism
   C. Fibromyalgia
   D. Ankylosing spondylitis

   C is the correct answer. Fibromyalgia is characterized by widespread pain accompanied by fatigue, sleep, memory and mood issues. Scientists believe that fibromyalgia amplifies painful sensations by affecting the way your brain processes pain signals. Fibromyalgia can be effectively managed through medications, lifestyle changes and stress management.

4. An 89-year-old woman with a history of hypertension and osteoporosis presents to the clinic owing to a 1-week history of right-sided pleuritic chest pain. The pain started after she was kicked in the chest by her 2-year-old grandson while changing his diaper. She is hemodynamically stable, and her O_2 saturation is 98% on room air. Physical examination reveals tenderness along the fifth rib. Laboratory tests were unremarkable other than low calcium and vitamin D levels. What imaging modality should be ordered on this patient?

   A. MRI chest
   B. CT chest
   C. Chest X-ray
   D. Ultrasound chest

   C is the correct answer. Older women with osteoporosis are more prone to fractures, and this patient's history and physical both suggest a rib fracture. It is reassuring to know that her saturation is 98% on room air, making the diagnosis of flail chest less likely. A chest X-ray is the best choice of imaging in this case given the high likelihood of a rib fracture. It is a quick and cost-effective way to confirm the diagnosis. Ultrasound can be useful in the right hands; however, it can be painful when compressing a fractured rib and is highly operator dependent.

5. A 55-year-old man presents with chest pain and gradually increasing swelling over the chest for the past 3 months. Physical examination reveals swelling and discomfort over the right chest that seems to extend deep into the chest. A CT scan reveals a chest wall tumor. What is the most classification of this tumor?

continued

    A. Sarcoma
    B. Myeloma
    C. Lymphoma
    D. Carcinoma

A is the correct answer. Chondrosarcoma is the most common malignant chest wall tumor. The most common benign chest wall tumor is an osteochondroma, which usually presents as a painless mass in young men.

REFERENCES

1. Woo KM, Schneider JI. High-risk chief complaints I: chest pain–the big three. *Emerg Med Clin North Am.* 2009;27(4):685-712.
2. Bösner S, Becker A, Hani MA, et al. Chest wall syndrome in primary care patients with chest pain: presentation, associated features and diagnosis. *Fam Pract.* 2010;27:363.
3. Verdon F, Herzig L, Burnand B, et al. Chest pain in daily practice: occurrence, causes and management. *Swiss Med Wkly.* 2008;138:340.
4. Scott EM, Scott BB. Painful rib syndrome–a review of 76 cases. *Gut.* 1993;34:1006.
5. Pluijms WA, Steegers MA. Chronic post-thoracotomy pain: a retrospective study. *Acta Anaesthesiol Scand.* 2006;804-808.
6. Ramonda R, Lorenzin M, Lo Nigro A, et al. Anterior chest wall involvement in early stages of spondyloarthritis: advanced diagnostic tools. *J Rheumatol.* 2012;1844-1849.
7. Whiting PF, Smidt N, Sterne JA, et al. Systematic review: accuracy of anti–citrullinated peptide antibodies for diagnosing rheumatoid arthritis. *Ann Intern Med.* 2010;152(7):456-464.
8. Benito-Garcia E, Schur PH, Lahita R, et al. Guidelines for immunologic laboratory testing in the rheumatic diseases: anti-Sm and anti-RNP antibody tests. *Arthritis Rheum.* 2004;51(6):1030-1044.
9. Pan LT, Tin SK, Boey ML, Fong KY. The sensitivity and specificity of autoantibodies to the Sm antigen in the diagnosis of systemic lupus erythematosus. *Ann Acad Med Singapore.* 1998;27(1):21-23.
10. Miller TL, Harris JD, Kaeding CC. Stress fractures of the ribs and upper extremities: causation, evaluation, and management. *Sports Med.* 2013;43:665-674.
11. Arendt EA, Griffiths HJ. The use of MR imaging in the assessment and clinical management of stress reactions of bone in high-performance athletes. *Clin Sports Med.* 1997;16:291-306.

18

ABDOMINAL PAIN

Joshua Lee, MD and Jon Zhou, MD

OVERVIEW
DEFINITION
MECHANISMS AND PAIN PATHWAYS
CLINICAL PRESENTATIONS OF ABDOMINAL PAIN
APPROACH TO CHRONIC ABDOMINAL
   PAIN DISORDERS
THE PEDIATRIC PATIENT
MANAGEMENT OF ABDOMINAL PAIN
   DISORDERS IN PEDIATRICS
WHEN TO REFER
   References

FAST FACTS

- Most patients with chronic abdominal pain have functional GI disorders such as functional dyspepsia or irritable bowel syndrome.
- Chronic abdominal pain syndromes can be subdivided into 2 categories: intra-abdominal and abdominal wall origin.
- Chronic abdominal pain may coexist with other medical and psychological syndromes such as obesity, depression, and anxiety.
- Abdominal pain is the second most common recurrent pain condition in children after headaches.

DEFINITION

Abdominal pain disorders are common and can be particularly challenging given the myriad of possible underlying etiologies: ranging from the life-threatening to chronic functional disorders. The International Association for the Study of Pain (IASP) defines chronic pain as "pain which has persisted beyond normal tissue healing time".[1] Both can be seen within the office-based primary care setting, each presenting with its own set of challenges.

The continuum of abdominal pain also includes somatic complaints relating to chronic functional abdominal pain, which may be difficult to manage. The challenge in the diagnosis and management of abdominal pain syndromes results in higher usage of health care resources primarily due to investigative workup, producing higher health care costs.

A structured approach to the evaluation, assessment, and investigation of abdominal pain allows for appropriate triaging and management. Although the focus of this section will be primarily on chronic abdominal pain, an overview of acute abdominal pain syndromes pertinent to primary care practices will also be reviewed.

MECHANISMS AND PAIN PATHWAYS

Anatomical abdominal pain pathways are complex owing to the presence of and possible coexistence of different types of nociceptive pain: visceral, somatic, and referred pain.

Somatic pain is defined as "pain arising from tissues such as the skin, muscle, joint capsules, and bone." Stimuli from somatic pain are primarily mediated by the C and A-delta afferent fibers, which also innervate the mesentery. Direct damage to the gastrointestinal tissue, such as ischemia, triggers firing of C and A-delta afferents that are present within the serosal layer of the gastrointestinal (GI) tract.

Visceral pain is defined as "pain arising from visceral organs." Visceral pain can often be diffuse, vague, and difficult to localize in some cases. Abdominal pain is mediated by the dual supply of visceral sensory information received by the splanchnic nerves and somatic information from cerebrospinal innervations. The splanchnic pathway innervates the visceral organs, where pain signals are transmitted by free afferent nerve endings through the spinal cord to the thalamus via the paleospinal and archispinal thalamic tracts. These afferent receptors are primarily located within the mucosal epithelium of the gastrointestinal tract and are mechanosensitive, receiving information from physical alterations in the tissue due to stretch and spasms[2] (Figure 18-1). Caustic agents and extreme changes in intraluminal pH can also cause firing of these visceral afferents (Table 18-1).

CLINICAL PRESENTATIONS OF ABDOMINAL PAIN

According to the CDC report, acute abdominal pain was the most common presenting complaint to emergency departments in the United States between 1998 and 2008.[3] Although less common in the office-based setting, abdominal pain remains a common reason for primary care visits.[4] Appropriate triaging and timely referrals by the primary physician could be potentially life-saving, especially in a practice far removed from a major facility with the capacity to intervene on major vascular emergencies.

In the primary care setting, the presentation of acute abdominal pain is most likely to be acutely atraumatic in nature (Figure 18-2).

The first immediate step in evaluating acute abdominal pain in an office-based practice should be a focused and general assessment of the patient's appearance and vital signs, with an emphasis on any objective evidence of possible hemodynamic instability. The goal of this very first step is to determine whether emergent interventions and resuscitative measures are required before transport to the higher level-of-care and to reduce overall morbidity and mortality.

APPROACH TO CHRONIC ABDOMINAL PAIN DISORDERS

Chronic abdominal pain syndromes can be subdivided into two categories: intra-abdominal and abdominal wall origin. Evaluation of chronic abdominal pain can be complex given the myriad of possible causes, some possibly overlapping in presentation. It is also important to keep in mind that pain syndromes, regardless of their etiologies, often coexist with other medical and psychological syndromes such as obesity, depression, and anxiety.

Malabsorptive Conditions	Inflammatory Bowel Disease

Postsurgery
  Gastrectomy
Intestinal disease
  Sprue
Pancreatic insufficiency
	Crohn disease
	Ulcerative colitis
	Other microscopic
	  colitis
	  Collagenous colitis
	  Mast cell disease

Dietary Factors	**Psychiatric Conditions**

Lactose intolerance
Caffiene
Alcohol
Fat-containing, gas-
  producing foods
  Cruciferous
    vegetables
	Panic disorder
	Depression
	Somatization disorders

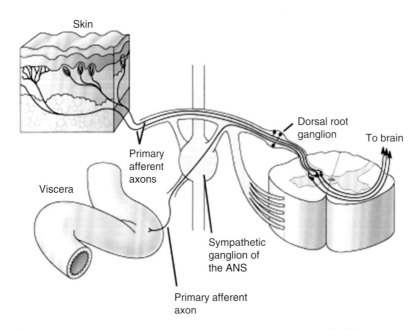

FIGURE 18-1 Neural pathways carrying pain information from visceral organs. ©2019 Lippincott Professional Development®.

Infections	Miscellaneous Conditions
Bacteria	Endometriosis
Campylobacter,	Endocrine tumors
Salmonella,	Cacinoid
Yersinia	Zollinger-Ellison
Parasites	syndrome
Giardia lamblia	VIPoma
	HIV disease

TABLE 18-1 General Characteristics of Pain due to Visceral Pathology

1. Is poorly localized with referral to somatic structures

2. Produces nonspecific regional or whole-body motor responses

3. Produces strong autonomic responses

4. Leads to sensitization of somatic tissues

5. Produces strong affective responses

Reprinted with permission from Sikandar S, Dickenson AH. Visceral pain: the ins and outs, the ups and downs. Curr Opin Support Palliat Care. 2012;6(1):17-26.

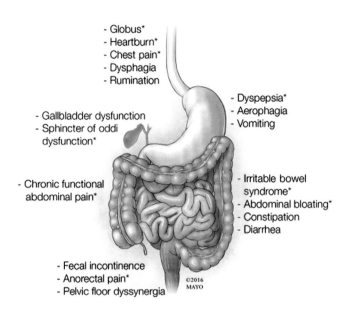

FIGURE 18-2 Common functional gastrointestinal disorders. * indicates conditions associated with pain. Reprinted from Bharucha AE, Chakraborty S, Sletten CD. Common functional gastroenterological disorders associated with abdominal pain. *Mayo Clin Proc.* 2016;91(8):1118-1132. Copyright © 2016 Elsevier. With permission.

Careful attention to reported or presenting signs and symptoms during a thorough history-taking should be of utmost importance, as physical findings may not be reproducible. Additionally, clues within the patient's presenting complaints may lead an astute clinician to a diagnosis without ordering otherwise unnecessary or costly radiologic imaging and laboratory tests.

The initial assessment of any abdominal pain during history-taking should the 6 following features:

1. Onset: *Rapid, sudden, slow onset.*
2. Quality: *Cramping, burning, sharpness, dullness, episodic.*
3. Intensity: *The severity of the pain perceived by the patient.*
4. Evolution: *Increasing, decreasing, or unchanged in intensity.*
5. Migration: *Radiation of the pain from a primary site, to another.*
6. Localization: *Involvement of the epigastrium, mid-abdominal, or lower abdominal areas.*

Diagnostic modalities can be considered if the outcomes were to be affected, significantly altering your clinical decision-making (Figure 18-3).

Abdominal wall pain, being somatic in origin, is distinct from visceral pain syndromes also with different anatomical considerations. In distinguishing abdominal wall pain from intra-abdominal sources, the abdominal examination could assess for Carnett sign: unchanged or an increase in abdominal pain with the abdomen tensed (Table 18-2).

Although opioids may be useful for acute intolerable pain including abdominal pain, it is often not the best first-line solution for chronic nonmalignant abdominal pain because of opioid-induced side effects including nausea/vomiting and constipation, which all may exacerbate the pain state. In patients with chronic abdominal pain, a multidisciplinary approach that includes cognitive behavioral therapy would be most ideal. Unless a recent intra-abdominal surgical history is present in the review of systems or history, surgical interventions are less likely to be of benefit as the first initial step. In these patients, diagnostic laparoscopies for chronic abdominal pain of unknown etiology have only been shown to result in symptomatic improvement in 50% of patients.[5] In this subset of patients, symptoms may be due to postsurgical development of adhesions, cholecystitis, internal hernias, or a defect in the mesentery. Although uncommon, abdominal wall abscess formation should also be considered in the differential diagnosis.

In female patients with recent pelvic or abdominal wall surgeries, most commonly low-transverse cesarean sections, presenting with chronic abdominal wall pain of unclear etiology can be challenging. After ruling out postsurgical and incision pain, one consideration can include the diagnosis of abdominal wall endometriosis with implantation of lesions within the wall, diagnosable using ultrasound. If patient habitus prevents appropriate visualization of suspected lesions, abdominal magnetic resonance imaging can be considered.

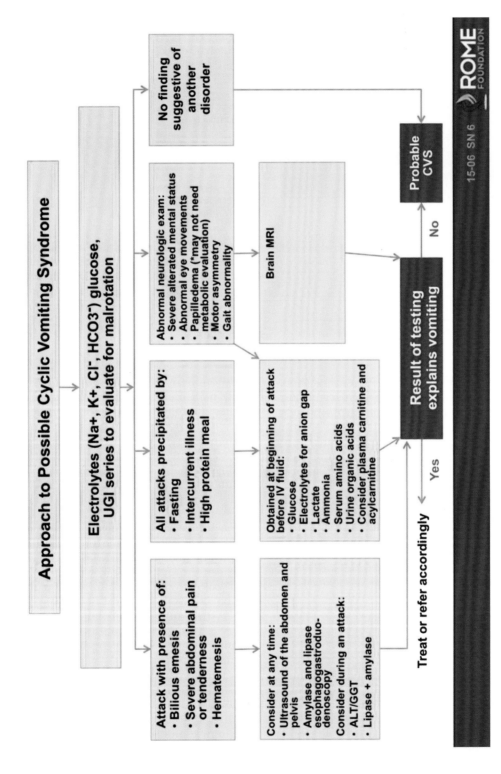

FIGURE 18-3 Approach to possible cyclic vomiting syndrome. Copyright © 2017 Rome Foundation, Inc. All Rights Reserved.

TABLE 18-2 Etiology of Abdominal Wall Pain		
ETIOLOGY	**COMMENTS**	**DIAGNOSIS**
Hernia	Protuberance in abdominal wall that usually decreases in size when patient is supine	Abdominal CT scanning, abdominal ultrasonography, herniography
Rectus nerve entrapment	Occurs along lateral edge of rectus sheath; worsening of pain with tensing of muscles	Injection of local anesthetic
Thoracic lateral cutaneous nerve entrapment	Occurs spontaneously, after surgery or during pregnancy	History and physical examination
Ilioinguinal and iliohypogastric nerve entrapment	Lower abdominal pain that occurs after inguinal hernia repair	History and physical examination
Endometriosis	Cyclic abdominal pain	Laparoscopy
Diabetic radiculopathy	Acute, severe truncal pain involving T6-T12 nerve roots	Paraspinal EMG
Abdominal wall tear	Occurs mainly in athletes	History and physical examination
Abdominal wall hematoma	Complication of abdominal laparoscopic procedures	Abdominal CT scanning, abdominal ultrasonography
Spontaneous rectus sheath hematoma	Presents as tender, usually unilateral mass that does not extend beyond midline	Abdominal CT scanning, abdominal ultrasonography
Desmoid tumor	Dysplastic tumor of connective tissue; occurs in young patients (women more often than men)	Surgical excision
Herpes zoster	Pain and hyperesthesia followed by vesicles along a dermatome	History and physical examination
Spinal nerve irritation	Caused by disorders of thoracic spine	CT scanning or MRI studies of thoracic spine
Slipping rib syndrome	Sharp, stabbing pain in upper abdomen caused by luxation of 8th to 10th ribs	Hooking maneuver to pull lower ribs anteriorly, which reproduces the pain and sometimes a click
Idiopathic	Myofascial pain	History and physical examination

Reprinted with permission from The Abdominal Wall: An Overlooked Source of Pain, August 1, 2001, Vol 64, No 3, American Family Physician. Copyright © 2001 American Academy of Family Physicians, All Rights Reserved.
CT, computed tomography; EMG, electromyography; MRI, magnetic resonance imaging.

Surgical excision of such isolated lesions has been reported to be successful, without very low recurrence rates.[6]

THE PEDIATRIC PATIENT

Abdominal pain is the second most common recurrent pain condition in children after headaches.[7] Abdominal pain is also the most common chief complaint requiring a pediatric referral to an emergency department, with nearly 800,000 patients presenting for acute care in 2012.[8] Furthermore, the Nationwide Emergency Department Sample spanning from the years 2008 to 2012 revealed that the highest incidence of emergency department (ED) visits for abdominal pain were in the 10- to 14-year age group.[9]

The impact of recurrent abdominal pain in the pediatric population can be significant, affecting up to 25% of school-age children in the United States. Chronic pain in the pediatric patient can have an immediate and significant detrimental impact on quality of life and the ability to function, often affecting school attendance, nutrition, sleep, and physical activity.[10] Interestingly, girls aged 10 years or older reported greater restrictions in function and higher medication use compared with age-matched boys.[11] Of note, it is also important to recognize that pain syndromes in children may be underdiagnosed and undertreated in African American, Hispanic, and American Indian children.[12]

On history-taking, the most common complaints from patients are nausea, headache, fullness, fatigue, and heartburn. The symptomatology may include complaints

TABLE 18-3 Differential Diagnosis of Acute Abdominal Pain by Predominant Age

YOUNGER THAN 2 YR	2-5 YR	5-12 YR	OLDER THAN 12 YR
Infantile colic	Gastroenteritis	Gastroenteritis	Appendicitis
Gastroenteritis	Appendicitis	Appendicitis	Gastroenteritis
Constipation	Constipation	Constipation	Constipation
UTI	UTI	Functional pain	Dysmenorrhea
Intussusception	Intussusception	UTI	Mittelschmerz
Volvulus	Volvulus	Trauma	PID
Incarcerated hernia	Trauma	Pharyngitis	Threatened abortion
Hirschsprung disease	Pharyngitis	Pneumonia	Ectopic pregnancy
	Sickle cell crisis	Sickle cell crisis	Ovarian/testicular torsion
	HSP	HSP	
	Mesenteric adenitis	Mesenteric adenitis	

Reprinted with permission from Yang WC, Chen CY, Wu HP. Etiology of non-traumatic acute abdomen in pediatric emergency departments. World J Clin Cases. 2013;1(9):276-284.
HSP, Henoch-Schonlein purpura; PID, pelvic inflammatory disease; UTI, urinary tract infection.

of anxiety and depression. Employing a multidimensional measure for recurrent abdominal pain (MM-RAP) in children may be useful.[13] Similar multidimensional systems have been created to aid in the evaluation of other pain and gastrointestinal disorders, such as the MM-GERD in 2008.[14]

The physical examination of the child should include thorough history-taking with a special focus on the child's behavior, interactions with other family members, and reaction to the presence of medical staff. Often, physical examination findings may be nonspecific (Table 18-3).

Diagnosis of functional gastrointestinal disorders in the pediatric population should follow the newly introduced ROME IV Criteria published in 2016.[15]

Proton-pump inhibitors (PPIs) and tricyclic antidepressants (TCAs) have been demonstrated to be effective in the treatment of epigastric pain syndrome in children.

Treatment for IBS will depend on the subtype present in the patient. Several new medications were recently approved for the treatment of IBS subtypes C and D in both adults and children. Linaclotide, a peptide agonist of guanylate cyclase 2C, was approved by the FDA in August 2012 for the treatment of IBS with constipation (IBS-C) in adults. Rifaximin and eluxadoline were approved by the FDA in May 2015 for the treatment of IBS-D (IBS with diarrhea) subtype.

Recall the high association between functional abdominal pain in childhood and coexisting anxiety and depression. There exists some evidence that cognitive behavioral therapy (CBT), and hypnotherapy may be of benefit in children and adolescents[16] with recurrent pain conditions.[17]

Early intervention should be pursued to reduce disability and development of visceral hyperalgesia.[18] The most recent evidence from the pediatric literature also suggests that nausea accompanying pediatric functional abdominal pain is associated with greater risk of long-term morbidity.[19]

MANAGEMENT OF ABDOMINAL PAIN DISORDERS IN PEDIATRICS

The end-goal of recognizing and treating pain in any individual is to ultimately improve the quality of life and overall function. The early steps of treatment involve validating the presence of the pain disorder and illness and expressing empathy. The pediatric patient may be vulnerable to external factors potentially influencing their pain behavior and augmenting pain perception.

In outlining a treatment plan, a goal should be clearly defined and established with the patient and their caretaker, if appropriate. For the pediatric patient, a reasonable goal, for example, would be the ability to return to school.

There is no "first-line" therapy for chronic abdominal pain in pediatric and adult patients. A discussion should be held to assess the level of comfort and understanding of therapeutic options before initiating any interventions or referrals.

In a review of patients with clinical features of abdominal wall pain syndromes by Kaiser Permanente Southern California in 2004, it was reported that approximately 80% of the affected patients were obese or morbidly obese.[20] If appropriate, incorporation of motivational interviewing techniques for weight loss could potentially improve symptomatology and candidacy for any surgical intervention that may be required in the future. Otherwise, treatment regimens reported in the review were: 60% patients receiving oral analgesics, 55% receiving topical heat application, 10% TCAs, and approximately 5% local anesthetic injections. Local anesthetic injections for chronic abdominal wall pain have been shown to have a mixed response (Table 18-4, Figure 18-4).

If conventional therapies are insufficient and/or declined, one can consider complementary therapies before invasive interventions. Acupuncture may be considered in the multimodality approach, given its relatively low risk-to-benefit ratio. No literature currently exists about the effect of acupuncture on modulation of GI visceral sensitivity and the GI-brain axis. Limited evidence exists on the use of transcutaneous electrical nerve stimulation (TENS) in children. Elective surgical procedures, such as lysis of adhesions, should be not be offered early unless there is a clear indication.

WHEN TO REFER

Chronic abdominal pain that persists or remains unresponsive or unimproved to conservative treatment after ruling out other medical conditions should be

TABLE 18-4 Pharmacological Treatments Options for Chronic Abdominal Pain

AGENTS	COMMENTS
TCAs	Low daily doses
	No evidence of efficacy in RCTs
	Loss effective than SNRIs in other chronic pain conditions
SSRI + SNRI combined agents	Venlafaxine, duloxetine
SSRIs	Useful when anxiety or depression coexist
Analgesics	Offer limited benefit
Narcotic analgesics	Should be avoided
Anticonvulsants	Gabapentin, carbamazepine, and lamotrigine
	Not specifically studied in FAPS
	Relatively safe and nonhabituating
	May interrupt the cycle between pain and depression

FAPS, functional abdominal pain syndrome; RCT, randomized controlled trial; SNRI, serotonin and norepinephrine reuptake inhibitors; SSRI, selective serotonin reuptake inhibitors; TCA, tricyclic antidepressant.

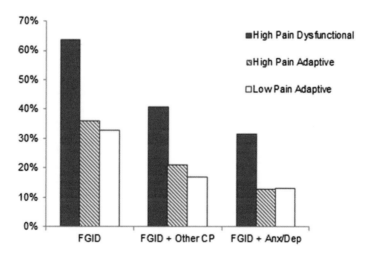

Percent of each FAP profile meeting criteria for various outcomes at follow-up

FIGURE 18-4 Percent of each functional abdominal pain profile (high pain dysfunctional, high pain adaptive, low pain adaptive) with incidences of several pain states. Anx/Dep, DSM-IV criteria for anxiety or depressive disorder; CP, chronic pain; FGID, functional gastrointestinal disorder w/ abdominal pain. Reprinted with permission from Walker LS, Sherman AL, Bruehl S, et al. Functional abdominal pain patient subtypes in childhood predict functional gastrointestinal disorders with chronic pain and psychiatric comorbidities in adolescence and adulthood. *Pain.* 2012;153(9):1798-1806.

referred to chronic pain providers. In a 2004 review, 43% of patients with chronic abdominal wall pain syndromes were eventually referred by gastroenterologists to chronic pain providers for continued management.[20] Patients with a well-defined underlying malignancy involving the solid organs or viscera could potentially benefit from referral for palliation. For example, a patient experiencing severe chronic abdominal pain as a result of a pancreatic adenocarcinoma could potentially benefit from a transaortic celiac plexus block.

Although the risks and benefits of the procedures will be discussed with the patient by the proceduralist, the primary physician should be aware of the most common and significant complications related to each intervention. Interventional pain management for refractory abdominal pain (typically due to malignancy) may include a celiac plexus (upper abdomen), ganglion impar (perineum), or a superior hypogastric plexus block (intra-abdominal). Any procedure involving needle manipulation has the potential for pain, bleeding, infection, and inadvertent intravascular access and injury to visceral organs, bowel, and nerves. When the procedure involves injection of local anesthetic(s) or neurolytic agents, the risk involves potential allergic reactions, nerve injury, tissue damage, arrhythmias, and even cardiac arrest if administered intravenously. Potentially life-threatening risks from the celiac block, in particular, also include hemorrhage from arterial or venous puncture and pneumothorax.

QUESTIONS

1. A 25-year-old man presents to your office with a chief complaint of abdominal pain lasting 6 months, accompanied with cyclical vomiting, temporarily relieved by hot showers. While providing the history, the patient is otherwise well-appearing. The intake vitals are within baseline. No medical records are available for review. Focused history-taking in which of the following is most likely to yield the diagnosis?

   A. Substance abuse history
   B. Surgical history
   C. Psychiatric history
   D. Family history

   A is the correct answer. The most likely diagnosis is cannaboid hyperemesis syndrome related to long-term heavy marijuana use. Patients classically report temporary relief with heat, hot showers, and baths. No diagnostic test is available and the history is made based on history and physical examination findings.

2. A 32-year-old sexually active woman scheduled for an office visit for abdominal pain suddenly becomes pale-appearing and complains of light-headedness while sitting in your waiting room. Medical transport is en-route and the local emergency department has been notified. Which of the following diagnosis is LEAST likely?

   A. Ruptured ectopic pregnancy
   B. Ruptured appendicitis with possible abscess formation
   C. Pyelonephritis progressing to septic shock
   D. Dissected abdominal aortic aneurysm

   D is the correct answer. All of the above are possible and considered life-threatening in nature. However, given the patient's age, a dissected abdominal aortic aneurysm alone is rare within the stated age group. Sexually active women of reproductive age are at the highest risk of developing an ectopic pregnancy. Additionally, women are at higher risk of developing pyelonephritis as a result of the anatomically shortened urethral length and predisposition to genitourinary flora changes.

3. Which of the following is the most likely cause of chronic abdominal pain in a long-time diabetic patient?

   A. Gastroparesis
   B. Thoracic polyradiculopathy
   C. Visceral polyradiculopathy
   D. Chronic pancreatic dysfunction

   A is the correct answer. Gastroparesis is common among diabetics, affecting approximately half of patients. With decreased gastric motility, patients are at higher risk of developing gastroesophageal reflux disease (GERD). Neuropathic pain affects approximately a quarter of diabetics, developing later in the course of the disease. Chronic pancreatic dysfunction can occur in poorly controlled diabetics and is unlikely to be a common cause of abdominal pain.

4. Which of the following conditions is MOST likely to coexist celiac disease and predispose patients to developing chronic abdominal pain?

   A. Chronic pancreatic insufficiency
   B. Gastroesophageal reflux disease
   C. Sphincter of Oddi dysfunction
   D. Small bowel dysmotility

   B is the correct answer. GERD is present in approximately 17% of patients with celiac disease. Chronic pancreatic insufficiency is more commonly seen in patients with cystic fibrosis, not celiac disease. Sphincture of Oddi and small bowel dysmotility are not features typically associated with celiac disease.

5. A 43-year-old man with irritable bowel syndrome with anxiety and depression returns to your clinic for a 3-week follow-up since starting fluoxetine 10 mg PO daily. The patient reports being compliant with the medication without any significant side effects thus far; however, his gastrointestinal symptoms persist, worsening his underlying anxiety. What would be the most effective step in management?

   A. Reassurance; no changes in fluoxetine dose
   B. Increase the fluoxetine dose to 20 mg PO daily and follow up in 3 weeks
   B. Start alprazolam 0.5 mg PO twice daily as needed and follow up in 1 week
   B. Discontinue fluoxetine and start a tricyclic antidepressant

   C is the correct answer. Recall that abdominal pain syndromes often coexist with psychiatric disorders, which also require medical management. Simple reassurance would not be appropriate, as it appears that the patient's underlying anxiety has not been treated and affects the patient's quality of life. Patients should also be informed that SSRIs (selective serotonin reuptake inhibitors) may take between 4 and 6 weeks before beneficial effects are experienced. Therefore, changes to dosages and discontinuation should not be made prematurely, unless there are significant side effects. It would be appropriate to start a short-term low-dose benzodiazepine for anxiolysis.

6. The same patient reports undesirable sexual side effects and wishes to discontinue fluoxetine. You discuss the risk and benefits of starting a tricyclic antidepressant, amitriptyline. Which of the following is the most appropriate initial test to order?

   A. 12-lead electrocardiography
   B. Serum transaminases
   C. Serum metabolic panel
   D. Complete blood count
   E. Transthoracic echocardiography
   F. PT/INR

   A is the correct answer. Remember that tricyclic antidepressants can have significant adverse cardiac effects, notably QT prolongation. Additionally, preexisting arrhythmias and myocardial infarctions are contraindications to amitriptyline. A baseline ECG is the most important initial test to obtain from list before initiating amitriptyline.

7. A 27-year-old woman with endometriosis status-post laparoscopic hysterectomy returns to your clinic with abdominal pain unrelieved by antiacids, nonsteroidal inflammatory analgesics, and conservative management. She denies other changes in her health and her bowel habits are within normal limits. You strongly suspect that she may be suffering from postsurgical adhesions. Which of the following statement is the least accurate?

   A. Over 50% of patients report significant sustained relief of pain after adhesiolysis.
   B. The risk of negative laparoscopy is approximately 20%.
   C. There is little evidence to support the routine use laparoscopy and adhesiolysis for chronic pain management.
   D. Approximately half of patients will require chronic pain management despite laparoscopic interventions.

   A is the correct answer. Risks and benefits of any intervention should always be discussed with the patient, including a negative diagnostic laparoscopy. The current medical literature demonstrates short-term pain relief with adhesiolysis in patients with positive findings on laparoscopy. The long-term benefits are not clear at this time. Larger series of studies reveals that regardless of the intervention, between 40 and 57% of patients will eventually be referred to chronic pain providers for management.

8. A 69-year-old man with Parkinson disease and chronic diabetes with abdominal pain due to severe gastroparesis would like to discuss possible pharmacologic agents that would improve gastric motility. Which of the following would be MOST appropriate as a promotility agent for diabetic gastroparesis?

   A. Metoclopramide
   B. Cisaperide
   C. Domperidone
   D. Erythryomycin

   C is the correct answer. Domperidone, a dopamine-agonist and promotility agent, would be the most appropriate in this case. Metoclopramide would be the least appropriate given its antidopaminergic activity. Cisaperide is currently not available in the United States because of the risk of QT prolongation and pro-arrhythmic effects. Erythromycin is an effect promotility agent, best delivered intravenously.

9. A 49-year-old previously healthy man presents with recurrent episodes of intermittent upper abdominal pain not associated with position. Previous workup for GERD returned negative. From your physical examination and history-taking, you narrow your diagnosis to pain of somatic origin. You order an abdominal CT scan for further evaluation of the ongoing pain. What is the most likely diagnosis?

continued

A. Ventral hernia
B. Chronic pancreatitis
C. Biliary dyskinesia
D. Peptic ulcer disease
E. Inguinal hernia
F. Superior mesenteric artery syndrome

A is the correct answer. The stem of the question hinted at a somatic source of pain, originating from the abdominal wall. The intermittent nature of the pain suggests a process involving the upper abdominal wall. The only diagnosis fitting of this pattern would be a ventral hernia that could be seen by CT imaging.

10. A 31-year-old woman returns to your office with unimproved localized abdominal pain without any other associated symptoms. The patient appears worried and reports that she recently read an article online about "peritoneal carcinomatosis." Your physical examination reveals multiple, discrete points on the abdominal exam where, when pressure was applied, the patient reported sensitivity and pain. The pain is reproducible. Which of the following interventions would most be appropriate?

A. Order a CT abdomen to evaluate for intra-abdominal processes and reassure the patient
B. Trial of local anesthetic injections
C. Ultrasound of the tender points to rule out peritoneal lesions
D. Trial of simethicone and probiotics, and discuss starting an antidepressant if symptoms are not improved
E. Discuss the risks and benefits of a celiac plexus block for analgesia
F. Order a complete blood count, metabolic panel, liver panel, CA 19-9, and consider a gastroenterology referral based on the results
G. Reassure the patient that your findings are normal and return to follow-up in 1 to 2 weeks

B is the correct answer. The patient most likely has myofascial pain, as evidenced by the multiple tender points that are reproducible with palpation. A trial of local anesthetic injections can be performed safely in the office setting, and also prove to be helpful in ruling in or out a diagnosis. Despite the patient's concern, an objective evaluation should be made by the physician without proceeding toward potentially expensive and low-yield diagnostic tests.

REFERENCES

1. Task Force on Taxonomy of the International Association for the Study of Pain. Merskey H, Bogduk N, eds. *Classification of Chronic Pain Descriptions of Chronic Pain Syndromes and Definitions of Pain Terms*. 2nd ed. Seattle: IASP Press; 2002.

2. Sengupta JN. Visceral pain: the neurophysiological mechanism. *Handb Exp Pharmacol*. 2009;(194):31-74. doi:10.1007/978-3-540-79090-7_2.

3. Bhuiya FA, Pitts SR, McCaig LF; Division of Health Care Statistics. *Emergency Department Visits for Chest Pain and Abdominal Pain: United States, 1999–2008*. NCHS Data Brief No. 43; 2010.

4. Hing E, Rui P, Palso K. National Ambulatory Medical Care Survey: 2013 State and National Summary Tables. Available from: http://www.cdc.gov/nchs/ahcd/ahcd_products.htm.

5. Alsulaimy M, Punchai S, Ali FA, et al. The utility of diagnostic laparoscopy in post-bariatric surgery patients with chronic abdominal pain of unknown etiology. *Obes Surg*. 2017;27(8):1924-1928. doi:10.1007/s11695-017-2590-0.

6. Rindos NB, Mansuria S. Diagnosis and management of abdominal wall endometriosis: a systematic review and clinical recommendations. *Obstet Gynecol Surv*. 2017;72(2):116-122. doi:10.1097/OGX.0000000000000399.

7. Huguet A, Olthuis J, McGrath PJ, et al. Systematic review of childhood and adolescent risk and prognostic factors for persistent abdominal pain. *Acta Paediatr*. 2017;106(4):545-553.

8. Olympia RP, Wilkinson R, Dunnick J, Dougherty BJ, Zauner D. Pediatric referrals to an emergency department from urgent care centers. *Pediatr Emerg Care*. 2016. [Epub ahead of print].

9. Pant C, Deshpande A, Sferra TJ, Olyaee M. Emergency department visits related to functional abdominal pain in the pediatric age group. *J Investig Med*. 2017;65(4):803-806. doi:10.1136/jim-2016-000300.

10. Friedrichsdorf SJ, Giordano J, Desai Dakoji K, Warmuth A, Daughtry C, Schulz CA. Chronic pain in children and adolescents: diagnosis and treatment of primary pain disorders in head, abdomen, muscles and joints. *Children (Basel)*. 2016;3(4):E42.

11. Roth-Isigkeit A, Thyen U, Stöven H, Schwarzenberger J, Schmucker P. Pain among children and adolescents: restrictions in daily living and triggering factors. *Pediatrics*. 2005;115(2):e152-e162.

12. Zook HG, Kharbanda AB, Flood A, Harmon B, Puumala SE, Payne NR. Racial differences in pediatric emergency department triage scores. *J Emerg Med*. 2016;50(5):720-727. doi:10.1016/j.jemermed.2015.02.056.

13. Malaty HM, Abudayyeh S, O'Malley KJ, et al. Development of a multidimensional measure for recurrent abdominal pain in children: population-based studies in three settings. *Pediatrics*. 2005;115(2):e210-e215.

14. Malaty HM, O'Malley KJ, Abudayyeh S, Graham DY, Gilger MA. Multidimensional measure for gastroesophageal reflux disease (MM-GERD) symptoms in children: a population-based study. *Acta Paediatr.* 2008;97(9):1292-1297. doi:10.1111/j.1651-2227.2008.00866.x.

15. Stanghellini V, Chan FK, Hasler WL, et al. Gastroduodenal disorders. *Gastroenterology.* 2016;150(6):1380-1392. doi:10.1053/j.gastro.2016.02.011.

16. Abbott RA, Martin AE, Newlove-Delgado TV, et al. Psychosocial interventions for recurrent abdominal pain in childhood (Protocol). *Cochrane Database Syst Rev.* 2017;1.

17. Eccleston C, Palermo TM, Williams AC, et al. Psychological therapies for the management of chronic and recurrent pain in children and adolescents. *Cochrane Database Syst Rev.* 2014;(5):CD003968. doi:10.1002/14651858.

18. Shelby GD, Shirkey KC, Sherman AL, et al. Functional abdominal pain in childhood and long-term vulnerability to anxiety disorders. *Pediatrics.* 2013;132(3):475-482. doi:10.1542/peds.2012-2191.

19. Russell AC, Stone AL, Walker LS. Nausea in children with functional abdominal pain predicts poor health outcomes in young adulthood. *Clin Gastroenterol Hepatol.* 2017;15(5):706-711. doi:10.1016/j.cgh.2016.07.006.

20. Costanza CD, Longstreth GF, Liu AL. Chronic abdominal wall pain: clinical features, health care costs, and long-term outcome. *Clin Gastroenterol Hepatol.* 2004;2:395-399.

19

LUMBAR SPINE

Morgan O'Connor, MD, Charles De Mesa, DO, MPH and Samir J. Sheth, MD

FAST FACTS

- Lower back pain is common with ~80% of the population having lower back pain at some point in their life.
- Most complaints of lower back pain are self-limiting and will resolve without intervention or imaging.
- Consideration of, and screening for, red flags is crucial for early identification and management of more serious diagnoses of lower back pain.
- Success of therapeutic procedures and surgeries relies heavily on appropriate patient identification/selection.

INTRODUCTION

Lower back pain is a common diagnosis with an estimated 80% of people having at least 1 episode of low back pain during their lifetime.[1] Furthermore, lower back is the fifth most common reason for all physician visits in the United States.[2] To define the scope of this chapter, lower back pain will be described as the perception of pain within the vertebrae, joints, tendons, and ligaments of the lumbosacral spine as well as the muscles, subcutaneous tissue, and skin overlying this region. Most patients (~85%) who present to primary care with a chief complaint of lower back pain have symptoms that cannot be reliably attributed to a specific disease or anatomic abnormality (thus termed nonspecific low-back pain),[3] and most patients recover without significant medical intervention within a few weeks.[4]

HISTORY

As with all musculoskeletal complaints it is important to include in the location, duration, details of any prior back pain, severity of the pain and any palliative or provocative features. Although the majority of patients presenting to primary care with a chief complaint of lower back pain will not have a serious condition, it is important to ensure consideration of more concerning causes in your evaluation. For example, pain that fails to improve with 1 month of therapy, unexplained weight loss, and previous history of cancer are associated with high specificity (90%) for cancer.[5] In patient with a history of cancer, sudden onset, severe pain should raise concern for a pathologic fracture. Spinal infections such as vertebral osteomyelitis or epidural abscess are modestly associated with a history of intravenous drug use or urinary tract or skin infections (sensitivity of 40%)[6] and may have associated symptoms such as fever and malaise. Other concerning findings by history include diminished sensation, weakness, and/or bowel/bladder incontinence, as these raise the threshold of suspicion for neurologic injury such as an acute radiculopathy or cauda equina syndrome. Bladder incontinence, in particular, is very sensitive for the detection of cauda equina syndrome (90%).[7]

MECHANISM/TIMING OF INJURY

The mechanism of injury for lower back pain can provide insight into possible pain generators in lower back pain. Acute pain after a lifting injury may indicate a soft tissue sprain or strain or possibly an acute disc herniation. An elderly/osteoporotic individual reporting acute-onset back pain after a bumpy car ride, coughing/sneezing, or mild trauma would be concerning for vertebral compression fracture. Conversely, chronic lower back pain in overweight individuals who spend most of their time at work sitting with poor posture may indicate discogenic pain (see Table 19-1).

LOCATION

Pain location and radiation characteristics may help in making an accurate diagnosis (Figure 19-1). Patients with lumbosacral spondylosis (zygapophysial or facet joint arthropathy) may report a deep achy pain radiating in a band across the lower back and/or radiation into the buttock or thigh, with radiation below the knee being rare.[8]

TABLE 19-1 Possible Lower Back Pain Diagnoses Based on Timing/Onset of Pain

ACUTE	INSIDIOUS	CHRONIC
Vertebral fracture		Vertebral fracture
• Compression • Traumatic • Pathologic		• Compression
Myofascial/ ligamentous	Myofascial/ ligamentous	Myofascial/ ligamentous
• Muscle strain • Muscle spasm • Ligamentous sprain	• Myofascial pain/ trigger points	• Myofascial pain/ trigger points
Infectious	Infectious	Infectious
• Vertebral osteomyelitis • Discitis • Epidural abscess	• Vertebral osteomyelitis • Discitis • Epidural abscess	• Vertebral osteomyelitis • Discitis
Intervertebral disc	Intervertebral disc	Intervertebral disc
• Herniation/ extrusion	• Degenerative disc disease	• Degenerative disc disease
Facet joint	Facet joint	Facet joint
• Dislocation, traumatic	• Arthropathy	• Arthropathy
Sacroiliac joint	Sacroiliac joint	Sacroiliac joint
• Dislocation, traumatic • Ligamentous sprain	• Inflammatory (sacroiliitis) • Arthropathy • Ligamentous sprain	• Inflammatory (sacroiliitis) • Arthropathy • Ligamentous sprain
Neurologic	Neurologic	Neurologic
• Lumbosacral radiculopathy • Cauda equina syndrome	• Lumbosacral radiculopathy • Spinal stenosis • Cauda equina syndrome	• Lumbosacral radiculopathy • Spinal stenosis • Cauda equina syndrome

Sacroiliac joint pain, a common source of nonradicular axial back pain, tends to be located at the lumbosacral-gluteal junction with referral into the ipsilateral lower extremity and/or groin. In general, sacroiliac joint pain causes pain at and below the waistline, whereas those with lumbar facet arthropathy will tend to localize their pain at and above the waistline.

Lumbar or sacral radicular pain is described as sharp/shooting/lancinating pain felt both superficially and deep that radiates down the leg.[9] In the absence of objective neurologic deficits this pain is called radiculitis. Radicular pain may occur secondary to mechanical factors causing impingement upon a nerve root (such as neural foraminal stenosis or a disc bulge) or owing to chemical irritation secondary to exposure of the nerve roots to herniated nucleus pulposus (which is enzymatically active and irritating to the nerve roots). This pain, with the possible exception of the S1 nerve root, does not reliably follow a specific dermatomal pattern when patients describe their symptoms.[10] Conversely, a lumbar or sacral radiculopathy is characterized by objective signs of neurologic deficits such as diminished sensation, strength, or reflexes in a dermatomal and/or myotomal pattern congruent with a nerve root distribution.

In any complaint of lower back pain, it is important to evaluate for any objective findings of neurologic deficit with examination of strength, sensation, and reflexes in the lower extremities. This can be accomplished efficiently but thoroughly with an understanding of lumbosacral dermatomes, myotomes, and reflexes. A sufficient examination for screening strength would include assessment of hip flexion (L2), knee extension (L3), ankle dorsiflexion (L4), great toe extension (extensor hallucis longus, L5), and ankle plantar flexion (S1). A screening sensory examination should include the L2-S2 dermatomes (see Figure 19-2 for reference). Reflex examination should include patellar reflexes (primarily L4), medial hamstring reflexes (L5), and Achilles reflexes (S1), with particular attention being paid to asymmetry from side to side. In addition, assessment for upper motor neuron signs in the lower extremity should be included, as injury at/above the level of the conus medullaris (generally ~L1) may cause an up going great toe on plantar response (Babinski sign) and/or clonus on ankle jerk.

Pain primarily located in the soft tissues of the lower back/buttock region may represent myofascial pain. This is conventionally defined as regional pain originating from exquisitely tender taut bands of muscle (trigger points) and may exist in isolation or as a response to postural or muscular accommodations for an underlying anatomic process such as degenerative disc disease, lumbar facet arthropathy, or scoliosis.[11]

Alleviating and Exacerbating Factors

Identification of movements and positions that exacerbate or alleviate pain can provide clues for diagnosing and treating lower back pain (see Table 19-2). For example, the zygapophyseal (facet) joints are synovial joints and, like other arthritic joints, pain may

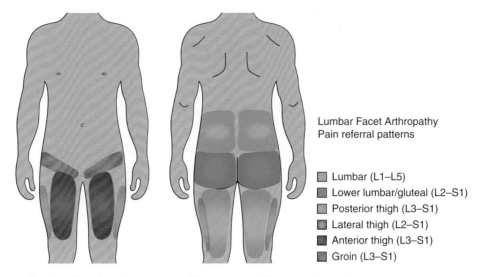

FIGURE 19-1 Generalized pain referral patterns of lumbosacral facet arthropathy.

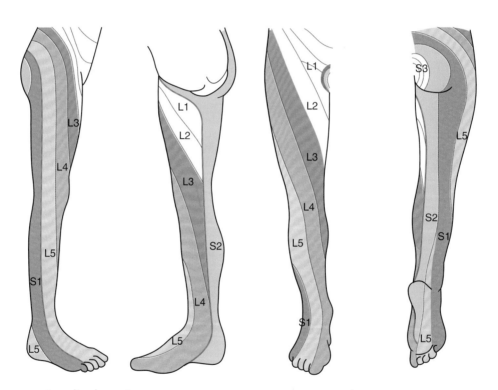

FIGURE 19-2 Lower extremity dermatomes.

be exacerbated with joint loading. Lumbar extension loads these zygapophyseal joints and causes an exacerbation of pain.[12]

Discogenic pain, or rather pain secondary to disc degeneration/annular derangement is often characterized as a dull midline pain or feeling of instability that may radiate to the buttocks; however, as compared with zygapophyseal joint pain, discogenic pain tends to be exacerbated by forward flexion of the lumbar spine or postures/positioning that can increase intradiscal pressures (such as sitting). This is due to the degenerative changes of the disc causing abnormal motion provoking

mechanical stimulus of local nociceptors[13] or disruption of the inner portions of the anulus fibrosus allowing the neuroirritating nucleus pulposus access to the outer one-third of the anulus fibrosus, which is innervated by the sinuvertebral nerves (Figure 19-3).

Lumbar spinal stenosis may also be described as a dull lower back pain with some degree of radiation to the sides or buttocks; however, unlike most other types of back pain, spinal stenosis tends to be exacerbated by standing and improved with sitting. Furthermore, a key feature of lumbar spinal stenosis is neurogenic claudication. Like vascular claudication, neurogenic claudication

TABLE 19-2 Suspected Lower Back Pain Diagnoses Based on Alleviating Versus Exacerbating Factors

DIAGNOSIS	ALLEVIATING FACTORS	EXACERBATING FACTORS
Lumbar spondylosis (facet arthropathy)	Changing positions, rest	Lumbar extension biased postures (such as standing)
Lumbar discogenic pain	Lying supine with legs elevated/supported	Lifting, coughing, Valsalva, lumbar flexion biased postures (such as sitting)
Lumbar radicular pain	Rest, lying supine with or without knees flexed	Increased neural tension (postures with increased lumbar or hip flexion with straight leg). Lifting, coughing, sneezing, Valsalva
Lumbar spinal stenosis	Sitting, spinal flexion	Walking, spinal extension
Sacroiliac joint pain	Unloading affected side	Prolonged sitting, forward flexion of the trunk/hip, transitional activities (i.e., sit to stand)
Myofascial pain	Gentle stretching of affected soft tissues, changing positions	Rapid activation or stretching of affected soft tissues, being in a single position for a prolonged time

is a progressively worsening aching/fatigued sensation in the legs (anterior thigh or calves being the most common) with standing and walking. In contrast to vascular claudication, the lower extremity discomfort in lumbar spinal stenosis is often eased by forward flexion of the trunk.[14] A common description that patients may provide is that they find themselves leaning over handle of a shopping cart as it eases their pain, a so-called shopping cart sign.

Although uncommon, vascular causes of lower back pain are important to be cognizant of and consider in your differential diagnosis in individuals with risk factors (such as obesity, diabetes mellitus, hypertension, hyperlipidemia, smoking). These vascular causes include peripheral arterial disease that may manifest as axial lower back pain with radiation into the lower extremities with exacerbation by activity with claudication symptoms as discussed earlier.[15]

Physical examination of these patients may be notable for absence of local lower back symptoms such as tenderness to palpation or exacerbation with flexion/extension and positive for decreased peripheral pulses or color/temperature changes in the lower extremities.

Another vascular cause of lower back pain that is critical to recognize is an arterial aneurysm (such as that of the abdominal aorta or iliac arteries). A patient with an abdominal aortic aneurysm may complain of vague abdominal or lower back pain that is described as deep/throbbing/pulsing and difficulty finding a comfortable position. Physical examination may be notable for a pulsating abdominal mass.[16] If patients complain of acute/tearing pain or hypotension is present, they should be taken immediately to an emergency room; otherwise the patient should be evaluated with an abdominal ultrasound and referred to vascular surgery.

Neurologic Symptoms

When evaluating a patient for a complaint of back pain, it is important to assess for symptoms or examination findings that might suggest neurologic injury. This includes both subjective symptoms of numbness, weakness, and tingling as well as objective findings on a thorough neurologic examination that includes manual motor testing, dermatomal sensory examination, and reflex testing. As the spinal cord generally transitions into the cauda equina at the level of the first lumbar vertebrae if a neurologic injury is present, it will most commonly follow a lower motor neuron pattern with some constellation of decreased strength, sensation, and diminished reflexes. If upper motor neuron signs such as increased reflexes or spasticity are present, it would raise concern for a pathologic process at/above the level of the conus medullaris.

In addition to the sensorimotor symptoms discussed earlier, it is also important to assess for any symptoms of neurogenic bowel or bladder. These symptoms may be either urine/fecal retention or incontinence and could indicate spinal cord, nerve/nerve root, or lumbosacral plexus compression/injury and need to be thoroughly investigated if present.

Associated Symptoms

Some extra-axial conditions may also cause pathologic changes in lumbar spine leading to back pain. For example, some estimated 5% to 36% of individuals with psoriatic arthritis develop axial symptoms. Axial back pain secondary to psoriatic arthritis can be variable with similarly variable radiographic changes. This radiographic variability can be beneficial, as it often does not follow a distinct caudocranial progression that is seen in ankylosing spondylitis.[17] Rheumatoid arthritis is another inflammatory arthropathy generally known for peripheral findings that may also cause axial lower back pain. The prevalence of chronic lower back pain in individuals with rheumatoid arthritis is slightly higher than in the general population (ranging from 19% to 40%)[18]; however, the lower back pain associated with rheumatoid arthritis tends to be milder than that from other spondyloarthropathies, with patients with rheumatoid arthritis reporting less pain and fatigue.[19]

Ankylosing spondylitis is another inflammatory disorder that can lead to bony fusion of vertebral joints causing pain, stiffness, and restricted range of motion. Although ankylosing spondylitis is an uncommon cause

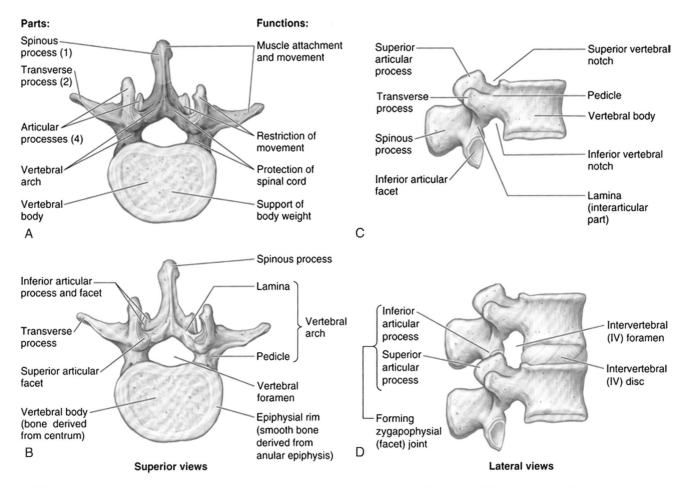

FIGURE 19-3 Lumbar anatomy. Reprinted with permission from Moore KL, Agur AMR, Dalley AF. *Clinically Oriented Anatomy.* 7th ed. Philadelphia, PA: Lippincott Williams & Wilkins; 2013.

of lower back pain, consideration of this diagnosis should be given in a patient under the age of 45 years who has greater than 3 months of back pain. In this patient population, there should be additional evaluation for other symptoms such as heel pain, dactylitis, uveitis, or personal/family history of syndromes associated with HLA B27 positivity: inflammatory bowel diseases, psoriatic arthritis, ankylosing spondylitis, or reactive arthritis. Diagnosis can be established with evidence of sacroiliitis on plain radiograph; however, even if negative, consideration should be made for magnetic resonance imaging (MRI) to identify any active inflammatory lesions of the sacroiliac joints.[20]

Inflammatory bowel diseases (Crohn disease and ulcerative colitis) are also associated with ankylosing spondylitis and other forms of inflammatory spondyloarthropathies, with as many as 10% to 15% cases of inflammatory bowel disease complicated by a spondyloarthropathy. Furthermore, ileal inflammation that resembles an inflammatory bowel disease has been reported in as many as two-thirds of cases of spondyloarthropathy.[21] Given the earlier discussion it may be prudent to consider earlier imaging for diagnosis in individuals with a personal or family history of psoriasis, inflammatory bowel disease, or ankylosing spondylitis.

There is an interesting association between psychologic factors and lower back pain. It is not uncommon to find that individuals with depression and anxiety tend to report subjectively worse lower back pain and lower quality of life than similar patients without these conditions.[22] There is some evidence to suggest that not only mood contributes to subjective worsening of lower back pain but also chronic lower back pain may be a risk factor for the development of psychiatric disorders such as depression or anxiety.[23]

PHYSICAL EXAMINATION

The physical examination for lower back pain can be broken into subcomponents of inspection/observation, palpation, range of motion, sensorimotor/reflex testing, and provocative tests.

When inspecting the lower back, it is important to evaluate the patient from a posterior viewpoint where observation may be made regarding coronal symmetry (evaluation for scoliosis), bony deformity, muscular atrophy/imbalance, or significant hip height difference (sometimes this may be demonstrated by a slanted waist band/belt line). In addition, the patient should be observed from a lateral view where it may be easier to appreciate abnormalities in sagittal alignment such as exaggerated or diminished lumbar lordosis.

The palpatory examination for lower back pain should include palpation of the spinous processes and facet joints at each vertebral level assessing for discomfort or deformity as well as thorough palpation of the lumbar paraspinal and gluteal musculature again assessing for discomfort and trigger points. Additional structures that should be included in the palpatory examination of the lower back are the posterior superior iliac spines, sacroiliac joints, and the greater trochanters, as discomfort stemming from these areas are not uncommonly found in lower back pain and may help guide further evaluation/treatment.

When assessing range of motion of the lower back, it is important to assess not only how far the patient is able to move but also if/where they feel discomfort and what they feel limits them if a diminished range of motion is present. In general, range of motion should be assessed with forward flexion, extension, lateral flexion/bending to each side, and axial rotation. If patients report discomfort with forward flexion, it may be suggestive a myofascial cause, as this stretches the posterior musculature, or a discogenic cause, as this position increases intradiscal pressures. Discomfort with extension or oblique extension may be suggestive of facetogenic pain, as this position increases pressure through the facet joints.

A neurologic examination of the lower extremities is important to include in your evaluation of lower back pain, as abnormalities may be secondary to a lumbar or sacral radiculopathy. Manual muscle testing of the lower extremities should include hip flexion, knee extension/flexion, ankle dorsiflexion, great toe extension, and ankle plantar flexion, as this will evaluate the motor component of spinal nerves from L2-S1. Screening sensory testing should include light touch and/or pinprick sensation testing of dermatomes from L2-S2, as this will screen for the most common nerve roots involved in radiculopathy. Deep tendon reflex testing in the lower extremities should include the patella (primarily L4), medial hamstring (primarily L5), and Achilles (primarily S1). While performing these neurologic examinations it is important to compare with the contralateral side, as asymmetry may be indicative of a radiculopathy.

Provocative tests employed during the lower back examination may be tailored based on clinical history, available imaging, and the results of the above examination maneuvers. If concerned for radicular pain, then tests of neural tension, such as a straight leg raise, crossed straight leg raise, or seated slump test, may be employed. The straight leg raise test is performed by having the patient supine on the examination table while the examiner passively raises the patient's leg while keeping the knee fully extended. The seated slump test has the patient positioned in a seated position on the examination table then assume a forward slumping posture by forward flexing the neck and upper back (exaggerating kyphosis), then the examiner gently lifts the patient's lower leg so that the knee moves into extension. If the patient's radicular symptoms radiate to the groin or thigh rather than to the lower leg, then inclusion of a reverse straight leg test may be appropriate to evaluate for nerve impingement in the upper lumbar region. To perform a reverse straight leg test, the patient is placed in a prone position on the examination table, then the examiner lifts the patient's leg creating hip extension while keeping the knee straight.

If evaluating for facet arthropathy, then use of maneuvers that stress these joints can be helpful if the patient's pain is replicated. One maneuver is an assessment of oblique extension (also described as extension and rotation or Kemp/lumbar quadrant test). This maneuver is performed by having the patient standing and facing away from the examiner. The examiner assists the patient into full lumbar extension; then, while still in extension, the examiner aides the patient in axially rotating so that they end in an oblique extension position. Another maneuver that may be employed is Yeoman test, which, although classically used to evaluate for sacroiliac joint pain, may be helpful in diagnosing lumbar facetogenic pain if the patient reports pain in the lumbar rather than in the sacroiliac joint region. To perform the Yeoman test, the patient is placed supine on the table; then the examiner flexes the patient's knee to 90° and lifts the leg moving the hip into extension. Pain in the lumbar region may be indicative of facet-mediated pain, whereas pain in the sacroiliac joint region may increase your suspicion for the sacroiliac joint as the pain generator.

There are numerous tests that can be used for the assessment of the sacroiliac joint as the source of the patient's pain, including Yeoman test, FABER (Flexion, Abduction, External Rotation), sacral distraction, sacral compression, thigh thrust, and sacral thrust tests. The FABER test, also known as Patrick test, begins with the patient in supine position. The examiner then asks the patient to make a figure 4 position with the leg, which essentially provides flexion, abduction, and external rotation of the tested leg. The examiner then places downward pressure on the knee of the tested leg while stabilizing the anterior superior iliac spine on the nontested side. To perform the sacroiliac distraction test, the patient is placed in a supine position and the examiner places his/her hands on the patient's anterior superior iliac spine and applies a steady force. The sacral compression test is performed with the patient in a side-lying position, and the examiner places his/her hands over the iliac crest and applies a downward pressure. The thigh thrust test is performed by starting with the patient in the supine position, and the leg of the side to be tested is placed in 90° of hip flexion. The examiner places one hand underneath the patient's sacrum for stabilization while an axial force is applied through the femur toward the examination table. The final sacroiliac joint maneuver we will describe is the sacral thrust test. For this maneuver, the patient is placed in a prone position and the examiner applies a downward force through the patient's sacrum. As some of these maneuvers can be uncomfortable, in general, it is important to ask the patient if the maneuver is reproducing their typical pain to avoid false positive. When evaluating the sacroiliac joint as the source of the patient's pain, it is important to note that, to achieve adequate specificity, you have at least 3 positive sacroiliac joint maneuvers.[24,25]

Diagnostic Studies and Therapeutic Interventions

If possible, it is helpful to evaluate a patient's prior diagnostic studies and therapeutic interventions, as these may guide your treatment plan and, possibly, spare the patient the expense of potentially unneeded repetition. Review of prior x-ray/MRI imaging and electrodiagnostic studies may help narrow your differential diagnosis and guide your diagnostic and treatment plan. A large proportion of individuals will have abnormalities on imaging but be asymptomatic. For example, an estimated 37% of 20-year-olds and 97% of 80-year-olds have asymptomatic disc degeneration[26]. For this reason, it is important to correlate a patient's symptoms with the imaging findings to provide appropriate treatment.

Evaluation of prior treatments may be helpful in guiding your treatment plan. It is important to understand response to prior medications (both oral and topical), therapies, procedures, surgeries, and alternative treatments such as chiropractic adjustment, massage therapy, and acupuncture. If a particular treatment was not effective, it is important to know what that treatment consisted of before eliminating it as a possible management strategy. For example, physical therapy may "fail" if an incorrect diagnosis was previously made and the treatment did not address the likely pathology. Alternatively, the patient's pain may have been significantly worse acutely, thus therapy was not tolerable at the time and with medication or procedural optimization the patient may be able to better participate.

Given that most episodes of lower back pain will resolve without the need for imaging or other diagnostics, the American Academy of Family Physicians recommendation is to not obtain imaging for lower back pain for the first 6 weeks unless red flags are present.[27] Red flags prompting the need for early imaging would be history or examination findings concerning for malignancy, infection, or progressive neurologic deficits. Initial imaging choice for back pain with suspicion for bony cause without neurologic involvement such as trauma or compression fracture, or spondylosis, should be standard anteroposterior and lateral lumbosacral plain radiography, as this is widely available and is low cost with subsequent follow-up with computed tomographic (CT) scan if indicated. If there is suspicion for ankylosing spondylitis, radiographs with the addition of angled views of the sacrum to assess the sacroiliac joints would be beneficial.[6] Symptoms of transient, position-based neurologic symptoms or radicular pain may be secondary to an unstable spondylolisthesis (translation of one vertebral segment as compared with another), and the addition of flexion and extension views would allow this to be identified.

Some less common causes of lower back pain may be readily identified on standard x-ray imaging. These include Baastrup disease (sometimes known as kissing spine syndrome) and Bertolotti syndrome. Baastrup disease refers to a close approximation of adjacent spinous processes leading to increased shearing forces and development of an adventitious bursitis (Figure 19-4). This generally occurs because of degenerative changes of the spine. This most commonly occurs in the lumbar spine with the L4-L5 level being the most likely to be affected. Pain secondary to Baastrup disease may be difficult to separate from that due to lumbar facet arthropathy, as both will be manifest as midline back pain with or without referral that is exacerbated by lumbar extension and alleviated by lumbar flexion. Furthermore, as the spinous processes come into approximation owing to degenerative changes it is not uncommon for facet arthropathy to be present. It is important to recognize this diagnosis, as it does allow for consideration of additional treatment

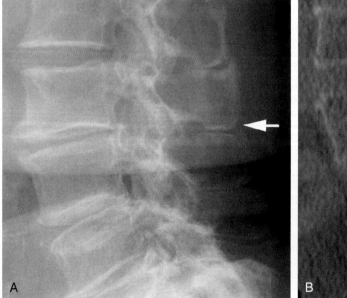
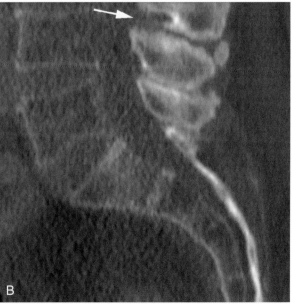

FIGURE 19-4 Baastrup disease (kissing spine syndrome). Reprined with permission from Chew FS. *Musculoskeletal Imaging: The Essentials*. 1st ed. Philadelphia: Wolters Kluwer; 2019.

strategies (such as injection or surgery) that differ from those that would be implemented for facet arthropathy alone.[28]

Lumbosacral transitional vertebrae (Bertolotti syndrome) may lead to altered biomechanical and degenerative changes that can cause lower back pain. A lumbosacral transitional vertebra is a congenital spinal abnormality in which there is a transitional vertebra that has resulted in varying degrees of fusion in the lumbosacral segment and represents a range from partial/complete L5 sacralization (yielding 4 lumbar vertebrae) to incomplete fusion of S1 to the sacrum (yielding 6 lumbar vertebrae) (Figure 19-5). These transitional vertebrae may have enlarged transverse processes and some degree of pseudoarticulation with the sacrum, which is susceptible to degeneration/arthritic changes and may become painful. These pseudoarticulations may be an incidental finding in your evaluation of lower back pain, and other potential explanations should be considered before attributing patient's symptoms exclusively to a transitional vertebral pseudarthrosis.

Advanced imaging for lower back pain (CT vs. MRI) as the initial imaging choice is indicated in cases in which a serious underlying pathology is suspected (such as cancer, infection, cauda equina syndrome, or other progressive neurologic symptoms). In addition, investigation with MRI is indicated in cases of radicular lower back pain or suspected stenosis with symptoms present for greater than 1 month.[29] CT scan is preferable for evaluation of bony anatomy (such as trauma patient in whom fracture is a concern); however, for evaluation of nonbony pathology MRI is generally the optimal imaging modality. For individuals with contraindication to MRI (generally owing to implanted device or similar) with suspected central canal or neuroforaminal stenosis one could consider CT myelogram; however, this is not entirely benign, as it does involve a lumbar puncture and thus carries risks such as infection, bleeding into the spinal canal, and postpuncture headache in addition to the radiation dose associated with the scan. If thought to be nonurgent, one could consider discussion with/referral to a spine specialist before obtaining a CT myelogram owing to these risks (see Table 19-3).

As discussed earlier, the majority of acute and subacute back pain complaints that present to a primary care clinic will be self-limited in nature. The 2017 American College of Physicians guidelines recommend initial management with noninvasive, nonpharmacologic treatment with modalities such as superficial heat, massage, and/or acupuncture.[31] If you desire to add pharmacologic management, the recommendation is to select nonsteroidal anti-inflammatories or skeletal muscle relaxants. For individuals with chronic lower back pain, it is also recommended to begin with nonpharmacologic treatment with modalities discussed earlier as well as exercise, rehabilitation, and mindfulness-based stress reduction strategies. If the above-mentioned strategies are not effective, then use pharmacologic management with nonsteroidal anti-inflammatory medications (first line) or tramadol/duloxetine as second-line therapy. Opioids should be reserved for recalcitrant pain and only initiated after

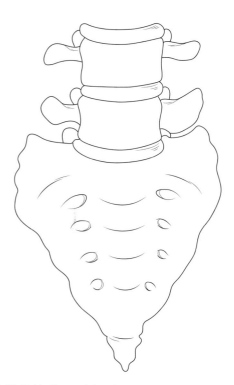

FIGURE 19-5 Unilateral lumbosacral transitional vertebrae with pseudarthrosis.

TABLE 19-3 Indications for Imaging in Lower Back Pain[30]	
X-RAY	**MRI**
• Trauma	• Suspected metastasis, tumor, osteomyelitis, discitis, or paraspinal abscess
• Presence of red flag symptoms (concern for fracture, infection, malignancy)	• Congenital/traumatic spinal deformities
• Clinical suspicion for ankylosing spondylitis or rheumatoid arthritis	• Severe pain
• Suspicion of spinal deformity	• Progressively severe symptoms or neurologic dysfunction
• Suspicion of instability (include flexion and extension views)	• Suspected cauda equina or conus medullaris compression
• Atypical presentation or history (such as prolonged corticosteroid use)	• Persistent radicular pain (~6-8 wk) that fails to improve with conservative management
	• Suspected vascular malformation
	• Compression fracture in elderly

carefully weighing the risks and potential functional benefits of opioid medications with discussion of expectations/realistic benefits with the patient.[31] For patients with a significant contribution from radicular-type pain consideration for use such as gabapentin or pregabalin is indicated. Some antidepressant medications (such as tricyclics and serotonin norepinephrine reuptake inhibitors) have also been found to have some benefit when treating neuropathic pain. Additional adjunctive measures that may provide some benefit include topical agents such as a methyl salicylate/menthol combination, lidocaine cream or patches, or use of a transcutaneous electrical nerve stimulation unit.

If your patient fails to improve with conservative measures as discussed earlier, it may be appropriate to consider referral for procedural or surgical intervention. Benefit from the procedure will depend greatly on making the correct diagnosis and addressing the appropriate anatomy.

For pain that is felt to primarily be derived from the zygapophyseal joints procedural interventions include intraarticular corticosteroid of the zygapophyseal joints directly or by disrupting the innervation of these joints. Initially, this would be accomplished by injecting local anesthetic in the area where the median branches of the nerves that supply the suspected joints generally are found (a medial branch block). As might be expected, this injection provides only temporary relief; however, if adequate improvement is made, then pursuit of an ablation of these nerves may be considered (radiofrequency ablation). Even though the nerve has ablated, the symptoms may return as the nerve regrows and restores innervation to the painful joint. For pain that is secondary to central canal stenosis or radicular in character, an epidural steroid injection may be considered. The route of injection (interlaminar, transforaminal, or caudal) is variable and will depend on your patient characteristics and clinical judgment of the pain medicine provider. Other, more invasive procedures that a pain medicine provider may consider for your patient include placement of an intrathecal pain pump or spinal cord stimulator unit. Given that these procedures require an implant of a device or leads and are more invasive than injection procedures

listed earlier these are generally reserved for pain that cannot be resolved through other measures. It is important to recognize that the above-mentioned procedures do not alter the underlying anatomy that is causing the patient discomfort and that use of therapy for stretching, strengthening, and biomechanical education will likely extend the benefit of these procedures. These pain procedures are described in more detail in other chapters.

Similar to injection-based procedures, the surgical options and the results of such for lower back pain vary depending on the underlying anatomic diagnosis. In the absence of progressive neurologic deficits, careful consideration should be made before surgical referral. As with procedural interventions, outcomes with surgery depend on careful patient selection. Generally, for chronic nonradicular back pain secondary to zygapophyseal or intervertebral disc degenerative changes, surgical results tend to be similar to that of an intensive rehabilitation program.[32] For patients with subacute radiculopathy secondary to a herniated lumbar disc, an open or minimally invasive microdiscectomy procedure likely offers symptomatic improvement short-term benefit as compared with nonoperative treatment.[33,34] In addition, those who do receive surgery may have greater improvement with long-term follow-up.[34-36] For symptomatic spinal stenosis, a decompressive surgery (that may also include fusion) is a viable treatment option that may provide greater improvement than nonsurgical management for patients with symptoms persisting for greater than 6 to 12 weeks.[37] This benefit, however, may equalize with nonoperative management long term.[38]

Lower back pain is a common complaint seen in primary care practices, and although most cases of lower back pain will be self-limited, it is important to evaluate for causes of lower back pain that may necessitate early imaging or referral. There are many treatment options available for lower back pain ranging from therapy to surgery, and it is important to understand the underlying pathology when selecting treatment so that the best option is chosen. See Table 19-4 for discussion of various diagnoses of back pain with common associated history/physical findings and recommended diagnostic/therapeutic considerations.

TABLE 19-4 Features, Diagnostics, Treatment, and Referral Recommendations for Various Causes of Lower Back Pain

DIAGNOSIS	HISTORY AND PHYSICAL	DIAGNOSTICS	TREATMENT	WHEN TO REFER
Myofascial pain	Pain/stiffness with prolonged positioning Tenderness to palpation of soft tissues often with taut bands of skeletal muscles ± muscle twitch and reproduction of referred pain	None initially. If refractory may consider screening laboratory evaluation for metabolic or rheumatologic cause: complete blood count (CBC), complete metabolic panel, thyroid stimulating hormone, creatine kinase (CK), 25-hydroxyvitamin D	Stretching, exercise, heat, ice, massage, acupuncture, physical therapy, NSAIDs, topicals (lidocaine, menthol, and/or salicylate based) If no improvement with above, consider trigger point injections or dry needling	Consider referral to rheumatology if suspicious for rheumatologic cause such as polymyalgia rheumatica or myositis

TABLE 19-4 Features, Diagnostics, Treatment, and Referral Recommendations for Various Causes of Lower Back Pain   (Continued)

DIAGNOSIS	HISTORY AND PHYSICAL	DIAGNOSTICS	TREATMENT	WHEN TO REFER
Lumbar facet arthropathy	Pain worse with standing more than sitting Reproduction of patient's pain with extension maneuvers	None initially If refractory, consider lumbar x-ray If considering a procedure, the interventionalist may request advanced imaging (usually MRI without contrast)	Stretching, exercise, heat, ice, massage, acupuncture, physical therapy, NSAIDs, topicals (lidocaine, menthol, and/or salicylate based) If no improvement with above, may consider intraarticular facet joint injection or lumbar medial branch blocks	Referral to pain management specialist for refractory pain with consideration for injection
Lumbar spondylolisthesis	If unstable may have positional-based radicular pain	X-ray with inclusion of lumbar flexion and extension views	Stretching, exercise, heat, ice, massage, acupuncture, physical therapy, NSAIDs, topicals (lidocaine, menthol, and/or salicylate based)	Referral to spine surgery if signs of myelopathy, severe/progressive radiculopathy, or instability on imaging
Sacroiliac joint pain	Pain with prolonged sitting, weight bearing through affected side Tenderness to palpation of posterior superior iliac spine and/or sacroiliac joint At least 3 positive provocative sacroiliac joint maneuvers	None initially unless concern for ankylosing spondylitis then consider lumbar x-rays with angled sacral views (if negative and still strongly suspicious, obtain MRI of lumbar spine with extension through sacroiliac joints) and obtain laboratory testing: erythrocyte sedimentation rate (ESR), C-reactive protein (CRP), alkaline phosphatase, CK, HLA-B27	Stretching, exercise, heat, ice, massage, acupuncture, physical therapy, NSAIDs, topicals (lidocaine, menthol, and/or salicylate based) If no improvement with above, consider sacroiliac joint steroid injection For severe pain refractory to injection patient may possibly benefit from sacroiliac joint fusion	Referral to pain management specialist for refractory pain for consideration of sacroiliac joint steroid injection Referral to rheumatology if imaging and/or laboratory findings concerning for ankylosing spondylitis
Degenerative disc disease (DDD) without neurologic involvement	Pain worse with sitting than standing, morning pain, pain worse with coughing, sneezing, lifting Pain worse with flexion	None initially If refractory may consider lumbar x-ray If considering a procedure, the interventionalist may request advanced imaging (usually MRI without contrast)	Stretching, heat, exercise, ice, massage, acupuncture, physical therapy, NSAIDs, topicals (lidocaine, menthol, and/or salicylate based) Typically, procedural intervention is not indicated for DDD without neurologic involvement; however, some providers may offer epidural steroid injection or lumbar fusion	Referral to pain management specialist for refractory pain may be considered
Lumbar radiculitis (secondary to disc bulge, disc herniation, or other cause of neural foraminal stenosis)	As above with addition of pain radiating into lower extremity (anterior thigh/groin for upper lumbar nerve root impingement, below the knee for lower lumbar nerve root impingement) without objective sensorimotor deficits Positive straight leg raise or seated slump for lower lumbar lesions Positive reverse straight leg raise for upper lumbar lesions	None initially If refractory, severe pain, OR onset of sensorimotor deficits, obtain lumbar MRI without contrast Could consider EMG; however, in presence of pain only this may be normal	Stretching, heat, exercise, ice, massage, acupuncture, physical therapy, NSAIDs For refractory or severe pain (that precludes participation in therapy/exercise) consider lumbar epidural steroid injection	Referral to management specialist for severe or refractory radicular pain Referral to spine surgeon for consideration of decompressive surgery if pain refractory to injection

TABLE 19-4 Features, Diagnostics, Treatment, and Referral Recommendations for Various Causes of Lower Back Pain (Continued)

DIAGNOSIS	HISTORY AND PHYSICAL	DIAGNOSTICS	TREATMENT	WHEN TO REFER
Lumbar radiculopathy (secondary to disc bulge, disc herniation, or other cause of neural foraminal stenosis)	May have subjective sensorimotor deficits (may describe difficulty going up stairs/catching toes or numbness/tingling in dermatomal distribution). Pain may or may not be present Abnormalities on strength, sensory, or reflex testing	If sensorimotor deficits are chronic and nonprogressive, imaging not necessary. EMG/NCS for localization If sensorimotor deficits are acute, progressive, or there is presence of other red flag symptoms (change in bowel/bladder function), obtain MRI. Depending on clinical scenario administration of IV contrast may be indicated: i.e., personal history of cancer, symptoms concerning for malignancy (unintentional weight loss, night sweats etc.), or history/examination findings concerning for spinal infection (hx IV drug use, fevers/chills, etc.)	If sensorimotor deficits are chronic and nonprogressive, then treatment may be conservative with stretching, heat, exercise, ice, massage, acupuncture, physical therapy, NSAIDs. If pain present and refractory to above, patient may benefit from epidural steroid injection If sensorimotor deficits are acute, progressive, or there is presence of red flag symptoms, then surgical intervention may be indicated	For chronic sensorimotor deficits with pain that is refractory to conservative treatment refer to pain management specialist for injection For acute/progressive neurologic deficits patient should be evaluated urgently by a spine surgeon
Cauda equina or conus medullaris syndrome	Lower extremity sensorimotor deficits, change in bowel/bladder function (incontinence or retention) Abnormalities on strength, sensory, or reflex testing. May have impaired rectal sensation/tone	Emergent lumbar MRI	Emergent surgical decompression	Patient should be sent to emergency department for facilitation of imaging and surgical intervention
Lumbar spinal stenosis	Bilateral claudicatory leg pain with ambulation/lumbar extension that improves upon sitting or with lumbar flexion (bending over shopping cart or a counter). May also have subjective and/or objective sensorimotor deficits	Lumbar MRI is beneficial for determining degree of spinal canal stenosis and procedural planning If unable to differentiate between neurogenic and vascular claudication (or presence of both) vascular studies (usually an ankle/brachial index) may help differentiate	Cardiovascular exercise (such as seated cycling), physical therapy, physical therapy, NSAIDs For severe symptoms or symptoms refractory to the above, patient may benefit from epidural steroid injection. May also consider surgical decompression	Referral to pain management specialist for consideration of injection Referral to spine surgeon for severe or refractory symptoms
Vertebral compression fracture	History of osteoporosis or risk factors for osteoporosis (elderly, history of chronic steroids, history of malignancy). Acute onset pain after coughing, sneezing, bumpy car ride, or other (potentially minor) trauma Bony tenderness to palpation	Lumbar x-ray. If concern for pathologic fracture or neurologic involvement obtain advanced imaging (MRI or CT)	Rest, ice, oral analgesic medications, lumbar brace, topicals (lidocaine, menthol, and/or salicylate based). If refractory to above, patient may derive pain relief with a bisphosphonate or calcitonin Severe, refractory pain may benefit from vertebroplasty or kyphoplasty	Referral to pain management specialist or spine surgeon if consideration for vertebroplasty/kyphoplasty

TABLE 19-4 Features, Diagnostics, Treatment, and Referral Recommendations for Various Causes of Lower Back Pain (Continued)

DIAGNOSIS	HISTORY AND PHYSICAL	DIAGNOSTICS	TREATMENT	WHEN TO REFER
Malignancy—primary or bony metastasis	History of cancer or red flag symptoms concerning for malignancy (failure of back pain to improve with conservative management, unintentional weight loss, night sweats, etc.) May or may not have significant bony tenderness on palpation	X-ray and advanced imaging (MRI or CT). CBC, alkaline phosphatase, and tumor-specific markers (such as prostate specific antigen) if clinically appropriate (i.e., history of prostate cancer)	Likely biopsy (by interventional radiology vs. open with spine surgery) Dependent on primary cancer and staging. For lumbar component treatment options may involve surgical resection, chemotherapy, or radiation therapy	Referral to hematology/oncology and possibly spine surgery or interventional radiology for biopsy
Lumbar infection (discitis/osteomyelitis or epidural abscess)	History of IV drug use, tuberculosis, skin, or urinary tract infection. Infectious symptoms (i.e., fevers, chills, weight loss) May have localized tenderness to palpation	MRI with contrast CBC, ESR, CRP, urinalysis, blood culture, basic metabolic panel (BMP) Biopsy or aspiration with culture	IV antibiotics—broad spectrum initially, narrow if able based on culture results Potentially surgery for source control	Referral to infectious disease physician for antibiotic therapy. Interventional radiology or spine surgery for biopsy and potentially spine surgery if other surgical intervention necessary

EMG, electromyography; IV, intravenous; MRI, magnetic resonance imaging; NASID, nonsteroidal anti-inflammatory drug; NCS, nerve conduction study.

REFERENCES

1. Hart LG, Deyo RA, Cherkin DC. Physician office visits for low back pain. Frequency, clinical evaluation, and treatment patterns from a U.S. national survey. *Spine.* 1995;20:11-19.
2. Deyo RA, Mirza SK, Martin BI. Back pain prevalence and visit rates: estimates from U.S. national surveys. *Spine.* 2002;2006(31):2724-2727.
3. van Tulder MW, Assendelft WJ, Koes BW, Bouter LM. Spinal radiographic findings and nonspecific low back pain. A systematic review of observational studies. *Spine (Phila Pa 1976).* 1997;22(4):427-434.
4. Maher C, Underwood M, Buchbinder R. Non-specific low back pain. *Lancet.* 2017;389(10070):736-747.
5. Deyo R, Diehl A. Cancer as a cause of back pain: frequency, clinical presentation, and diagnostic strategies. *J Gen Intern Med.* 1988;3(3):230-238.
6. Jarvik JG, Deyo RA. Diagnostic evaluation of low back pain with emphasis on imaging. *Ann Intern Med.* 2002;137:586-597.
7. Deyo RA Rainville J Kent DL What can the history and physical examination tell us about low back pain? *JAMA.* 1992;268:760-765.
8. Gellhorn AC, Katz JN, Suri P. Osteoarthritis of the spine: the facet joints. *Nat Rev Rheumatol.* 2013;9(4):216-224.
9. Govind J. Lumbar radicular pain. *Aust Fam Physician.* 2004;33(6):409-412.
10. Murphy DR, Hurwitz EL, Gerrard JK, Clary R. Pain patterns and descriptions in patients with radicular pain: Does the pain necessarily follow a specific dermatome? *Chiropr Osteopat.* 2009;17:9. doi:10.1186/1746-1340-17-9.
11. Saleet Jafri M. Mechanisms of myofascial pain. *Int Sch Res Notices.* 2014;2014:523924, 16 p. doi:10.1155/2014/523924.
12. Kalichman L, Hunter DJ. Lumbar facet joint osteoarthritis: a review. *Semin Arthritis Rheumatism,* 2007;37(2):69-80.
13. Brisby H. Pathology and possible mechanisms of nervous system response to disc degeneration. *J Bone Joint Surg Am.* 2006;88(suppl 2):68-71.
14. Genevay S, Atlas SJ. Lumbar spinal stenosis. *Best Pract Res Clin Rheumatol.* 2010;24(2):253-265.
15. Villacorta J, Kortebein P. Peripheral arterial disease masquerading as low back pain. *Am J Phys Med Rehabil.* 2012;(12):1104-1105.
16. Patel S, Kettner N. Abdominal aortic aneurysm presenting as back pain to a chiropractic clinic: a case report. *J Manipulative Physiol Ther.* 2006;29:409.e1-409.e7.
17. Cantini F, Niccoli L, Nannini C, Kaloudi O, Bertoni M, Cassara E. Psoriatic arthritis: a systemic review. *Int J Rheum Dis.* 2010;13(4):300-317.
18. Neva M, Hakkinen A, Isomaki P, Sokka T. Chronic back pain in patients with rheumatoid arthritis and in a control population: prevalence and disability–a 5-year follow-up. *Rheumatology.* 2011;50(9):1635-1639.
19. Michelsen B, Fiane R, Diamantopoulos AP, et al. A comparison of disease burden in rheumatoid arthritis, psoriatic arthritis and axial spondyloarthritis. *PLoS One.* 2015;10(4):e0123582.
20. Taurog J, Chhabra A, Colbert R. Ankylosing spondylitis and axial spondyloarthritis. *N Engl J Med.* 2016;374:2563-2574.
21. Colombo E, Latiano A, Palmieri O, Bossa F, Andriulli A, Annese V. Enteropathic spondyloarthropathy: a common genetic background with inflammatory bowel disease? *World J Gastroenterol WJG.* 2009;15(20):2456-2462.

22. Toshinaga T, Matsudaira K, Sato H, Vietri J. The impact of depression among chronic low back pain patients in Japan. *BMC Musculoskeletal Disorders.* 2016;17(1):447.

23. van't Land H, Verdurmen J, ten Have M, van Dorsselaer S, de Graaf R. The association between chronic back pain and psychiatric disorders; results from a longitudinal population-based study. In: Szirmai Ã, ed. *Anxiety and Related Disorders.* 2011. ISBN:978-953-307-254-8.

24. van der Wurff P, Buijs EJ, Groen GJ. A multitest regimen of pain provocation tests as an aid to reduce unnecessary minimally invasive sacroiliac joint procedures. *Arch Phys Med Rehabil.* 2006;87(1):10-14.

25. Laslett M Evidence-based diagnosis and treatment of the painful sacroiliac joint. *J Man Manip Ther.* 2008;16(3):142-152.

26. Brinjikji W, Luetmer PH, Comstock B, et al. Systematic literature review of imaging features of spinal degeneration in asymptomatic populations. *AJNR Am J Neuroradiol.* 2015;36(4):811-816.

27. Casazza BA. Diagnosis and treatment of acute low back pain. *Am Fam Physician.* 2012;85(4):343-350.

28. Filippiadis DK, Mazioti A, Argentos S, et al. Baastrup's disease (kissing spines syndrome): a pictorial review. *Insights Imaging.* 2015;6(1):123-128.

29. Chou R, Qaseem A, Snow V, et al. Diagnosis and treatment of low back pain: a joint clinical practice guideline from the American College of Physicians and the American Pain Society. *Ann Intern Med.* 2007;147:478-491.

30. Chou R, Qaseem A, Owens DK, Shekelle P. Diagnostic imaging for low back pain: advice for high-value health care from the American College of Physicians. *Ann Intern Med.* 2011;154(3):181-198.

31. Qaseem A, Wilt TJ, McLean RM, Forciea MA; for the Clinical Guidelines Committee of the American College of Physicians. Noninvasive treatments for acute, subacute, and chronic low back pain: a clinical practice guideline from the American College of Physicians. *Ann Intern Med.* 2017;166:514-530.

32. Chao R, Baisden J, Carragee EJ, Resnick DK, Shaffer WO, Loeser JD. Surgery for low back pain: a review of the evidence for an American Pain Society Clinical Practice Guideline. *Spine.* 2009;34(10):1094-1109.

33. Weinstein JN, Tosteson TD, Lurie JD, et al. Surgical vs non-operative treatment for lumbar disk herniation: the spine patient outcomes research trial (SPORT): a randomized trial. *JAMA.* 2006;296(20):2441-2450.

34. Weinstein JN, Lurie JD, Tosteson TD, et al. Surgical vs non-operative treatment for lumbar disk herniation: the spine patient outcomes research trial (SPORT) observational cohort. *JAMA.* 2006;296(20):2451-2459.

35. Weinstein JN, Lurie JD, Tosteson TD, et al. Surgical versus non-operative treatment for lumbar disc herniation: four-year results for the spine patient outcomes research trial (SPORT). *Spine.* 2008;33(25):2789-2800. doi:10.1097/BRS.0b013e31818ed8f4.

36. Lurie JD, Tosteson TD, Zhao W, et al. Surgical versus non-operative treatment for lumbar disk herniation: eight-year results for the spine patient outcomes research trial (SPORT). *Spine.* 2014;39(1):3-16.

37. Weinstein JN, Tosteson TD, Lurie JD, et al. Surgical versus nonsurgical therapy for lumbar spinal stenosis. *N Engl J Med.* 2008;358:794-810.

38. Lurie JD, Tosteson TD, Tosteson ANA, et al. Long-term outcomes of lumbar spinal stenosis: eight-year results of the spine patient outcomes research trial (SPORT). *Spine.* 2015;40(2):63-76.

20

HIP PAIN

Kevin Burnham, MD, Brian Toedebusch, MD and Charles De Mesa, DO, MPH

FAST FACTS

- Overlapping anatomic structures may present challenges in the differential diagnoses of hip pain.
- Hip pain can be caused by referred pain from the lumbar spine.
- Hip pain can be a result of a problem in the hip joint itself (intra-articular) or from the surrounding soft tissues (extra-articular).
- A systematic approach is essential for effective management of hip pain.

INTRODUCTION

Hip pain is a common presenting symptom for primary care visits. Among adults older than 60 years, nearly 15% reported some hip pain when followed over a period of 6 weeks.[1,2] The hip is a complex area of anatomy where underlying pain generators can range from the femoral-acetabular joint and capsule to overlying tendons, muscles, ligaments, nerves, and vascular structures. In addition, overlapping anatomic structures may complicate a differential diagnosis, including perineal, abdominal, and lumbosacral pathology. A systematic approach is essential to effective pain management and treatments. The purpose of this chapter is to review common causes of hip pain and emphasize key aspects of history and physical examination to aid in correct diagnosis and treatment.

HISTORY

A comprehensive history is vital to determining the cause of hip pain. Acquire information such as age, onset of pain, mechanism of injury, description of severity and location, associated symptoms such as numbness and tingling, and aggravating and relieving factors. Carefully review past medical and surgical histories, especially congenital or childhood hip deformities, underlying rheumatologic conditions, history of cancer, or previous trauma involving the lower extremity.

Inquire about previous treatments, and document the response to each treatment. This will help guide your next step in management. The next few sections further describe important aspects of the history and how they correlate to underlying hip pain generators, as well as corresponding physical examination findings.

ONSET AND AGE

Acute onset of pain is often associated with an inciting traumatic event or athletic injury. In contrast, chronic hip pain is usually insidious and related to degenerative conditions.[3] It is useful to consider the more common causes of hip pain with increasing age.

Epidemiology of Common Causes of Hip Pain

Septic arthritis may occur at any age, although it may peak at 0 to 6 years. The male to female ratio is 1:1. The patient presents with acute onset of fever pain, malaise, and refusal to stand.[3,4] Infants may exhibit poor feeding and irritability.

Transient synovitis usually occurs at age 3 to 8 years. The male to female ratio is 2:1. It mostly occurs in the fall and winter seasons and often follows viral illness. For this reason, it is believed to be a postinfectious reactive arthritis. Although the child does not appear to be ill, he or she may refuse to bear weight on the affected lower limb.[3–5]

Perthes disease typically affects children aged 3 to 12 years. The male to female ratio is 4:1. It is rare in African American children. Pain onset is insidious, starting with a painless limp and then developing hip, groin, lateral thigh, or knee pain over time. Physical observation may reveal a leg length discrepancy, decreased internal rotation, and abduction of the affected hip.[3,4]

Slipped capital femoral epiphysis typically affects individuals in early adolescence with a mean age of 12 years for girls and 13.5 years for boys. The male to female ratio is approximately 2:1. This medical condition may be observed in children who are overweight affected by endocrinopathy in 8% and also with African American ethnicity more so than Caucasian and Hispanic American ethnicity.[3,4,6] The patient complains of pain in the hip or knee, and an obligate external rotation of the hip can be seen with passive hip flexion.

Once an individual becomes skeletally mature, hip pain is often a result of musculotendinous strain, ligamentous sprain, contusion, or bursitis. In older adults, degenerative osteoarthritis and fractures should be considered first.

MECHANISM OF INJURY

In general, the mechanism of injury has less importance regarding etiology of hip pain especially because the majority of hip pain is attributed to chronic conditions. However, there are a few notable injuries with characteristic mechanisms.

Traumatic and high-energy injury to the hip region can cause fracture or dislocation. Direct impact or axial loads to the pelvis or femur from a fall or motor vehicle accident can lead to fractures.[2,7] If a fracture is present, pain will be severe and physical examination will typically reveal deformities. On inspection, the affected limb may appear shortened compared with the uninjured extremity.

A common nontraumatic cause of hip dislocation is following hip replacement surgery. Patients are instructed to avoid specific postoperative range of motion, especially excessive hip flexion and adduction for several months if a posterior surgical approach was used. Nearly 90% of all hip dislocations occur in the posterior direction. A posterior dislocation will present with the affected limb in flexion, adduction, and internal rotation. In contrast, an anterior dislocation will present with limb in flexion, abduction, and external rotation.

Muscle strains are another common cause of acute hip pain with notable mechanism of injury, especially when related to physical activity. Acute onset of groin pain after injury is most often caused by an adductor muscle strain. This injury occurs in sports owing to sudden changes of lateral direction and is characterized by the patient as a "pull" in the groin region. The adductor group is composed of 6 muscles, but the most commonly injured muscle is the adductor longus. Acute anterior hip pain located lateral to the groin can reflect strain of the hip flexor, rectus femoris, or iliopsoas muscles. These muscles are frequently injured during eccentric quadriceps contraction such as bringing the hip into extension during kicking activities. A patient with a recent hip flexor strain will often have pain and difficulty with an active straight leg raise. Hamstring strains are a common cause of acute posterior gluteal or thigh pain. The mechanism of hamstring injury can be from explosive sprinting activity, which causes excessive eccentric stretch of the muscle group. The patient may note a "pop" or "pull" in the posterior thigh and will have difficulty with walking.

Repetitive activities may make certain individuals prone to specific hip conditions. One such condition is athletic pubalgia or sports hernia, which is caused by repetitive hyperabduction of the abdominal muscles on the pubis. The repetitive rotation of the upper leg and torso common in athletes playing ice hockey, soccer, and rugby causes a higher risk of athletic pubalgia. Dancers also represent a distinct population. Owing to extreme range of motion of the hip, dancers are vulnerable to labral tears. Finally, people who play sports that require repeated single leg stance are at high risk of developing posterior hip pain because of sacroiliac joint dysfunction.[5]

LOCATION

Asking the patient to identify the pain location will help narrow the differential diagnosis. A simple test to specifically isolate location is to have the patient point with one finger where pain is the most intense. Location of hip pain can be generally categorized as anterior, lateral, or posterior. However, there can be considerable overlap in location for several common causes of hip pain.

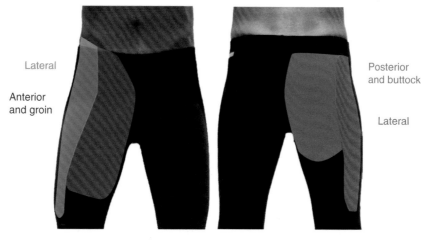

Front and Lateral Hip   Back and Lateral Hip

Traditionally, pain localizing to the anterior hip or groin suggests primary involvement of the hip joint or intra-articular pathology. Patients may indicate hip pain by cupping the anterolateral hip with their thumb and forefinger in the shape of a "C." This is referred to as the "C sign" (Figure 20-1). Common causes of intra-articular hip pain include osteoarthritis, labral tears, femoroacetabular impingement (FAI), avascular necrosis, septic arthritis, fracture, chondral lesions, loose bodies, and ligamentum teres tears.[8] Associated mechanical symptoms such as snapping, popping, locking, and reduced range of motion are more often associated with intra-articular pathology.[8,9] Other causes of anterior groin pain may be from extra-articular hip pathology. These include sports hernia (athletic pubalgia), osteitis pubis, adductor strain, or abdominal/pelvic viscera conditions such as hernia, genitourinary pathology, and abdominal strains. A notable cause of extra-articular anterior pain with mechanical symptoms is internal snapping hip or snapping of the iliopsoas tendon.[6]

Unlike anterior hip or groin pain, lateral hip is more likely to be extra-articular in origin. Common causes of lateral hip pain include greater trochanteric pain syndrome (which includes greater trochanteric bursitis, gluteal muscle tear, or tendinopathy), iliotibial band snapping (external snapping hip), and iliac crest apophysis avulsion (hip pointer). Lateral hip pain with a burning quality that radiates into the anterior thigh may be meralgia paresthetica (lateral femoral cutaneous nerve entrapment) or an upper lumbar nerve root radiculopathy.

The least common location of hip pain is the posterior region or along the gluteal region. Similar to lateral hip pain, posterior hip pain is typically related to extra-articular hip pathology. Posterior hip pain occurs between the posterior iliac crests and the gluteal fold. Common causes of posterior hip pain include proximal hamstring strain, tendinopathy, or avulsion, ischial

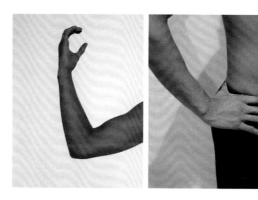

FIGURE 20-1 Example of "C sign," which indicates intra-articular hip pathology. The patient complains of anterior (groin) or lateral hip pain usually cupping their lateral hip with their hand creating a "C" with their hand.

apophysis bursitis or avulsion, ischiofemoral impingement, piriformis syndrome, lumbar osteoarthritis or radiculopathy, or sacroiliac joint dysfunction.[5,6,8] Posterior hip pain may be accompanied by radicular pain of varying degrees depending on the cause. For example, referred pain from sacroiliac joint dysfunction rarely travels below the knee, whereas piriformis syndrome travels distally to the calf muscles and to the undersurface of the foot.

Certainly, patients with hip pain often complain of several locations of pain, which poses diagnostic challenges. For instance, even though intra-articular hip pathology most commonly causes anterior groin pain, coexisting pain locations include the lateral and posterior hip, thigh, and, in some cases, knee. The reason for overlapping pain is the innervation of hip structures. Therefore, the clinician must consider several possibilities in the differential diagnosis.

ALLEVIATING AND EXACERBATING FACTORS

Intra-articular hip pain is usually exacerbated with activity and relieved with rest. Other clues that suggest intra-articular hip pathology include pain becoming worse with prolonged sitting, rising from a seated position, walking on inclined surfaces, and pivoting activities.[10-12] Patients may also describe that pain increases with prolonged standing or weight bearing. Young patients with FAI may mention pain with prolonged sitting or transitioning from sitting to standing.[11] Patients with intra-articular hip disease experience a constant dull and achy pain with episodic periods of sharp pain on pivoting and kicking. Lateral hip pain from greater trochanteric pain syndrome is increased when lying down on the affected side, climbing stairs, or crossing the affected legs.

Other notable exacerbating factors include thigh numbness and/or pain due to meralgia paresthetica related to a tight waistband on pants or clothing. Posterior hip pain can be increased by prolonged sitting on the ischial tuberosity, which can aggravate ischial bursitis and proximal hamstring tendinopathy.

ASSOCIATED SYMPTOMS

Paresthesias are an important symptom to note when evaluating hip pain. Burning pain is more likely neuropathic, whereas dull, achy pain is more descriptive of intra-articular musculotendinous causes. In addition, associated symptoms such as clicking, locking, and popping are important to recognize and usually indicate an intra-articular source of pain. An exception is a "snapping hip" or *coxa sultans* caused by a muscle or tendon temporarily catching on a bony projection.

Nerve entrapments around the hip will cause predictable neurologic pain patterns. The most common is lateral femoral cutaneous nerve entrapment known as meralgia paresthetica (Figure 20-2). It is characterized by a localized area of burning pain and paresthesia in the lateral hip and anterior thigh. These sensations are not exacerbated by palpation or special tests of the hip. Conversely, lumbar radicular pain usually has a broader distribution of radiating symptoms, which can be provoked with neural stretch tests, such as straight leg raise, slump test, or femoral nerve stretch test. Radiculopathy may classically follow a dermatomal distribution in the lower extremity. For example, L4/L5 radiculopathy causes lateral hip pain radiating down the leg sometimes into the ankle.

Physical examination maneuvers can be used to exacerbate intra-articular and extra-articular causes of hip pain.[13]

Log roll test

Steps

- The patient is in the supine position with knee extended.

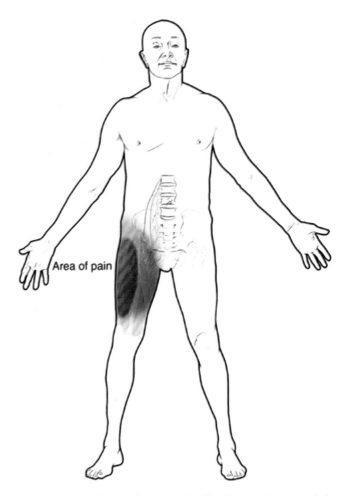

FIGURE 20-2 Illustration of pain distribution for meralgia paresthetica. Reprinted with permission from Waldman SD. *Waldmans comprehensive atlas of diagnostic ultrasound of painful conditions*. 1st ed. Philadelphia, PA: Wolters Kluwer; 2016.

- The examiner grasps the patient's ankle and internally and externally rotates the entire leg including the hip joint.

Positive test

- Ipsilateral hip pain

Positive test implication

- Intra-articular hip pathology
- Synovitis
- Septic hip joint
- Trauma

Stinchfield test

Steps

- The patient lies supine and flexes the hip (with knee fully extended) 15° off of the table.
- The examiner then performs gentle downward resistance to hip flexion.

Positive test

- Pain in the groin or anteriorly in the hip

Positive test implications

- Intra-articular hip pathology
- Iliopsoas bursitis

FABER (Flexion, Abduction, External Rotation) (Patrick's) examination

Steps

- The examiner flexes, abducts, and externally rotates the patient's leg and rests the ipsilateral ankle of the leg on the contralateral thigh.
- The examiner then compresses posteriorly on the ipsilateral knee while stabilizing contralateral anterior superior iliac spine.

Positive test

- Pain in the groin of the ipsilateral hip joint

Positive test implication

- Intra-articular hip pathology
- Osteoarthritis

Note: contralateral buttock pain signifies sacroiliac joint pathology.

FADIR (Flexion, Adduction, Internal Rotation)

Steps

- The patient is in the supine position, and the hip and knee are flexed greater than or equal to 90°.
- The femur is then internally rotated and flexed until an endpoint.

Positive test

- Pain in the groin or anteriorly in the hip

Positive test implications

- Anterior/superior labral pathology
- Femoral acetabular impingement syndrome (FAI)

Note: The FADIR maneuver may simply cause a stretching sensation or pain along the buttock area. This is an indication of tight gluteal muscles and can reproduce piriformis pain, and therefore stretching the affected muscles would respond with favorable outcomes (Figure 20-3).

Hip scour maneuver

Steps

- With the patient laying supine and hip flexed to 90° and knee flexed to >90°, the examiner places a downward compressive force through the femur with pressure applied at the knee.
- The examiner then circumducts the hip maintaining the downward pressure.

Positive test

- Indicated by pain in the groin, anteriorly in the hip with this maneuver

Positive test implications

- Intra-articular hip pathology
- Osteoarthritis
- Osteochondral defect

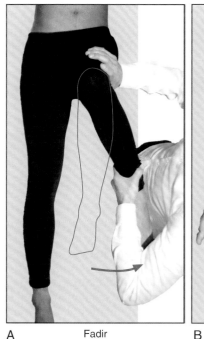 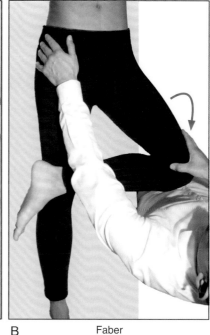

A   Fadir   B   Faber

FIGURE 20-3 Example A illustrates FADIR (flexion, adduction, internal rotation) maneuver for intra-articular pain. Example B illustrates FABER (flexion, abduction, external rotation) maneuver for posterior hip pain.

- Avascular necrosis
- Acetabular labrum defect
- Joint capsule tightness

Tenderness to palpation of greater trochanter

Steps

- Palpation of the tissues overlying the greater trochanter.

Positive test

- Pain is consistent with patient's typical pain

Positive test implication

- Greater trochanteric pain syndrome (gluteus medius tendinopathy, gluteal muscle tears, and/or greater trochanteric bursitis)

  Note: A true bursitis is rare.

  Ober test

Steps

- The patient is positioned with the unaffected hip on the examination table.
- The examiner stands behind the patient with one hand on the patient's hip and the other hand supporting the lower leg.
- Evaluate the following:
  - Tensor fasciae latae (TFL): The hip and knee are held at 0° extension and allowed to passively adduct below and behind the examination table.
  - Gluteus medius: The hip is held at 0° extension and 45° to 90° of knee flexion.
  - Gluteus maximus: The hip is rotated back toward the table with the hip in flexion and knee in extension.

Positive test

- Patient cannot adduct the leg

Positive test implications

- TFL tightness
- Gluteus medius tightness
- Gluteus maximus tightness

Snapping hip maneuver

Steps

- The examiner places one hand over the inguinal area.
- With the other hand, position the hip into flexion, abduction, and external rotation.
- The lower extremity is then moved into extension.

Positive test

- Audible and/or palpable snap in the groin

Positive test implications

- Iliopsoas bursitis

Lateral hip pain due to greater trochanteric pain syndrome can be increased with a single leg stance. Greater trochanteric pain with single leg stance has been shown to be highly specific for this diagnosis.[14]

Single leg stance may also cause a drop of the contralateral pelvis when standing on the affected side. This Trendelenburg effect is due to weakness or tear of the hip abductors with greater trochanteric pain syndrome. Hip abduction strength is more accurately determined by having the patient abduct the affected side against resistance. Palpation of snapping tendon with extension and external rotation is indicative of external snapping hip.

DIAGNOSTIC STUDIES AND THERAPEUTIC INTERVENTIONS

Radiographs should be obtained for any patient with trauma, acute hip pain, or concern for intra-articular pathology. This imaging modality is useful for detecting bony disease around the hip, including fracture, degenerative changes, and loose bodies. A weight-bearing anteroposterior (AP) view of the pelvis and lateral view of the proximal femur will assess for osteoarthritic changes such as articular joint space narrowing, osteophytes, and sclerosis of the joint space margins. "CAM" and "pincer" deformities are hip morphologic changes that can be seen on radiographs associated with FAI (Figures 20-4 and 20-5). Another indication of FAI is a crossover or posterior wall sign on AP radiograph indicating acetabular retroversion (Figure 20-6). This makes the hip prone to acetabular impingement and labral injury. Although pelvis and femur fractures are usually readily identified on radiograph, stress fractures are not well visualized on radiograph and often require advanced diagnostic studies.[15]

Advanced imaging includes magnetic resonance imaging (MRI) with or without arthrography, computed tomography, or nuclear medicine bone scanning. MRI is the most sensitive and specific imaging modality for hip pathology. However, it is expensive and may identify asymptomatic pathology. Soft tissue injuries such as muscle tears, tendinopathy, and bursitis are identified using MRI. In addition, stress fractures are best seen on MRI or bone scan. The use of arthrography with MRI, known as magnetic resonance arthrography, increases sensitivity to 90% for the detection of labral tears.[16] If athletic pubalgia, osteitis pubis, or adductor strain is suspected, MRI of the pelvis rather than hip should be obtained.

Ultrasonography is an increasingly used technology among experienced musculoskeletal clinicians. Ultrasound imaging has fewer side effects compared with radiography and MRI. However, the diagnostic yield is more heavily operator dependent. Soft tissue disorders such as tendinopathy, bursitis, joint effusions, and functional causes of hip pain such as snapping hip syndrome are particularly well suited to evaluation with ultrasound imaging. Ultrasound imaging can also safely be used to accurately perform image-guided injections and aspiration around the hip by the experienced practitioner.[17]

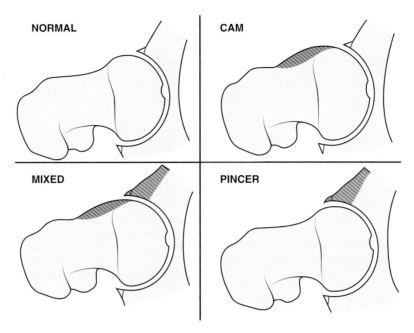

FIGURE 20-4 Illustration of CAM and pincer abnormalities in femoroacetabular impingement.

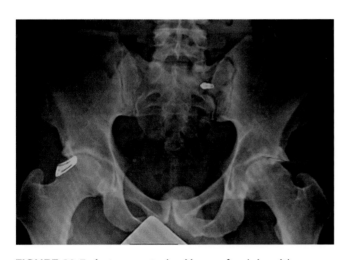

FIGURE 20-5 Anteroposterior X-ray of pelvis with right femoral head with green highlighted area noting location of CAM deformity. Left acetabular coverage in red highlighted area noting location of pincher deformity.

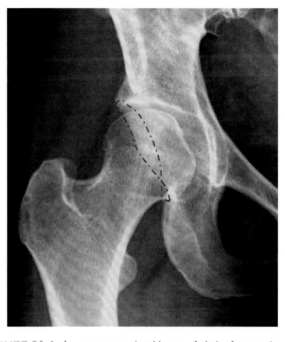

FIGURE 20-6 Anteroposterior X-ray of right femoral acetabular joint with "crossover" sign that indicates acetabular retroversion.

Finally, electrodiagnostic studies which include Nerve Conduction Studies/Electromyography (NCS/EMG) are occasionally used to provide diagnostic information for hip pain. If there is radiating paresthesia associated with hip pain, NCS/EMG would be helpful in diagnosing a radiculopathy, plexopathy, or mononeuropathy. A notable exception is meralgia paresthetica, which is often difficult to accurately detect on NCS/EMG.

CONCLUSION

The hip is a complex structure because of the various pain generators. Overlapping anatomic structures may present challenges in the differential diagnoses. Therefore, a systematic approach is essential for effective management of hip pain.

REFERENCES

1. Christmas C, Crespo CJ, Franckowiak SC, Bathon JM, Bartlett SJ, Andersen RE. How common is hip pain among older adults? Results from the Third National Health and Nutrition Examination Survey. *J Fam Pract.* 2002;51(4):345-348.

2. Berry SD, Miller RR. Falls: epidemiology, pathophysiology, and relationship to fracture. *Curr Osteoporos Rep.* 2008;6(4):149-154.

3. Hollingworth P. Differential diagnosis and management of hip pain in childhood. *Br J Rheumatol.* 1995;34(1):78-82.

4. Frick SL. Evaluation of the child who has hip pain. *Orthop Clin North Am.* 2006;37(2):133-140.

5. Prather H, Cheng A. Diagnosis and treatment of hip girdle pain in the athlete. *PM R.* 2016;8(3 suppl):S45-S60.

6. Wilson JJ, Furukawa M. Evaluation of the patient with hip pain. *Am Fam Physician.* 2014;89(1):27-34.

7. Arneson TJ, Melton LJ, Lewallen DG, O'Fallon WM. Epidemiology of diaphyseal and distal femoral fractures in Rochester, Minnesota, 1965–1984. *Clin Orthop Relat Res.* 1988;(234):188-194.

8. Tibor LM, Sekiya JK. Differential diagnosis of pain around the hip joint. *Arthroscopy.* 2008;24(12):1407-1421.

9. Carreira D, Bush-Joseph CA. Hip arthroscopy. *Orthopedics.* 2006;29(6):517-523; quiz 524-5.

10. Beck M, Kalhor M, Leunig M, Ganz R. Hip morphology influences the pattern of damage to the acetabular cartilage: femoroacetabular impingement as a cause of early osteoarthritis of the hip. *J Bone Joint Surg Br.* 2005;87(7):1012-1018.

11. Byrd JW, Jones KS. Prospective analysis of hip arthroscopy with 2-year follow-up. *Arthroscopy.* 2000;16(6):578-587.

12. Ganz R, Parvizi J, Beck M, Leunig M, Nötzli H, Siebenrock KA. Femoroacetabular impingement: a cause for osteoarthritis of the hip. *Clin Orthop Relat Res.* 2003;(417):112-120.

13. Hoppenfeld S. *Physical Examination of the Spine and Extremities.* New York: Appleton-Century-Crofts; 1976.

14. Grimaldi A, Mellor R, Nicolson P, Hodges P, Bennell K, Vicenzino B. Utility of clinical tests to diagnose MRI-confirmed gluteal tendinopathy in patients presenting with lateral hip pain. *Br J Sports Med.* 2017;51(6):519-524.

15. Silvis ML, Mosher TJ, Smetana BS, et al. High prevalence of pelvic and hip magnetic resonance imaging findings in asymptomatic collegiate and professional hockey players. *Am J Sports Med.* 2011;39(4):715-721.

16. Robertson WJ, Kadrmas WR, Kelly BT. Arthroscopic management of labral tears in the hip: a systematic review of the literature. *Clin Orthop Relat Res.* 2007;455:88-92.

17. Rowbotham EL, Grainger AJ. Ultrasound-guided intervention around the hip joint. *Am J Roentgenol.* 2011;197(1):W122-W127.

21

KNEE, ANKLE, AND FOOT PAIN

Jesse Goitia, MD and Kevin Burnham, MD

FAST FACTS

- Osteoarthritis of the knee is the most common cause of disability in the elderly.
- Pain in the foot and ankle affects 1 in 5 adults 58 years and older.
- Stroke should be included in the differential for a patient with acute lower extremity weakness or loss of sensation.
- Diabetic neuropathy and ischemia-related nerve damage in peripheral artery disease results in lower limb pain.

INTRODUCTION

Lower extremity pain is a common patient encounter in primary care.[1] The prevalence of knee pain is estimated to be as high as 20% in the general population of adults and can be associated with significant disability.[2] Similarly, pain in the foot and ankle affects approximately 1 in 5 adults 58 years and older.[3] In this chapter, we will discuss important causes of pain at, or around, the knee, leg, ankle, and foot. Pain associated with hip pathology will be discussed separately.

HISTORY

An accurate history can help a physician to focus the physical examination appropriately and guides the diagnostic process.[4] The goal of the clinical interview should be to characterize the chief complaint, evaluate the impact on patient function, and attempt to establish a cause.[5] Key elements of the history include localizing the area of pain, exploring the characteristics of the pain, defining the time course, inquiring about any recent trauma or prior interventions, exploring associated symptoms, and uncovering the mechanism of injury[5–7] (Table 21-1).

MECHANISM OF INJURY

Having a clear understanding of the mechanism by which an injury took place increases the ability to make an accurate diagnosis. A thorough description of the mechanism of injury must account for the events leading to the injury and a description of the body/joint biomechanics at the time of injury. This description should include information regarding the environment where the injury took place, physical characteristics of the patient, the involvement of any forces external to the patient, including direct blows to the patient's body and the presence of accelerating or decelerating forces.[46]

Classically, anterior cruciate ligament (ACL) injuries are described as a twisting injury of the knee that is accompanied by an audible pop and rapid swelling of the knee joint.[47] It is also helpful to note if the injury occurred with acceleration or deceleration, a directional change, presence or absence of joint loading, a varus or valgus force through the joint, and the degree of knee extension.[48] It is valuable to understand that, in overuse injuries, the inciting injury may not be a single memorable event the patient will be able to recall.

TABLE 21-1 Differential Diagnosis by Timing

ACUTE/ABRUPT	CHRONIC/INSIDIOUS
Knee	
ACL rupture[8]	
Baker cyst, rupture causes acute pain[9]	Baker cyst[9]
Dislocations[10]	
Hamstring tendonitis[11]	Hamstring tendonitis[11]
Medial plica syndrome[12]	IT band syndrome[13]
Meniscal tear[14]	Meniscal tear[14]
Monoarthritis (septic arthritis, gout, pseudogout, or inflammatory arthritis)[15,16]	
Patellar fracture[17,18]	Patellar tendinopathy[19]
Patellar tendon rupture[20,21]	Patellofemoral pain syndrome[22]
Pes anserine bursitis[23]	Pes anserine bursitis[23]
Prepatellar bursitis[24]	Prepatellar bursitis[25]
Quadriceps tendon rupture[21]	
Lower Leg	
Baker cyst, rupture causes acute pain[9]	Chronic exertional compartment syndrome[26]
DVT[27]	DVT[27]
Maisonneuve fracture[28]	Medial tibial stress syndrome[29]
	Popliteal artery entrapment syndrome[30]
	Tibial bone stress injuries[29]
Ankle and Foot	
Achilles tendon rupture[31]	Achilles tendinopathy[32]
Acute compartment syndrome[33]	
Ankle sprain[34]	
Calcaneal stress fracture[35]	Calcaneal stress fracture[35]
First MTP joint sprain[36]	
Metatarsal fractures[37]	Metatarsal fractures[37]
Os trigonum (posterior impingement)[38,39]	Os trigonum (posterior impingement)[38,39]
Plantar fasciitis[40]	Plantar fasciitis[40]
Sinus tarsi syndrome[41]	Sinus tarsi syndrome[41]
Stress fractures[42]	Stress fractures[42]

ACUTE/ABRUPT	CHRONIC/INSIDIOUS
Syndesmotic ("high") ankle sprain[43]	
Tarsal tunnel syndrome[44]	Tarsal tunnel syndrome[45]

IT, iliotibial; MTP, metatarsophalangeal.

LOCATION

Musculoskeletal pain may be well localized, occur in a particular anatomical region, or be widespread.[49] The localization of pain is often poor in deep-tissue structures, and it can be difficult to differentiate pain from bones, muscles, tendons, or ligaments.[49] For the knee, determining the general region from which pain is arising (anterior, medial, lateral, or posterior) can be useful when establishing a differential diagnosis.[12] For example, anterior knee pain may be suggestive of patellar or patellofemoral pathology, whereas medial knee pain may be more suggestive of meniscal or degenerative joint disease.[12]

Similarly, the location of pain within the foot and ankle can help formulate a differential diagnosis.[50] Pain in the rear foot could be brought on by Achilles tendon injury, plantar fasciitis, calcaneal stress fracture, heel contusion, or posterior tibial tendinopathy.[40] Pain along the medial aspect of the mid-foot may be a symptom of tarsal tunnel syndrome, whereas pain at the lateral mid-foot may be brought about by sinus tarsi syndrome.[51]

ALLEVIATING AND EXACERBATING FACTORS

Assessment of aggravating and alleviating factors aids diagnosis and development of a management strategy[52,53] (Table 21-2). Patellofemoral pain is described as a diffuse, aching anterior knee pain, without clear inciting injury.[22,59] There may be mechanical symptoms, such as the knee catching or popping while walking, but not locking of the knee.[22,59] Swelling is uncommon but may be reported along with stiffness.[22] Patellofemoral pain is exacerbated by activities that increase stress on the patellofemoral joint, such as prolonged knee flexion ("theater sign"), walking down stairs, squatting, running, or jumping.[22,59] Always ask about recent changes in physical activity that could cause repetitive overload at the patellofemoral joint, particularly exercise routines.[22,59] Pain from pes anserine bursitis is exacerbated by going up and down stairs and is worse in the morning.[65] Meniscus pain is worse on torsional knee movements during weight bearing, such as pivoting about the knee while walking or running.[66] Plantar fasciitis is a common cause of heel pain in adult primary care setting. Pain is believed to be due to microtears at the calcaneal enthesis caused by biomechanical overuse from prolonged standing or running. Patients typically report heel pain and tightness on rising from bed in the morning or

TABLE 21-2 Alleviating and Exacerbating Factors of Painful Lower Extremity Conditions

	EXACERBATING	ALLEVIATING
Knee		
Baker cyst	• End-range knee extension[54]	
Hamstring tendonitis	• Repetitive activities with the leg or hamstrings, including running, cycling, or stairs • Sudden knee flexion[11]	
IT band syndrome	• Running downhill • Increasing stride length • Prolonged knee flexion, such as sitting[55]	
Medial plica syndrome	• Walking up or down stairs • Squatting • Rising from a chair after prolonged sitting[56]	
Meniscal tear	• Walking • Standing • Twisting motions • Nighttime[57]	
Patellar tendinopathy	• Repetitive activities with the leg or quadriceps • Prolonged sitting or squatting[58]	• Pain may improve after a certain "warm-up" period[58]
Patellofemoral pain syndrome	• Prolonged sitting • Walking down stairs • Squatting • Running • Jumping[22,59]	
Pes anserine bursitis	• Walking up or down stairs[23] • Repetitive flexion and extension[12]	
Prepatellar bursitis	• Direct pressure over the bursa • End-range knee flexion[60]	
Septic arthritis	• Range of motion, particularly flexion[15]	
Lower Leg		
Chronic exertional compartment syndrome	• Pain increases in relation to intensity or duration of exertion[26]	• Rest[26]
Medial tibial stress syndrome	• Pain at the start of activity or exercise[26]	
Ankle and Foot		
Achilles tendinopathy	• Pain at the start of exercise[61] • Running • Jumping	
First MTP joint sprain	• First MTP motion, particularly with walking or running[62]	
Morton neuroma	• Ambulation • Footwear with narrow toe box[63]	• Rest[63] • Wide toe-box footwear
Os trigonum	• Running downhill • End-range ankle dorsiflexion[38]	
Plantar fasciitis	• Weight bearing immediately out of bed or after prolonged rest[40] • Prolonged walking or standing[40]	• Moderate ambulation typically improves pain[40]

(Continued)

TABLE 21-2 Alleviating and Exacerbating Factors of Painful Lower Extremity Conditions (Continued)

	EXACERBATING	ALLEVIATING
Sinus tarsi syndrome	• Running or sprinting • Stepping off a curb or walking on uneven ground may worsen the sensation of instability[41]	
Tarsal tunnel syndrome	• Prolonged sitting or standing[64] • Nighttime symptoms are commonly reported[64]	• Rest and leg elevation[64]

IT, iliotibial; MTP, metatarsophalangeal.

after prolonged sitting. The pain typically improves with ambulation but can intensify toward the end of the day if patients had been on their feet most of the time.[40]

NEUROLOGIC SYMPTOMS

Damage to nerve tissue of the lower extremities is not uncommon and can lead to poor functional outcomes.[67] Symptoms of nerve injury include pain, loss of motor function, loss of sensation, and abnormal sensations.[68] Stroke should be included in the differential for a patient with acute lower extremity weakness or loss of sensation.[69] Other possible nonmechanical causes of lower extremity neurologic symptoms include diabetic neuropathy and ischemia-related nerve damage in peripheral artery disease.[70,71]

Trauma is an obvious example of an acute cause of lower extremity neurologic symptoms. For instance, traumatic dislocation of the knee can cause damage to the local neurovascular structures, particularly the tibial or peroneal nerve, which can lead to chronic pain and progressive weakness.[72] Common peroneal nerve injury impairs dorsiflexion and eversion of the foot.[73] Absence of the ability to dorsiflex the foot results in foot drop, and unopposed inversion of the foot exacerbates this by making it even more difficult for a patient to clear their toes from hitting the ground during the swing phase of walking.[73] Deep peroneal nerve entrapment results in impairment of foot dorsiflexion and toe extension.[74] Superficial peroneal nerve damage affects ankle eversion.[74]

Morton neuroma is a common cause of chronic foot pain. It is actually proliferative fibrosis of perineural tissue rather than a true nerve tumor. The underlying cause is not clear. Patients classically report a burning pain at the plantar aspect of the foot, between the third and fourth metatarsal heads. The pain may radiate to the toes and be associated with paresthesias. Walking in high heels or in shoes with a narrow toe box exacerbates the pain. The pain may be relieved with a change in footwear or foot massage.[75]

ASSOCIATED SYMPTOMS

Inquiring about the related symptoms and features associated with a patient's pain can be crucial in deriving a diagnosis. A patient with pain due to meniscal damage may describe insidious knee pain without identifiable injury that is associated with mechanical symptoms such as painful clicking, locking, and painless giving way.[76] Medial tibial stress syndrome is a common cause of exertional leg pain, particularly in runners, and is often described as absent at rest and subsiding after a period of continued exertion.[26] In contrast, pain due to a tibial stress fracture is more likely to be associated with increasing intensity with exertion and, possibly, pain at rest.[26] Another cause of exertional lower extremity pain is chronic exertional compartment syndrome. This disorder is often characterized as a cramping sensation that can affect any of the lower leg compartments and can be associated with numbness, weakness, and paresthesias.[26] An Achilles tendon rupture is associated with weakness, unsteady gait, limping, and difficulty climbing a step.[77]

PRIOR DIAGNOSTIC STUDIES AND THERAPEUTIC INTERVENTIONS

Musculoskeletal imaging can be a powerful diagnostic tool for a wide variety of conditions. Review of prior images can provide a great deal of insight into a patient's existing injury that history and examination may not be able to provide.[78] It is important to know about past treatments a patient may have received, not only to document efficacy but also to recognize the possibility of additional pathology brought about by those interventions.[79] For instance, the Achilles tendon is vulnerable to rupture following corticosteroid injection; knowledge of prior injections may raise suspicion for rupture in a patient presenting with rear-foot and ankle pathology.[80] In fact, patients may be at risk for tendon rupture even without a history of local steroid injections.[79] Systemic corticosteroid use can also place a person at risk for Achilles rupture, as can a history of fluoroquinolone use.[79,81]

The history of prior surgical interventions is similarly essential when evaluating a patient. For instance, patients with a history of ACL repair are at increased risk of graft rupture within the first 5 years following surgery, compared with individuals with no history of reconstruction.[82]

Consider obtaining a physical medicine and rehabilitation consult when treating musculoskeletal injuries that do not improve with simple conservative measures such as rest, ice, compression, and elevation. Surgical referrals are necessary depending on the diagnosis; appropriate referral time is further delineated in Table 21-3.

TABLE 21-3 Examination and Management of Painful Lower Extremity Conditions				
	EXAMINATION	**WORKUP**	**TREATMENT**	**WHEN TO REFER**
MSK				
ACL injury	Hemarthrosis likely present. May be unable to fully extend knee. Lachman, anterior drawer, and pivot shift tests are the most accurate[8]	MRI is study of choice[8]	Conservative if no major instability, normal range of motion, and minimal/ no meniscal or collateral ligament damage[8] Will need surgery if tear and if person is active	Active, young athletes, additional meniscal or collateral ligament injuries[8]
Patellofemoral pain syndrome	Look for J-sign on single-leg squat. Patellar glide, tilt, grind, and apprehension tests may be positive[59]	Clinical diagnosis[22,59]	Physical therapy with activity modification, foot orthoses may be helpful[59]	Symptoms longer than 6-12 mo despite treatment.[59] Refer to PM&R
Meniscal tear	Effusion is common.[14] Joint line tenderness is fairly sensitive, McMurray test is specific[14,83]	MRI is the imaging test of choice[83]	Conservative treatment if asymptomatic or small and stable, and most chronic degenerative tears[84]	Large complex tears, tears associated with ACL rupture, and symptoms that fail to resolve with conservative treatment.[84] Refer to Orthopedic Surgery
Patellar tendinopathy	Pain on palpation of inferior pole of patella or reproduced on resisted knee extension[85]	Clinical diagnosis but US can be helpful[19]	Eccentric physical therapy with activity modification[19,86,87]	After failing 3 mo of conservative treatment.[88] Refer to PM&R
IT band syndrome	Tenderness at lateral knee approximately 2 cm above joint line, can be increased by standing with 30° of knee flexion[55]	Clinical diagnosis but MRI may be helpful[55]	Activity modification, physical therapy, ice and NSAIDs[55]	If poor response to conservative treatment.[55] Refer to PM&R
Patellar dislocation	Usually reduces spontaneously; often large effusion, hemarthrosis, and tenderness near medial retinaculum[44,89]	Weight-bearing radiographs in AP view in extension, in 45° flexion, and lateral view in 30° flexion.[44] MRI is usually obtained[90]	2-3 wk of immobilization with 20° of knee flexion, weight bearing as tolerated as soon as possible, followed by physical therapy[44]	Inaugural dislocation, athletic patients without predisposing factors, bone avulsion, risk factors for recurrence, and recurrent dislocation[44] Refer to Orthopedic Surgery
Maisonneuve fracture	Tenderness over deltoid ligament, syndesmosis, and proximal fibula near fracture[28]	Ankle series and dedicated films of proximal tibia[28]	6-8 wk of casting if intact ankle mortise[91]	If mortise is not in anatomic alignment.[91] Refer to Orthopedic Surgery
Achilles tendon rupture	Palpable gap in tendon may be present. Thompson test positive in complete rupture[32]	Clinical diagnosis, but MRI or US may be helpful[31,32]	Casting and immobilization for 8-12 wk[31] or functional bracing with early rehabilitation[92]	Younger and more active patients[31] Refer to Orthopedic Surgery
Medial tibial stress syndrome	May have tenderness along distal 2/3 of posteromedial tibia. Navicular drop test may be positive[26]	MRI can help differentiate medial tibial stress syndrome from tibial bone stress injury[26]	Relative rest with gradual increases in activity[26]	If conservative measures fail.[26] Refer to PM&R
Tibial bone stress injury	Tenderness at site of reported pain with possible swelling[26]	MRI is study of choice[26]	Immobilization, followed by nonimpact activities[26]	In cases of delayed healing and in athletes[26] Refer to PM&R and/or Ortho (Sports)

(Continued)

TABLE 21-3 Examination and Management of Painful Lower Extremity Conditions (Continued)

	EXAMINATION	WORKUP	TREATMENT	WHEN TO REFER
Ankle sprains	Swelling may be present. Perform anterior drawer, inversion stress, squeeze, and external rotation tests[93]	Use Ottawa ankle rules to determine need for radiographs. If symptomatic >6 wk, CT or MRI should be considered[34]	Rest, ice, compression, and elevation but no prolonged immobilization[93]	Diastasis of the syndesmosis[43] Prolonged pain Refer to PM&R and/or Orthopedic Surgery
First MTP joint sprain	May have swelling, ecchymosis, malalignment, and tenderness at the joint[36]	Weight bearing AP, lateral, and sesamoid axial radiographs. MRI may be helpful[36]	Rest, ice, compression, elevation, and NSAIDs. Short leg cast with toe spica extension in slight plantar flexion may be helpful[36]	MTP joint instability, associated fractures, chondral injury, and failed conservative treatment.[36] Refer to Orthopedic Surgery
Fifth metatarsal fracture	Tenderness with surrounding ecchymosis and swelling[94]	AP, lateral, and 45° oblique radiographs and should be repeated 10-14 d after onset symptoms[37]	Conservative if nondisplaced, depending on fracture location and individual patient factors[37]	Dependent on displacement, angulation, and when closed reduction is insufficient.[37] Refer to Orthopedic Surgery
Lisfranc injury	Plantar ecchymosis and tenderness at the mid-foot[95]	Weight bearing AP, lateral, and 30° oblique radiographs. MRI if clinical suspicion persists despite normal XR and CT images[95]	Immobilization, rest, ice, and elevation with progression to mobility as tolerated with walking cast or controlled ankle motion boot[95]	If displacement present on imaging.[95] Refer to Orthopedic Surgery
Vascular				
PAD	Cool extremities, absent distal pulses, audible bruit over iliac, femoral, or popliteal arteries, and nonhealing ulcers may be present[96]	ABIs are inexpensive and noninvasive[96]	Lifestyle modification, statin, antiplatelet therapy, cilostazol, and graduated exercise[96]	Emergent revascularization for acute limb ischemia. May be appropriate for symptomatic chronic PAD.[96] Refer to Vascular Surgery
DVT	Edema, erythema, warmth, and tenderness may be present[97]	US when pretest probability is intermediate or high, D-dimer if low[97]	Anticoagulation, determined according to specific patient factors[98]	IVC filter placement may be needed if anticoagulation is contraindicated. Mechanical/pharmacomechanical treatment may be appropriate in certain patients[98]
Acute compartment syndrome	Involved compartment may appear full and tense, but this is unreliable. Distal pulses may not be affected until pressure in the compartment overcomes systemic blood pressure[33]	Clinical diagnosis but intracompartmental pressure monitoring may be helpful[33]	Initial temporizing measures: removal of constrictive devises or wraps and leg elevation[33]	Fasciotomy is definitive treatment.[33] Refer to Surgery
Chronic exertional compartment syndrome	Normal examination at rest. Sensorimotor deficits may be appreciated after exercise and passive stretching may be painful[26]	Preexertional and postexertional intracompartmental pressure testing[26]	May be as simple as avoiding offending activity. Forefoot running may help anterior chronic exertional compartment syndrome. Botulinum toxin A intramuscular injections may be effective[26]	Surgical fasciotomy is the mainstay of treatment[26] Refer to Surgery

TABLE 21-3 Examination and Management of Painful Lower Extremity Conditions (Continued)

	EXAMINATION	WORKUP	TREATMENT	WHEN TO REFER
Neuro				
Morton neuroma	Observe footwear and gait and note any soft tissue abnormalities. Web space tenderness may be appreciable and plantar percussion test over affected webspace may elicit pain or paresthesia[75]	US and MRI are the most commonly used imaging modalities[75]	Footwear modifications and local injections with steroids, alcohols, and anesthetic agents may be effective[75]	If symptoms are not improving with conservative treatment.[75] Refer to PM&R
Peripheral neuropathy	Symptoms/findings typically are asymmetric, sensory symptoms are dermatomal, with possible loss of vibratory, proprioceptive, temperature, and pinprick sensation and decreased ankle reflexes[99]	CBC, CMP, fasting glucose, B$_{12}$ and TSH, EMG or nerve biopsy may be needed[99]	Treat underlying disease process. Gabapentin, topirimate, carbamazepine, pregabalin, or amitriptyline may improve pain[99]	Lower extremity peripheral nerve decompression may help diffuse diabetic polyneuropathy.[99] Refer to PM&R

ABI, ankle-brachial indices; AP, anteroposterior; CBC, complete blood count; CMP, complete metabolic panel; CT, computed tomography; DVT, deep vein thrombosis; EMG, electromyography; IT, Iliotibial; IVC, inferior vena cava; MRI, magnetic resonance imaging; MTP, metatarsophalangeal; NSAID, nonsteroidal anti-inflammatory drug; PM&R, physical medicine and rehabilitation; TSH, thyroid stimulating hormone; US, ultrasound; XR, X-ray.

Common Differential Diagnosis Affecting the Lower Extremity

Pain in the lower extremity can generally be divided into 4 categories musculoskeletal, vascular, neurologic, and radicular/referred pain. A common musculoskeletal cause, and the most common cause of visits to a primary care physician for knee pain, is patellofemoral pain syndrome.[22,59] It is the result of excess stress at the patellofemoral joint, but the exact cause of this stress is not well understood (Figure 21-1).[22]

Iliotibial (IT) band syndrome occurs frequently in runners and cyclists. The proposed mechanism of injury is repetitive flexion and extension of the knee leading to friction between the distal portion of the IT band and the lateral femoral condyle, causing inflammation. It is associated with diffuse pain over the lateral knee initially, which progresses to more localized and intense, sharp pain at the lateral femoral condyle and/or the lateral tibial ("Gerdy") tubercle. Pain typically comes several minutes into or following activity, but, as time goes on, the symptoms begin earlier and can even occur at rest. Pain is worsened by running downhill, increasing one's stride length, or having the knee flexed for long periods, such as prolonged sitting.[19]

Osteoarthritis of the knee is the most common cause of disability in the elderly.[100] Morning stiffness may be present but usually lasts for less than 30 minutes.[101] There may be a history of swelling or crepitus on squatting or kneeling[102–104] or a sensation of locking at the knee joint.[102] Climbing or going down stairs, rising from a seated position, squatting, or kneeling makes the pain worse.[103] Pain typically progresses from mild discomfort during a high amount of use of the knee and is relieved with rest, to constant pain during use to finally pain at rest and at night.[105]

Meniscal tears are common and associated with osteoarthritis of the knee.[57,106] Traumatic tears are more common in younger patients (under 40 y old), and degenerative tears tend to occur in older patients.[106] Acute traumatic tears are most often due to noncontact forces such as sudden acceleration or deceleration while rotating, causing the meniscus to catch between the tibia and femur.[84] Patients report recurrent knee pain, classically with episodic catching, popping, and locking of the knee, particularly during squatting or twisting of the knee.[14] Patients generally report a variable amount of pain and swelling; the swelling usually develops within the first 24 hours after injury (Figure 21-2).[84]

The ACL is a primary stabilizer of the knee and acts to prevent anterior displacement and internal rotation of the tibia. Most ACL tears occur from noncontact injuries, usually during deceleration of the lower extremity while the quadriceps are maximally contracted and the knee is near full extension. Such injuries can be seen in soccer players during sudden cutting maneuvers and basketball players who land on an internally rotated knee that is not fully flexed. Contact ACL injuries require a planted lower leg and enough torque to tear the ligament. Patients often describe a popping sound that occurs at the time of injury, immediately followed by pain and swelling of the knee. After the injury, patients may describe a sensation of knee instability or giving-way (Figure 21-3)[8].

Pes anserine bursitis is inflammation at the conjoined insertion points of the sartorius, gracilis, and semitendinosus tendons along the proximal medial aspect of the tibia.[23] It is believed to be due to friction at the bursa from overuse due to excessive valgus stress or rotary stress on the knee, or by direct blow.[23] The classic symptoms include swelling and tenderness along the proximal medial tibia, and patients may report vague medial knee pain.[23] Pain is worse when going up and down stairs and with repetitive flexion and extension of the knee.[12,23]

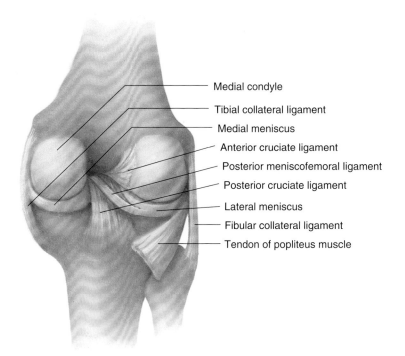

FIGURE 21-1 Ligaments of the knee. Asset provided by Anatomical Chart Co.

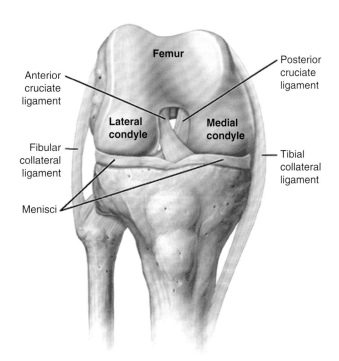

Flexed knee, anterior view

FIGURE 21-2 Meniscal injuries. Reprinted with permission from Williams A. *Study Guide to Accompany Massage Mastery: Theory and Technique.* 1st ed. Philadelphia, PA: Wolters Kluwer Health/Lippincott William & Wilkins; 2012. Figure 22.9.

Medial plica syndrome is a source of knee pain more commonly seen in younger patients and is believed to occur when the medial synovial plica glides over the anteromedial aspect of the medial femoral condyle on flexion and extension of the knee, producing pain. Patients often describe a dull, aching sensation at the medial aspect of the knee that is made worse with activity and is particularly bothersome at night. Patients may report crepitus, pseudolocking, and catching at the anteromedial aspect of the knee on rising from a seated position after a prolonged period. History of knee trauma is uncommon, but there usually is a history of activity involving repetitive knee flexion and extension.[56]

Hamstring injuries can involve the muscles or tendons.[11,107,108] Hamstring muscle injuries are usually strains, and hamstring muscle tears are usually partial, often occurring during jumping or sprinting.[108] Hamstring tendinopathy tends to occur in young endurance athletes, and these injuries can be acute and severe following a sudden increase in the volume of endurance activity, such as running or cycling.[11,107] The hamstrings are particularly vulnerable to injury as they cross both the hip and knee joints, and excessive stretching across these joints leads to injury.[108] The presentation of hamstring injuries will therefore be variable, depending on whether the injury occurs closer to the hip or the knee joint.[108] Injuries involving the proximal portion of the hamstring muscle are the most common and will be discussed in the hip pain chapter.[109] Pain associated with biceps femoris tendinopathy is described as an insidious,

Normal knee anatomy
(Patella removed)

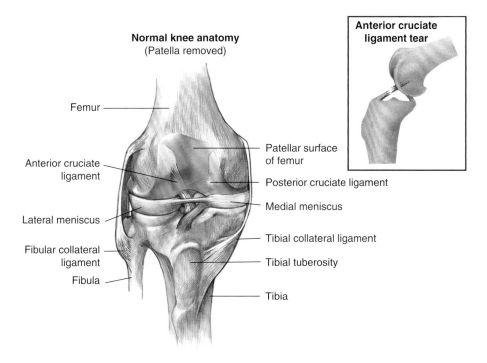

Anterior cruciate
ligament tear

Femur

Patellar surface
of femur

Anterior cruciate
ligament

Posterior cruciate ligament

Medial meniscus

Lateral meniscus

Tibial collateral ligament

Fibular collateral
ligament

Tibial tuberosity

Fibula

Tibia

FIGURE 21-3 Anterior cruciate ligament tear. Asset provided by Anatomical Chart Co.

progressive ache in the posterior knee.[11,107] Pain is often worse with activities such as running, cycling, going up and down stairs, or sudden knee flexion.[11]

A Baker cyst is a synovial fluid–filled mass in the popliteal fossa that can compress local structures, the popliteal vein most frequently.[110] Patients will typically have a history of inflammatory or degenerative joint disease or other internal derangement of the knee leading to excess synovial fluid production.[110,111] Meniscal tears are commonly associated with these cysts.[110] Complications of Baker cysts can include compression of the popliteal vein leading to thrombophlebitis or cyst rupture, which can mimic deep vein thrombosis or thrombophlebitis[110].

Knee dislocations are rare injuries but carry the potential for significant functional impairment for the patient.[112] Any of the 3 articulations of the knee can be involved: the patellofemoral, tibiofemoral, and/or proximal tibiofibular joints.[10] The peroneal nerve is at risk for injury in all types of knee dislocation.[10]

Traumatic dislocation of the proximal tibiofibular joint tends to occur in young patients and is often self-limited.[10] Anterolateral dislocation of the proximal tibiofibular joint is most common and typically occurs during a fall onto a flexed knee with an inverted foot, as the leg becomes adducted by the weight of the falling body. This is classically seen in parachuting drops.[10] Anterior dislocation of the tibiofibular joint may result in paresthesias along the distribution of the peroneal nerve and the potential for "foot drop" if the damage is extensive enough.[10,113]

Tibiofemoral dislocations are rare but often devastating and associated with significant soft tissue and neurovascular damage. Most tibiofemoral dislocations are high-energy injuries, usually seen in motor vehicle collisions, falls from height, and industrial accidents. Rapid reduction and careful assessment of neurovascular structures, typically with advanced imaging, is critical to avoid severe complications.[10]

Patellofemoral dislocations typically occur in younger patients during sports activities, with recurrence rates as high as 40%.[10] By far, the leading cause of acute traumatic patellar dislocation involves a noncontact knee sprain while in flexion and valgus.[10,114] A patellar dislocation may be transient, and the young athlete may not even know the dislocation took place.[10] Patients often report the sensation of knee slippage, followed by severe pain and effusion.[10,114] Dislocations usually resolve spontaneously.[10]

Patellar tendon rupture is rare, and patients are likely to have a history of chronic microtrauma and degeneration of the tendon.[20,21] The injury is often the result of indirect trauma due to the sudden contraction of the quadriceps with the knee in moderate flexion, which can occur during sprinting or during an attempt to avoid a fall.[115] The pain is described as an acute tearing sensation, and patients report the inability to bear weight (Figure 21-4).

Medial tibial stress syndrome is common among runners and is most commonly defined as exertional pain along the posteromedial border of the tibia that is not due to ischemia or stress fracture. The exact

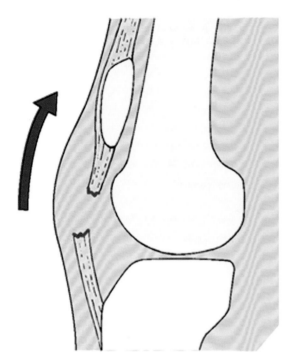

FIGURE 21-4 Patellar tendon rupture. Reprinted with permission from Greenspan A. *Orthopeadic Imaging: A Practical Approach.* 5th ed. Philadelphia, PA: Wolters Kluwer Health/Lippincott Williams & Wilkins; 2010.

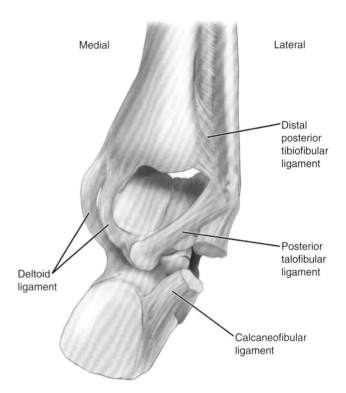

FIGURE 21-5 Inversion ankle sprain. Reprinted with permission from Anderson, MK. *Foundations of Athletic Training.* 6th ed. Philadelphia, PA: Wolters Kluwer; 2016.

mechanism is unclear, but it is believed to be related to decreased bone density or inability to adapt to increased tibial loading. Often, pain is absent at rest, starts with the initiation of activity, and then subsides with continued exertion. Pain with continued exertion is possible but should raise suspicion for a tibial bone stress injury.[26]

Tibial bone stress injuries can occur proximally or distally and include fractures and nonfractures. The exact mechanism of injury is not known, but it is believed to involve an altered bone remodeling response to repetitive microtrauma, which results in a weakening of the tibia bone. Athletes typically present with the insidious onset of pain, which is made worse with weight-bearing activities. Initially, there is pain after exertion, but this progresses to pain during exertion. It is important to inquire about recent increases in intensity of exercise routines.[26]

Acute ankle sprain is extremely common and occurs most often in young patients during athletic events. Lateral sprains are the most common, which occur owing to inversion of the ankle, usually with some degree of plantar flexion, damaging the lateral ankle ligaments. Patients describe sudden onset of pain along with swelling and ecchymosis (Figure 21-5).[34]

A syndesmotic sprain, or "high ankle sprain," occurs when the ligaments that support the joint formed by the distal ends of the tibia and fibula are damaged.[34] Syndesmotic sprains are more often seen in patients participating in sports such as football or downhill skiing; the most common mechanism of injury is believed to be external rotation, hyperdorsiflexion, and talar

eversion.[34,116] Patients may report anterior and posteromedial ankle pain, as well as pain with weight bearing or attempting to push off the ground.[43]

Maisonneuve fracture is a spiral fracture involving the proximal one-third of the fibula with significant associated injury to the distal tibiofibular syndesmosis, often including a concomitant fracture of the medial malleolus or the posterior margin of the distal tibia. These injuries are usually the result of violent internal rotation of the leg while on a planted foot with relative external rotation of the talus. Most patients report significant ankle pain with inability to bear weight on the involved extremity. Pain in the proximal tibia region is usually not reported.[28]

Achilles tendon ruptures occur most frequently in men, aged 30 to 50 years, and often during strenuous physical activity.[31] Patients commonly report the sensation of being struck in the posterior ankle and an audible pop during strenuous exercise.[31] A chronic rupture, defined as an untreated rupture of at least 4 weeks, usually presents with some degree of posterior ankle pain, swelling, and difficulty with pushing off with the affected limb.[32]

Plantar fasciitis is a common cause of heel pain in the adult primary care setting. Pain is believed to be due to microtears at the calcaneal enthesis caused by biomechanical overuse from prolonged standing or running. Patients typically report heel pain and tightness on rising from bed in the morning or after prolonged sitting. The pain typically improves with

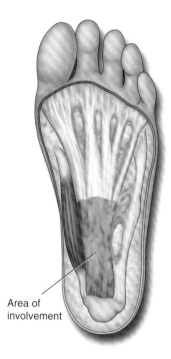

FIGURE 21-6 Plantar fascitis. Reprinted with permission from Werner R. *Massage Therapist's Guide to Pathology: Critical Thinking and Practical Application.* 6th ed. Philadelphia, PA: Wolters Kluwer; 2015. Figure 3.40.

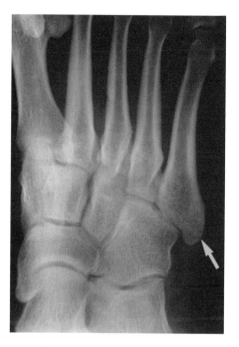

FIGURE 21-7 Nondisplaced Jones fracture (arrow). Reprinted with permission from Bittle MM, Gunn ML, Gross JA, Stern EJ. *Trauma Radiology Companion.* 2nd ed. Philadelphia, PA: Wolters Kluwer Health/Lippincott William & Wilkins; 2011. Figure 5.52B.

ambulation but can intensify toward the end of the day if the patient had been on his or her feet most of the time (Figure 21-6).[40]

"Turf toe," or first metatarsophalangeal (MTP) joint sprain, is usually the result of an injury involving an axial load being delivered to a foot with ankle in fixed equinus position while the great toe is in extension. This results in hyperextension of the first MTP joint and disrupts the capsular ligamentous complex of the joint. Patients are likely to present with pain and swelling of the first MTP joint after an acute injury.[36]

Metatarsal fractures are common, accounting for 5% to 6% of all fractures encountered in the primary care setting, and fifth metatarsal fractures, including Jones fractures, account for approximately 68% of metatarsal fractures. The proximal fifth metatarsal is known for poor healing; fifth metatarsal injuries generally present with acute or repetitive trauma to the forefoot, typically causing a transverse or slightly oblique fracture (Figure 21-7).[37]

Stress fractures of the foot and ankle can cause significant disability in all types of athletes, but particularly in runners. They are due to repetitive exposure to submaximal forces of energy that ultimately alter the balance between bone reabsorption and formation. Military recruits are at particular risk given the abrupt increase in physical activity. Patients often describe an insidious and progressive onset of pain and swelling of the foot or ankle.[42]

A Lisfranc injury involves damage to the bones or ligaments of the tarsometatarsal joints of the foot.[117] These injuries are rare, but failure to treat appropriately can lead to significant physical impairment and dysfunction.[117] Often subtle and occurring at low energy, the mechanism of injury typically involves excessive plantar flexion and abduction with associated longitudinal forces acting on the forefoot.[95] The presentations seen in Lisfranc injuries are broad, and patients may present with a benign history or a history of high-energy trauma.[95] Patients with more subtle presentations will usually report some degree of swelling in the mid-foot and almost invariably report pain on bearing weight.[95]

Hallux rigidus refers to osteoarthritis of the first MTP joint, which is one of the most common problems affecting the great toe.[101,118] Pain may occur on ambulation, and there may be a limited range of motion.[101] Hallux valgus deformity may be appreciable.[101]

Hallux valgus is a lateral deviation of the great toe at the first MTP joint and is the most common forefoot problem in adults.[119,120] It can cause pain, trouble walking, and difficulty fitting into shoes.[119] Patients report plantar foot pain, medial joint pain at the first MTP joint, and pain with weight bearing and poor-fitting shoes.[120]

Acute prepatellar bursitis is often caused by a bacterial infection, *Staphylococcus aureus* being the most commonly identified organism.[24] Approximately one-third of cases of prepatellar bursitis are known as septic bursitis, with the remaining being nonseptic bursitis.[121] Septic and nonseptic bursitis are both usually the result of some form of trauma, with introduction of bacteria into the bursal space.[60] Patients who experience repetitive trauma to their knees, such as wrestlers, gardeners, mechanics, or carpet layers, are at increased risk.[60] Patients report anterior knee pain, made worse by direct pressure over the bursa or compression of the bursa via extreme flexion at the knee.[60]

Septic arthritis must be considered in the differential for a patient presenting with monoarticular arthropathy, with the knee being the most commonly affected joint. Pathogens may enter the joint through direct inoculation (during trauma invasive procedure), from the spread of a local infection (osteomyelitis, abscess, septic bursitis), or through hematogenous spread during bacteremia (most common). Patients report acute onset of pain, swelling, warmth, erythema, impaired joint mobility, and possibly fever.[15]

Gout is the most common inflammatory arthropathy and is due to the deposition of monosodium urate crystals in a joint space.[16,122] Patients report rapid development of pain, swelling, and erythema, often involving the first MTP joint.[16] Attacks typically begin at night and peak within 24 hours of onset.[16] History may be notable for obesity, high calorie or high alcohol intake, or the use of loop or thiazide diuretic.[16] Trauma is also important to recognize as an antecedent to a gout flare and can present similarly to septic arthritis.[16]

Pseudogout (inflammatory arthropathy related to calcium pyrophosphate deposition) can present similarly to gout or osteoarthritis and may even be confused with rheumatoid arthritis, as joint involvement can be symmetric.[123] Pseudogout most commonly affects the knee.[123] Pseudogout can mimic gout in clinical presentation, and synovial fluid analysis may be needed to differentiate.[16,122]

Venous thromboembolic disease is common in the United States and manifests mainly as deep vein thrombosis (DVT) or pulmonary embolism (PE). According to Virchow triad, DVT is the result of hypercoagulability, blood flow alteration, and endothelial damage or dysfunction. Risks for DVT include surgery, trauma, hip fracture, spinal cord injury, malignancy, hormone therapy, oral contraceptives, pregnancy, previous DVT, thrombophilia, and immobility. Classically, patients describe pain, swelling, warmth, and erythema in the lower extremity, although it is possible for a patient to be completely asymptomatic.[97]

Acute compartment syndrome is a surgical emergency, and the leg is the most common location. The complications of delayed or ineffective treatment include muscle dysfunction, ischemic contractures, permanent dysesthesia, loss of limb, or even loss of life. It is often due to acute trauma but can have many other causes, including burn injuries, casts or other circumferential constrictive devices, bleeding disorders, and infection. Severe pain, out of proportion to a patient's injury, should be the first sign of acute compartment syndrome. Clinicians should not focus on the presence of pallor, paresthesias, pulselessness, or paralysis but should instead key in on the severity of pain as a trigger to consider the diagnosis. Patients may report resting pain or pain on passive stretching. Symptoms tend to progress and evolve over time.[33]

In contrast to acute compartment syndrome, chronic exertional compartment syndrome is an exertional pain syndrome that resolves with rest. About 95% of cases affect the lower leg. The mechanism is not entirely clear, but what is known is that intracompartmental pressures increase following exertion. Patients often describe pain after a specific amount of physical activity involving any or all of the compartments of the leg and may report bilateral symptoms in up to 82% of cases. The pain is described as a cramping sensation that increases with the intensity of exertion. Pain generally resolves on cessation of activity, almost immediately at first, but recovery time can gradually increase. Weakness, numbness, and paresthesias can occur.[26]

Morton neuroma is a common cause of chronic foot pain. It is actually proliferative fibrosis of perineural tissue rather than a true nerve tumor. The underlying cause is not clear. Patients classically report a burning pain at the plantar aspect of the foot, between the third and fourth metatarsal heads. The pain may radiate to the toes and be associated with paresthesias. Walking in high heels or in shoes with a narrow toe box exacerbates the pain. The pain may be relieved with a change in footwear or foot massage.[75]

Pain that is located distant to the actual source of pain is known as "referred pain" and can occur in musculoskeletal as well as visceral pain syndromes.[49] For instance, knee pain may be the manifestation of injury located at the hip, ankle, foot, or sacroiliac joint.[124] Hip pain more commonly refers to the groin and anterior thigh but may refer to the foot and knee in up to 6% and 2% of patients with symptomatic hip joint pathology, respectively.[125] Pain occurring at or below the knee can also be a symptom of radicular pain in patients with sciatica and can be accompanied by numbness, tingling, and weakness in the foot, leg, or groin.[126] Lower extremity pain localized to the anterior thigh, leg, or foot can also be caused by radicular pain from the lumbosacral spine, and this pain may also be accompanied by weakness and paresthesias.[127]

REFERENCES

1. Cecchi F, Mannoni A, Molino-Lova R, et al. Epidemiology of hip and knee pain in a community based sample of Italian persons aged 65 an older. *Osteoarthritis Cartilage.* 2008;16(9):1039-1046.

2. Jackson JL, O'Malley PG, Kroenke K. Evaluation of acute knee pain in primary care. *Ann Intern Med.* 2003;139(7):575-588.

3. Thomas MJ, Roddy E, Zhang W, Menz HB, Hannan MT, Peat GM. The population prevalence of foot and ankle pain in middle and old age: a systematic review. *Pain.* 2011;152(12):2870-2880.

4. Lichstein PR. Chapter 3 the medical interview. In: Hall WD, Walker HK, Hurst JW, eds. *Clinical Methods: the History, Physical and Laboratory Examinations.* Boston, MA: Butterworths; 1990:29-36.

5. Woolf AD, Akesson K. Primer: history and examination in the assessment of musculoskeletal problems. *Nat Clin Pract Rheumatol.* 2008;4(1):26-33.

6. Rossi R, Federico D, Bruzzone M, Cottino U, D'Elicio DG, Bonasia DE. Clinical examination of the knee: know your tools for diagnosis of knee injuries. *Sports Med Arthrosc Rehabil Ther Technol.* 2011;25(3).

7. FitzSimmons CR, Wardrope J. 9 assessment and care of musculoskeletal problems. *Emerg Med J.* 2005;22(1):68-76.

8. Cimino F, Volk BS, Setter D. Anterior cruciate ligament injury: diagnosis, management, and prevention. *Am Fam Physician.* 2010;82(8):917-922.

9. Macfarlane DG, Bacon PA. Popliteal cyst rupture in normal knee joints. *Br Med J.* 1980;281(6249):1203-1204.

10. Kapur S, Wissman RD, Robertson M, Verma S, Kreeger MC, Oostveen RJ. Acute knee dislocation: review of an elusive entity. *Curr Probl Diagn Radiol.* 2009;38(6):237-250.

11. Bylund WE, de Weber K. Semimembranosus tendinopathy: one cause of chronic posteromedial knee pain. *Sports Health.* 2010;2(5):380-384.

12. Calmbach WL, Hutchens M. Evaluation of patients presenting with knee pain: Part II. Differential diagnosis. *Am Fam Physician.* 2003;68(5):917-922.

13. Ellis R, Hing W, Reid D. Iliotibial band friction syndrome—a systematic review. *Man Ther.* 2007;12(3): 200-208.

14. Calmbach WL, Hutchens M. Evaluation of patients presenting with knee pain: part I. history, physical examination, radiographs, and laboratory tests. *Am Fam Physician.* 2003;68(5):907-912.

15. Horowitz DL, Katzap E, Horowitz S, Barilla-LaBarca ML. Approach to septic arthritis. *Am Fam Physician.* 2011;84(6):653-660.

16. Becker JA, Daily JP, Pohlgeers KM. Acute monoarthritis: diagnosis in adults. *Am Fam Physician.* 2016;94(10):810-816.

17. Bhatt J, Montalban AS, Wang KH, Lee HD, Nha KW. Isolated osteochondral fracture of the patella without patellar dislocation. *Orthopedics.* 2011;34(1):54.

18. Della Rocca GJ. Displaced patella fractures. *J Knee Surg.* 2013;26(5):293-299.

19. Fredberg U, Bolvig L. Jumper's knee. Review of the literature. *Scand J Med Sci Sports.* 1999;9(2):66-73.

20. Roudet A, Boudissa M, Chaussard C, Rubens-Duval B, Saragaglia D. Acute traumaic patellar tendon rupture: early and late results of surgical treatment of 38 cases. *Orthop Traumatol Surg Res.* 2015;101(3):307-311.

21. Lee D, Stinner D, Mir H. Quadriceps and patellar tendon ruptures. *J Knee Surg.* 2013;26(5):301-308.

22. Dutton RA, Khadavi MJ, Fredericson M. Patellofemoral pain. *Phys Med Rehabil Clin N Am.* 2016;27(1):31-52.

23. Rennie WJ, Saifuddin A. Pes anserine bursitis: incidence in symptomatic knees and clinical presentation. *Skeletal Radiol.* 2005;34(7):395-398.

24. Mathieu S, Prati C, Bossert M, Toussirot E, Valnet M, Wendling D. Acute prepatellar and olecranon bursitis. Retrospective observational study in 46 patients. *Joint Bone Spine.* 2011;78(4).

25. Wilson-MacDonald J. Management and outcome of infective prepatellar bursitis. *Postgrad Med J.* 1987;63(744):851-853.

26. Rajasekaran S, Finnoff JT. Exertional leg pain. *Phys Med Rehabil Clin N Am.* 2016;27(1):91-119.

27. Karande GY, Hedgire SS, Sanchez Y, et al. Advanced imaging in acute and chronic deep vein thrombosis. *Cardiovascular Diagn Ther.* 2016;6(6):493-507.

28. Taweel NR, Raikin SM, Karanjia HN, Ahmad J. The proximal fibula should be examined in all patients with ankle injury: a case series of missed maisonneuve fractures. *J Emerg Med.* 2013;44(2):e251-e255.

29. Brewer RB, Gregory AJ. Chronic lower leg pain in athletes: a guide for the differential diagnosis, evaluation, and treatment. *Sports Health.* 2012;4(2):121-127.

30. Igolnikov I, Santiago MJ, Gollotto KT. Poster 137 delayed diagnosis of popliteal artery entrapment mistaken for exertional compartment syndrome, novel use of MSK US to improve diagnostic sensitivity: a case report. *PM R.* 2016;8(9S):S206.

31. Mazzone MF, McCue T. Common conditions of the Achilles tendon. *Am Fam Physician.* 2002;65(9): 1805-1810.

32. Weinfeld SB. Achilles tendon disorders. *Med Clin North Am.* 2014;98(2):331-338.

33. von Keudell AG, Weaver MJ, Appleton PT, et al. Diagnosis and treatment of acute extremity compartment syndrome. *Lancet.* 2015;386(10000):1299-1310.

34. Tiemstra JD. Update on acute ankle sprains. *Am Fam Physician.* 2012;85(12):1170-1176.

35. Serrano S, Figueiredo P, Pascoa Pinheiro J. Fatigue fracture of the calcaneus: from early diagnosis to treatment: a case report of a triathlon athlete. *Am J Phys Med Rehabil.* 2016;95(6):e79-e83.

36. McCormick JJ, Anderson RB. Turf toe: anatomy, diagnosis, and treatment. *Sports Health.* 2010;2(6):487-494.

37. Bowes J, Buckley R. Fifth metatarsal fractures and current treatment. *World J Orthop.* 2016;7(12):793-800.

38. Brown GP, Feehery RV, Grant SM. Case study: the painful os trigonum syndrome. *J Orthop Sports Phys Ther.* 1995;22(1):22-25.

39. Giannini S, Buda R, Mosca M, Parma A, Di Caprio F. Posterior ankle impingement. *Foot Ankle Int.* 2013;34(3):459-465.

40. Goff JD, Crawford R. Diagnosis and treatment of plantar fasciitis. *Am Fam Physician.* 2011;84(6):676-682.

41. Helgeson K. Examination and intervention for sinus tarsi syndrome. *N Am J Sports Phys Ther.* 2009;4(1):29-37.

42. Greaser MC. Foot and ankle stress fractures in athletes. *Orthop Clin North Am.* 2016;47(4):809-822.

43. Williams GN, Jones MH, Amendola A. Syndesmotic ankle sprains in athletes. *Am J Sports Med.* 2007;35(7):1197-1207.

44. Duthon VB. Acute traumatic patellar dislocation. *Orthop Traumatol Surg Res.* 2015;101(1):S59-S67.

45. Hudes K. Conservative management of a case of tarsal tunnel syndrome. *J Can Chiropr Assoc.* 2010;54(2): 100-106.

46. Bahr R, Krosshaug T. Understanding injury mechanisms: a key component of preventing injuries in sport. *Br J Sports Med.* 2005;39(6):324-329.

47. Heard WM, VanSice WC, Savoie FH. Anterior cruciate ligament tears for the primary care sports physician: what to know on the field and in the office. *Phys Sportsmed.* 2015;43(4):432-439.

48. Shimokochi Y, Shultz S. Mechanisms of noncontact anterior cruciate ligament injury. *J Athl Train.* 2008;43(4): 396-408.

49. Graven-Nielsen T, Arendt-Nielsen L. Assessment of mechanisms in localized and widespread musculoskeletal pain. *Nat Rev Rheumatol.* 2010;6(10):599-606.

50. Sizer PS, Phelps V, Dedrick G, James R, Matthijs O. Diagnosis and management of the painful ankle/foot. Part 2: examination, interpretation and management. *Pain Pract.* 2003;3(4):343-374.

51. Tu P, Bytomski J. Diagnosis of heel pain. *Am Fam Physician.* 2011;84(8):909-916.

52. Fink R. Pain assessment: the cornerstone to optimal pain management. *Proc (Bayl Univ Med Cent).* 2000;13(3):236-239.

53. Austermuehle PD. Common knee injuries in primary care. *Nurse Pract.* 2001;26(10):32-45.

54. Frush TJ, Noyes FR. Baker's cyst: diagnostic and surgical considerations. *Sports Health.* 2015;7(4):359-365.

55. Khaund R, Flynn SH. Iliotibial band syndrome: a common source of knee pain. *Am Fam Physician.* 2005;71(8):1545-1550.

56. Griffith CJ, LaPrade RF. Medial plica irritation: diagnosis and treatment. *Curr Rev Musculoskeletal Med.* 2008;1(1):53-60.

57. Kamimura M, Umehara J, Takahashi A, Aizawa T, Itoi E. Medial meniscus tear morphology and related clinical symptoms in patients with medial knee osteoarthritis. *Knee Surg Sports Traumatol Arthrosc.* 2015;23(1)158-163.

58. Malliaras P, Cook J, Purdam C, Rio E. Patellar tendinopathy: clinical diagnosis, load management, and advice for challenging case presentations. *J Orthop Sports Phys Ther.* 2015;45(11):887-898.

59. Dixit S, DiFiori JP, Burton M, Mines B. Management of patellofemoral pain syndrome. *Am Fam Physician.* 2007;75(2):194-202.

60. McAfee JH, Smith DL. Olecranon and prepatellar bursitis. Diagnosis and treatment. *West J Med.* 1988;149(5):607-610.

61. Maffulli N, Via AG, Oliva F. Chronic Achilles tendon disorders: tendinopathy and chronic rupture. *Clin Sports Med.* 2015;34(4):607-624.

62. Drakos MC, Fiore R, Murphy C, DiGiovanni CW. Plantar-plate disruptions: "The severe turf-toe injury." Three cases in contact athletes. *J Athl Train.* 2015;50(5):553-560.

63. Richardson DR, Dean EM. The recurrent Morton neuroma: what now? *Foot Ankle Clin.* 2014;19(3): 437-449.

64. Ahmad M, Tsang K, Mackenney PJ, Adedapo AO. Tarsal tunnel syndrome: a literature review. *Foot Ankle Surg.* 2012;18(3):149-152.

65. Helfenstein M, Kuromoto J, Anserine syndrome. *Rev Bras Reumatol.* 2010;50(3):313-327.

66. Shiraev T, Anderson SE, Hope N. Meniscal tear–presentation, diagnosis and management. *Aust Fam Physician.* 2012;41(4):182-187.

67. Immerman I, Price AE, Alfonso I, Grossman JA. Lower extremity nerve trauma. *Bull Hosp Jt Dis.* 2013;72(1):43-52.

68. Grant GA, Goodkin R, Kliot M. Evaluation and surgical management of peripheral nerve problems. *Neurosurgery.* 1999;44(4):825-839.

69. Sato S, Uehara T, Ohara T, Suzuki R, Minematsu K. Factors associated with unfavorable outcome in minor ischemic stroke. *Neurology.* 2014;83(2):174-181.

70. Sun P, Guo J, Xu N. Correlation between diabetic lower-extremity arterial disease and diabetic neuropathy in patients with type II diabetes: an exploratory study. *Int J Clin Exp Med.* 2015;8(1):1396-1400.

71. MM M. Lower extremity manifestations of peripheral artery disease: the pathophysiologic and functional implications of leg ischemia. *Circ Res.* 2015;116(9):1540-1550.

72. Krych AJ, Giuseffi SA, Kuzma SA, Stuart MJ, Levy BA. Is peroneal nerve injury associated with worse function after knee dislocation? *Clin Orthop Relat Res.* 2014;472(9):2630-2636.

73. Moore KL, Dalley AF, Agur AMR. *Clinically Oriented Anatomy.* 6th ed. Philadelphia: Wolters Kluwer|Lippincott Williams & Wilkins; 2010:1134.

74. Baima J, Krivickas L. Evaluation and treatment of peroneal neuropathy. *Curr Rev Musculoskeletal Med.* 2008;1(2):147-153.

75. Jain S, Mannan K. The diagnosis and management of Morton's neuroma: a literature review. *Foot Ankle Spec.* 2013;6(4).

76. Howell R, Kumar NS, Patel N, Tom J. Degenerative meniscus: pathogenesis, diagnosis, and treatment options. *World J Orthop.* 2014;5(5):597-602.

77. Bussewitz BW. How to address the neglected Achilles tendon rupture. *Podiatry Today.* 2011;24(11).

78. Dean Deyle G. The role of MRI in musculoskeletal practice: a clinical perspective. *J Man Manip Ther.* 2011;19(3):152-161.

79. van der Linden PD, Sturkenboom MC, Herings RM, Leufkens HM, Rowlands S, Stricker BH. Increased risk of Achilles tendon rupture with quinolone antibacterial use, especially in elderly patients taking oral corticosteroids. *Arch Intern Med.* 2003;163(15):1801-1807.

80. Turmo-Garuz A, Rodas G, Balius R, et al. Can local corticosteroid injection in the retrocalcaneal bursa lead to rupture of the Achilles tendon and the medial head of the gastrocnemius muscle? *Musculoskeletal Surg.* 2014;98(2):121-126.

81. Kotnis RA, Halstead J, Hormbrey PJ. Atraumatic bilateral Achilles tendon rupture: an association of systemic steroid treatment. *J Accid Emerg Med.* 1999;16(5):378-379.

82. Salmon L, Russell V, Musgrove T, Pinczewski L, Refshauge K. Incidence and risk factors for graft rupture and contralateral rupture after anterior cruciate ligament reconstruction. *Arthroscopy.* 2005;21(8):948-957.

83. Grover M. Evaluating acutely injured patients for internal derangement of the knee. *Am Fam Physician.* 2012;85(3):247-252.

84. Morelli V, Braxton TM. Meniscal, plica, patellar, and patellofemoral injuries of the knee: updates, controversies and advancements. *Prim Care.* 2013;40(2):357-382.

85. Rutland M, O'Connell D, Brismee JM, Sizer P, Apte G, O'Connell J. Evidence-supported rehabilitation of patellar tendinopathy. *N Am J Sports Phys Ther.* 2010;5(3):166-178.

86. Schwartz A, Watson JN, Hutchinson MR. Patellar tendinopathy. *Sports Health.* 2015;7(5):415-420.

87. Reinking MF. Current concepts in the treatment of patellar tendinopathy. *Int J Sports Phys Ther.* 2016;11(6):854-866.

88. Rodriguez-Merchan EC. The treatment of patellar tendinopathy. *J Ortho Traumatol.* 2013;14(2):77-81.

89. Jain NP, Khan N, Fithian DC. A treatment algorithm for primary patellar dislocation. *Sports Health.* 2011;3(2):170-174.

90. Petri M, Ettinger M, Stuebig T, et al. Current concepts for patellar dislocation. *Arch Trauma Res.* 2015;4(3):e29301.

91. Millen JC, Lindberg D. Maisonneuve fracture. *J Emerg Med.* 2009;41(1):77-78.

92. Egger AC, Berkowitz MJ. Achilles tendon injuries. *Curr Rev Musculoskelet Med.* 2017;10(1):72-80.

93. Wolfe MW, Uhl T, Mattacola CG, McCluskey LC. Management of ankle sprains. *Am Fam Physician.* 2001;63(1):93-104.

94. Strayer SM, Reece SG, Petrizzi MJ. Fractures of the proximal fifth metatarsal. *Am Fam Physician.* 1999;59(9):2516-2522.

95. Reissig J, Bitterman A, Lee S. Common foot and ankle injuries: what not to miss and how best to manage. *J Am Osteopath Assoc.* 2017;117(2):98-104.

96. Hennion DR, Siano K. Diagnosis and treatment of peripheral artery disease. *Am Fam Physician.* 2013;88(5):306-310.

97. Wilbur J, Shian B. Diagnosis of deep venous thrombosis and pulmonary embolism. *Am Fam Physician.* 2012;86(10):913-919.

98. Behravesh S, Hoang P, Nanda A, et al. Pathogenesis of thromboembolism and endovascular management. *Thrombosis.* 2017;2017.

99. Azhary H, Farooq M, Bhanushali M, Majid A, Kassab MY. Peripheral neuropathy: differential diagnosis and management. *Am Fam Physician.* 2010;81(7):887-892.

100. Mazzuca SA, Brandt KD, Katz BP, Ding Y, Lane KA, Buckwalter KA. Risk factors for progression of tibiofemoral osteoarthritis: an analysis based on fluoroscopically standardised knee radiography. *Ann Rheum Dis.* 2006;65(4):515-519.

101. Sinusas K. Osteoarthritis. *Am Fam Physician.* 2012;85(1):49-56.

102. Peat G, Duncan RC, Wood LR, Thomas E, Muller S. Clinical features of symptomatic patellofemoral joint osteoarthritis. *Arthritis Res Ther.* 2012;14(2):R63.

103. Kim YM, Joo YB. Patellofemoral osteoarthritis. *Knee Surg Relat Res.* 2012;24(4):193-200.

104. Schiphof D, van Middelkoop M, de Klerk BM, et al. Crepitus is a first indication of patellofemoral osteoarthritis (and not of tibiofemoral osteoarthritis). *Osteoarthritis Cartilage.* 2014;22(5):631-638.

105. Swagerty DL, Hellinger D. Radiographic assessment of osteoarthritis. *Am Fam Physician.* 2001;64(2):279-286.

106. McDermott I. Meniscal tears, repairs and replacement: their relevance to osteoarthritis of the knee. *Br J Sports Med.* 2011;45(4):292-297.

107. Longo UG, Garau G, Denaro V, Maffulli N. Surgical management of tendinopathy of biceps femoris in athletes. *Disabil Rehabil.* 2008;30(20-22):1602-1607.

108. Kujala UM, Orava S, Jarven M. Hamstring injuries. Current trends in treatment and prevention. *Sports Med.* 1997;23(6):397-404.

109. Aldebeyan S, Boily M, Martineau PA. Complete tear of the distal hamstring tendons in a professional football player: a care report and review of the literature. *Skeletal Radiol.* 2016;45(3):427-430.

110. Fritschy D, Fasel J, Imbert JC, Bianchi S, Verdonk R, Wirth CJ. The popliteal cyst. *Knee Surg Sports Traumatol Arthrosc.* 2006;14(7):623-628.

111. Bennett RM, Haleem AM, Bywaters EG, Holt PJ. Studies of a popliteal synovial fistula. *Ann Rheum Dis.* 1972;31(6):482-486.

112. Khamaisy S, Haleem AM, Williams RJ, Rozbruch SR. Neglected rotary knee dislocation: a case report. *Knee.* 2014;21(5):975-978.

113. Myers RJ, Murdock EE, Farooqi M, Van Ness G, Crawford DC. A unique case of common peroneal nerve entrapment. *Orthopedics.* 2015;38(7):e644-e646.

114. Longo UG, Ciuffreda M, Locher J, Berton A, Salvatore G, Denaro V. Treatment of primary acute patellar dislocation: systematic review and quantitative synthesis of the literature. *Clin J Sport Med.* 2017;27:511-523.

115. Larsen P, Court-Brown CM, Vedel JO, Vistrup S, Elsoe R. Incidence and epidemiology of patellar fractures. *Orthopedics.* 2016;39(6):1154-1158.

116. Schnetzke M, Vetter SY, Beisemann N, Swartman B, Grutzner PA, Franke J. Management of syndesmotic injuries: what is the evidence? *World J Orthop.* 2016;7(11):718-725.

117. Lewis JS, Anderson RB. Lisfranc injuries in the athlete. *Foot Ankle Int.* 2016;37(12):1374-1380.

118. Polzer H, Polzer S, Brumann M, Mutschler W, Regauer M. Hallux rigidus: joint preserving alternatives to arthrodesis - a review of the literature. *World J Orthop.* 2014;5(1):6-13.

119. Mortka K, Lisiński P. Hallux valgus-a case for a physiotherapist or only for a surgeon? Literature review. *J Phys Ther Sci.* 2015;27(10):3303-3307.

120. Hecht PJ, Lin TJ. Hallux valgus. *Med Clin North Am.* 2014;98(2):227-232.

121. Baumbach SF, Lobo CM, Badyine I, Mutschler W, Kanz KG. Prepatellar and olecranon bursitis: literature review and development of a treatment algorithm. *Arch Orthop Trauma Surg.* 2014;134(3):359-370.

122. Hainer BL, Matheson E, Wilkes RT. Diagnosis, treatment, and prevention of gout. *Am Fam Physician.* 2014;90(12):831-836.

123. Choy G. An update on the treatment options for gout and calcium pyrophosphate deposition. *Expert Opin Pharmacother.* 2005;6(14):2443-2453.

124. Vaughn DW. Isolated knee pain: a case report highlighting regional interdependence. *J Orthop Sports Phys Ther.* 2008;38(10):616-623.

125. Lesher JM, Dreyfuss P, Hager N, Kaplan M, Furman M. Hip joint pain referral patterns: a descriptive study. *Pain Med.* 2008;9(1):22-25.

126. Grovle L, Haugen AJ, Keller A, Natvig B, Brox JI, Grotle M. The bothersomeness of sciatica: patients' self-report of paresthesia, weakness and leg pain. *Eur Spine J.* 2010;19(2):263-269.

127. Van Boxem K, Cheng J, Patijn J, van Kleef M, Lataster A, Mekhail N, Van Zundert J. 11. Lumbosacral pain. *Pain Pract.* 2010;10(4):339-358.

22

PELVIC PAIN

Rachel Worman, PT, DPT, MPT and Samir J. Sheth, MD

FAST FACTS

- Chronic pelvic pain (CPP) can affect males as well as females, and the worldwide estimated prevalence is 2.1% to 24%.
- When determining the cause of CPP, a thorough account of past surgical, psychological, and sexual history, including sexual abuse, should be identified.
- CPP can arise from many different organ systems and as such, multidisciplinary management (gynecology, urology, gasteroenterology, pain medicine) is not uncommon.

- Treatment usually begins with pelvic floor physical therapy, which is combined with behavioral health strategies. Pharmacologic and nonpharmacologic procedural interventions should be considered in patients with treatment-resistant CPP.

INTRODUCTION

Pelvic pain is a common disorder defined as a "pain located at the level of the lower abdomen, pelvis, or pelvic structures, which persists either intermittently or continuously for at least 3 to 6 months unassociated with menstrual cycle or pregnancy."[1] Although much of the literature focuses on chronic pelvic pain (CPP) in females, it is a disorder that commonly affects males as well. The prevalence of CPP is thought to be anywhere from 2.1% to 24% of the worldwide population.[2,3] Despite its high prevalence, the exact diagnosis is unknown in up to two-thirds of patients[4] owing to the complex nature of CPP and the various causes.

HISTORY

When taking a history of patients with CPP, it is important to be comprehensive. In addition to asking standard questions such as about pain intensity, quality, radiation, pain interference, and timing, it is important to ask the patient's past surgical, psychological, and sexual history (including any sexual abuse history) (see later discussion). Patients with CPP have a rate of depression that may be 3 times higher than that of the general population.[5] Surgical history also aids the initial workup and/or etiology. The International Pelvic Pain Society (IPPS) has a Pelvic Pain Assessment questionnaire available at http://pelvicpain.org/professional/documents-and-forms.aspx. Other surveys include the National Institutes of Health-Chronic Prostatitis Symptom Index (NIH-CPSI). The IPPS assessment questionnaire is more comprehensive and includes questions regarding surgical history and sexual history, along with mental health problems and/or history of sexual abuse. Prior surgery and history of falls greatly facilitate etiology of the patient's pain. For example, patients with prior inguinal herniorrhaphy can develop scar tissue, including neuroma, which can cause severe neuropathic pain. Patients who had surgery and/or trauma to the pelvic floor may have compression of the pudendal nerve, which leads to pain with sitting along with pain in perineum (see later discussion). If a questionnaire is not used, a thorough history as detailed later should be considered.

SUBJECTIVE

In the subjective interview, it is essential to focus on standard assessment models of pain (i.e., onset, quality, radiation, severity, and timing), especially the aggravating and alleviating factors. In pelvic pain, it is important to determine the changes occurring throughout the day as well as the cyclical nature on a monthly and/or seasonal basis.

Special questions in a pelvic pain interview include a thorough bowel, bladder, and dietary history. For the sake of time, it may be useful to have an intake form that can be completed by the patient before the visit.

Chief Complaints

Specifying the location of pelvic pain can be difficult, as visceral sensation is difficult to describe. When patients describe pain, it may be diffuse and poorly localized to areas such as the abdomen, groin, low back, and buttock. This information will support physical examination findings.

Aggravating factors in pelvic pain include activities, movements, positions, and dietary intake that trigger the pain. Alleviating factors in pelvic pain commonly include avoidance of certain foods, improved fiber intake, medications, positional changes, and rest.

Bowel, Bladder, and Diet Logs

Bowel, bladder, and diet logs can be completed via intake forms or interview. Bowel questions are outlined in Box 22-1, Bladder questions are outlined in Box 22-2 and Diet questions are outlined in Box 22-3.

Psychosocial History

High-quality studies exploring the psychosocial aspects of pelvic pain are limited. The current literature associates psychological factors such as stress, pain catastrophizing, personality factors, and social factors with the development of chronic prostatitis/chronic pelvic pain syndrome in men.[12] Moreover, psychologic factors including catastrophizing, hypervigilance, depression, fear of pain, and anxiety are correlated with provoked vestibulodynia in women.[13,14] Indeed, impaired sexual function is a frequent finding among women with vestibulodynia.[13]

Assessment and treatment of psychosocial factors is part of a multimodal pain management approach to pelvic pain. Box 22-4 outlines a list of potential questions for the interview.

Box 22-1 Bowel Interview Questions

1. Do you have any change in your bowel function?
2. What do you eat/drink for breakfast, lunch, dinner, and snacks?
3. How many bowel movements do you have per day or per week?
4. Do you have pain before, during, and/or after bowel movements?
5. How do you describe your stool on the Bristol stool scale?
6. Do you use any of the following (fiber supplements, stool softeners, stimulant laxatives, probiotics)?
7. Do you have any bowel incontinence (fecal smearing; mucous, watery stool; soft stool; pebbles)?
8. Does a strong urge precede any bowel disorder?
9. What is your position when defecating?
10. Do you have a history of irritable bowel syndrome? Type (constipated and/or loose)?
11. Do you have a history of irradiation in the pelvic region?

Box 22-2 Bladder Interview Questions

1. Do you have any change in bladder function?
2. How many times per day do you void?
   a. Is it frequent in the morning or afternoon?
3. How many times do you void at night?
4. Do you have urinary incontinence?
   a. With coughing, sneezing, lifting, and laughing was leaking unavoidable?
   b. How many episodes of incontinence per day or per week do you experience?
   c. Do you wear pads? (Depends, B-sure, Always incontinence pads)
      i. Are the pads saturated (minimal [drops], moderate [50%], or maximal [100%])?
5. Fluid intake
   a. How many glasses of water do you drink every day?
   b. How much of each of the following do you drink? Coffee, tea (herbal or caffeinated), alcohol, soda, juice, milk?

Etiology

There are many potential causes to CPP. The overlap between somatic and visceral pain can be a diagnostic challenge. Therefore, it is important to be systematic

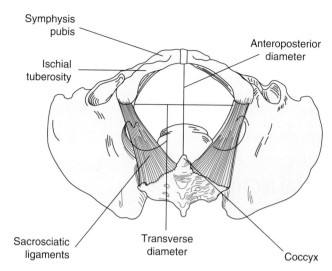

FIGURE 22-1 Pelvic anatomy. Reprinted with permission from Pillitteri A, Silbert-Flagg J. *Maternal and Child Nursing*. 4th ed. Philadelphia, PA: Lippincott, Williams & Wilkins; 2003.

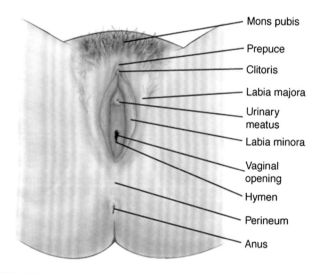

FIGURE 22-2 Female external genitalia. Reprinted with permission from Smith NE. *Introductory Medical-Surgical Nursing*. 12th ed. Philadelphia, PA: Wolters Kluwer; 2017.

when assessing pelvic pain. The European Association of Urology recommends assessing multiple anatomical regions (urologic, gynecologic, colorectal, myofascial, and neurologic) when developing a differential diagnosis in patients with CPP.[6]

Anatomy and Physical Examination

Anatomy

The anatomical structures of the pelvis and its interconnections to the spine, trunk, and lower extremity make it a unique and complex relay center for function. Pelvic pain may arise from bone, joint, ligament, fascia, muscle, arterial, venous or lymphatic vessels, and visceral or nerve structures. Although pain may arise from one structure, other structures may respond and develop further dysfunction. Specialty clinicians must consider these functional anatomical interconnections when approaching the diagnostic and treatment process for pelvic pain.[7]

The pelvic perineum is the area overlying the pelvic outlet and includes the genitalia, perineal body, and urogenital and anal triangles. It is contained by bony and ligamentous borders between the pubic symphysis anteriorly, the pubic ramus anterolaterally, ischioramus laterally, sacrotuberous ligament posterolaterally, and the coccyx posteriorly (Figure 22-1).

In females, the perineum includes the vulva (female genitalia), which contains the labia majora and minora. Anteriorly, labia majora and labia minora form the hood of the clitoris, or prepuce and frenulum of the clitoris and its tissues may be implicated and must be tested in painful conditions such as clitorodynia. The labia minora contains sweat glands and joins posteriorly to become the posterior fourchette of the vagina, which is

often torn during child delivery and may be a source of pain or dyspareunia due to decreased mobility with scar tissue (see Figure 22-2).

In males, the perineum has the same bony borders, with the external genitalia comprising the scrotum and penis.

Figure 22-3 details the visceral as well as muscular components for the pelvis and perineum in both males and females, respectively. These figures are especially helpful when performing a pelvic floor physical examination or when reading a report from a pelvic floor physical therapist.

Finally, Hart line (Figure 22-4) is an important female anatomical landmark for clinicians. It is the line between the labia minora and the vestibule. This is where the cotton swab test is performed (see section on pelvic examination). The vestibule is a space outlined by the urethra, inner labia minora, vagina, and Bartholin gland

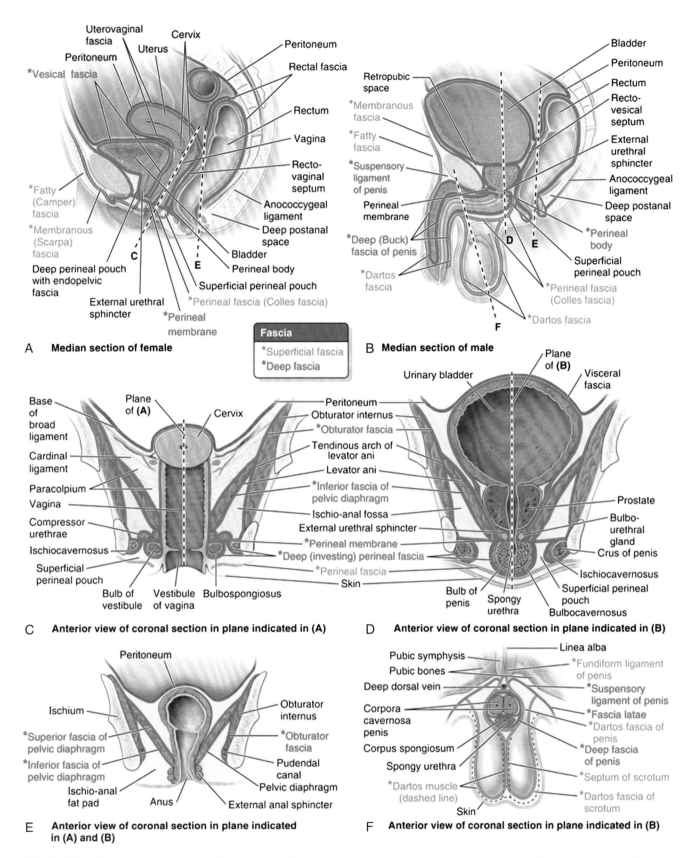

FIGURE 22-3 Fasciae of perineum. **A and B,** Median sections, viewed from left, demonstrate the fasciae in the female (A) and male (B). The planes of the sections shown in parts (C)–(F) are indicated. **C,** This coronal section of the female urogenital triangle is in the plane of the vagina. Fibroareolar components of the endopelvic fascia (cardinal ligament and paracolpium) are shown. **D,** This coronal section of the male urogenital triangle is in the plane of the prostatic urethra. **E,** This coronal section of the anal triangle is in the plane of the lower rectal and anal canals. **F,** This coronal section demonstrates the subcutaneous tissue of the proximal penis and scrotum. Reprinted with permission from Moore KL, Dalley AF, Agur AM. *Moore Clinically Oriented Anatomy.* 7th ed. Philadelphia, PA: Lippincott Williams & Wilkins; 2014.

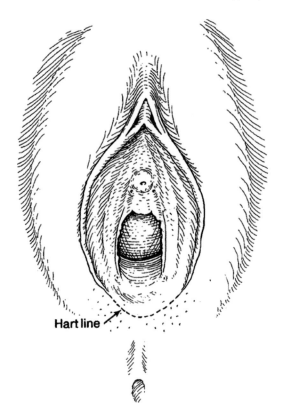

FIGURE 22-4 Hart line. The vulvar vestibule and the position of Hart line. Hart line can be found on the medial aspect of the labia majora, extending in a curvilinear manner from the most inferior posterior portion of the labia minora to the vaginal fourchette. Reprined with permission from Mills SE. *Histology for Pathologists.* 4th ed. Philadelphia, PA: Wolters Kluwer Health/Lippincott Williams & Wilkins; 2012.

posteriorly. Pain that is medial to Hart line yet distal to the introitus indicates the diagnosis of vestibulodynia. Lateral to Hart line sensation is normal (without pain).

The neurovascular supply to the pelvic region arises from multiple different spinal levels. Blood is supplied to the external genitalia via the internal and external pudendal arteries, bilaterally. The bulb of the penis and the vestibule and labia drain to the internal pudendal vein.

Two main nerves provide the innervation to the external genitalia. Their course from the spine may provide the practitioner with information about other suspect structures.

The ilioinguinal nerve is mainly derived from the anterior rami of L1 nerve with contributions from T12. It pierces the psoas muscle before traversing laterally and anterior to the quadratus lumborum. It pierces the transverse abdominus at the anterior iliac crest and lies between the transverse abdominus and internal oblique muscle. Branches of the ilioinguinal nerve innervate the skin of anterior scrotum and base of the penis in males and the skin of the mons pubis and upper labia majora in females.[29]

The genitofemoral nerve is derived from the L1-L2 nerve roots and travels inferior to pierce through psoas major muscle at the L3-4 intervertebral disc level and then runs along its anterior surface. It branches to become the femoral and genital nerves.[29]

The femoral branch courses posterior to the inguinal ligament and innervates the skin of superior anterior thigh.[29]

The genital nerve enters the inguinal canal by passing through the deep inguinal ring.[29] The genital branch provides sensory innervation to posterior scrotum in males as well as motor supply to the cremasteric muscle in males. In females, the nerve provides sensory innervation to the ipsilateral mons pubis and labia majora.[33]

The pudendal nerve derives from the anterior rami of the sacral 2 to 4 nerve roots. The nerve travels through the greater sciatic foramen anteriorly before turning posteriorly to pass between the sacrospinous and sacrotuberous ligaments. The pudendal nerve then travels anteriorly through the lesser sciatic foramen into the perineal region via Alcock canal (obturator internus fascia) before giving off its 3 major branches: deep perineal, superficial perineal, and inferior rectal nerves (see Figure 22-5). The pudendal nerve supplies the skin of the penis and clitoris, the sensory innervation to the perineum along with the posterior aspect of the scrotum, and labia majora. It also provides motor innervation to the deep muscles of the pelvic floor along with the external anal sphincter.[29,30]

Physical Examination

The physical examination of the pelvic floor is distinct and requires special training to perform properly. It can be uncomfortable for patients, and if the patient has a lot of pain with the maneuvers, the physical examination may have to be done in subsequent appointments. In general, collaborating with a pelvic floor physical therapist or specialist who is trained in pelvic floor physical examination is advantageous given the complex nature of pelvic floor dysfunction.

OBJECTIVE

Observation

View the perineum in lithotomy position. Note any asymmetry in gluteal muscles and adductor muscles. Note any sign of skin breakdown or tissue dehydration. In females, tissue dehydration may be present early in life with contraceptive medications or later in life following menopause. The vulva will present as wrinkled and atrophied and will not fall back into place when mobilized, as the skin turgor is altered. The perineal body in men and women should lie approximately 1 cm above the level of the ischial tuberosities. If it is elevated greater than 1 cm, the practitioner may note possible signs of hypertonicity of the pelvic floor muscles. If it is descended below the level of ischial tuberosities, the practitioner may be concerned about hypotonicity, muscle weakness, fascial or ligamentous laxity, and/or prolapse that can all be contributing to pain.

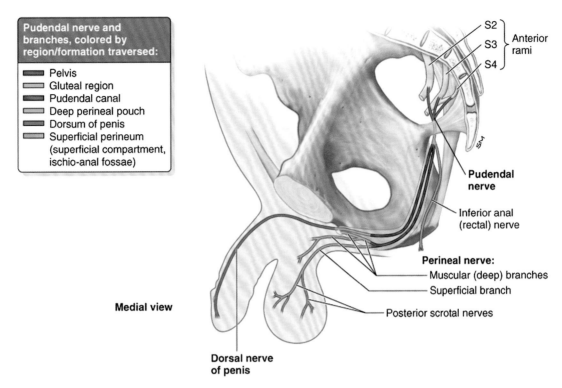

Pudendal nerve and branches, colored by region/formation traversed:

- Pelvis
- Gluteal region
- Pudendal canal
- Deep perineal pouch
- Dorsum of penis
- Superficial perineum (superficial compartment, ischio-anal fossae)

S2
S3 } Anterior rami
S4

Pudendal nerve

Inferior anal (rectal) nerve

Perineal nerve:
Muscular (deep) branches
Superficial branch

Posterior scrotal nerves

Medial view

Dorsal nerve of penis

FIGURE 22-5 Pudendal nerve. Reprinted with permission from Moore KL, Dalley AF, Agur AM. *Moore Clinically Oriented Anatomy.* 7th ed. Philadelphia, PA: Lippincott Williams & Wilkins; 2014.

On observation, signs of genital or perineal disease or lesion must either be ruled out or referred to gynecology, urology, urogynecology, or vulvar dermatology for further testing. In the absence of genital and perineal lesions, the neuromusculoskeletal examination can proceed.

Patchy erythema is commonly observed distal to the vaginal opening in patients with vestibulodynia.[15] Friedrich's criteria (Box 22-5) are used to diagnose vulvar vestibulitis syndrome and includes in its criteria vulvar erythema.[16] If signs of vestibulitis are present, patients should be referred to urogynecology for proper medical management. Once the inflammation is under control, a referral to pelvic health physical therapy should follow to address any related muscle, fascia, and residual nerve sensitivity problems.

Function

Functional testing allows the therapist to observe movement patterns without manually provoking pain. In cases in which the patient chooses not to have a manual examination, but will allow for perineal observation, this can offer some information to assess and initiate a treatment program. In the lithotomy position, the practitioner will ask the patient to contract his or her pelvic floor muscles. Normal function is an independent lift of the perineal body that appears symmetric on the first attempt.

Box 22-5 Friedrich's Criteria for Vulvar Vestibulitis Syndrome[16]

1. Vulvar erythema
2. Severe pain over vulvar vestibule upon touch or attempted vaginal entry
3. Tenderness to pressure of the vulvar vestibule

Abnormal patterns to document may be perineal body lift with accessory muscle (gluteal, abdominal), overactivity such as gluteal, abdominal or adductor activity, asymmetries in pelvic floor muscle activity, and paradoxical contraction (patient either eccentrically lengthens or performs a Valsalva maneuver causing the perineal body to drop instead of lift). The practitioner will gain a sense of coordination of the pelvic floor. Reports of pain with attempts to contract should be documented as well. Observation of breathing patterns on attempts to contract is important to note.

Muscle Testing

Standard guidelines for the testing of pelvic floor muscles as a source of pain do not exist. Yet, in the presence of other disease, muscles can be affected and eventually become their own source of pain. Especially in the absence of other disease, muscle testing should be pursued. Testing techniques for pelvic floor muscles are generally borrowed from studies assessing other body regions.[17] These include palpation of muscles for quality of tissue. Quality of muscle tissue can be defined by its ability to yield to, dissipate, resist, or withstand force of palpation. Other features such as boggy, stiff, fibrous, dense, and atrophy can describe the quality of the tissue. Muscle tone can be palpated as having hypertonic, hypotonic, or intermittent spasms. Palpation may also give information about local muscle tender points or trigger points that are tender and perceived as referred pain elsewhere.[18,19]

Laycock's Modified Oxford Grading System is a reliable manual muscle test of pelvic floor strength (Box 22-6).[20] On digital vaginal examination, the patient is asked to contract the pelvic floor muscles. Muscle endurance is the ability to sustain the contraction at 50% or greater effort.[17] This is clinically tested for 10 seconds.

First Layer

Externally, the bulbospongiosus, ischiocavernosus, superficial transverse perineal, iliococcygeal, and coccygeal muscles can all be palpated through the skin in a clockwise manner (Figure 22-6). At each muscle palpated, the practitioner notes the tissue quality and requests the patient report their pain level and where they feel pain, noting if it is felt local or referred (Table 22-1).

Cotton Swab Test

Chronic unexplained vulvar pain in females is a highly prevalent disorder often misdiagnosed.[21] The cotton swab test is part of the workup for vulvodynia or vestibulodynia and uses a cotton swab to systematically instill light pressure distal to the introitus superficial to the vestibule over the Hart line (Figure 22-4), in a clockwise fashion to test sensitivity or pain. In women with vulvodynia, pressure-pain sensitivities tested over the vulvar region and peripheral regions were both elevated, suggesting possible central sensitization.[22] The cotton swab test may underestimate pain levels compared with reports of symptoms in studies and is therefore not necessary diagnosis of vulvodynia or vestibulodynia.[16,23]

Second Layer

The second testing layer requires digital palpation to the compressor urethra and sphincter urethrae muscles. These muscles are found when the practitioner aims the pad of the finger anteriorly to the posterior pubic bone. At midline, the urethra is found and urethral sphincter can be palpated approximately 1 inch from the introitus in females. In males, the prostatic urethra cannot be palpated, as the prostate surrounds it at approximately 3 to 3.5 inches from the anus. To confirm location of the compressor urethra in females, the patient can be asked to contract. The practitioner will feel a slight contraction around the urethra. He or she will move the palpating finger from the urethral sphincter just lateral to feel for the compressor urethra. This can be palpated in females alongside the urethra and in males alongside the prostate. To confirm, the patient can contract and the urethra should be felt moving anterior toward the pubic bone in females and a thickening of the muscle in males.

Third Layer

With the pad of the practitioner's digit aiming directly posterior, at approximately 2 to 2.5 inches from the introitus in females or the anus in males (and females if testing muscles through the rectum), the coccyx can be palpated. This will be through or lateral to the rectum if testing from the vaginal canal. Once the lateral border of the coccyx and lower sacrum is palpated, the coccygeal muscle can be followed as it narrows laterally toward the ischial spine. Return to mid belly of the coccygeal muscle, move anteriorly and inferiorly to find the iliococcygeal muscle. Pubococcygeal muscle is palpated further anteriorly and can be followed to its attachments at the posterior pubic bone. The muscles are then palpated on the opposite side for comparison.

Fourth Layer

The clinical fourth layer or pelvic wall is formed by the obturator internus laterally and piriformis posteriorly. The obturator internus is found by palpating directly lateral from the vaginal canal and anterior of lateral from

---

Box 22-6 Laycock Modified Oxford Grading System for Pelvic Floor Muscle Strength[20]

0—No active muscle contraction
1-
1—Very slight muscular contraction
1+
2-
2—Full-motion overcome the force of gravity
2+
3-
3—Full-motion against gravity
3+
4-
4—Full-motion against slight resistance
4+
5-
5—Full-motion against strong resistance
5+

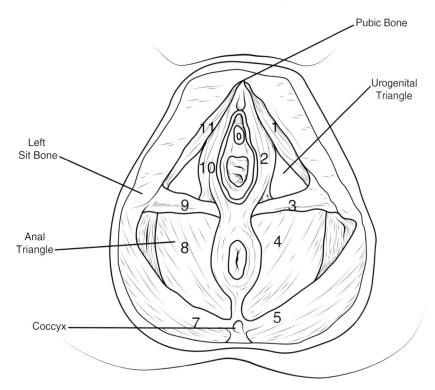

FIGURE 22-6 Pelvic testing clock.

TABLE 22-1 Documentation Chart for Layer 1 Palpation

MUSCLE	RIGHT PAIN/NOTES	LEFT PAIN/NOTES
Bulbospongiosus		
Ischiocavernosus		
Superficial transverse perineal		
Iliococcygeal		
Coccygeal		

the rectal canal. The practitioner follows the iliococcygeal superiorly until a thickened "ledge" is felt. This is the tendinous arch of levator ani. The palpating finger moves superiorly to the tendinous arch to find obturator internus. To confirm, the patient is asked to abduct the knee into the practitioner's available hand and the obturator muscle will thicken. Obturator muscle can be followed anteriorly to its attachment on posterior pubic bone or posteriorly before it passes below the ischial spine.

To identify the piriformis muscle, first locate the sacrococcygeal joint by palpation. Further palpation is done along the superolateral border to confirm the piriformis attachment to the anterior surface of the sacrum. The piriformis functions as a hip abductor in hip flexion. The piriformis will contract with this action.

TESTING LAYERS

Testing layers of the pelvic floor are listed in Table 22-2.

Pudendal Nerve Testing

Pudendal neuralgia is the result of chronic compression of the pudendal nerve.[24] Nante's criteria (Box 22-7) aid the diagnostic process.[25]

Common chief complaints from patients with pudendal neuralgia, which will lead the practitioner to consider testing the pudendal nerve, are reports of pain with sitting, pain with wearing tight clothing and relief with wearing loose clothing or no undergarments and/or preference of wearing skirts, or complaints of feeling like there is a "golf ball" or "rock" inside of the rectum. There may be a history of obstetric trauma, chronic constipation or defecatory straining, or chronic stress (that may have triggered pelvic floor muscle spasms).

Internally, it can be tested by palpating at 2 points. The first point is at the convergence of S2, S3, and S4 nerve roots when they become the pudendal nerve. The practitioner finds coccygeal muscle at its sacrococcygeal attachment and moves laterally about two-thirds of the way toward its attachment to the ischial spine. By gently applying pressure and reaching superiorly, the examiner

TABLE 22-2 Testing Layers of the Pelvic Floor

LAYERS	MUSCLES	NERVE SUPPLY	COMMENTS
Superficial layer (urogenital triangle layer; layer 1)	Ischiocavernosus, bulbospongiosus, and the superficial transverse perineal muscle	Sacral nerve roots 2-4	From recent dissection studies, the bulbospongiosus appears to interdigitate medially with superficial transverse perineal muscle and may share innervation with the external anal sphincter, with possible clinical implications in testing for pain[8] The superficial transverse perineal muscle originates on ischial tuberosities and inserts at the perineal body and functions support the urogenital diaphragm
Intermediate layer (urogenital diaphragm layer; layer 2)	Deep transverse perineal, compressor urethrae, urethral sphincter (rhabdosphincter), and puborectalis	Perineal branch of the pudendal nerve	Urethral sphincter is a ring of muscle around the urethra inferior to the bladder in females and prostate in males
Deep layer (levator ani layer; layer 3)	Pubococcygeal and iliococcygeal muscles and in some texts the puborectalis[9]	S3-4 nerve roots	The iliococcygeus muscles play an important role in supporting the levator ani muscles and in stabilizing the coccyx anteriorly. Unilateral muscle spasm will place a rotatory force on the coccyx. The iliococcygeus muscle receives posterior stabilizing support from the gluteus maximus, which attaches to the dorsal lateral borders of the coccyx[10]
Pelvic wall muscle layer (layer 4)	Obturator internus and piriformis	L5, S1, and S2— obturator internus; S1 and S2 for piriformis	The obturator internus fascia forms a tunnel, Alcock canal, for the pudendal nerve, artery, and vein at the lower third of the medial obturator internus The sciatic nerve passes anteriorly to the piriformis in 87% of the population, known as type I conventional anatomy. About 13% of the population have a type II variation where the sciatic nerve splits and one nerve passes anteriorly, whereas the other pierces the piriformis muscle[11]

Box 22-7 Nante's Criteria for Pudendal Neuralgia[25]

1. Pain in the anatomical territory of the pudendal nerve
2. Made worse by sitting
3. Not awaken by pain at night
4. No objective sensory loss on clinical examination
5. Positive response to anesthetic pudendal nerve block

will then feel the pulse of the pudendal artery with which the pudendal nerve travels. Slight application of pressure on the pudenal nerve will cause local or referred pain. Nerve entrapment has been found surgically in 70% of the cases.[26]

The pudendal nerve can also be palpated internally over Alcock canal, found inferior to the tendinous arch of levator ani.

Externally, the pudendal nerve is palpated deep to the perianal fossa. The perineal branch is palpated medial to the pubic rami.

Nerve tension testing of the pudendal nerve is performed by flexing the hip and looking for reproduction of symptoms. In healthy subjects, hip flexion will cause the pudendal nerve to move caudally and laterally. Unfortunately, hip flexion will stress many other structures, decreasing the accuracy of the test. To confirm, the nerve can be lightly palpated internally and the hip slowly flexed to feel for increased nerve tension. The nerve can be gently pushed to look for reproduction of symptoms under tension. A positive sign would be pain locally, proximal or distal along the nerve line, or reports of referred pain. Caution is advised when palpating the nerve.

Clinical Presentation and Therapeutic Interventions

Because this table represents only a brief overview of common pelvic pain presentations, it is helpful to employ a systematic organ systems approach.

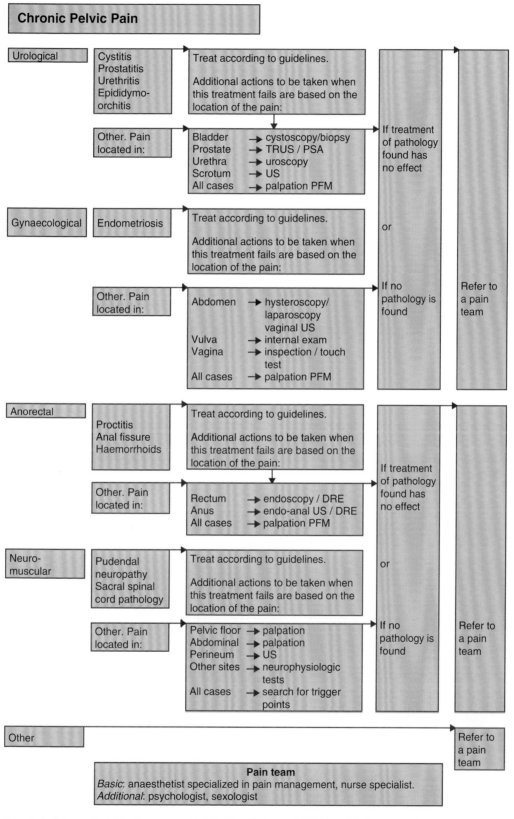

Reprinted from Fall M, Baranowski AP, Elneil S, et al. EAU guidelines on chronic pelvic pain. *Eur Urol.* 2010;57(1):35-48. Copyright © 2009 European Association of Urology. With permission.

A Brief List of Common Clinical Presentations With Treatments[29-32]

PATIENT COMPLAINT LOCATION	PATIENT HISTORY	PROPOSED MECHANISM	DIAGNOSIS	TREATMENT
Rectal pain or sacrococcygeal pain	Severe pain in rectal area that is worse with sitting than with standing and is >30 min	Hypertonic or spasms of levator ani (puborectalis)	Levator ani syndrome	Multifactorial—CBT, sitz bath, electrogalvanic stimulation, muscle relaxants, physical therapy
Rectal pain, sacrococcygeal pain Severe, episodic	Severe pain in rectal area that is infrequent, but can wake patients up at night. Up to 30 min, but usually only minutes to seconds	Smooth muscle dysfunction	Proctalgia fugax	As episodes are short lived, education about the disease process
Patient with pain over groin region with radiation to the scrotum or labia	Patient with prior hernia surgery presenting with allodynia/hyperalgesia to palpation over the inguinal canal and burning pain into scrotum/penis	Scar tissue over ilioinguinal nerve from prior surgery; tumor; trauma	Ilioinguinal neuralgia	Topical analgesic medications (e.g., lidocaine), neuropathic medications, neuromodulation
Vaginal pain	Pain in the vulvar region; dyspareunia; burning, itching in vulvar area	Contact irritation, stretching of the vulvar muscles, and/or hormonal changes	Vulvar vestibulitis syndrome	Biofeedback; neuropathic pain medications; topical analgesic medications (e.g., lidocaine)
Perineal pain	Pain in the perineum that is worse with sitting (see earlier text for Nantes criteria)	Prolonged sitting or bike riding; obstetric and nonobstetric trauma, pelvic floor surgery; chronic defecatory straining	Pudendal neuralgia	Pelvic floor physical therapy; biofeedback; pudendal nerve blocks; surgery; neuromodulation

CBT, cognitive behavioral therapy.

As the flow diagram suggests, when conventional treatments fail, diagnostic studies are inconclusive and/or surgery is not recommended, a referral to a multidisciplinary pain management team should be considered.

The pain specialist should have knowledge regarding medication management, psychological-based therapies, and interventional blocks as well as neuromodulation. It is first important to determine if the pain has neuropathic characteristics (see chapter on neuropathic pain). When neuropathic pain is suspected, one should consider neuropathic agents such as gabapentin, duloxetine, and pregabalin. As tricyclic antidepressants (TCAs) have also been shown to be helpful for patients with neuropathic pain, it is reasonable to also consider TCA medications for CPP.[6] However, there is no consensus on which neuropathic medication should be chosen first. To be sure, opioids should never be first-line treatment of CPP.[6,27,28] In our experience, the use of compounding creams and medications can be considerably effective for patients. These medications must be made by specialized compounding pharmacies but can include a variety of different medications such as gabapentin, lidocaine, and ketamine.

Interventional pain procedures can include trigger points and neuroablative procedures and can also involve more involved procedures such as nerve blocks using local anesthetic and steroids under fluoroscopic or ultrasound guidance.[28] Experimental therapies that have shown some promise include botulinum toxin and neuromodulation-based therapies, such as spinal cord stimulation and sacral nerve stimulation. As these are investigational and can carry substantial expense and procedural risk, they are not routinely recommended and should be used in treatment refractory cases.[6,28]

It is extremely important to combine pharmacologic and procedural interventions with behavioral health management and routine pelvic floor physical therapy. Indeed, an integrated, multidisciplinary approach for treating CPP has shown superiority over a nonmultidisciplinary approach.[28] Examples of behavioral health management can include cognitive behavioral therapy and biofeedback. Experienced pelvic floor physical therapists can aid in biofeedback as well.

CONCLUSION

Although CPP can be very difficult to treat, a systematic approach can be helpful when developing a differential diagnosis. Take a careful medical, psychological, and sexual history. Physical examination maneuvers can be complicated and uncomfortable for the patient. Therefore, early referral to a pelvic floor physical therapist and pain medicine specialist is recommended. As with many chronic pain disorders, developing a multidisciplinary treatment plan can improve long-term outcomes.

REFERENCES

1. Díaz-Mohedo E, Hita-Contreras F, Luque-Suárez A, Walker-Chao C, Zarza-Luciáñez D, Salinas-Casado J, Prevalence and risk factors of pelvic pain. *Actas Urol Esp Engl Ed.* 2014;38(5):298-303. doi:10.1016/j.acuroe.2014.01.006.

2. Speer LM, Mushkbar S, Erbele T. Chronic pelvic pain in women. *Am Fam Physician.* 2016;93(5):380-387.

3. Chiarioni G, Asteria C, Whitehead WE. Chronic proctalgia and chronic pelvic pain syndromes: new etiologic insights and treatment options. *World J Gastroenterol.* 2011;17(40):4447-4455. doi:10.3748/wjg.v17.i40.4447.

4. Udoji MA, Ness TJ. New directions in the treatment of pelvic pain. *Pain Manag.* 2013;3(5):387-394. doi:10.2217/pmt.13.40.

5. Vercellini P, Somigliana E, Viganò P, Abbiati A, Barbara G, Fedele L. Chronic pelvic pain in women: etiology, pathogenesis and diagnostic approach. *Gynecol Endocrinol.* 2009;25(3):149-158. doi:10.1080/09513590802549858.

6. Fall M, Baranowski AP, Elneil S, et al. EAU guidelines on chronic pelvic pain. *Eur Urol.* 2010;57(1):35-48. doi:10.1016/j.eururo.2009.08.020.

7. Gorniak G, Conrad W. An anatomical and functional perspective of the pelvic floor and urogenital organ support system. *LWW.* 2015;39(2):65-82.

8. Plochocki JH, Rodriguez-Sosa JR, Adrian B, Ruiz SA, Hall MI. A functional and clinical reinterpretation of human perineal neuromuscular anatomy: application to sexual function and continence. *Clin Anat.* 2016;29(8):1053-1058. doi:10.1002/ca.22774.

9. Moore KL, Dalley AF. *Clinically Oriented Anatomy.* 4th ed. Philadelphia, PA: Lippincott Williams & Wilkins; 1999.

10. Woon JTK, Stringer MD. Clinical anatomy of the coccyx: a systematic review. *Clin Anat.* 2012;25(2):158-167. doi:10.1002/ca.21216.

11. Varenika V, Lutz AM, Beaulieu CF, Bucknor MD. Detection and prevalence of variant sciatic nerve anatomy in relation to the piriformis muscle on MRI. *Skeletal Radiol.* 2017;46(6):751-757. doi:10.1007/s00256-017-2597-6.

12. Riegel B, Bruenahl CA, Ahyai S, Bingel U, Fisch M, Löwe B. Assessing psychological factors, social aspects and psychiatric co-morbidity associated with chronic prostatitis/chronic pelvic pain syndrome (CP/CPPS) in men – a systematic review. *J Psychosom Res.* 2014;77(5):333-350. doi:10.1016/j.jpsychores.2014.09.012.

13. Desrochers G, Bergeron S, Landry T, Jodoin M. Do psychosexual factors play a role in the etiology of provoked vestibulodynia? A critical review. *J Sex Marital Ther.* 2008;34(3):198-226. doi:10.1080/00926230701866083.

14. Desrochers G, Bergeron S, Khalifé S, Dupuis MJ, Jodoin M. Fear avoidance and self-efficacy in relation to pain and sexual impairment in women with provoked vestibulodynia. *Clin J Pain.* 2009;25(6):520-527. doi:10.1097/AJP.0b013e31819976e3.

15. Edwards L, Lynch PJ. *Genital Dermatology Atlas.* 2nd ed. Lippincott Williams & Wilkins; 2012.

16. Dargie EE, Chamberlain SM, Pukall CF. Provoked vestibulodynia: diagnosis, self-reported pain, and presentation during gynaecological examinations. *J Obstet Gynaecol Can.* 2017;39(3):145-151. doi:10.1016/j.jogc.2017.01.001.

17. Bo K, Berghmans B, Morkved S, Van Kampen M. *Evidence Based Physical Therapy for the Pelvic Floor: Bridging Science and Clinical Practice.* Elsevier; 2008.

18. Travell JG, Simons DG. *Myofascial Pain and Dysfunction: The Trigger Point Manual.* Vol. 1. 2nd ed. Philadelphia: Lippincott Williams & Wilkins; 1999.

19. Travell JG, Simons DG. *Myofascial Pain and Dysfunction: The Trigger Point Manual.* Vol. 2. 1st ed. Philadelphia: Lippincott Williams & Wilkins; 1999.

20. Chevalier F, Fernandez-Lao C, Cuesta-Vargas AI. Normal reference values of strength in pelvic floor muscle of women: a descriptive and inferential study. *BMC Womens Health.* 2014;14:143. doi:10.1186/s12905-014-0143-4.

21. Harlow BL, Stewart EG. A population-based assessment of chronic unexplained vulvar pain: have we underestimated the prevalence of vulvodynia? *J Am Med Womens Assoc (1972).* 2003;58(2):82-88.

22. Giesecke J, Reed BD, Haefner HK, Giesecke T, Clauw DJ, Gracely RH. Quantitative sensory testing in vulvodynia patients and increased peripheral pressure pain sensitivity. *Obstet Gynecol.* 2004;104(1):126-133. doi:10.1097/01.AOG.0000129238.49397.4e.

23. Reed BD, Plegue MA, Harlow SD, Haefner HK, Sen A. Does degree of vulvar sensitivity predict vulvodynia characteristics and prognosis? *J Pain Off J Am Pain Soc.* 2017;18(2):113-123. doi:10.1016/j.jpain.2016.10.006.

24. Charlotte W, Sebastian D, Viviane T, Luc B. Selection criteria for surgical treatment of pudendal neuralgia. *Neurourol Urodyn.* 2017;36(3):663-666. doi:10.1002/nau.22988.

25. Labat J-J, Riant T, Robert R, Amarenco G, Lefaucheur J-P, Rigaud J. Diagnostic criteria for pudendal neuralgia by pudendal nerve entrapment (Nantes criteria). *Neurourol Urodyn.* 2008;27(4):306-310. doi:10.1002/nau.20505.

26. Ploteau S, Perrouin-Verbe M-A, Labat J-J, Riant T, Levesque A, Robert R. Anatomical variants of the pudendal nerve observed during a transgluteal surgical approach in a population of patients with pudendal neuralgia. *Pain Physician.* 2017;20(1):E137-E143.

27. Dowell D, Haegerich TM, Chou R. CDC guideline for prescribing opioids for chronic pain – United States, 2016. *MMWR Recomm Rep Morb Mortal Wkly Rep Recomm Rep.* 2016;65(1):1-49. doi:10.15585/mmwr.rr6501e1.

28. Stein SL. Chronic pelvic pain. *Gastroenterol Clin North Am.* 2013;42(4):785-800. doi:10.1016/j.gtc.2013.08.005.

29. Peng PW, Tumber PS. Ultrasound-guided Interventions for patients with chronic pelvic pain – a description of techniques and review of the literature. *Pain Physician.* 2008;11(2):215-224.

30. Khoder W, Hale D. Pudendal neuralgia. *Obstet Gynecol Clin N Am.* 2014;41:443-452.

31. Cho H, Park D, Kim DH, Nam HS. Diagnosis of ilioinguinal nerve injury based on electromyography and ultrasonography: a case report. *Ann Rehabil Med.* 2017;41(4):705-708.

32. Rao S, Bharucha AE, Chiarioni G., et al. Functional Anorectal Disorders. *Gastroenterology.* 2017. doi: 10.1053/j.gastro.2016.02.009. pii: S0016–5085(16)00175-X.

33. Waldman S. *Pain Review.* Elsevier; 2017.

IV

CHRONIC PAIN TREATMENT

23

PHYSICAL THERAPIES IN THE MANAGEMENT OF PAIN

Kathryn Schopmeyer, DPT, Richard Jacob Boyce, DPT and Rebecca Vogsland, PT, DPT

OVERVIEW

Chronic, or persistent, pain is a complex condition with varied genetic, environmental, psychosocial, and cultural factors, each having disparate manifestations in patients both in terms of pain experience and impact on function.[1] Treatment of persistent pain in the United States has been pendular during the past half century, with rehabilitation and nonpharmacological approaches shifting into and out of focus. Beginning in the 1970s and continuing through the 1990s, multidisciplinary pain rehabilitation—specifically work-hardening and operant conditioning models—gained in popularity.[2-5] Although research demonstrated the benefits of multidisciplinary care, the use of rehabilitative and interdisciplinary treatment approaches for persistent pain declined from the late 1990s through the first decade of the 21st century,[6] while prescriptions of opioid analgesics increased.[7] Between 1999 and 2013, the amount of prescription opioids sold in the United States nearly quadrupled,[8] yet there was no overall change in how much pain Americans reported or how successfully it was managed.[9-11] The medical profession increasingly relied on pharmaceuticals to treat pain because there was (1) consensus that chronic opioid therapy was safe,[12,13] (2) a perception that pain was being undertreated in the United States,[14] and (3) aggressive marketing by large synthetic opioid manufacturers.[4,6,7,15-17]

Giordano and Schatman discussed the ethical implications of these trends[18-20] and called for a return to a multidisciplinary and integrative approach to pain care in 2008.[20] The Veterans Health Administration issued a national directive in 2009, mandating the implementation of at least 1 interdisciplinary pain rehabilitation program for each of the 21 Veterans Integrated Service Networks.[21] Another rapid change occurred after the Centers for Disease Control and Prevention released its Guideline for Prescribing Opioids for Chronic Pain in March 2016, with a greater emphasis placed back on behavioral and rehabilitation approaches to managing persistent pain.[22,23] Both the National Institutes for Health and Centers for Disease Control and Prevention guidelines now recommend nonpharmacological physical therapy (PT) as a primary approach for the treatment of chronic, noncancer pain.[1,22]

PHYSICAL THERAPISTS AND PHYSICAL THERAPY PRACTICE

Physical therapists are collaborative professionals working across the health care system in the United States. They are active in primary, secondary, and tertiary level clinical settings and have a scope of practice that allows for direct treatment of illness states as well as disease prevention and health promotion via wellness and fitness consultation, education, research, and health policy administration.[24] As of January 2015, all graduates of accredited PT programs are awarded a doctoral degree with training that readies them to deliver front-line health care services. In addition, curriculum content for graduate programs has been evolving to meet the demand of persistent pain problems in the United States.[25] All US states, including the District of Columbia, Puerto Rico, and the US Virgin Islands, now have "direct access" to physical therapy,[26] meaning that patients are afforded some level of access to PT services without a physician referral. The Guide to Physical Therapy Practice (2014) describes PT as "a dynamic profession with an established theoretical and scientific base and widespread clinical applications in the restoration, maintenance, and promotion of optimal physical function" (Figure 23-1). The enhancement of physical function allows the individual to regain or maintain health and optimize participation in valued activities, thus maximizing quality of life despite persisting pain.

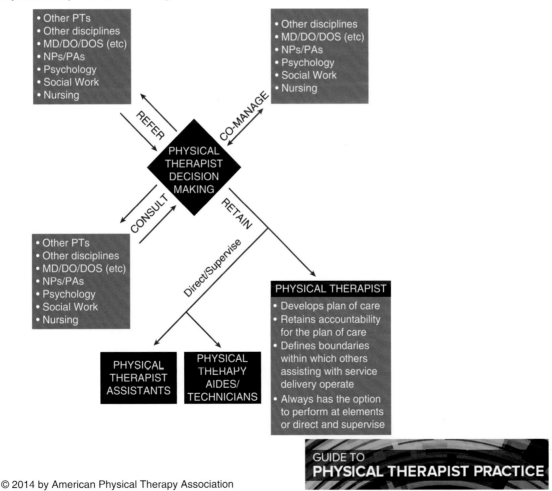

Physical therapist decision making related to the involvement of other providers.

© 2014 by American Physical Therapy Association

FIGURE 23-1 APTA guide to physical therapy practice. From Guide to Physical Therapist Practice 3.0. Alexandria, VA: American Physical Therapy Association; 2014. Available at: http://guidetoptpractice.apta.org/. Accessed December 18, 2018.

PHYSICAL THERAPY FOR PERSISTENT PAIN

Physical therapists have sought to develop treatment-based classification systems for the diagnosis and treatment of musculoskeletal conditions[27-29] and clinical practice guidelines (CPG) to inform patient care.[30-37] Practice that is congruent with CPG generally leads to improved outcomes and decreased health care costs.[38-41] A subset of patients with persistent pain, however, respond poorly to PT interventions designed to address mechanically reproducible peripheral symptoms. A noted deficit in the existing guidelines and classification systems is a robust category for centrally mediated pain (central sensitization [CS]). Smart et al. (2010) proposed a classification system surrounding the underlying neurophysiological mechanisms of pain based on clinical findings. In this system, patients are classified based on clinical assessment findings into 1 of 3 categories: nociceptive pain, peripheral neuropathic pain, or CS (Table 23-1). Nociceptive pain refers to pain directly linked to afferent input from the periphery in response to noxious mechanical, chemical, or thermal stimuli.[42] Peripheral

neuropathic pain refers to pain directly resulting from a problem or lesion in the peripheral nervous system.[43] CS refers to pain arising from neurophysiologic changes in the central nervous system that leads to an amplification of neural signaling and ultimately hypersensitivity to afferent input.[44] People with chronic pain can fall into any of these 3 categories and may also present with a mix of symptoms, with 1 category being dominant. Using a mechanism-based approach may result in more accurate clinical reasoning and more effective treatment selections.[1,45] Physical therapists have knowledge and skills to manage patients in any of these categories. Primary aims of PT intervention are identifying and diagnosing movement impairments, facilitating recovery of function, teaching patients active self-management strategies, and increasing patients' confidence so they can independently and successfully cope with recurrent acute or sustained chronic conditions, including pain, in the long term.

PASSIVE VERSUS ACTIVE APPROACHES TO PAIN MANAGEMENT

Passive treatments are those *done to a patient*, delivered by either a practitioner or a device, without cognitive or physical engagement by the patient. Persistent pain poses a treatment challenge because of the multidimensional complexity of the problem.[46,47] Health care professionals' desire to alleviate pain and suffering for patients often means they recommend treatments designed to quell symptoms with minimal side effects, such as massage, electrical or thermal modalities, dry needling, or manual joint manipulations. The use of passive treatment interventions designed to reduce suffering may compromise long-term outcomes if psychosocial factors are not first considered when developing a pain care plan. There is an inherent risk of worsening outcomes if passive strategies are the primary elements of a care plan for patients with persistent pain and avoidant behavior or pain-related fear of movement.[48,49]

Passive treatments are often used to create short-term results[37,50,51] and may indeed have the potential for negative outcomes with prolonged use.[52,53] However, owing to the potential to decrease nociceptive input, and the likely central nervous system modulation that occurs with passive treatments,[54,55] it is reasonable to consider passive interventions as an option; there is evidence showing that various passive interventions can positively affect pain and function in the short term.[56,57] Ideally, passive interventions are utilized as "bridge therapies," intended to create an opportunity to implement active strategies while pain symptoms are somewhat reduced. Finding ways for patients to apply passive treatments to themselves may afford them with a greater sense of control and self-efficacy regarding their own pain management.

In contrast, active treatments are those in which the patient is physically and/or cognitively engaged as a participant. The self-application of a passive modality

TABLE 23-1 Overview of Pain Mechanism Classifications

MECHANISM	CLUSTER OF CLINICAL FINDINGS
Primary Nociceptive	Pain is: • Proportionate anatomical response to aggravating/alleviating factors • Intermittent and sharp with mechanical provocation • Constant dull ache at rest • Localized to the area of concern Absence of: • Other dysesthesias • Night pain • Burning or electric pain • Antalgic movement patterns
Peripheral neuropathic	• History of nerve pathology, injury, or compromise • Pain provocation with mechanical/movement examination procedures • Dermatomal or cutaneous distribution of pain
Central sensitization	• Disproportionate to injury/pathology • Associated with maladaptive psychosocial factors • Disproportionate, unpredictable response to many ill-defined aggravating/alleviating factors • Diffuse, nonanatomic distribution

Reprinted from Smart KM, Blake C, Staines A, Thacker M, Doody C. Mechanisms-based classifications of musculoskeletal pain: part 1 of 3: symptoms and signs of central sensitisation in patients with low back (±leg) pain. Man Ther. 2012;17(4):336-344. Copyright © 2012 Elsevier. With permission.

can be considered active, because the patient is taking ownership of the process. Active cognitive coping and self-management skills appear to be the most significant mediators of positive outcomes for those who participate in multidisciplinary pain rehabilitation programs.[47,58,59] Active strategies employed by physical therapists include education, adaptations, facilitation, graded motor imagery, exercise-based interventions, and graded exposure techniques.

Self-Efficacy and Persistent Pain

A psychosocial factor that is tightly correlated with disability due to pain is self-efficacy.[60] Self-efficacy is characterized as the belief in one's own ability to achieve a specific goal or bring about a desired outcome.[61] A strong sense of self-efficacy is a powerful mediator between pain and disability.[60,62-65] According to Bandura (1997), self-efficacy is impacted by the following: (1) past performances, (2) verbal persuasion, (3) vicarious experiences, and (4) physiologic feedback. Physical therapists are uniquely suited to positively impact the 4 components of self-efficacy in patients with persistent pain through education, facilitation of successful experiences, coaching/encouragement, behavior modeling, and exercise instruction. Physical activity and exercise increase self-efficacy in patients with pain.[62,66] Providing patients with the tools to implement active self-management strategies can help bolster their self-efficacy by improving successful performance of functional tasks and modulating physiologic feedback. The literature suggests a reciprocal relationship between high self-efficacy and ability to engage in valued physical activity.[62] In addition, specialized education about pain, known as Pain Neuroscience Education, can act as verbal persuasion and also help mediate the interpretation of physiologic feedback, thereby positively impacting self-efficacy.

The remainder of this chapter will outline the prominent nonpharmacological, PT treatment elements with the strongest empirical support for the treatment of persistent pain conditions. Table 23-2 summarizes some main points.

ACTIVE TREATMENTS

Pain Neuroscience Education

Teaching patients the principles of pain physiology and neuroplasticity as a therapeutic intervention is now termed "Pain Neuroscience Education" (PNE).[67-69] PNE aims to reconceptualize pain as the nervous system's response to perceived threat of danger, rather than a direct reflection of tissue injury.[70,71] Patients living in pain want to know about their pain and why it persists,[72] yet common frameworks to explain pain use a biomechanical or structural model. Traditional models of patient education that focus on pathoanatomy are not helpful for patients with chronic pain[73,74] and can even worsen both fear and pain.[75] A modern view of pain science rejects a strict biomechanical (nociception = pain)

TABLE 23-2 Physical Therapies for Persistent Pain

Common physical therapies for persistent pain care with little or no empirical support:

- Ultrasound (Desmeules et al., 2015; Wong et al., 2007; Robertson and Baker, 2001; Nussbaum, 1997; Gam and Johanssen, 1995)
- Mechanical traction for axial spine pain (Young et al., 2009; Graham et al., 2008; Clarke et al., 2006; Guild, 2012; Madson and Hollman, 2016; Macario and Pergolizzi, 2006; Wegner et al., 2013)
- Back braces (Chou and Huffman, 2007)

Effective physical therapies for persistent pain care (best used in combination and prescribed based on shared decision making, patient values, and SMART goals):

- Individualized therapeutic exercise (Falla and Hodges, 2017) EULAR revised recs for FM
- Manual and manipulative therapies
- Graded motor imagery
- Dry needling
- Pain neuroscience education
- Electrical stimulation (TENS, LLLT)
- Classification-based cognitive functional therapy (Vibe Fersum et al., 2013)

model and embraces the biological, psychological, and social impacts of pain on our physiology.[70,76-78] Cortical changes are likely more influential to ongoing pain than are structural tissue impairments for common persistent pain problems such as nonspecific low back pain, headache, neuropathic pain, postsurgical pain, osteoarthritis, whiplash, shoulder impingement syndromes, and elbow pain, so using a biomechanical/structural model is not only inaccurate but also incomplete.[73,77,79-82]

There are now several resources available for clinicians to increase knowledge and teaching skills.[73,83-86] PNE has demonstrated efficacy for reducing pain and improving function and movement while decreasing disability, catastrophization, and health care utilization.[71,87,88] Physical therapists have been the primary contributors to the body of evidence surrounding the development and use of PNE.

PNE can be delivered in various settings using different mediums, and some of the key components are in Table 23-3.[73,89] Although clinicians generally assume that patients will not comprehend the neurophysiology of pain, research shows that clinicians can learn to teach it and patients can understand the material with good effect.[90] PNE can have a direct impact on the element of self-efficacy related to interpretations of physiologic feedback processed by the brain. If the threat-value of such input can be decreased, it would follow that self-efficacy can be bolstered in relation to activity and pain management.

THE POWER OF LANGUAGE AND PERSISTENT PAIN

The major aims of PNE are to *explain pain* to people (rather than pathoanatomy) and to do so in a way that does not induce or promote fear in patients. Clinicians commonly explain pain problems using anatomy references or in terms of pathoanatomy or disease states. Clinicians are likely unaware of how their word choice influences the cognitions and actions of patients, and having a deeper understanding of this might improve health care delivery.[91-93] Metaphors help people understand and express experience through language,[94] although the metaphors we choose in health care could have unforeseen nocebo effects on patients, particularly if they evoke images of vulnerability, frailty, or damage. For example, a popular way to explain functions of the human body is by comparing it with a mechanical object with parts that break down after too much use or that the body must follow specific rules of alignment to function well and without pain. "Wear and tear" is considered benign by many health care providers, yet when patients describe their conditions in terms of degeneration, they demonstrate a poor self-prognosis.[95] Stress associated with fear, anxiety, and threat triggers a cascade of neurophysiological events, including systemic endocrine upregulation, enhanced immune response, and localized neurogenic inflammation.[96,97] Patients with chronic pain can exist in this state of perpetual stress and threat related to bodily sensations. The resultant biochemical cascade can negatively impact the body and mind, affecting cognition, endocrine function, sleep, and the experience of pain.[96-98] People who exist in a state of perpetual threat frequently develop maladaptive catastrophic thought patterns and/or kinesiophobia. They tend to avoid activity and are more likely to have poor long-term outcomes for pain and overall health. Choosing words with limited threat value and teaching about pain physiology, rather than strictly anatomy, can reduce fear-induced stress and improve the lives of patients suffering with persistent pain conditions.[99-101]

TABLE 23-3 PNE Curriculum Contents

Nociception and nociceptive pathways

Neurons, synapses, and action potentials

No reference to anatomical/pathoanatomical descriptions

Spinal inhibition and facilitation

Peripheral and central sensitization

Contribution of psychosocial factors and beliefs

Plasticity of the nervous system

Neurophysiology of pain

Modified from Nijs J, Paul van Wilgen C, Van Oosterwijck J, van Ittersum M, Meeus M. How to explain central sensitization to patients with "unexplained" chronic musculoskeletal pain: practice guidelines. Man Ther. 2011;16(5):413-418. doi:10.1016/j.math.2011.04.005; Louw A, Zimney K, Puentedura EJ, Diener I. The efficacy of pain neuroscience education on musculoskeletal pain: a systematic review of the literature. Physiother Theory Pract. 2016;3985:1-24. http://www.ncbi.nlm.nih.gov/pubmed/27351541; Louw A, Zimney K, O'Hotto C, Hilton S. The clinical application of teaching people about pain. Physiother Theory Pract. 2016;32(5):385-395. doi:10.1080/09593985.2016.119 4652; and Louw A, Puentedura E, Zimney K. Teaching patients about pain: it works, but what should we call it? Physiother Theory Pract. 2016;32(5):328-331. doi:10.1080/095 93985.2016.1194669.

PHYSICAL THERAPY AND PAIN NEUROSCIENCE EDUCATION

PNE is best used in conjunction with other PT interventions. Table 23-4 outlines some of the interventions paired with PNE; one or more may be combined within a given episode of care or single treatment session. Physical therapists conduct highly skilled evaluations including subjective interviews and physical examinations, while taking into account several psychosocial concomitant factors, and are trained to screen out red flag symptoms or other signs of health impairments that require medical attention. The result of this detailed subjective and objective evaluation will help with categorization of the patient into 1 (or more) of the 3 pain mechanism types, which allows the therapist to more accurately explain a patient's pain and help address pain-related fear. Physical therapists are able to apply their knowledge of anatomy, physiology, and pathophysiology to demystify symptoms and synthesize clinical and diagnostic medical imaging findings to explain ongoing pain states while normalizing the patient's experiences. PNE would be an applicable active treatment approach for patients in all 3 pain mechanisms categories, especially as pain persists beyond normal tissue healing time and becomes chronic. The application of PNE early in an episode of care may be helpful to allow for deeper understanding of the plan of care and decreased fear of pain to promote engagement in movement-based approaches.[71]

Exercise Recommendations and Considerations for the Patient With Persistent Pain

When appropriately prescribed, regular exercise improves the majority of chronic medical conditions and provides substantial benefit to overall health.[102-104] In the presence of chronic pain conditions, however, patients and providers are often apprehensive regarding engagement in regular exercise and reasonably ask the

TABLE 23-4 PNE as Adjunct Therapy

• Manual therapy (Moseley, 2002; Ryan et al., 2010; Puentedura and Flynn, 2016)

• Trigger point dry needling (Tellez-Garcia et al., 2014)

• Aerobic exercise, including circuit training (Ryan et al., 2010)

• Stabilization exercise/motor control (Moseley, 2002, 2003; Ryan et al., 2010; Beltran-Alacreu et al., 2015)

• Aquatic exercise (Pires et al., 2015)

• Movement exercise (Vibe Fersum et all., 2013)

• Graded exposure and pacing strategies for daily tasks (Meeus et al., 2010; Vibe Fersum et al., 2013) following questions: Will exercise cause harm? Is exercise beneficial as treatment of chronic pain? How should exercise be prescribed if it hurts to move?

A movement and exercise plan for patients with chronic pain should take into consideration the following factors:

- the neurobiological adaptations present in persistent pain states
- patient expectations and goals
- a patient's past experiences with exercise
- exercise mode accessibility

Exercise-based interventions are active interventions and may help promote self-efficacy in patients with persistent pain. Physical therapists can create a plan that meets the needs of the individual.

EXERCISE IS SAFE AND EFFECTIVE

Many musculoskeletal and degenerative conditions, such as osteoarthritis and degenerative disc disease, are commonly associated with persistent pain. Commonly held beliefs about the body based on the outdated biomechanical model influence behavior and medical advice that is either confusing or inconsistent with research: running after age 50 years should be avoided; exercise is not appropriate for arthritic conditions or will not be tolerated; "move through the pain no matter what"; "don't move it if hurts." Based on our current understanding of pain processing, we now know that the presence or absence of pain is not an accurate representation of the state of the tissues,[70,81,82,105] and that the presence of a chronic degenerative condition is not an accurate predictor of pain.[106] We also know that exercising does not accelerate degenerative or chronic inflammatory conditions.[107-112] In fact, when properly prescribed, engaging in regular exercise and activity is not only safe but also improves function, mood, physical fitness, self-efficacy, and quality of life and reduces pain, even in the presence of most degenerative conditions.[102,107-114] Physical therapists create exercise prescriptions for complex patient populations and are excellent resources when patients are fearful of movement because of pain.

SPECIAL CONSIDERATIONS REGARDING PERSISTENT PAIN AND EXERCISE

Pain-Related Fear and Avoidance Behaviors

Pain-related fear of movement (kinesiophobia), avoidance behaviors, and pain-related catastrophic thoughts and beliefs can become significant barriers to exercise adherence and progression and should be addressed when present.[115,116] Using PNE to explain that "hurt does not equal harm" can improve pain-related fear avoidance, catastrophic beliefs, and kinesiophobia.[68,71,115,117-120] Decreased fear and catastrophizing

allows patients to accept that some amount of discomfort is expected and not representative of new injury. The reconceptualization of discomfort with movement serves to increase willingness to engage in therapy programs.

Impairment of the Endogenous Analgesic Mechanism: Considerations for Exercise Prescription

Moderately challenging and vigorous exercise stimulate activation of the body's endogenous endorphin analgesic and supraspinal inhibitory mechanisms, resulting in reduced sensitivity to nociceptive input.[121] The phenomenon, known as exercise-induced analgesia, is present in most pain-free adults. This endogenous analgesic mechanism is impaired in those with chronic pain conditions, specifically those with evidence of CS, which can negatively affect exercise tolerance.[81,122,123]

CS is not exclusively a feature of fibromyalgia and chronic fatigue syndrome but can be present in other chronic pain conditions with a mix of pain mechanisms, such as knee osteoarthritis (nociceptive and central).[81,124] Individuals with features of CS do not exhibit the same analgesic response to exercise compared with either the general population or patients with persistent pain who do not have features of CS.[125,126] Coaching patients with persistent pain to initiate exercise at tolerable levels and progress more gradually over time correlates to better outcomes.[127,128]

Adherence to a Movement Program

Exercise adherence is a significant issue for the population with persistent pain.[129-132] Although no singular exercise mode (e.g., walking, aquatics, strength training, biking) is superior to any other,[129] certain characteristics of a program are predictive of higher rates of adherence. These include:

- personalizing the exercise program to the patient's own goals and preferences
- using an instructor who specializes in chronic pain
- being encouraging and supportive
- emphasizing and cultivating self-efficacy
- assuring the mode of exercise is accessible to the patient
- using individual supervised sessions when available[129,133,134]

Adherence to the continuation of exercise over the longer term can be improved by:

- using behavioral strategies such as positive reinforcement, an exercise contract, self-monitoring strategies, and goal setting
- allowing intermittent supervised follow-up sessions over longer periods of time for reinforcement of behavior change
- using instructional reinforcement materials when face-to-face follow-up is not possible[129]

Exercise Modes for Persistent Pain

Patients with chronic pain may have complex biopsychosocial presentations and are best managed by a trained physical therapist in the initial phase of exercise prescription. Maintenance programs can be continued independently or with the guidance of exercise instructors.

AEROBIC EXERCISE

Aerobic exercise is defined as sustained movement involving rhythmic contraction of large muscle groups leading to an increase in oxygen demand.[130,131,135,136] In addition to the benefits of pain reduction,[130,136,137] aerobic exercise modes are accessible to most individuals and involve simple movement patterns requiring minimal supervision or equipment, including walking, jogging, upper extremity ergometry, cycling, dancing, and swimming. Forms of aerobic exercise can be modified by the physical therapist to accommodate disabilities or other barriers. Aerobic exercise should be considered a key ingredient of a balanced program for patients with persistent pain.

Low-Intensity Activity and Movement

Low-intensity activity, such as tai chi, yoga, walking in the pool, slow land-based walking, Qi Gong, and light cycling, have been shown to decrease pain and anxiety, improve balance and mobility, and reduce depression and are generally well tolerated in patients with chronic pain with or without signs of CS.[130] Although low-intensity activity has not been associated with the same overall health benefits and functional improvements as moderate and vigorous levels of exercise, it may be a good starting point for those patients who cannot yet tolerate moderate-intensity activity.[130,131,133,136] It should be emphasized here that the mode of exercise or activity is important only in terms of accessibility, patient interest, and tolerance. Prescribing pool therapy or yoga for patients who do not have access to these resources in the long term, for example, is not recommended, as this would likely sabotage patient self-efficacy and a patient's ability to adhere to an exercise program.

Strength Training

The clinical benefits of strength training for patients with chronic pain include increased and maintained muscle strength, pain relief, reduced disability, decreased depression, increased self-efficacy, and increased quality of life.[130,133,138] Individuals with evidence of CS and no prior experience with strength training can harness these outcomes in as few as 2 training sessions per week.[133,139-141] However, to ensure tolerance, it is best to manage the intensity of strength training sessions for patients with chronic pain during the initial phases of implementation. The program must be well tolerated with no adverse events before progression.[130,133] This can be done by:

- allowing the patient to define volitional fatigue with each set of strengthening exercise

- starting with exercises that are simple and easy to understand and perform correctly
- guiding patients to perform slow, controlled repetitions to decrease the likelihood of tendon or muscle strain or irritation[130,131,133,141]

Flexibility

Exercises designed to address subjective feelings of stiffness or tightness and improve joint range of motion are modestly beneficial for pain and more efficacious for anxiety, depression, and quality of life. When stretching is included as part of an overall fitness program, optimal outcomes ensue.[130,138,142]

Exercise Guidelines for Patients With Persistent Pain

Some patients may benefit from more specifically targeted exercise prescription addressing the previously mentioned classifications of persistent pain: CS, peripheral neuropathic, and nociceptive. As people living with persistent pain re-engage in movement programs, disruptive flare up cycles are expected, so working with a physical therapist familiar with treating persistent pain can help patients avoid common pitfalls. PT professionals who specialize in treatment of persistent pain conditions use motivational interviewing communication strategies, address pain-related fear of movement, and train patients in self-treatment strategies. Figures 23-2 and 23-3, and Table 23-5 provide general clinical decision guidelines regarding exercise for people with persistent pain conditions.

PASSIVE MODALITIES

Electrical Stimulation Therapies

Electrostimulation has been used for the treatment of pain since the time of the Egyptians[143] and became part of modern medicine in 1967,[144] after the gate control theory by Melzack and Wall was published.[145] Various forms of electrotherapy have been applied to treat pain symptoms, including transcutaneous electrical nerve stimulation (TENS), interferential stimulation, electrical muscle stimulation, and low-level laser therapy. The forms of electrostimulation with the strongest empirical support (moderate) for use with persistent pain are included here. When a modality is applied by a practitioner without the physical or cognitive engagement of the patient, it is considered a completely passive intervention. However, if a patient is taught how and when to thoughtfully apply a modality independently, the meter moves this more toward the active self-management end of the spectrum. Electrical stimulation modalities can be useful for modulating pain in all categories of pain mechanisms (i.e., nociceptive, neuropathic, CS). Some clinical considerations are listed in the TENS Clinical Application Table 23-6.

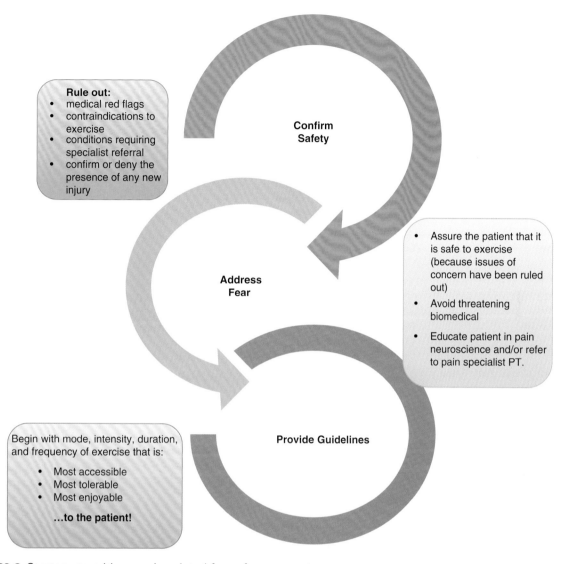

FIGURE 23-2 Strategy to address pain-related fear of movement.

Patient Guidance

- Start low, go slow.

- Begin with what's most tolerable, most enjoyable, and most accessible.

- Rest as needed.

- Touch the barrier but don't push through it.

- Some discomfort with exercise is ok.

- Be patient, positive changes will occur over time with regular daily activity.

- Symptom flare ups are not likely a sign of new tissue damage, modify rather than abandon activity

- Consult a physical therapist who specializes in management of chronic pain conditions for the best

FIGURE 23-3 Patient self-treatment strategy.

Transcutaneous Electrical Nerve Stimulation

TENS is a form of electrical stimulation that involves a portable, small format device with adhesive electrodes that are placed on the surface of the skin. TENS delivers electrical stimulation through the skin and is used for the treatment of acute and chronic pain. TENS is favored over interferential current or other electrical stimulation modalities for the treatment of chronic pain because it is low cost and can be applied independently. TENS has been shown to be beneficial when applied in conjunction with active treatment interventions such as therapeutic exercise[146] and thus is often introduced by and used in PT sessions. However, it does not require instruction by a skilled physical therapist and these devices are now readily available over the counter.

TENS is applied at varied frequencies, intensities, and pulse durations and works by muting central neuronal excitability[147-151] and activating descending inhibitory pathways.[146,147,150,152-154] There is an abundance of research on the use of TENS for a multitude of pain

TABLE 23-5 Clinical Decision Guidelines for Exercise: Exercise Guidelines for Patients With Chronic Pain

INTENSITY	MODE	FREQUENCY	DURATION
• Start with the most tolerable level of intensity • Even low-intensity activity can provide some benefit (Jones, 2006) • Progress intensity when you are confidently tolerating current level well for 4 wk (Rooks, 2008) • Positive health benefits can be attained at moderate levels. Vigorous intensity is not necessary (Rooks, 2008)	• Begin with what you know, like, can tolerate, and have access to • Consulting a physical therapist who is a specialist in pain management is the best way get started • Set reasonable goals and keep track of how you progress (Jones, 2006; Jordan, 2010)	**Low and moderate intensity:** 3-5×/wk to equal 150-300 min for each week (USDHHS, 2008) Strength exercise should be performed 2-3×/wk with 24-72 h rest between sessions (Rook, 2008; USDHHS, 2008).	Start at what is tolerable and increase slowly until sessions of >=10 min are achieved. The goal is to try to achieve 30-45 total minutes per day (Rook, 2008; Jones, 2006). A good rule of thumb could be to increase time 10% after 1 wk at current duration is tolerated well (Rooks, 2008).
Low intensity: • <50% age predicted HRmax (Jones, 2006) • <=11 on Borg RPE (Muyor, 2013)	**Low intensity:** Qi Gong, yoga, stretching, Tai Chi, slow walking, water walking, light cycling, darts (Haskell, 2007; Jones, 2006; Rooks, 2008)		
Moderate intensity: • Intense enough to cause breathing changes to occur, but able to carry on a conversation (Jones, 2006; Foster, 2008) • 50%-60% of age-predicted HRmax (Rook, 2008; USDHHS, 2008) • 12-13 on Borg RPE(Muyor, 2013)	**Moderate intensity:** Walking, water aerobics, heavy cleaning, badminton, basketball (shooting around), cycling flat surface, light weight lifting, slow dancing, table tennis, leisurely swim (USDHHS, 2008; Haskell, 2007; Rooks, 2008)		
Vigorous intensity: • Intense enough to cause not only breathing changes but also an inability to speak more than a few words at a time (Foster, 2008) • 60%-80% of age-predicted HRmax (USDHHS, 2008; Haskell, 2007) • 14-19 on Borg RPE (Muoyr, 2013)	**Vigorous intensity:** Jogging/running, high speed/hill walking, shoveling, carrying heavy load, casual soccer, heavy weight lifting, basketball, high-paced swimming, singles tennis (USDHHS, 2008; Haskell, 2007)	**Vigorous intensity:** >=20 min/d to 2-5×/wk to equal >=75 min/wk (USDHHS, 2008)	

RPE, rate of perceived exertion.

conditions, including acute and chronic low back pain, osteoarthritis, fibromyalgia, dysmenorrhea, postoperative pain, chronic musculoskeletal pain, cancer, and complex regional pain syndrome type, but its efficacy remains equivocal.[155-159] Conflicting research findings are suspected to be the result of inconsistent methodology and heterogeneous subgrouping in clinical trials, so considerations for use of TENS should include cost-effectiveness and its potential to support self-efficacy in patients with persistent pain.[160,161] Moreover, it is the opinion of these authors that TENS in isolation relies on the pain gate theory and thus is not sufficient to address the complex nature of chronic pain as it ignores the cognitive components of the pain experience. Use of TENS as an adjunctive modality to help dampen nociceptive input may be of value, and the idea of the patient being able to employ a tool without the direct involvement of a health care professional likely increases the sense of self-efficacy of the patient.

Low-Level Laser Therapy

Light therapy is used for the treatment of multiple painful conditions, including rheumatoid arthritis, lateral epicondylitis, low back pain, neck pain, osteoarthritis, and myofascial pain syndromes.[162-168] Although it has been implemented clinically for over 30 years, much of the research has not been published in academic journals.[168] Lasers that are considered therapeutic are known as "3A or 3B," or commonly termed low-level laser therapy (LLLT) and low-intensity laser therapy (LILT),[169] and are typically administered at a nonthermal dose to the treated tissue. LLLT devices generate light with a wavelength between 600 and 1000 nm, which lies in the near-infrared and red visible bands of the electromagnetic spectrum.[168] Doses measured at 820 to 830 nm are most effective in the range of 0.8 to 9.0 J per point, with irradiation times of 15 to 180 s.[168]

TABLE 23-6 TENS Clinical Application	
TENS: Clinical Application Considerations	
• High frequency (>50 Hz)	
• Low frequency (<10 Hz)	
• Intensity is based on sensory experience of user	
• Sensory level = "tingling" (high), "tapping" (low)	
• Motor level = muscle contraction	
• Conventional TENS = high frequency applied at low intensity	
• Acupuncture-like TENS = low frequency applied at high intensity (w/motor contraction)	
Chronic opioid therapy affects TENS efficacy	With morphine-tolerant patients, high-frequency TENS is more effective than low-frequency TENS (Solomon et al., 1980; Sluka et al., 2000; Leonard et al., 2011)
Presence of primary hyperalgesia dictates parameters	High-frequency TENS partially reduces primary analgesia (King and Sluka, 2001) Low-frequency TENS is *ineffective* on primary analgesia (King and Sluka, 2001; Kalra et al., 2001)
Dosage frequency	Effects occur only *during* treatment and wane within 30 min after removal of the electricity (Chesterson et al., 2002) Application should be intermittent. Humans become habituated to TENS so efficacy decreases within 4-5 d if used incessantly (Chandran and Sluka, 2003; Liebano et al., 2011)
Dosage intensity	TENS intensity should be titrated to achieve the strongest possible intensity without adding bothersomeness (Moran et al., 2011)

LLLT is thought to work by reducing inflammatory responses, oxidative stress, and effecting nerve action potentials that modulate pain signals.

See Tables 23-7 and 23-8 for summaries of research for TENS and LLLT.

Manual Therapy

Manual therapy used by physical therapists, osteopathic physicians, and chiropractors encompasses techniques intended to improve tissue extensibility; increase range of motion; induce relaxation; mobilize or manipulate soft tissue and joints; modulate pain; and reduce soft tissue swelling, inflammation, or restriction.[24] Manual techniques are directed at the joints (mobilization/manipulation), soft tissue, and nervous system (see chapter 24 Osteopathic Manipulative Medicine).[170] The skilled practitioner will be able to identify the scenarios in which to apply manual techniques and how to maximize impact with timing and in combination with other treatments (see Table 23-9). It should be noted that manual therapy is considered a passive treatment (one that is done to a patient) and thus should not be used as the sole treatment modality within an episode of care. Manual techniques that are geared toward facilitation of movement, activation, or localization could be considered active interventions, as the patient must be physically and/or cognitively engaged in those processes.

Bialosky et al (2009) proposed a framework for the mechanisms of manual therapy to include a mix of biomechanical, neurophysiological, peripheral, spinal, and supraspinal mechanisms. They suggested that the application of techniques at the tissue level created a cascade of events that facilitate changes via the other mechanisms. This framework was expanded upon to include placebo effects that are likely influenced by a host of other factors.[171,172] A narrative review by Puentedura and Flynn (2016) suggested that manual therapy and tactile information may help restore or improve body schema maps citing several studies supporting pain modulation via cortical reorganization. The authors believed that manual intervention along with verbal cues from the therapist "could link sensory and proprioceptive neural circuits within the brain and help to refresh its representational body maps." It is practical to conclude that the biomechanical and peripheral neurophysiological impacts of manual therapy could serve to decrease nociceptive afferent input and thus decrease the bombardment of the central nervous system that has been linked with CS. Based on the actions across the proposed mechanisms it is reasonable to suggest that, if applied early in the pain experience, manual therapy could be an element in prophylaxis for pain chronification.[173]

Manual Therapy in Chronic Pain Care

Manual therapy has the potential to impact chronic pain from both top-down (supraspinal/cortical and spinal mechanisms) and bottom-up (biomechanical and peripheral neurophysiological). Manual therapy techniques can be applied with patients who present with any of the 3 categories, although with patients who are predominantly categorized as having CS, techniques should be modified to respect the altered processing of sensory input that is present in those individuals so as not

TABLE 23-7 Research Summary TENS

TENS	NUMBER OF STUDIES INCLUDED IN SYSTEMATIC REVIEW	CONCLUSIONS	AUTHORS/PUBLICATION YEAR
Chronic pain	19	Inconclusive	Carroll et al. (2000)
CLBP	9	No evidence to support use of TENS	Brosseau et al. (2002) Khadilkar et al. (2008)
Neurological disorders	11	• Not recommended for the treatment of chronic low back pain • Should be considered in the treatment of painful diabetic neuropathy	Dubinsky and Miyasaki (2010)
Primary dysmenorrhea	9	• High-frequency TENS more effective than placebo • Low-frequency TENS no more effective than placebo	Proctor et al. (2001)
Labor pain	10	No significant effect	Carroll et al. (1997)
Knee OA	7	Conventional and acupuncture-like TENS more effective than placebo	Osiri et al. (2001)
Knee OA	11	Inconclusive owing to high heterogeneity of studies	Rutjes et al. (2010)
Lower extremity OA	6	TENS (high or low frequency) useful for knee/hip pain over placebo	Brosseau et al. (2004)
Poststroke shoulder pain	4	Inconclusive	Price and Pandyan (2000)
Postoperative pain	21	TENS, administered with a strong, subnoxious intensity at an adequate frequency in the wound area, can significantly reduce analgesic consumption for postoperative pain. Mean reduction across trials: 26.5% (range 6% to +51%) better than placebo	Bjordal et al. (2002)
Musculoskeletal pain	38	TENS is effective for chronic, musculoskeletal pain	Johnson and Martinson (2007)
Cancer pain	3	Inconclusive owing to a lack of suitable RCTs	Hurlow et al. (2012)

CLBP, chronic low back pain; OA, osteoarthritis; RCT, randomized controlled trial; TENS, transcutaneous electrical nerve stimulation.

TABLE 23-8 Research Summary LLLT

LOW-LEVEL LASER THERAPY	NUMBER OF STUDIES INCLUDED IN SYSTEMATIC REVIEW	CONCLUSIONS	AUTHORS/PUBLICATION YEAR
Nonspecific low back pain	7	Effective method for relieving pain, but there is still a lack of evidence supporting its effect on function	Huang et al. (2015)
Chronic neck pain	5	Modest reduction in pain levels with CNP	Chow and Barnsley (2005)
Neck pain (acute or chronic)	16	Reduces pain immediately after treatment in acute neck pain and up to 22 wk after completion of treatment in patients with chronic neck pain	Chow et al. (2009)

CNP, chronic neck pain.

TABLE 23-9 Manual Therapy Research Summary		
CONDITION	**ARTICLE TYPE**	**AUTHORS/PUBLICATION YEAR**
Manual Therapy is Recommended as an Adjunct to Other Interventions in the Conditions Below		
Chronic low back pain	Clinical Practice Guideline	Wong et al. (2007)
	Clinical Practice Guideline	Delitto et al. (2012)
	Clinical Practice Guideline	NICE (2016)
	Clinical Practice Guideline Comparative	Oaseem et al. (2017)
	Effectiveness Review	Chou et al. (2016)
Chronic neck pain	Systematic Review	Schmid et al. (2008)
	Systematic Review	Gross et al. (2010)
	Systematic Review	Gross et al. (2015)
	Systematic Review	Wong et al. (2016)
	Clinical Practice Guideline	Childs et al. (2009)
Chronic headache	Clinical Practice Guideline	Childs et al. (2009)
	Systematic Review	Bronfort et al. (2004)
	Systematic Review	Varatharajan et al. (2016)
Shoulder pain	Systematic Review	Brantingham (2013) (lateral epicondylopathy, & carpal tunnel syndrome)
	Clinical Practice Guideline	Kelly et al. (2013) (Frozen shoulder)
	Systematic Review	Brantingham (2011)
	Systematic Review	Page et al. (2016) (Rotator cuff)
Lower extremity (hip, knee, ankle/foot)	Systematic Review	Brantingham (2014)
	Clinical Practice Guideline	Robroy et al. (2014) (Heel pain)
	Clinical Practice Guideline	Cibulka et al. (2009) (Hip OA)
	Clinical Practice Guideline	Enseki et al. (2014) (Hip nonarthritic)
Temporomandibular dysfunction	Systematic Review	Brantingham (2013)
	Systematic Review	Calixtr et al. (2015)
	Systematic Review	Martins et al. (2016)
	Systematic Review	Armijo-Olivo et al. (2016)

to perpetuate the cycle.[173] Manual therapy is best used in combination with other interventions and not as a stand-alone treatment of persistent pain symptoms.[174,175] In cases of chronic pain, using manual therapy alone does not promote self-efficacy. Instead, manual therapy can be used as a bridge or adjuvant to modulate pain so that patients can meaningfully engage in other active interventions.[57,176-179]

Table 23-10 is a summary table of the research for manual therapy with chronic pain.

TABLE 23-10 Manual Therapy Research Summary		
CONDITION	**ARTICLE TYPE**	**AUTHORS/PUBLICATION YEAR**
Manual Therapy is Recommended as an Adjunct to Other Interventions in the Conditions Below		
Chronic low back pain	Clinical Practice Guideline	Wong et al. (2007)
	Clinical Practice Guideline	Delitto et al. (2012)
	Clinical Practice Guideline	NICE (2016)
	Clinical Practice Guideline	Oaseem et al. (2017)
	Comparative Effectiveness Review	Chou et al. (2016)
Chronic neck pain	Systematic Review	Schmid et al. (2008)
	Systematic Review	Gross et al. (2010)
	Systematic Review	Gross et al. (2015)
	Systematic Review	Wong et al. (2016)
	Clinical Practice Guideline	Childs et al. (2009)
Chronic headache	Clinical Practice Guideline	Childs et al. (2009)
	Systematic Review	Bronfort et al. (2004)
	Systematic Review	Varatharajan et al. (2016)
Shoulder pain	Systematic Review	Brantingham (2013) (lateral epicondylopathy, & carpal tunnel syndrome)
	Clinical Practice Guideline	Kelly et al. (2013) (Frozen shoulder)
	Systematic Review	Brantingham (2011)
	Systematic Review	Page et al. (2016) (Rotator cuff)
Lower extremity (hip, knee, ankle/foot)	Systematic Review	Brantingham (2014)
	Clinical Practice Guideline	Robroy et al. (2014) (Heel pain)
	Clinical Practice Guideline	Cibulka et al. (2009) (Hip OA)
	Clinical Practice Guideline	Enseki et al. (2014) (Hip nonarthritic)
Temporomandibular dysfunction	Systematic Review	Brantingham (2013)
	Systematic Review	Calixtr et al. (2015)
	Systematic Review	Martins et al. (2016)
	Systematic Review	Armijo-Olivo et al. (2016)

SUMMARY

Many health, wellness, and fitness professionals are legally authorized to work with clients to improve painful conditions, but physical therapists have a unique knowledge base, skillset, and scope of practice that make them ideal resources for the nonpharmacological management of patients with persistent pain. Physical therapists are trained to take a holistic approach to patient care and have a strong foundation in anatomy and physiology of the human body and have begun pursuing training and conducting research on "psychologically informed" PT interventions.[180,181] Physical therapists are now more commonly incorporating principles and techniques of cognitive behavioral therapy, motivational interviewing, and health coaching as a routine part of patient care and are vital participants in the rehabilitation of patients with persistent pain.[59,181-184] Persistent pain is a condition of the nervous system, extending beyond tissue or movement dysfunction.[185-187] Management of this multidimensional, individual, and complex condition is best done using a multimodal, interdisciplinary, and biopsychosocial approach.[188-192]

REFERENCES

1. Reuben DB, Alvanzo AA, Ashikaga T, et al. National Institutes of Health Pathways to Prevention Workshop: the role of opioids in the treatment of chronic pain. *Ann Intern Med.* 2015;162(4):295-300. doi:10.7326/M14-2775.

2. Fordyce WE. An operant conditioning method for managing chronic pain. *Postgrad Med.* 1973;53(6):123-128. doi:10.1080/00325481.1973.11713462.

3. Cairns D, Mooney V, Crane P. Spinal pain rehabilitation: inpatient and outpatient treatment results and development of predictors for outcome. *Spine (Phila PA 1976).* 1984;9(1). http://journals.lww.com/spinejournal/Abstract/1984/01000/Spinal_Pain_Rehabilitation__Inpatient_and.20.aspx. Accessed 2 April 2017.

4. Flor H, Fydrich T, Turk DC. Efficacy of multidisciplinary pain treatment centers: a meta-analytic review. *Pain.* 1992;49(2):221-230. doi:10.1016/0304-3959(92)90145-2.

5. Chapman SL, Brena SF, Bradford AL. Treatment outcome in a chronic pain rehabilitation program. *Pain.* 1981;11(2):255-268. doi:10.1016/0304-3959(81)90011-7.

6. Guzmán J, Esmail R, Karjalainen K, Malmivaara A, Irvin E, Bombardier C. Multidisciplinary rehabilitation for chronic low back pain: systematic review. *BMJ.* 2011;322:1511-1516. https://www.researchgate.net/profile/Emma_Irvin/publication/11920686_Multidisciplinary_rehabilitation_for_chronic_low_back_pain_Systematic_review/links/0f31753cd842b25bb4000000.pdf. Accessed 8 April 2017.

7. Van Zee A. The promotion and marketing of oxycontin: commercial triumph, public health tragedy. *Am J Public Health.* 2009;99(2):221-227. doi:10.2105/AJPH.2007.131714.

8. Dowell D, Haegerich TM, Chou R. CDC guideline for prescribing opioids for chronic pain—United States, 2016. *JAMA.* 2016;315(15):1624-1645. doi:10.1001/jama.2016.1464.

9. Mularski RA, White-Chu F, Overbay D, Miller L, Asch SM, Ganzini L. Measuring pain as the 5th vital sign does not improve quality of pain management. *J Gen Intern Med.* 2006;21(6):607-612. doi:10.1111/j.1525-1497.2006.00415.x.

10. Daubresse M, Chang H-Y, Yu Y, et al. Ambulatory diagnosis and treatment of non-malignant pain in the United States, 2000–2010. *Med Care.* 2013;51(10). doi:10.1097/MLR.0b013e3182a95d86.

11. Morone NE, Weiner DK. Pain as the fifth vital sign: exposing the vital need for pain education. *Clin Ther.* 2013;35(11):1728-1732. doi:10.1016/j.clinthera.2013.10.001.

12. Quality improvement guidelines for the treatment of acute pain and cancer pain. American Pain Society Quality of Care Committee. *JAMA.* 1995;274:1874-1880.

13. Sayers M, Marando R, Fisher S, Aquila A, Morrison B, Dailey T. No need for pain. *J Healthc Qual.* 2000;22(3):10-15.

14. Administration VH. *Pain as the 5th Vital Sign Toolkit.* Washington, DC; 2000.

15. Guzmán J, Esmail R, Karjalainen K, Malmivaara A, Irvin E, Bombardier IE. Multidisciplinary bio-psycho-social rehabilitation for chronic low-back pain (review). *Cochrane Database Syst Rev.* 2002;(1):CD000963. http://www.thecochranelibrary.com. Accessed 8 April 2017.

16. Hatzakis MJ, Schatman ME. The impact of interventional approaches when used within the context of multidisciplinary chronic pain management. In: Schatman ME, Campbell A, eds. *Chronic Pain Management: Guidelines for Multidisciplinary Program Development–Google Books.* CRC Press; 2007:101-113. https://books.google.com/books?hl=en&lr=&id=oGhTBPtq0JEC&oi=fnd&pg=PA101&dq=Hatzakis+and+Schatman,+2007&ots=rq2hvu9xuY&sig=GgtBGjNOM4V4B8fwuUOL9o4QDNc#v=onepage&q=Hatzakis and Schatman%2C 2007&f=false. Accessed 12 April 2017.

17. Hoffman BM, Papas RK, Chatkoff DK, Kerns RD. Meta-analysis of psychological interventions for chronic low back pain. *Heal Psychol.* 2007;26(1):1-9. doi:10.1037/0278-6133.26.1.1.

18. Giordano J, Schatman ME. An ethical analysis of crisis in chronic pain care: facts, issues and problems in pain medicine; part I. *Pain Physician.* 2008;11:483-490. https://www.researchgate.net/profile/Michael_Schatman/publication/23159030_An_Ethical_Analysis_of_Crisis_in_Chronic_Pain_Care_Facts_Issues_and_Problems_in_Pain_Medicine_Part_I/links/53ea369f0cf28f342f418a3a/An-Ethical-Analysis-of-Crisis-in-Chronic-Pain-Ca. Accessed 8 April 2017.

19. Giordano J, Schatman ME. A crisis in chronic pain care: an ethical analysis. Part two: proposed structure and function of an ethics of pain medicine. *Pain Physician.* 2008;11(5):589-595. http://www.ncbi.nlm.nih.gov/pubmed/18850024. Accessed 8 April 2017.

20. Giordano J, Schatman ME. A crisis in chronic pain care: an ethical analysis. Part three: toward an integrative, multi-disciplinary pain medicine built around the needs of the patient. *Pain Physician.* 2008;11(6):775-784. www.painphysicianjournal.com. Accessed 26 March 2017.

21. Veterans Health Administration. *VHA Pain Management Directive (2009-053).* Washington, DC; 2009.

22. Dowell D, Haegerich TM, Chou R. CDC guideline for prescribing opioids for chronic pain—United States, 2016. *MMWR Recomm Rep.* 2016;65(1):1-49. doi:10.15585/mmwr.rr6501e1er.

23. Rosenberger P, Philip E, Lee A, Kerns R. The VHA's national pain management strategy: implementing the stepped care model. *Fed Pract.* 2011;8:39-42.

24. Guide to Physical Therapist Practice 3.0. Alexandria, VA: American Physical Therapy Association. http://guidetoptpractice.apta.org/. Published 2014. Accessed 4 April 2017.

25. Hoeger Bement MK, Sluka KA. The current state of physical therapy pain curricula in the United States: a faculty survey. *J Pain.* 2015;16(2):144-152. doi:10.1016/j.jpain.2014.11.001.

26. Bellamy J. Direct Access at the State Level. http://www.apta.org/StateIssues/DirectAccess/. Accessed 19 March 2017.

27. Fritz JM, Cleland JA, Brennan GP. Does adherence to the guideline recommendation for active treatments improve the quality of care for patients with acute low back pain delivered by physical therapists? *Med Care.* 2007;45(10):973-980. doi:10.1097/MLR.0b013e318070c6cd.

28. Fritz JM, Brennan GP. Preliminary examination of a proposed treatment-based classification system for patients receiving physical therapy interventions for neck pain. *Phys Ther.* 2007;87(5):513-524. doi:10.2522/ptj.20060192.

29. Burns SA, Foresman E, Kraycsir SJ, et al. A treatment-based classification approach to examination and intervention of lumbar disorders. *Sports Health.* 2011;3(4):362-372. doi:10.1177/1941738111410378.

30. Martin RL, Davenport TE, Reischl SF, et al. Heel pain—plantar fasciitis: revision 2014. *J Orthop Sport Phys Ther.* 2014;44(11):A1-A33. doi:10.2519/jospt.2014.0303.

31. Martin RL, Davenport TE, Paulseth S, et al. Ankle stability and movement coordination impairments: ankle ligament sprains. *J Orthop Sport Phys Ther.* 2013;43(9):A1-A40. doi:10.2519/jospt.2013.0305.

32. Cibulka MT, White DM, Woehrle J, et al. Hip pain and mobility deficits – hip osteoarthritis: clinical practice guidelines linked to the international classification of functioning, disability, and health from the orthopaedic section of the American Physical Therapy Association. *J Orthop Sport Phys Ther.* 2009;39(4):A1-A25. doi:10.2519/jospt.2009.0301.

33. Kelley MJ, Shaffer MA, Kuhn JE, et al. Shoulder pain and mobility deficits: adhesive capsulitis. *J Orthop Sport Phys Ther.* 2013;43(5):A1-A31. doi:10.2519/jospt.2013.0302.

34. Carcia CR, Martin RL, Wukich DK, et al. Achilles pain, stiffness, and muscle power deficits: achilles tendinitis. *J Orthop Sport Phys Ther.* 2010;40(9):A1-A26. doi:10.2519/jospt.2010.0305.

35. Logerstedt DS, Snyder-Mackler L, Ritter RC, et al. Knee pain and mobility impairments: meniscal and articular cartilage lesions. *J Orthop Sport Phys Ther.* 2010;40(6):A1-597. doi:10.2519/jospt.2010.0304.

36. Childs JD, Cleland JA, Elliott JM, et al. Neck pain. *J Orthop Sport Phys Ther.* 2008;38(9):A1-A34. doi:10.2519/jospt.2008.0303.

37. Delitto A, George SZ, Van Dillen LR, et al. Low back pain. *J Orthop Sports Phys Ther.* 2012;42(4):A1-A57. doi:10.2519/jospt.2012.42.4.A1.

38. Hanney WJ, Masaracchio M, Liu X, Kolber MJ. The influence of physical therapy guideline adherence on healthcare utilization and costs among patients with low back pain: a systematic review of the literature. *PLoS One.* 2016;11(6):e0156799. doi:10.1371/journal.pone.0156799.

39. Childs JD, Fritz JM, Wu SS, et al. Implications of early and guideline adherent physical therapy for low back pain on utilization and costs. *BMC Health Serv Res.* 2015;15:150. doi:10.1186/s12913-015-0830-3.

40. Rutten GM, Degen S, Hendriks EJ, Braspenning JC, Harting J, Oostendorp RA. Adherence to clinical practice guidelines for low back pain in physical therapy: do patients benefit? *Phys Ther.* 2010;90(8):1111-1122. doi:10.2522/ptj.20090173.

41. Fritz JM, Cleland JA, Speckman M, Brennan GP, Hunter SJ. Physical therapy for acute low back pain: associations with subsequent healthcare costs. *Spine (Phila PA 1976).* 2008;33(16):1800-1805. doi:10.1097/BRS.0b013e31817bd853.

42. Smart KM, Blake C, Staines A, Thacker M, Doody C. Mechanisms-based classifications of musculoskeletal pain: part 3 of 3: symptoms and signs of nociceptive pain in patients with low back (±leg) pain. *Man Ther.* 2012;17:352-357. doi:10.1016/j.math.2012.03.002.

43. Smart KM, Blake C, Staines A, Thacker M, Doody C. Mechanisms-based classifications of musculoskeletal pain: part 2 of 3: symptoms and signs of peripheral neuropathic pain in patients with low back (±leg) pain. *Man Ther.* 2012;17:345-351. doi:10.1016/j.math.2012.03.003.

44. Smart KM, Blake C, Staines A, Thacker M, Doody C. Mechanisms-based classifications of musculoskeletal pain: part 1 of 3: symptoms and signs of central sensitisation in patients with low back (±leg) pain. *Man Ther.* 2012;17(4):336-344. doi:10.1016/j.math.2012.03.013.

45. Nijs J, Malfliet A, Ickmans K, Baert I, Meeus M. Treatment of central sensitization in patients with "unexplained" chronic pain: an update. *Expert Opin Pharmacother.* 2014;15(12):1671-1683. doi:10.1517/14656566.2014.925446.

46. Gaskin DJ, Richard P, Dekker J, Sorbi MJ, Bensing JM. The economic costs of pain in the United States. *J Pain.* 2012;13(8):715-724. doi:10.1016/j.jpain.2012.03.009.

47. Edwards RR, Dworkin RH, Sullivan MD, Turk DC, Wasan AD. The role of psychosocial processes in the development and maintenance of chronic pain. *J Pain.* 2016;17(9):T70-T92. doi:10.1016/j.jpain.2016.01.001.

48. Ramond A, Bouton C, Richard I, et al. Psychosocial risk factors for chronic low back pain in primary care–a systematic review. *Fam Pract.* 2011;28(1):12-21. doi:10.1093/fampra/cmq072.

49. Litt MD, Shafer DM, Ibanez CR, Kreutzer DL, Tawfik-Yonkers Z. Momentary pain and coping in temporomandibular disorder pain: exploring mechanisms of cognitive behavioral treatment for chronic pain. *Pain.* 2009;145(1-2):160-168. doi:10.1016/j.pain.2009.06.003.

50. Wiangkham T, Duda J, Haque S, Madi M, Rushton A, Alonso-Coello P. The effectiveness of conservative management for acute Whiplash Associated Disorder (WAD) II: a systematic review and meta-analysis of randomised controlled trials. Eldabe S, ed. *PLoS One.* 2015;10(7):e0133415. doi:10.1371/journal.pone.0133415.

51. Chou R, Deyo R, Friedly J, et al. *Noninvasive Treatments for Low Back Pain.* Rockville, MD: Agency for Healthcare Research and Quality (US); 2016. http://www.ncbi.nlm.nih.gov/pubmed/26985522. Accessed 19 March 2017.

52. Carlson H, Carlson N. An overview of the management of persistent musculoskeletal pain. *Ther Adv Musculoskelet Dis.* 2011;3(2):91-99. doi:10.1177/1759720X11398742.

53. Snow-Turek AL, Norris MP, Tan G. Active and passive coping strategies in chronic pain patients. *Pain.* 1996;64:455-462.

54. Schmid A, Brunner F, Wright A, Bachmann LM. Paradigm shift in manual therapy? Evidence for a central nervous system component in the response to passive cervical joint mobilisation. *Man Ther.* 2008;13(5):387-396. doi:10.1016/j.math.2007.12.007.

55. Bialosky JE, Bishop MD, Price DD, Robinson ME, George SZ. The mechanisms of manual therapy in the treatment of musculoskeletal pain: a comprehensive model. *Man Ther.* 2010;14(5):531-538. doi:10.1016/j.math.2008.09.001.

56. ACPA Resource Guide to Chronic Pain Treatment an Integrated Guide to Physical, Behavioral and Pharmacologic Therapy.

57. Low Back Pain and Sciatica in Over 16s: Assessment and Management | Recommendations | Guidance and Guidelines | NICE. https://www.nice.org.uk/guidance/NG59/chapter/Recommendations. Accessed 19 March 2017.

58. de Rooij A, de Boer MR, van der Leeden M, Roorda LD, Steultjens MPM, Dekker J. Cognitive mechanisms of change in multidisciplinary treatment of patients with chronic widespread pain: a prospective cohort study. *J Rehabil Med.* 2014;46(2):173-180. doi:10.2340/16501977-1252.

59. Burns JW, Nielson WR, Jensen MP, Heapy A, Czlapinski R, Kerns RD. Specific and general therapeutic mechanisms in cognitive behavioral treatment of chronic pain. *J Consult Clin Psychol.* 2015;83(1):1-11. doi:10.1037/a0037208.

60. Costa Lda C, Maher CG, McAuley JH, Hancock MJ, Smeets RJ. Self-efficacy is more important than fear of movement in mediating the relationship between pain and disability in chronic low back pain. *Eur J Pain.* 2011;15(2):213-219. doi:10.1016/j.ejpain.2010.06.014.

61. Bandura A. *Self-Efficacy: The Exercise of Control.* W.H. Freeman/Times Books/Henry Holt & Co; 1997. http://psycnet.apa.org/psycinfo/1997-08589-000. Accessed 1 April 2017.

62. McAuley E, Szabo A, Gothe N, Olson EA. Self-efficacy: implications for physical activity, function, and functional limitations in older adults. *Am J Lifestyle Med.* 2011;5(4). doi:10.1177/1559827610392704.

63. Arnstein P, Caudill M, Mandle CL, Norris A, Beasley R. Self efficacy as a mediator of the relationship between pain intensity, disability and depression in chronic pain patients. *Pain.* 1999;80(3):483-491. doi:10.1016/S0304-3959(98)00220-6.

64. Asghari A, Nicholas MK. Pain self-efficacy beliefs and pain behaviour. A prospective study. *Pain.* 2001;94(1):85-100. doi:10.1016/S0304-3959(01)00344-X.

65. Denison E, Åsenlöf P, Lindberg P. Self-efficacy, fear avoidance, and pain intensity as predictors of disability in subacute and chronic musculoskeletal pain patients in primary health care. *Pain.* 2004;111(3):245-252. doi:10.1016/j.pain.2004.07.001.

66. Li F, Harmer P, McAuley E, Fisher KJ, Duncan TE, Duncan SC. Tai Chi, self-efficacy, and physical function in the elderly. *Prev Sci.* 2001;2(4):229-239. http://www.ncbi.nlm.nih.gov/pubmed/11833926. Accessed 1 April 2017.

67. Louw A, Puentedura E, Zimney K. Teaching patients about pain: it works, but what should we call it? *Physiother Theory Pract.* 2016;32(5):328-331. doi:10.1080/09593985.2016.1194669.

68. Ryan CG, Gray HG, Newton M, Granat MH. Pain biology education and exercise classes compared to pain biology education alone for individuals with chronic low back pain: a pilot randomised controlled trial. *Man Ther.* 2010;15(4):382-387. doi:10.1016/j.math.2010.03.003.

69. Van Oosterwijck J, Nijs J, Meeus M, et al. Pain neurophysiology education improves cognitions, pain thresholds, and movement performance in people with chronic whiplash: a pilot study. *J Rehabil Res Dev.* 2011;48(1):43-58. doi:10.1682/JRRD.2009.12.0206.

70. Moseley GL. A pain neuromatrix approach to patients with chronic pain. *Man Ther.* 2003;8(3):130-140. doi:10.1016/S1356-689X(03)00051-1.

71. Louw A, Diener I, Butler DS, Puentedura EJ. The effect of neuroscience education on pain, disability, anxiety, and stress in chronic musculoskeletal pain. *Arch Phys Med Rehabil.* 2011;92(12):2041-2056. doi:10.1016/j.apmr.2011.07.198.

72. Diener I, Kargela M, Louw A. Listening is therapy: patient interviewing from a pain science perspective. *Physiother Theory Pract.* 2016;32(5):356-367. doi:10.1080/09593985.2016.1194648.

73. Nijs J, Paul van Wilgen C, Van Oosterwijck J, van Ittersum M, Meeus M. How to explain central sensitization to patients with "unexplained" chronic musculoskeletal pain: practice guidelines. *Man Ther.* 2011;16(5):413-418. doi:10.1016/j.math.2011.04.005.

74. Nijs J, Roussel N, Paul van Wilgen C, Köke A, Smeets R. Thinking beyond muscles and joints: therapists' and patients' attitudes and beliefs regarding chronic musculoskeletal pain are key to applying effective treatment. *Man Ther.* 2013;18(2):96-102. doi:10.1016/j.math.2012.11.001.

75. Greene L, Appel AJ, Reinert SE, Palumbo MA. Lumbar disc herniation: evaluation of information on the internet. *Spine (Phila PA 1976).* 2005;30(7):826-829. http://ovidsp.uk.ovid.com/sp-3.24.1b/ovidweb.cgi?QS2=434f4e1a73d37e8cdfd212f0e7c8b84c2f1268b-b4a7c84cfd40fc3830aded143a5d8e6c710c3b02b-482c619e4feaa984d564ff36f1a7307eee268f64ac-14ce8b63d55ff74a24d7e2cd693fa698e6b9aab2d-2247603b6c72301cfe204342d785e16dad7a435. Accessed 4 April 2017.

76. Moseley GL. Reconceptualising pain according to modern pain science. *Phys Ther Rev.* 2007;12(3):169-178. doi:10.1179/108331907X223010.

77. Lederman E. The fall of the postural-structural-biomechanical model in manual and physical therapies: exemplified by lower back pain. *J Bodyw Mov Ther.* 2011;15(2):131-138. doi:10.1016/j.jbmt.2011.01.011.

78. O'Sullivan P. It's time for change with the management of non-specific chronic low back pain. *Br J Sport Med.* 2012;46(4):224-227. doi:10.1136/bjsm.2010.081638.

79. Spielmann AL, Forster BB, Kokan P, Hawkins RH, Janzen DL. Shoulder after rotator cuff repair: MR imaging findings in asymptomatic individuals–initial experience. *Radiology.* 1999;213(3):705-708. doi:10.1148/radiology.213.3.r99dc09705.

80. Nijs J, Van Houdenhove B, Oostendorp RA. Recognition of central sensitization in patients with musculoskeletal pain: application of pain neurophysiology in manual therapy practice. *Man Ther.* 2010;15(2):135-141. doi:10.1016/j.math.2009.12.001.

81. Woolf CJ. Central sensitization: implications for the diagnosis and treatment of pain. *Pain.* 2011;152(suppl 3). doi:10.1016/j.pain.2010.09.030.

82. Puentedura EJ, Louw A. A neuroscience approach to managing athletes with low back pain. *Phys Ther Sport.* 2011:1-11. doi:10.1016/j.ptsp.2011.12.001.

83. Louw A, Puentedura E. *Therapeutic Neuroscience Education: Teaching Patients About Pain. A Guide for Clinicians.* First. (OPTP, ed.). International Spine and Pain Institute; 2013.

84. Louw A, Puentedura EJ. Therapeutic neuroscience education, pain, physiotherapy and the pain neuromatrix. *Int J Health Sci.* 2014;2(3):33-45. doi:10.15640/ijhs.v2n3a4.

85. Van Wilgen CP, Keizer D. The sensitisation model: a method to explain chronic pain to a patient. *Ned Tijdschr Geneeskd.* 2004;148(51):2535-2538. doi:10.1016/j.pmn.2010.03.001.

86. Butler DS, Moseley GL. *Explain Pain*. Adelaide, Australia: Noigroup Publications.

87. Moseley GL, Butler DS. Fifteen years of explaining pain: the past, present, and future. *J Pain*. 2015;16(9):807-813. doi:10.1016/j.jpain.2015.05.005.

88. Louw A, Zimney K, Puentedura EJ, Diener I. The efficacy of pain neuroscience education on musculoskeletal pain: a systematic review of the literature. *Physiother Theory Pract*. 2016;3985:1-24. http://www.ncbi.nlm.nih.gov/pubmed/27351541.

89. Louw A, Zimney K, O'Hotto C, Hilton S. The clinical application of teaching people about pain. *Physiother Theory Pract*. 2016;32(5):385-395. doi:10.1080/09593985.2016.1194652.

90. Moseley L. Unraveling the barriers to reconceptualization of the problem in chronic pain: the actual and perceived ability of patients and health professionals to understand the neurophysiology. *J Pain*. 2003;4(4):184-189. doi:10.1016/S1526-5900(03)00488-7.

91. Loftus S. Pain and its metaphors: a dialogical approach. *J Med Humanit*. 2011;32(3):213-230. doi:10.1007/s10912-011-9139-3.

92. Bedell SE, Graboys TB, Bedell E, Lown B. Words that harm, words that heal. *JAMA*. 2004;164(13):1365-1368. doi:10.1001/archinte.164.1365.

93. Darlow B, Dowell A, Baxter GD, Mathieson F, Perry M, Dean S. The enduring impact of what clinicians say to people with low back pain. *Ann Fam Med*. 2013;11(6):527-534. doi:10.1370/afm.1518.

94. Lakoff G, Johnson M. *Metaphors We Live by*. London: The University of Chicago Press; 2003.

95. Sloan TJ, Walsh DA. Explanatory and diagnostic labels and perceived prognosis in chronic low back pain. *Spine (Phila PA 1976)*. 2010;35(21):E1120-E1125. doi:10.1097/BRS.0b013e3181e089a9.

96. Black PH. Stress and the inflammatory response: a review of neurogenic inflammation. *Brain Behav Immun*. 2002;16(6):622-653. doi:10.1016/S0889-1591(02)00021-1.

97. Chapman CR, Tuckett RP, Song CW. Pain and stress in a systems perspective: reciprocal neural, endocrine, and immune interactions. *J Pain*. 2008;9(2):122-145. doi:10.1016/j.jpain.2007.09.006.

98. Littlejohn G. Neurogenic neuroinflammation in fibromyalgia and complex regional pain syndrome. *Nat Rev Rheumatol*. 2015;11(11):1-10. doi:10.1038/nrrheum.2015.100.

99. Picavet HSJ, Vlaeyen JWS, Schouten JS. Pain catastrophizing and kinesiophobia: predictors of chronic low back pain. *Am J Epidemiol*. 2002;156(11):1028-1034. doi:10.1093/aje/kwf136.

100. Domenech J, Sánchez-Zuriaga D, Segura-Ortí E, Espejo-Tort B, Lisón JF. Impact of biomedical and biopsychosocial training sessions on the attitudes, beliefs, and recommendations of health care providers about low back pain: a randomised clinical trial. *Pain*. 2011;152(11):2557-2563. doi:10.1016/j.pain.2011.07.023.

101. Poiraudeau S, Rannou F, Baron G, et al. Fear-avoidance beliefs about back pain in patients with subacute low back pain. *Pain*. 2006;124(3):305-311. doi:10.1016/j.pain.2006.04.019.

102. Kujala UM. Evidence on the effects of exercise therapy in the treatment of chronic disease. *Br J Sports Med*. 2009;43(8):550-555. doi:10.1136/bjsm.2009.059808.

103. Hoffmann TC, Maher CG, Briffa T, et al. Prescribing exercise interventions for patients with chronic conditions. *CMAJ*. 2016;188(7):510-518. doi: 10.1503/cmaj.150684.

104. Hordern MD, Dunstan DW, Prins JB, Baker MK, Singh MAF, Coombes JS. Exercise prescription for patients with type 2 diabetes and pre-diabetes: a position statement from Exercise and Sport Science Australia. *J Sci Med Sport*. 2012. 15(1):25-31. doi:10.1016/j.jsams.2011.04.005.

105. Garland EL. Pain processing in the human nervous system: a selective review of nociceptive and biobehavioral pathways. *Prim Care*. 2012;39(3):561-571. doi:10.1016/j.pop.2012.06.013.

106. Brinjikji W, Luetmer PH, Comstock B, et al. Systematic literature review of imaging features of spinal degeneration in asymptomatic populations. *Am J Neuroradiol*. 2015;36(4):811-816. doi:10.3174/ajnr.A4173.

107. Bennell KL, Hinman RS. A review of the clinical evidence for exercise in osteoarthritis of the hip and knee. *J Sci Med Sport*. 2011;14(1):4-9. doi:10.1016/j.jsams.2010.08.002.

108. Millner JR, Barron JS, Beinke KM, et al. Exercise for ankylosing spondylitis: an evidence-based consensus statement. *Semin Arthritis Rheum*. 2016;45(4):411-427. doi:10.1016/j.semarthrit.2015.08.003.

109. Hughes SL, Seymour RB, Campbell RT, et al. Long-term impact of fit and strong! On older adults with osteoarthritis. *Gerontologist*. 2006;46(6):801-814.

110. Hurkmans E, van der Giesen FJ, Vliet Vlieland TP, Schoones J, Van den Ende EC. Dynamic exercise programs (aerobic capacity and/or muscle strength training) in patients with rheumatoid arthritis. *Cochrane Database Syst Rev*. 2009;(4):CD006853. doi:10.1002/14651858.CD006853.pub2.

111. Roddy E, Zhang W, Doherty M, et al. Evidence-based recommendations for the role of exercise in the management of osteoarthritis of the hip or knee—the MOVE consensus. *Rheumatology*. 2005;44:67-73. doi:10.1093/rheumatology/keh399.

112. Ageberg E, Link A, Roos EM. Feasibility of neuromuscular training in patients with severe hip or knee OA: the individualized goal-based NEMEX-TJR training program. *BMC Musculoskelet Disord*. 2010;11. http://www.biomedcentral.com/1471-2474/11/126.

113. Fiatarone MA, O'Neill EF, Ryan ND, et al. Exercise training and nutritional supplementation for physical frailty in very elderly people. *N Engl J Med*. 1994;330(25):1769-1775.

114. Fiatarone MA, Marks EC, Ryan ND, Meredith CN, Lipsitz LA, Evans WJ. High-intensity strength training in nonagenarians. Effects on skeletal muscle. *JAMA*. 1990;263(22):3029-3034.

115. Brox JI, Storheim K, Grotle M, Tveito TH, Indahl A, Eriksen HR. Systematic review of back schools, brief education, and fear-avoidance training for chronic low back pain. *Spine J*. 2008;8(6):948-958. doi:10.1016/j.spinee.2007.07.389.

116. Vlaeyen JW, Crombez G. Fear of movement/(re)injury, avoidance and pain disability in chronic low back pain patients. *Man Ther*. 1999;4(4):187-195. doi:10.1054/math.1999.0199.

117. Vlaeyen J., Linton S. Fear avoidance and its consequences in chronic musculoskeletal pain: a state of the art. *Pain*. 2000;85:317-332.

118. Moseley GL. Evidence for a direct relationship between cognitive and physical change during an education intervention in people with chronic low back pain. *Eur J Pain*. 2004;8(1):39-45. doi:10.1016/S1090-3801(03)00063-6.

119. Zimney K, Louw A, Puentedura EJ. Use of therapeutic neuroscience education to address psychosocial factors associated with acute low back pain: a case report. *Physiother Theory Pract.* 2014;30(3). doi:10.3109/09593985.2013.856508.

120. Dolphens M, Nijs J, Cagnie B, et al. Efficacy of a modern neuroscience approach versus usual care evidence-based physiotherapy on pain, disability and brain characteristics in chronic spinal pain patients: protocol of a randomized clinical trial. *BMC Musculoskelet Disord.* 2014;15:149. doi:10.1186/1471-2474-15-149.

121. Nijs J, Kosek E, Vanoosterwijck J, et al. Dysfunctional endogenous analgesia during exercise in patients with chronic pain: to exercise or not to exercise? *Pain Physician.* 2012;15(suppl 3):ES205-ES213. http://www.ncbi.nlm.nih.gov/pubmed/22786458.

122. Nijs J, Kosek E, Van Oosterwijck J, Meeus M. Dysfunctional endogenous analgesia during exercise in patients with chronic pain: to exercise or not to exercise? *Pain Physician.* 2012;15(suppl 3):ES203-ES213.

123. Nijs J, Torres-Cueco R, van Wilgen CP, et al. Applying modern pain neuroscience in clinical practice: criteria for the classification of central sensitization pain. *Pain Physician.* 2014;17(12):447-457. https://biblio.ugent.be/publication/5710382/file/5710391.pdf. Accessed 28 March 2017.

124. Phillips K, Clauw DJ. Central pain mechanisms in chronic pain states–maybe it is all in their head. *Best Pract Res Clin Rheumatol.* 2011;25(2):141-154. doi:10.1016/j.berh.2011.02.005.

125. Meeus M, Roussel NA, Truijen S, Nijs J. Reduced pressure pain thresholds in response to exercise in chronic fatigue syndrome but not in chronic low back pain: an experimental study. *J Rehabil Med.* 2010;42(9):884-890. doi:10.2340/16501977-0595.

126. Meeus M, Hermans L, Ickmans K, et al. Endogenous pain modulation in response to exercise in patients with rheumatoid arthritis, patients with chronic fatigue syndrome and comorbid fibromyalgia, and healthy controls: a double-blind randomized controlled trial. *Pain Pract.* 2015;15(2):98-106. doi:10.1111/papr.12181.

127. Häuser W, Klose P, Langhorst J, et al. Efficacy of different types of aerobic exercise in fibromyalgia syndrome: a systematic review and meta-analysis of randomised controlled trials. *Arthritis Res Ther.* 2010;12(3):R79. doi:10.1186/ar3002.

128. Larun L, Brurberg K, Odgaard-Jensen J, Price J. Exercise therapy for chronic fatigue syndrome (review). *Cochrane Database Syst Rev.* 2015;(2):1-116. doi:10.1002/14651858.CD003200.pub3.

129. Jordan JL, Holden MA, Mason EE, et al. Interventions to improve adherence to exercise for chronic musculoskeletal pain in adults. *Cochrane Database Syst Rev.* 2010;(1):CD005956. doi:10.1002/14651858.CD005956.pub2.

130. Ambrose KR, Golightly YM. Physical exercise as non-pharmacological treatment of chronic pain: why and when. *Best Pract Res Clin Rheumatol.* 2015;29(1):120-130. doi:10.1016/j.berh.2015.04.022.

131. Jones KD, Adams D, Winters-Stone K, et al. A comprehensive review of 46 exercise treatment studies in fibromyalgia (1988–2005). *Health Qual Life Outcomes.* 2006;4:67. doi:10.1186/1477-7525-4-67.

132. Giannotti E, Koutsikos K, Pigatto M, Rampudda ME, Doria A, Masiero S. Medium-/long-term effects of a specific exercise protocol combined with patient education on spine mobility, chronic fatigue, pain, aerobic fitness and level of disability in fibromyalgia. *Biomed Res Int.* 2014;2014. doi:10.1155/2014/474029.

133. Brosseau L, Wells GA, Tugwell P, et al. Ottawa panel evidence-based clinical practice guidelines for strengthening exercises in the management of fibromyalgia: part 2. *Phys Ther.* 2008;88(7):873-886. doi:10.2522/ptj.20070115.

134. Jones KD, Burckhardt CS, Clark SR, Bennett RM, Potempa KM. A randomized controlled trial of muscle strengthening versus flexibility training in fibromyalgia. *J Rheumatol.* 2002;29(5):1041-1048.

135. Dimeo FC. Effects of exercise on cancer-related fatigue. *Cancer.* 2001;92(suppl 6):1689-1693. doi:10.1002/1097-0142(20010915)92:6+<1689::AID-CNCR1498>3.0.CO;2-H.

136. Busch AJ, Webber SC, Brachaniec M, et al. Exercise therapy for fibromyalgia. *Curr Pain Headache Rep.* 2011;15(5):358-367. doi:10.1007/s11916-011-0214-2.

137. Dupree Jones K, Adams D, Winters-Stone K, Burckhardt CS. A comprehensive review of 46 exercise treatment studies in fibromyalgia (1988–2005). *Health Qual Life Outcomes.* 2006;4:67. doi:10.1186/1477-7525-4-67.

138. Sañudo B, Carrasco L, de Hoyo M, McVeigh JG. Effects of exercise training and detraining in patients with fibromyalgia syndrome: a 3-yr longitudinal study. *Am J Phys Med Rehabil.* 2012;91(7):561-569. quiz 570-573. doi:10.1097/PHM.0b013e31824faa03.

139. Häkkinen A, Häkkinen K, Hannonen P, Alen M. Strength training induced adaptations in neuromuscular function of premenopausal women with fibromyalgia: comparison with healthy women. *Ann Rheum Dis.* 2001;37(6):21-26.

140. Valkeinen H, Hakkinen K, Pakarinen A, et al. Muscle hypertrophy, strength development, and serum hormones during strength training in elderly women with fibromyalgia. *Scand J Rheumatol.* 2005;34(4):309-314. doi:10.1080/03009740510018697.

141. Valkeinen H, Alén M, Häkkinen A, Hannonen P, Kukkonen-Harjula K, Häkkinen K. Effects of concurrent strength and endurance training on physical fitness and symptoms in postmenopausal women with fibromyalgia: a randomized controlled trial. *Arch Phys Med Rehabil.* 2008;89(9):1660-1666. doi:10.1016/j.apmr.2008.01.022.

142. Gavi MBRO, Vassalo DV, Amaral FT, et al. Strengthening exercises improve symptoms and quality of life but do not change autonomic modulation in fibromyalgia: a randomized clinical trial. *PLoS One.* 2014;9(3). doi:10.1371/journal.pone.0090767.

143. Walsh DM. The evolution of tens. *Hong Kong Physiother J.* 2003;21. doi:10.1016/S1013-7025(09)70033-8.

144. 144Wall PD, Sweet WH. Temporary abolition of pain in man. *Science.* 1967;155(3758):108-109.

145. Melzack R, Wall PD. Pain mechanisms: a new theory. *Surv Anesthesiol.* 1967;11(2):89-90.

146. Vance CG, Dailey DL, Rakel BA, Sluka KA. Using TENS for pain control: the state of the evidence. *Pain Manag.* 2014;4(3):197-209. doi:10.2217/pmt.14.13.

147. Kalra A, Urban MO, Sluka KA. Blockade of opioid receptors in rostral ventral medulla prevents antihyperalgesia produced by Transcutaneous Electrical Nerve Stimulation (TENS). *J Pharmacol Exp Ther.* 2001;298(1).

148. Sluka KA, Lisi TL, Westlund KN. Increased release of serotonin in the spinal cord during low, but not high, frequency transcutaneous electric nerve stimulation in rats with joint inflammation. *Arch Phys Med Rehabil.* 2006;87(8):1137-1140. doi:10.1016/j.apmr.2006.04.023.

149. Ma YT, Sluka KA. Reduction in inflammation-induced sensitization of dorsal horn neurons by transcutaneous electrical nerve stimulation in anesthetized rats. *Exp Brain Res.* 2001;137(1):94-102. doi:10.1007/s002210000629.

150. Sluka KA, Deacon M, Stibal A, Strissel S, Terpstra A. Spinal blockade of opioid receptors prevents the analgesia produced by TENS in arthritic rats. *J Pharmacol Exp Ther.* 1999;289(2):840-846.

151. Sluka KA, Vance CGT, Lisi TL. High-frequency, but not low-frequency, transcutaneous electrical nerve stimulation reduces aspartate and glutamate release in the spinal cord dorsal horn. *J Neurochem.* 2005;95(6):1794-1801. doi:10.1111/j.1471-4159.2005.03511.x.

152. Maeda Y, Lisi TL, Vance CGT, Sluka KA. Release of GABA and activation of GABAAA in the spinal cord mediates the effects of TENS in rats. *Brain Res.* 2007;1136(1):43-50. doi:10.1016/j.brainres.2006.11.061.

153. DeSantana JM, Walsh DM, Vance C, Rakel BA, Sluka KA. Effectiveness of transcutaneous electrical nerve stimulation for treatment of hyperalgesia and pain. *Curr Rheumatol Rep.* 2008;10(6):492-499. doi:10.1007/s11926-008-0080-z.

154. Fang J-F, Liang Y, Du J-Y, Fang J-Q. Transcutaneous electrical nerve stimulation attenuates CFA-induced hyperalgesia and inhibits spinal ERK1/2-COX-2 pathway activation in rats. *BMC Complement Altern Med.* 2013;13(1):134. doi:10.1186/1472-6882-13-134.

155. Melzack R, Vetere P, Finch L. Transcutaneous electrical nerve stimulation for low back pain a comparison of TENS and massage for pain and range of motion. *Phys Ther.* 1983;63(4).

156. 156Poitras S, Brosseau L. Evidence-informed management of chronic low back pain with transcutaneous electrical nerve stimulation, interferential current, electrical muscle stimulation, ultrasound, and thermotherapy. *Spine J.* 2008;8(1):226-233. doi:10.1016/j.spinee.2007.10.022.

157. Khadilkar A, Odebiyi DO, Brosseau L, Wells GA. Transcutaneous electrical nerve stimulation (TENS) versus placebo for chronic low-back pain. In: Brosseau L, ed. *Cochrane Database of Systematic Reviews.* Chichester, UK: John Wiley & Sons, Ltd; 2008. doi:10.1002/14651858. CD003008.pub3.

158. Buchmuller A, Navez M, Milletre-Bernardin M, et al. Value of TENS for relief of chronic low back pain with or without radicular pain. *Eur J Pain.* 2012;16(5):656-665. doi:10.1002/j.1532-2149.2011.00061.x.

159. Bilgili A, Cakir T, Dogan S, Ercalik T, Filiz M, Toraman F. The effectiveness of transcutaneous electrical nerve stimulation in the management of patients with complex regional pain syndrome: a randomized, double-blinded, placebo-controlled prospective study. *J Back Musculoskelet Rehabil.* 2016;29(4):661-671.

160. Rutjes AW, Nüesch E, Sterchi R, et al. Transcutaneous electrostimulation for osteoarthritis of the knee. *Cochrane Database Syst Rev.* 2009;(4):CD002823. www.cochranelibrary.com. doi:10.1002/14651858.CD002823.pub2.

161. Bennett MI, Hughes N, Johnson MI. Methodological quality in randomised controlled trials of transcutaneous electric nerve stimulation for pain: low fidelity may explain negative findings. *Pain.* 2011;152:1226-1232. doi:10.1016/j.pain.2010.12.009.

162. Annaswamy TM, De Luigi AJ, O'Neill BJ, Keole N, Berbrayer D. Emerging concepts in the treatment of myofascial pain: a review of medications, modalities, and needle-based interventions. *PM R.* 2011;3(10):940-961. doi:10.1016/j.pmrj.2011.06.013.

163. Hakgüder A, Birtane M, Gürcan S, Kokino S, Tura FN. Efficacy of low level laser therapy in myofascial pain syndrome: an algometric and thermographic evaluation. *Lasers Surg Med.* 2003;33(5):339-343. doi:10.1002/lsm.10241.

164. Gur A, Karakoc M, Cevik R, Nas K, Sarac AJ, Karakoc M. Efficacy of low power laser therapy and exercise on pain and functions in chronic low back pain. *Lasers Surg Med.* 2003;32(3):233-238. doi:10.1002/lsm.10134.

165. Gur A, Cosut A, Jale Sarac A, Cevik R, Nas K, Uyar A. Efficacy of different therapy regimes of low-power laser in painful osteoarthritis of the knee: a double-blind and randomized-controlled trial. *Lasers Surg Med.* 2003;33(5):330-338. doi:10.1002/lsm.10236.

166. Gur A, Sarac AJ, Cevik R, Altindag O, Sarac S. Efficacy of 904 nm gallium arsenide low level laser therapy in the management of chronic myofascial pain in the neck: a double-blind and randomize-controlled trial. *Lasers Surg Med.* 2004;35(3):229-235. doi:10.1002/lsm.20082.

167. Maher S. Is low-level laser therapy effective in the management of lateral epicondylitis? *Phys Ther.* 2006;86(8):1161-1167. doi:10.1093/ptj/86.8.1161.

168. Chow RT, Johnson MI, Lopes-Martins RA, Bjordal JM. Efficacy of low-level laser therapy in the management of neck pain: a systematic review and meta-analysis of randomised placebo or active-treatment controlled trials. *Lancet.* 2009;374(9705):1897-1908. doi:10.1016/S0140-6736(09)61522-1.

169. Karu T. Low intensity laser light action upon fibroblasts and lymphocytes. In: Ohshiro T, Calderhead RG, eds. *Progress in Laser Therapy: Selected Papers From the October 1990 ILTA Congress;* 1991:175-179.

170. Bialosky JE, Bishop MD, Price DD, Robinson ME, George SZ. The mechanisms of manual therapy in the treatment of musculoskeletal pain: a comprehensive model. *Man Ther.* 2009;14(5):531-538. doi:10.1016/j.math.2008.09.001.

171. Bialosky JE, Bishop MD, George SZ, Robinson ME. Placebo response to manual therapy: something out of nothing? *J Man Manip Ther.* 2011;19(1):11-19. doi:10.1179/2042618610Y.0000000001.

172. Bishop MD, Bialosky JE, Cleland JA. Patient expectations of benefit from common interventions for low back pain and effects on outcome: secondary analysis of a clinical trial of manual therapy interventions. *J Man Manip Ther.* 2011;19(1):20-25. doi:10.1179/106698110X12804993426929.

173. Nijs J, Van Houdenhove B. From acute musculoskeletal pain to chronic widespread pain and fibromyalgia: application of pain neurophysiology in manual therapy practice. *Man Ther.* 2009;14(1):3-12. doi:10.1016/j.math.2008.03.001.

174. Lluch Girbés E, Meeus M, Baert I, Nijs J. Balancing "hands-on" with "hands-off" physical therapy interventions for the treatment of central sensitization pain in osteoarthritis. *Man Ther.* 2015;20(2):349-352. doi:10.1016/j.math.2014.07.017.

175. 175Page CJ, Hinman RS, Bennell KL. Physiotherapy management of knee osteoarthritis. *Int J Rheum Dis.* 2011;14(2):145-151. doi:10.1111/j.1756-185X.2011.01612.x.

176. Fritz J, Clelan JA, Childs J. Subgrouping patients with low back pain: evolution of a classification approach to physical therapy. *J Orthop Sport Phys Ther*. 2007;37(6):290-302.

177. Fritz JM, Lindsay W, Matheson JW, et al. Is there a subgroup of patients with low back pain likely to benefit from mechanical traction? Results of a randomized clinical trial and subgrouping analysis. *Spine (Phila PA 1976)*. 2007;32(26):E793-800. doi:10.1097/BRS.0b013e31815d001a.

178. Fritz JM, Cleland JA, Speckman M, Brennan GP, Hunter SJ. Physical therapy for acute low back pain. *Spine (Phila PA 1976)*. 2008;33(16):1800-1805. doi:10.1097/BRS.0b013e31817bd853.

179. Fritz JM, Childs JD, Wainner RS, Flynn TW. Primary care referral of patients with low back pain to physical therapy. *Spine (Phila PA 1976)*. 2012;37(25):2114-2121. doi:10.1097/BRS.0b013e31825d32f5.

180. Vibe Fersum K, O'Sullivan P, Skouen JS, Smith A, Kvale A. Efficacy of classification-based cognitive functional therapy in patients with non-specific chronic low back pain: A randomized controlled trial. *Eur J Pain*. 2013;17(6):916-928. doi:10.1002/j.1532-2149.2012.00252.x.

181. Hall A, Richmond H, Copsey B, et al. Physiotherapist-delivered cognitive-behavioural interventions are effective for low back pain, but can they be replicated in clinical practice? A systematic review. *Disabil Rehabil*. 2016:1-9. doi:10.1080/09638288.2016.1236155.

182. Beissner K, Henderson CR, Papaleontiou M, Olkhovskaya Y, Wigglesworth J, Reid MC. Physical therapists' use of cognitive-behavioral therapy for older adults with chronic pain: a nationwide survey. *Phys Ther*. 2009;89(5):456-469. doi:10.2522/ptj.20080163.

183. RMcHugh, VMcQuiddy. No Title. In: *"Use of Motivational Interviewing Techniques to Improve Self-Management in Physical Therapist Practice."* Charlotte, NC: PT in Motion. News@NEXT.

184. Nessen T, Opava CH, Martin C, Demmelmaier I. From clinical expert to guide: experiences from coaching people with rheumatoid arthritis to increased physical activity. *Phys Ther*. 2014;94(5):644-653. doi:10.2522/ptj.20130393.

185. Benini A, DeLeo JA. René Descartes' physiology of pain. *Spine (Phila PA 1976)*. 1999;24(20):2115. http://journals.lww.com/spinejournal/Citation/1999/10150/Ren__Descartes__Physiology_of_Pain.10.aspx. Accessed 17 April 2017.

186. Melzack R. From the gate to the neuromatrix. *Pain*. 1999;suppl 6(1):S121-S126. doi:10.1016/S0304-3959(99)00145-1.

187. Melzack R. Evolution of the neuromatrix theory of pain. The Prithvi Raj Lecture: presented at the third world Congress of World Institute of Pain, Barcelona 2004. *Pain Pract*. 2005;5:85-94. doi:10.1111/j.1533-2500.2005.05203.x.

188. Nahin RL. Estimates of pain prevalence and severity in adults: United States, 2012. *J Pain*. 2015;16(8):769-780. doi:10.1016/j.jpain.2015.05.002.

189. Nahin RL, Boineau R, Khalsa PS, Stussman BJ, Weber WJ. Evidence-based evaluation of complementary health approaches for pain management in the United States. *Mayo Clin Proc*. 2016;91(9):1292-1306. doi:10.1016/j.mayocp.2016.06.007.

190. Peppin JF, Cheatle MD, Kirsh KL, McCarberg BH. The complexity model: a novel approach to improve chronic pain care. *Pain Med*. 2015;16(4):653-666. doi:10.1111/pme.12621.

191. Jones M, Edwards I, Gifford L. Conceptual models for implementing biopsychosocial theory in clinical practice. *Man Ther*. 2002;7(1):2-9. doi:10.1054/math.2001.0426.

192. Blickenstaff C, Pearson N. Reconciling movement and exercise with pain neuroscience education: a case for consistent education. *Physiother Theory Pract*. 2016;32(5). doi:10.1080/09593985.2016.1194653.

24

OSTEOPATHIC MANIPULATIVE MEDICINE

Anthony Digirolamo, DO, Joshua Minori, DO and Karen Snider, DO

FAST FACTS

- Osteopathic manipulative medicine (OMM) can be used to treat a variety of painful conditions.
- The goal of OMM is to identify somatic dysfunction and reduce or remove the dysfunction.
- Osteopathic manipulative treatments improve pain by normalizing biomechanical function, removing structural impediments to vascular and lymphatic drainage, restoring nervous system tone, and decreasing the energetic demand on the body.

OSTEOPATHIC MANIPULATIVE MEDICINE IN THE TREATMENT OF ACUTE AND CHRONIC PAIN

History and Philosophy

Osteopathic manipulative medicine (OMM) is the use of hands-on structural diagnosis and osteopathic manipulative treatment (OMT). OMM is a therapeutic modality used by the osteopathic medical profession as part of a holistic approach to patient care governed by osteopathic principles and practice (OPP). Osteopathy was founded in the 19th century by Andrew Taylor Still, MD, DO, an American frontier physician who partially rejected the existing framework of medical practice that included toxic medicinal substances and questionable surgeries.[1] Still believed that the body had the inherent ability to heal itself, but this ability was adversely affected by abnormal musculoskeletal mechanics affecting nerve, vascular, and lymphatic functioning.[2] The effect of the musculoskeletal system on the natural healing potential of the body formed the basis of his philosophy.[2] Dr. Still applied the term "osteopathy" to this new medical philosophy to highlight how clinical pathology throughout the body was reflected within the skeletal system. The modern osteopathic medical profession is not a system that solely relies on a musculoskeletal-oriented diagnosis and treatment; it is a scientifically comprehensive school of medicine that embraces a holistic philosophy. This philosophy recognizes the whole person, the body's homeostatic mechanics, and its structure-function relationships. Osteopathic treatment focuses on health-oriented principles utilizing the full scope of treatment options including pharmaceuticals, surgery, lifestyle interventions, and OMM.[3]

OPP is summarized in the following 4 tenets[3]:

1. *The human being is a dynamic unit of function integrating mind, body, and spirit.*
2. *The body possesses self-regulatory mechanisms that are self-healing in nature.*
3. *Structure and function are reciprocally interrelated at all levels.*
4. *Rational treatment is based on these principles.*

Multidisciplinary pain programs are recognizing that many hands-on approaches to patient care and associated modalities, such as OMM, chiropractic manipulation, and massage, may provide solutions to treating persistent pain conditions.[4] The use of OMT by a practitioner trained in OMM has been viewed by many patients as highly effective.[5-8] Studies have shown OMM to be a safe method of reducing pain, increasing mobility, and ultimately improving function.[6-13]

Current Practice of Osteopathic Manipulative Medicine

OMM is taught at all colleges of osteopathic medicine within the United States. Licensure examinations taken by graduating doctors of osteopathic medicine (DO) ensure that all DOs are competent to practice OMM. Many residency programs will continue to provide OMM training and one specialty, osteopathic neuromusculoskeletal medicine (ONMM), focuses on OMM as the primary treatment modality within the specialty.

Many osteopathic physicians specializing in primary care provide OMM to their patients. Specialists who focus on the musculoskeletal system, such as physical medicine and rehabilitation (PM&R), sports medicine, and orthopedic surgery, may also provide OMM to their patients.

Osteopathic Models of Care

The osteopathic approach to patient care recognizes the multitude of interdependent functions within the body. The Educational Council on Osteopathic Principles (ECOP) of the American Association of Colleges of Osteopathic Medicine defined 5 diagnosis and treatment models that, when applied to patient care, guide a physician to consider these interdependent functions. The 5 osteopathic diagnosis and treatment models are the biomechanical, respiratory-circulatory, neurologic, metabolic-energy, and behavioral models.[3] These 5 models each focus on homeostatic mechanisms that affect the adaptability of the body to environmental stressors and can all be affected by or predispose a patient to persistent pain symptoms. The biomechanical model stresses optimization of structure-function relationships within the musculoskeletal system. The respiratory-circulatory model stresses optimization of respiratory mechanics and vascular and lymphatic drainage. The neurologic model stresses normalization of somatic and autonomic nervous tone. The metabolic-energetic model focuses on minimizing energetic demands on the body and optimizing metabolic and physiologic processes. The behavioral model focuses on the improving health through the effect of the mind and spirit on the body.[3,14] By applying these models to each patient, the physician considers a variety of avenues for diagnosis and management of conditions causing both acute and chronic pain.[3]

Treatment of the musculoskeletal system with OMM can play a role in each of the 5 osteopathic diagnosis and treatment models. The musculoskeletal system has a rich afferent input into the central nervous system and, through its effect on vascular and lymphatic drainage, has a multitude of mechanisms to interact with other organ systems. The interaction of the musculoskeletal, immune, neurologic, and endocrine (MINE) "supersystem" creates a collective network that can be dysregulated by nociception and attribute to chronic persistent pain.[14] The behavioral model recognizes the effect of persistent pain on the mind-body-spirit connection and its impact on quality of life. Similar to the biopsychosocial models that are incorporated into the multidisciplinary pain approach, the 5-model approach focuses on physical, mental, emotional, and spiritual functions often affected by chronic persistent pain. Therefore, it is reasonable to assume that structural and functional disturbances placed on the musculoskeletal system will have consequences on homeostatic processes throughout the body. The 5-model approach to diagnosis and treatment focuses on restoring health by influencing repair and recovery from illness, sickness, and disease via multiple mechanisms.[3]

PHYSIOLOGY OF OSTEOPATHIC MANIPULATIVE MEDICINE

Nociceptive Neuromuscular Reflexes

OMM reduces pain through several physiologic mechanisms. One such mechanism is known as the nociceptive neuromuscular reflex. During an injury to a muscle or tendon, muscle spindles composed of afferent sensory and gamma efferent nerves are rapidly stretched. Nociception afferents communicate with alpha motor neurons via excitatory interneurons within the spinal cord to cause a reflexive muscle contraction to avoid further injury. The reflexive contraction may cause localized muscle spasm, creating more nociception and additional spasm.[15,16] This cycle, known as the pain-spasm-pain cycle can persist leading to lowered firing thresholds of the neurons at the level of the dorsal horn of the spinal cord. This phenomenon known as sensitization or segmental facilitation can affect the somatic and visceral structures innervated from the sensitized area of the spinal cord. OMM is thought to disrupt these nociceptive neuromuscular reflexes by decreasing nociceptive input, thus reducing activation of the gamma motor neuron, which lessens the sensitivity of muscle spindles to stretch.

Somatic Dysfunction

Somatic dysfunction is defined as the impaired or altered function of interconnected components of the somatic system, including skeletal, arthrodial, and myofascial structures and related vascular, lymphatic, and neural elements.[17] Somatic dysfunction is diagnosed by the presence of one or more physical findings: excessive sensitivity (S) or tenderness (T), asymmetry (A), restrictive motion (R), and tissue texture abnormalities (T).[17] Collectively known as STAR or TART findings, the individual findings provide clues to the underlying mechanisms of a patient's injury and pathophysiologic status.[14] Collectively, somatic dysfunction findings reflect the peripheral and central physiological mechanisms that underlie the condition disrupting a patient's health and function.[18]

The presence of somatic dysfunction is the clinical indication for performing OMT.[19] The goal of OMT is to improve physiologic function and restore homeostatic mechanisms that have been altered by the somatic dysfunction.[17] OMT encompasses a variety of hands-on techniques, but the choice of techniques is based on the specific TART findings found on physical examination. Through palpation, the physician localizes the techniques to the somatic dysfunctions, monitors tissue texture changes during the treatment, and determines the effectiveness by assessing the tissue response.[20] OMT effects pain generators by reducing or removing somatic dysfunction and by modulating central and peripheral mechanisms responsible for producing or maintaining pain.

Pain Generators

Pain generators are commonly defined as the nociceptive sources of pain.[21] They are found by correlating anatomic location, quality, and referral distribution of the pain with well-studied dermatomal, sclerotomal, and myotomal pain maps.[1,22] The different pain generator types and associated structures have unique characteristics that can direct the physician into making an appropriate diagnosis and formulating a custom treatment plan. It is up to the physician to determine if the cause of pain is coming from a given structure and/or identified somatic dysfunction.

Dermatomal pain is pain that follows along the sensory distribution of a spinal nerve root. The character of the pain may vary depending on the cause. For example, herpetic neuralgia is often described as burning, whereas compression of the dorsal sensory root may cause a lightning or electric type of sensation. Sclerotomal tissues such as skeletal, arthrodial, and ligamentous structures produce pain that is often described as "deep and dull," and the pain patterns are usually located distal to the actual pain generators. Myotomal pain is often described as "cramping or stiffness," can be associated with certain movements, and may include active or latent myofascial

trigger points (MTrPs). Like sclerotomal pain, myotomal pain symptoms are usually located at a distance away from the pain generator and have predictable referral patterns.

Segmental facilitation within the dorsal horn of the spinal cord can contribute to pain referral through sensitization of nociceptive neurons of the affected tissues as well as neurons in adjacent areas of the spinal cord.[1] This central nervous system sensitization can lead to pain referral patterns into body areas that are not directly related to the origin of disease or insult as is seen with a myocardial infarction radiating pain into the left arm.[23]

Applying the 5 Models of Care

The 5 osteopathic diagnosis and treatment models help the osteopathic physician develop an appropriate plan for applying OMT and setting individualized treatment goals. Incorporating a mixture of these models into the plan of care allows the physician to view the patient holistically. Diagnosis and treatment of the musculoskeletal system with OMM can play a role in each of the 5 models. The osteopathic physician can use OMT to correct the somatic dysfunction in order to normalize biomechanical function, remove structural impediments to vascular and lymphatic drainage, normalize nervous system tone, decrease the energetic demand on the body, and improve pain.[20] Table 24-1 reviews the 5 models as they pertain to assessment and treatment.

COMMON CONDITIONS/DIAGNOSES TREATED WITH OMM AND ASSOCIATED EXAM FINDINGS IN PATIENTS WITH CHRONIC PAIN

Common Treatable Conditions/Diagnoses Causing Chronic Pain

Osteopathic manipulation has been utilized with success for a wide variety of pain conditions.[24] Pain conditions that are commonly treated with OMM are summarized in Table 24-2. In the primary care setting, OMT is most commonly used to treat pain in the low back and head.[25] Specific conditions include degenerative disk and joint disease (spondylosis), piriformis syndrome, sacroiliac joint pain, coccydynia, psoas syndrome, short leg syndrome, cervicogenic headache (CGH), occipital neuralgia, migraine, and tension-type headache.[26,27] Low back pain (LBP), CGH, and postural strain/sprain tend to have the highest occurrence rate with increased tendency for disability due to persistent pain and the strongest evidence for the successful application of diagnosis and treatment using OMM.[1,28-30]

Associated Exam Findings of Common Conditions/Diagnoses

A musculoskeletal examination that includes an assessment for TART/STAR findings is required for OMM.

TABLE 24-1 Five Osteopathic Models of Patient Care

MODEL	ANATOMICAL FOCUS	HOMEOSTATIC AND PHYSIOLOGICAL FUNCTIONS
Biomechanical	Skeletal muscle; connective tissue and ligaments; joints of the spine, extremities, and head	Postural balance, muscular function, connective tissue compliance, articular motion
Respiratory-circulatory	Thoracic cage; transitional areas between body cavities-thoracic inlet, abdominal diaphragm, pelvic diaphragms, and tentorium cerebelli	Mechanical respiratory motion; vascular and lymphatic flow; pulmonary and cardiovascular function
Neurologic	Central nervous system, peripheral nervous system including the sensory, somatic, and autonomic nervous systems	Regulation of visceral function; transmission of sensory input and motor control; proprioception; coordination of function between organ systems
Metabolic-energetic	Internal viscera, exocrine and endocrine glands	Biochemical and physiologic processes; energy demand and consumption; immunological and endocrinological regulatory processes; inflammation and repair; digestion and nutrition; waste removal and excretion; reproductive processes
Behavioral	Mentation, emotions, spirituality	Cognition and memory; psychological status including emotions, mood, motivations, and behaviors; lifestyle activities; spiritual beliefs

TABLE 24-2 Pain Conditions Commonly Treated With Osteopathic Manipulative Medicine Based on Anatomic Region

ANATOMIC REGION	CONDITION/DIAGNOSIS
Head	Headache Sinusitis Temporal mandibular joint dysfunction
Cervical region	Neck pain Cervical strain
Upper extremities	Carpal tunnel syndrome Shoulder pain Elbow pain
Thoracic spine and ribs	Thoracic strain Postural strain Postthoracotomy pain Thoracic outlet syndrome
Lumbar spine and abdomen	Back pain Lumbar strain Pancreatitis
Sacrum and pelvis	Sacroiliac pain Pelvic pain Sciatica
Lower extremities	Short-leg syndrome Knee pain Ankle pain Foot pain

TART/STAR findings can provide information for identifying the source of the pain generator. Conditions causing persistent pain may result in compensatory mechanisms, muscle spasms, and MTrPs. MTrPs are discrete, hypersensitive points in a muscle or fascia that can be felt as a nodule or band, and are associated with a localized twitch response and predicable pain referral elicited upon stimulation.[31,32] MTrPs are often associated with LBP, headaches, carpal tunnel syndrome, temporomandibular joint dysfunction, and pain perceived as angina.[33-35] A few examples of pain conditions with associated exam findings are described in the following sections.

Low Back Pain

Pain generators associated with LBP include the articular structures such as the lumbar facet and sacroiliac joints and soft-tissue structures such as muscle, fascia, and ligaments. Studies have shown that people with LBP have been found to have higher level of severity of somatic dysfunction in articular and soft-tissue structures than people without LBP.[28,36] Structures that can contribute to LBP include the thoracolumbar fascia; pelvic diaphragm; quadratus lumborum, hamstrings, and iliopsoas muscles; and the iliolumbar, interspinous, and sacrotuberous ligaments.[18,27]

A study assessing patients with chronic LBP found 6 common somatic dysfunction patterns in the lumbar spine, pelvis, and lower extremities. These common somatic dysfunction patterns included (1) shears at the pubic symphysis characterized by tenderness and a palpable step off between the right and left pubic rami; (2) shears at one of the sacroiliac joints characterized by significant asymmetry between the right and left anterior iliac spines, posterior iliac spines, and ischial tuberosities; (3) restricted sacral motion characterized by lack of permissible anterior motion at either the right or left sacral base; (4) presence of short leg; (5) postural muscle imbalance characterized by excessive tension in the thoracolumbar extensors and hip flexors, weakness in the abdominal and gluteal muscles, and excessive anterior pelvic tilt; and (6) individual lumbar vertebral segments caught in a flexed or extended position.[37] These 6 somatic dysfunction patterns were termed the "dirty half-dozen" with 55% of the studied patients exhibiting 3 or more of these 6 common somatic dysfunction patterns and only 2.7% failing to demonstrate any of the 6 patterns. After OMT, 75% of the dysfunctional group returned to work and/or activities of daily living. The outcome seen in this study was consistent with other studies that have found significant improvement with OMT in chronic LBP symptoms and related disability.[6,7,10,12,38,39]

The American Osteopathic Association (AOA) published guidelines for the utilization of OMM for the treatment of LBP.[40,41] These guidelines were based on a systematic literature review performed by the Task Force on the Low Back Pain Clinical Practice Guidelines. The Task Force concluded that there was a moderate quality of evidence suggesting significant relief of nonspecific acute and chronic LBP and improvements in function with OMT. These guidelines recommend that when somatic dysfunction is a contributing factor or cause of LBP, OMT is an indicated treatment.[40,41] Additionally, Prinsen et al found that OMT was associated with lowered utilization of analgesic pain medication and a reduction of days off work in patients with LBP.[42]

Cervicogenic Headaches and Associated Neck Pain

By definition, CGHs are headaches that are associated with dysfunction in the cervical region.[43] Pain is usually elicited by pressure on the cervical muscles or by neck movement. Asymmetry of musculoskeletal structures of the head and neck may be present. Active or passive neck motion restriction of the upper 3 cervical joints is a common finding, especially at the atlantoaxial (C1-2) joint.[44] Palpation of the neck, upper thoracic, or shoulder muscles may reveal tenderness, hypertonicity, or MTrPs that may refer pain to the ipsilateral head region. Neck pain and headaches may also arise from the intersegmental sympathetic innervation via the vertebral and sinuvertebral nerves and the trigeminovascular system arising from various levels encompassing C2-C7.[45] OMM as well as other manual medicine techniques directed to the head, cervical, upper thoracic, and shoulder articular and muscular dysfunctions have been shown to be beneficial for CGHs.[46-49] Somatic dysfunction at distant sites including the lumbar spine and pelvis has also been shown to contribute to CGH.[1,26]

Patterns Associated With Certain Pain Syndromes

Predictable pain referral patterns are associated with nociception and irritation to different tissue types. Facet joint pain has been shown to refer to the head or upper extremity, chest wall, and lower extremities depending on the spinal level.[50,51] Please refer to the *Neck and Back Pain chapters* of this text for information regarding the referral patterns of facet joint–mediated pain.

Postural stress and associated strains/sprains can often result in sclerotomal or myotomal pain. Figures 24-1 and 24-2 represent the referral distribution of specific structural pain generators. A failure to address excessive functional demands (ergonomics at work or play), patterns of postural imbalances, and other perpetuating factors may decrease the effectiveness of pain management interventions aimed at peripheral pain generators or increase the likelihood of recurrence following these interventions.

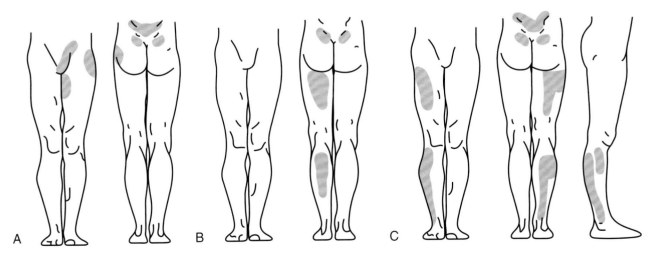

FIGURE 24-1 Sclerotomal pain referral regions from Ligaments: (A) iliolumbar ligament, (B) sacrospinous and sacrotuberous ligaments, (C) posterior sacroiliac ligaments. Redrawn from Kuchera ML. Applying osteopathic principles to formulate treatment for patients with chronic pain. *J Am Osteopath Assoc.* 2007;107(11):28-38.

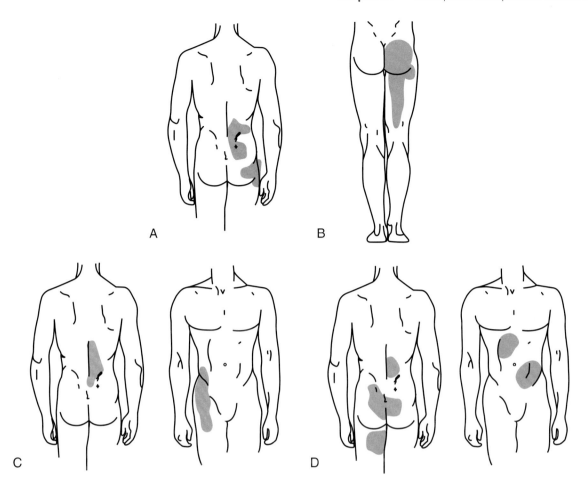

FIGURE 24-2 Myotomal pain referral regions from muscle trigger points: (A) quadratus lumborum, (B) piriformis, (C) iliopsoas, (D) rotatores and multifidi muscles. OMM, osteopathic manipulative medicine. Redrawn from Kuchera ML. Applying osteopathic principles to formulate treatment for patients with chronic pain. *J Am Osteopath Assoc.* 2007;107(11):28-38.

OSTEOPATHIC MANIPULATIVE TREATMENT

Indications and Contraindications

OMT is indicated for the treatment of pain conditions secondary to or in association with somatic dysfunction. These conditions may include but are not limited to back pain, joint pain from musculoskeletal injury or rheumatologic disease, musculoskeletal pain associated with pregnancy,[52,53] neck pain,[54] abdominal and pelvic pain,[55] headaches,[26,56] and cancer related pain. There are no general contraindications to OMT for chronic pain conditions; however, there are several absolute and relative contraindications to using specific techniques with certain diagnoses (see common treatment techniques). Following is an example of an initial visit note to an OMM provider:

Chief Complaint: Chronic Low Back Pain

History of present illness (HPI): Mr. Smith is a 54-year-old right hand–dominant man referred for evaluation and treatment of acute exacerbation of chronic low back pain. He states that symptoms started insidiously 7 years ago. His pain is characterized as a dull ache in a bandlike distribution across the low back. Occasionally, pain will radiate down his left buttock and posterior thigh. He occasionally has numbness and tingling in his lateral thigh, but rarely distal to the knee. His pain is typically 3-5/10 intensity and usually worse by the end of the day. He does have morning stiffness in his back, which usually improves after 15 to 20 minutes of activity. He has had multiple acute exacerbations over the years and had been to physical therapy several times which on occasion, caused worsening of symptoms. A few days ago, he was helping a friend move and lifted several heavy boxes. The next day, his pain worsened and is presently 8/10 in intensity localized to the low back with radiation into the left buttock. He denies saddle anesthesia, recent changes in bowel/bladder function, worsening of pain at night or systemic symptoms of fever, chills, night sweats, or weight loss. Exacerbating factors include extension and standing and sitting for longer than 15 minutes. Flexion is initially painful but provides temporary relief after a few seconds. He has been taking 600 mg of ibuprofen 3 times a day with minimal relief.

Review of systems: Significant for feeling depressed secondary to pain, otherwise negative unless mentioned in the HPI.

Diagnostics: He had an MRI of the lumbar spine 7 years ago, which revealed L5-S1 disk disease with left-sided foraminal narrowing but no nerve root involvement. An EMG 1 year ago revealed no signs of lumbar radiculopathy or peripheral neuropathy.

Past medical and surgical history: GERD, IBS, degenerative disk disease.

Social history: He is divorced and has 3 grown children. He denies a history of tobacco or illicit drug use. He drinks a few beers or glasses of wine nightly. He is employed as computer technician and has missed several weeks of work this year because of back pain.

Family history: Mother with depression. Father with alcohol abuse. No family history of neuromuscular or rheumatologic disease.

Medications: omeprazole, ibuprofen prn.

Physical exam:

General: He is well dressed and well groomed, appears uncomfortable.

HEENT: Head is NC/AT, mucous membranes moist.

Psych: somewhat anxious, affect flat.

Respiratory: breathing comfortably with no accessory muscle use.

Cardiovascular: extremities are warm with symmetric radial, dorsalis pedis, and posterior tibial pulses.

Musculoskeletal: Stands with flexed forward posture at waist, shoulder protracted with forward head carriage. Lumbar spine range of motion reduced in all directions. Hip range of motion within normal limits IR, ER but reduced in extension with positive Thomas test. Flexion, abduction, external rotation (FABER) test positive on left. Gaenslen and sacroiliac thrust tests positive on left.

Neurologic: Strength is 5/5 in the bilateral lower extremities; patellar and Achilles deep tendon reflexes are 2+/4 and bilaterally symmetric; light touch in dermatomes L1-S2 are intact and symmetric bilaterally. Straight leg test negative bilateral. Tenderness to palpation along lumbar paraspinal muscles and left sacroiliac joint. Restricted active range of motion in lumbar flexion to 40 degrees and extension to 5 degrees. L5 extended, rotated left and sidebent left; sacrum demonstrates a left, right-on-left sacral torsion. Pelvis demonstrates a left posteriorly rotated innominate.

Assessment: 54-year-old man with acute exacerbation of chronic low back pain with somatic dysfunction of the lumbar, sacral, and pelvic regions. Symptoms are most consistent with facet-mediated pain in setting with muscle spasm perpetuated by a maladaptive postural compensation pattern. In addition, other factors likely contributing to lack of success with previous interventions include depression and overall work dissatisfaction.

Plan:

1. Low back pain with somatic dysfunction secondary to degenerative disk and joint disease and poor postural compensation. Will follow up in 1 week for reevaluation. Home exercises given include titrated increase in activity level with walking, gentle range of motion, and breathing/relaxation technique.

2. Chronic pain with depressive symptoms: He reports many years of depressive symptoms. PHQ-9 depression scale obtained with score of 12 indicating moderate symptoms. Recommend referral to pain psychology with consideration of cognitive behavioral therapy and/or mindfulness-based therapy. Consider initiation of pharmacotherapy (may consider SNRI).

Treatment provided: OMT was recommend based on the physical findings on today's examination. Verbal consent obtained for trial of OMT. OMT performed to the lumbar, sacral, and pelvic regions using myofascial release, counterstrain and muscle energy to all regions, and balanced ligamentous tension and cranial technique to the sacrum. Patient tolerated treatment well and reported a 75% reduction in symptoms post treatment. Post OMT evaluation revealed increase in lumbar and pelvic range of motion with a reduction in tenderness to the involved soft-tissue structures.

The Osteopathic Referral: When to Refer

A referring provider should consider including OMT as part of a chronic pain treatment plan when TART/STAR findings of somatic dysfunction are found on physical examination. If the provider has not been trained in OMT, then referral to a trained OMM provider is appropriate. Timing of referral is dependent upon various factors. A provider may wish to refer for OMM sooner in a patient who reports responding well to manual therapies in the past or when a patient has poor tolerance to medications or is at risk of medication abuse. OMT is also a good treatment option if the patient previously had limited success with active modalities such as physical therapy. OMT may also be considered prior to therapeutic injections, but may also be of benefit when there has been limited success with interventional procedures (i.e., peripheral joint and/or epidural steroid injections). Additionally, OMT is a good option for adjunctive pain management in the acute postoperative period, or after soft-tissue healing has occurred to address myofascial adhesions that may be generating pain. When a referral is placed, the OMM provider should be informed of the current working diagnosis and prior workup including imaging and treatments already performed. An algorithm for consideration of OMT for common pain conditions is shown in Figure 24-3. An example of a typical referral for OMM is shown in Figure 24-4.

Who to Refer to

Depending on the geographic region, finding an OMM provider is sometimes challenging. There are several resources that may be of benefit to the referring provider. One resource is through the American Osteopathic Association (AOA) website www.osteopathic.org. Through this website, a physician can search by region and locate an osteopathic physician who specializes in ONMM. If no providers are mentioned for ONMM, a referring physician may also try contacting other specialists listed; although OMM may not be the primary focus of their specialty, it may be a significant part of their practice. Commonly, osteopathic family physicians provide OMM to patients. As mentioned earlier, other specialists such as osteopathic physiatrists (physical medicine and rehabilitation) and osteopathic sports medicine providers frequently treat with OMM. Other resources to

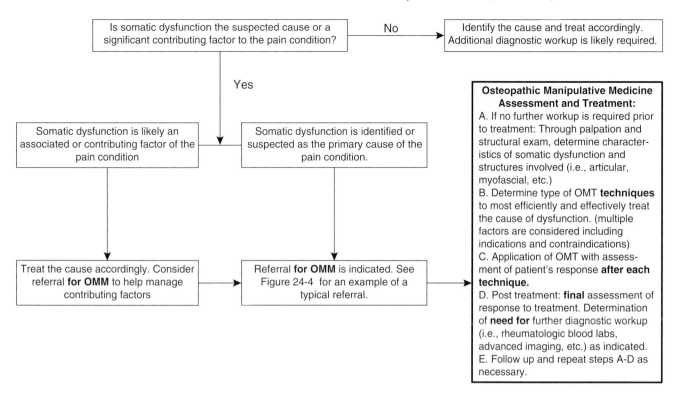

FIGURE 24-3 Algorithm for consideration of osteopathic manipulative treatment for common pain conditions.
Adapted from Nelson KE. The manipulative prescription. In: Nelson KE, Glonek T, eds. *Somatic Dysfunction in Osteopathic Family Medicine*. Baltimore, MD: Lippincott Williams & Wilkins; 2007:27-32.

Diagnosis: 1. Mechanical low back pain 2. Somatic dysfunction of the lumbar spine
Referral to: Osteopathic Manipulative Medicine Provider
Referral for: Osteopathic manipulative medicine. 54-year-old man with acute exacerbation of chronic low back pain. Physical exam reveals somatic dysfunction consisting of sensitivity to palpation, tissue texture changes and restrictive motion. MRI reveals degenerative changes in the lumbar spine without nerve root impingement.
Precautions: none
Referring physician recheck date: 3 mo

FIGURE 24-4 Example of typical referral for osteopathic manipulative treatment.

find OMM providers include the American Academy of Osteopathy (AAO) website at academyofosteopathy.org and the Osteopathic Cranial Academy website at cranialacademy.org.

The first appointment to an OMM provider is similar to that of other specialties. The physician will take a thorough history including review of prior diagnostic workup, imaging, treatments, medications in addition to review of past medical and surgical history. As discussed in earlier sections, a detailed social history is also obtained, which helps to identify any biopsychosocial impacts on the patient's health. A thorough neurologic and musculoskeletal exam is performed that includes assessment for STAR/TART findings. The goal of the exam is to identify somatic dysfunction within local structures that may be causing pain directly and to identify distant abnormalities that may be contributing factors

and/or compensation patterns leading to and maintaining somatic dysfunction and pain.

Goals of Treatment

The primary indication for OMT is the presence of somatic dysfunction found on physical examination. If somatic dysfunction is identified and there are no contraindications to treatment or further workup required, the osteopathic physician may proceed with OMT. The goal of OMM is to identify somatic dysfunction and then, to reduce or remove the dysfunction. In the context of chronic pain, the goal is also to modulate central and peripheral mechanisms generating pain. The osteopathic physician does this by utilizing a variety of approaches as further discussed in the following section common treatment techniques. OMT techniques vary greatly in the amount of force applied and thus the osteopathic physician has many tools that may benefit a variety of patient conditions and tolerance to manipulation. For example, a patient with articular somatic dysfunction who tolerates and responds well to more forceful techniques may benefit from high-velocity/low-amplitude (HVLA) technique, direct myofascial release, or muscle energy technique. A patient with chronic pain, who has severe allodynia, is unlikely to tolerate the aforementioned techniques and may respond better to counterstrain technique, balanced ligamentous tension techniques, or osteopathic cranial manipulative medicine techniques, which tend to use less force.

Patients suffering with chronic pain conditions often have central nervous system sensitization that results in autonomic dysregulation. Pain often ignites the sympathetic nervous system with a fight or flight response. Alterations in parasympathetic tone can also occur in the setting of pain. Autonomic dysfunction in response to pain is often witnessed in common comorbidities such as irritable bowel syndrome or as a cause of the pain condition itself, as is the case with chronic regional pain syndrome (i.e., regional sympathetic dystrophy).[14] For this reason, treatment often incorporates the 5 models of care. In the case of chronic LBP, a biomechanical model may address associated muscle imbalances or joint restriction. Associated gastrointestinal symptoms may be addressed through a neurologic model in which somatovisceral reflexes via sympathetic and parasympathetic nervous system are treated. A respiratory/circulatory model aims to improve blood supply and nutrition to the area being treated and may also relieve associated symptoms (such as gastrointestinal upset) by enhancing surrounding lymph drainage and venous return.[14] Touch alone is a powerful tool and has been shown to benefit patients suffering with pain, anxiety, and depression and is taken into consideration through the psychobehavioral model of osteopathic care. A metabolic-energetic model may be utilized to balance associated somatic dysfunction in the sacrum, affecting the central and autonomic nervous systems through the cranial rhythmic impulse.[57]

OMM aims to decrease peripheral nociception and central facilitation through hands-on treatment of somatic dysfunction.[58] The goal of treatment is to not only decrease biomechanical and biochemical stressors but also to improve a patient's homeostatic mechanisms and ultimately improve a patient's quality of life.[1] The comprehensive treatment plan, especially with chronic pain, must be personalized and may include pharmacotherapy and nonpharmacologic interventions such as exercise, biofeedback, cognitive behavioral therapy, and mindfulness based practices in addition to the application of osteopathic principles with OMT.[58]

Common Treatment Techniques

There are numerous types of OMT techniques that may be utilized during a treatment with OMM. The treating physician will decide which type of technique is appropriate based upon the condition being treated, the chronicity of the condition, the patient's age, the physical findings, and any contraindications. Other factors considered when deciding on techniques include risk/benefit ratio, ability of the patient to tolerate or cooperate with a technique, and the patient's response to previous treatment. General information and descriptions of techniques may be obtained through the Glossary of Osteopathic Terminology by the American Association of Colleges of Osteopathic Medicine (AACOM) at www.aacom.org. A brief description of commonly utilized techniques with indications and contraindications is listed below.

1. **Balanced ligamentous tension (BLT):** is a technique based on the principle that joints are balanced ligamentous articular mechanisms. Ligaments provide proprioceptive information that affects surrounding myofascial structures and tensions around the joint. To perform a BLT technique the joint treated is slowly brought into a position of ease where all directions of tension are in balance. This position of ease causes the surrounding dysfunctional tissues to reset, which may be experienced as a palpable relaxation response. Successful treatment should result in an increase in pain free range of motion of the dysfunctional structures.[59]

   Indications: muscular hypertonicity; myofascial tension or scarring; restricted joint motion; venous and lymphatic congestion.[59]

   Contraindications (relative): malignancy; local infection; severe osteoporosis; fracture, dislocation, or gross joint instability.[59]

2. **Counterstrain:** is a system of diagnosis and technique that uses specific body positioning to treat somatic dysfunction identified in the form of a myofascial tender point. The tender point is thought to be secondary injury resulting from altered muscle spindle and proprioceptive activity. The treatment position shortens the tissues containing the tender point until the tenderness is reduced by a least 70%, then the position is maintained for 90 seconds. After treatment the local tenderness should be significantly reduced. In general, counterstrain is well tolerated in most pain conditions.[60]

   Indications: localized, discrete tenderness typically associated with muscular hypertonicity, myofascial tension, restricted joint motion, or associated viscerosomatic reflexes.[60]

   Contraindications: acute trauma in which positioning may further damage the affected tissues; severe illness in which positioning is not possible; instability of the area treated with potential to injure neurovascular structures by positioning; inability of the patient to relax during treatment.[60]

3. **High-velocity, low-amplitude (HVLA):** is a technique in which a rapid thrust is applied over a short distance at a dysfunctional joint's restrictive barrier to improve articular motion. HVLA often results in an articular cavitation or "popping" sound.[61] The mechanism of action is believed to be restoration of normal articular mechanics along with a reflex relaxation of the surrounding muscles.[61]

Indications: restricted joint motion.[62]

Contraindications: acute sprain or strain; osteoporosis; severe osteoarthritis, spondylosis, ankylosis, or rheumatologic disease; hypermobile joint; local infection; joint replacement; congenital anomalies.[62]
Cervical spine HVLA contraindications include vertebrobasilar insufficiency, skeletal dysplasias such achondroplastic dwarfism, cervical joint or ligament instability such as that which may occur in Down syndrome and rheumatoid arthritis.[62]

4. **Myofascial release (MFR):** is a system of diagnosis and treatment that can range from gentle to forceful pressure application to the myofascial system. Myofascial release is aimed at releasing maladaptive patterns of soft tissue (muscle, fascia, tendon, and ligament) and associated joint restriction. Myofascial release techniques are performed by guiding the tissues to either the restrictive barrier (direct MFR) or along the path of least resistance (indirect MFR) until tissue motion is improved.[63,64]

Indications: muscular hypertonicity; myofascial tension or scarring; restricted joint motion; venous and lymphatic congestion.[64]

Contraindications (relative): acute sprain or strain; malignancy; local infection; severe osteoporosis; fracture, dislocation, or gross joint instability.[64]

5. **Muscle energy technique (MET):** is a technique in which the patient is placed in a precise position, then actively contracts muscles in a specific direction, against physician counterforce to correct somatic dysfunction. Types of MET include postisometric relaxation, joint mobilization, respiratory assistance, oculocephalogyric reflex, reciprocal inhibition, and crossed extensor reflex. MET utilizes the brief reflex relaxation period that occurs in both agonist and antagonist muscles after a muscle contraction. During the period of reflexive relaxation, the dysfunctional joint or muscle is repositioned repeatedly until normal motion is obtained. Amount of force used in the technique will vary depending on the type of MET, therefore indications and contraindications vary depending on which form of muscle energy is utilized.[65]

Indications: muscular hypertonicity, myofascial tension, restricted joint motion.[65]

Contraindications (relative): acute sprain or strain, severe osteoporosis, severe illness. (Absolute): fracture, dislocation, or gross instability.[65]

6. **Cranial osteopathic manipulative medicine (COMM):** (also known as osteopathy in the cranial field and craniosacral therapy) is a system of diagnosis and treatment using a variety of techniques to affect the primary respiratory mechanism. The primary respiratory mechanism is a term used to describe the interrelatedness of cellular processes and the interconnected movement of the tissues throughout the body. COMM is generally applied with very light touch and is typically well tolerated.[66]

Indications: headaches, whiplash, sinusitis, trigeminal neuralgia, TMJ dysfunction, vertigo, tinnitus, otitis media.[66]

Contraindications: increased intracranial pressure, status epilepticus, intracranial bleed, undiagnosed intracranial mass, acute skull fracture.[66]

Treatment Plan and Follow up

The OMT plan varies depending upon chronicity, severity, and response to treatment. Andrew Taylor Still, the founder of osteopathy, frequently stated "find it, fix it, and leave it alone." This statement refers to the osteopathic tenet that the "body is self-regulating and self-healing." When somatic dysfunction is identified and treated appropriately, it enhances the patient's ability to self-heal. During a single visit, OMT may be limited to a single technique to correct an isolated somatic dysfunction, or may include a wide variety of techniques to address somatic dysfunctions found throughout the body. Treatments may last a few minutes to an hour or more.[57] Frequency of treatments is dependent upon the number and severity of physical findings and their response to the initial treatment plan. For example, treatment of an acute lumbar strain may require a reevaluation within a few days of the initial treatment, while treatment for a recurrent or chronic condition may only require reevaluation every several months. Depending on the condition, an individual treatment may result in long-term relief, or short-term relief with need for regular follow-up. Chronic pain conditions may require reevaluations ranging from twice a month, to once or twice a year. The referring provider should discuss the cost-benefit ratio with the patient if long-term follow-up is recommended.[57]

DIFFERENCE AND SIMILARITIES BETWEEN OSTEOPATHIC MANIPULATIVE MEDICINE AND OTHER FORMS OF MANUAL MEDICINE TREATMENT

Osteopathic manipulation shares commonality with several other medical practices that utilize manual medicine. Chiropractic medicine began in the late 1800s and focused treatment around correcting vertebral "subluxations" that adversely affected nervous system function. Historically, chiropractic adjustments utilized spinal manipulation techniques similar to high-velocity, low-amplitude osteopathic techniques. Currently, doctors of chiropractic (DC) are taught and utilize a wide variety of techniques and lifestyle interventions in their treatment plans. Likewise, naturopathic manipulation or mechanotherapy is a form of manual medicine practiced by naturopathic doctors (ND), which utilizes techniques similar to osteopathic and chiropractic manipulation. Currently, many schools of physical therapy also teach a variety of manual medicine techniques including myofascial release, counterstrain, muscle energy technique, and soft-tissue techniques. Some states have expanded teaching and practice rights of doctors in physical therapy (DPT) to include spinal manipulation thrust techniques. A variety of manual therapy disciplines are also practiced throughout the United States with licensure status varying by state. A few of these therapists include massage therapists, craniosacral therapists, manual lymphatic drainage therapists, bodyworkers, and Rolfers®. Many of these therapists employ osteopathic-like techniques that focus on myofascial tissues.

Osteopathic physicians differ with the abovementioned practitioners in several ways. Osteopathic physicians are fully licensed in all 50 states. Their license is unrestricted, allowing them to provide comprehensive care for their patients including prescribing medications, performing surgery, performing and interpreting diagnostic testing, and performing office-based procedures such as trigger point and peripheral joint injections, in addition to OMM. This contrasts with the abovementioned manual practitioners who are generally limited to manual techniques. Chiropractic physicians have a limited licensed in all 50 states. Their scope of practice typically includes manual medicine and radiologic interpretation but may include gynecology and obstetrics depending on the state. In early 2017, NDs were licensed with a varying scope of practice in 17 of 50 states. Likewise, the scope practice of physical therapists varies by state, with some states requiring a physician's referral and oversight of the therapist's treatment plan.

The evidence base supports the efficacy of manual medicine techniques regardless of discipline. When referring for manual medicine treatments, the choice of provider should be based on several factors including the reputation of the individual provider, their location, and availability. Most medical insurance covers osteopathic and chiropractic manipulation, as well as physical therapy. However, coverage for naturopathic manipulation and massage therapy is less common. The financial burden of uncovered care must be considered when recommending a care plan to a patient. Irrespective of discipline, the philosophies of the various manual medicine disciplines discussed earlier share commonality of providing skilled care to the patient suffering from pain.

CONCLUSION

OMM is therapeutic modality used within the osteopathic medical profession as part of holistic patient care governed by the osteopathic principles. OMM specifically seeks to optimize structure-function relationships within the body using OMT to enhance the body's self-healing and self-regulatory mechanisms to improve a patient's function and all aspects of health including physical, mental, emotional, and spiritual well-being. In the presence of chronic pain, OMT works to reduce or remove identified somatic dysfunction to modulate central and peripheral mechanisms generating pain. OMM should be considered when developing a comprehensive care plan for chronic pain patients who demonstrate physical findings of somatic dysfunction that relate to their condition. OMM should be considered for patients suffering from back pain, joint pain from musculoskeletal

injury or rheumatologic disease, musculoskeletal pain associated with pregnancy, neck pain, abdominal and pelvic pain, postural strain, repetitive use injuries, and headaches. The goal of treatment is not only to decrease biomechanical and biochemical stressors but also to empower "patients to reduce the impact of persistent pain on quality of life."[1]

REFERENCES

1. Kuchera ML. Osteopathic considerations in neurology. In: Oken BS, ed. *Complementary Therapies in Neurology: An Evidence-Based Approach*. The Parthenon Publishing Group; 2004:59-112.

2. Gevitz NA. Degree of difference: the origins of osteopathy and first use of the "DO" designation. *J Am Osteopath Assoc*. 2014;114(1):30-40. doi:10.7556/jaoa.2014.005.

3. Seffinger MA, King HH, Ward RC, Jones JM III, Rogers FJ, Patterson MM. Osteopathic philosophy. In: Chila AG, et al. *Foundations of Osteopathic Medicine*. 3rd ed. Baltimore, MD: Lippincott Williams & Wilkins, A Wolters Kluwer Business; 2011:3-22.

4. Mann E. Managing pain. *BMJ*. 2003;326(7402):1320-1321.

5. Licciardone JC, Gamber R, Cardarelli K. Patient satisfaction and clinical outcomes associated with osteopathic manipulative treatment. *J Am Osteopath Assoc*. 2002;102(1):13-20.

6. Licciardone JC, Aryal S. Clinical response and relapse in patients with chronic low back pain following osteopathic manual treatment: results from the OSTEOPATHIC trial. *Man Ther*. 2014;19(6):541-548. doi:10.1016/j.math.2014.05.012.

7. Licciardone JC, Minotti DE, Gatchel RJ, Kearns CM, Singh KP. Osteopathic manual treatment and ultrasound therapy for chronic low back pain: a randomized controlled trial. *Ann Fam Med*. 2013;11(2):122-129. doi:10.1370/afm.1468.

8. Schwerla F, Kaiser AK, Gietz R, Kastner R. Osteopathic treatment of patients with long-term sequelae of whiplash injury: effect on neck pain disability and quality of life. *J Altern Complement Med*. 2013;19(6):543-549. doi:10.1089/acm.2012.0354.

9. Arienti C, Daccò S, Piccolo I, Redaelli T. Osteopathic manipulative treatment is effective on pain control associated to spinal cord injury. *Spinal Cord*. 2011;49(4):515-519. doi:10.1038/sc.2010.170.

10. Licciardone JC, Kearns CM, Crow WT. Changes in biomechanical dysfunction and low back pain reduction with osteopathic manual treatment: results from the OSTEOPATHIC trial. *Man Ther*. 2014;19(4):324-330. doi:10.1016/j.math.2014.03.004.

11. Schwerla F, Bischoff A, Nurnberger A, Genter P, Guillaume JP, Resch KL. Osteopathic treatment of patients with chronic non-specific neck pain: a randomised controlled trial of efficacy. *Forsch Komplementmed*. 2008;15(3):138-145. doi:10.1159/000132397.

12. Licciardone JC, Gatchel RJ, Aryal S. Recovery from chronic low back pain after osteopathic manipulative treatment: a randomized controlled trial. *J Am Osteopath Assoc*. 2016;116(3):144. doi:10.7556/jaoa.2016.031.

13. Andersson GB, Lucente T, Davis AM, Kappler RE, Lipton JA, Leurgans S. A comparison of osteopathic spinal manipulation with standard care for patients with low back pain [published correction appears in *N Engl J Med*. 2000;342:817]. *N Engl J Med*. 1999;341:1426-1431.

14. Elkiss ML, Jerome JA. Chronic pain management. In: Chila AG, et al, eds. *Foundations of Osteopathic Medicine.* 3rd ed. Baltimore, MD: Lippincott Williams & Wilkins, A Wolters Kluwer Business; 2011:253-275.

15. Wong CK. Strain counterstrain: current concepts and clinical evidence. *Man Ther.* 2012;17(1):2-8. doi:10.1016/j.math.2011.10.001.

16. Korr IM. Proprioceptors and somatic dysfunction. *J Am Osteopath Assoc.* 1975;74(7):638-650. http://www.ncbi.nlm.nih.gov/pubmed/124754. Accessed March 12, 2017.

17. Glossary of Osteopathic Terminology. 2011. https://www.aacom.org/docs/default-source/insideome/got2011ed.pdf?sfvrsn=2. Accessed March 12, 2017.

18. Hutson M, Ward A, eds. *Oxford Textbook of Musculoskeletal Medicine.* Oxford University Press; 2015. doi:10.1093/med/9780199674107.001.0001.

19. Snider KT, Jorgensen DJ. Billing and coding for osteopathic manipulative treatment. *J Am Osteopath Assoc.* 2009;109(8):409-413. http://www.ncbi.nlm.nih.gov/pubmed/19706830. Accessed March 12, 2017.

20. DiGiovanna EL. Goals, classifications and models of osteopathic manipulation. In: DiGiovanna EL, Schiowitz S, Dowling DJ, eds. *An Osteopathic Approach to Diagnosis and Treatment.* 3rd ed. Philadelphia, PA: Lippincott Williams & Wilkins; 2005:77-79.

21. Taub NS, Worsowicz GM, Gnatz SM, Cifu DX. Definitions and diagnosis of pain. *Arch Phys Med Rehabil.* 1998;79(3):S49-S53. http://www.archives-pmr.org/article/S0003-9993(98)90123-X/pdf. Accessed March 12, 2017.

22. Kuchera ML. Applying osteopathic principles to formulate treatment for patients with chronic pain. *J Am Osteopath Assoc.* 2007;107(11):28-38.

23. Patterson MM. A model mechanism for spinal segmental facilitation. *J Am Osteopath Assoc.* 1976;76(1):62-72. http://www.ncbi.nlm.nih.gov/pubmed/1048967. Accessed February 6, 2017.

24. Steel A, Sundberg T, Reid R, et al. Osteopathic manipulative treatment: a systematic review and critical appraisal of comparative effectiveness and health economics research. *Musculoskeletal Sci Pract.* 2017;27:165-175.

25. Johnson SM, Kurtz ME. Conditions and diagnoses for which osteopathic primary care physicians and specialists use osteopathic manipulative treatment. *J Am Osteopath Assoc.* 2002;102(10):527-532, 537-540.

26. Hruby RJ, Fraix MP, Giusti RE. Cervicogenic headache. In: Chila AG, et al, eds. *Foundations of Osteopathic Medicine.* 3rd ed. Baltimore, MD: Lippincott Williams & Wilkins, A Wolters Kluwer Business; 2011:939-945.

27. Fraix MP, Seffinger MA. Acute low back pain. In: Chila AG, et al, eds. *Foundations of Osteopathic Medicine.* 3rd ed. Baltimore, MD: Lippincott Williams & Wilkins, A Wolters Kluwer Business; 2011:1006-1020.

28. Licciardone JC, Brimhall AK, King LN. Osteopathic manipulative treatment for low back pain: a systematic review and meta-analysis of randomized controlled trials. *BMC Musculoskelet Disord.* 2005;6:43. doi:10.1186/1471-2474-6-43.

29. Kuchera ML. Osteopathic principles and practice/osteopathic manipulative treatment considerations in cephalgia. *JAOA.* 1998;98(4):14-19.

30. Van tulder M V, Koes BW, Bouter LM. Conservative Treatment of acute and chronic nonspecific low back pain. A systematic review of randomized controlled trials of the most common interventions. *Spine (Phila PA 1976).* 1997;22(1):2128-2156.

31. Dommerholt J, Bron C, Franssen J. Myofascial trigger points: an evidence-informed practice. *J Man Manip Ther.* 2006;14(4):203-221. doi:10.1179/106698106790819991.

32. Travell JG, Simons DG. *Myofascial Pain and Dysfunction: The Trigger Point Manual.* Williams & Wilkins; 1983.

33. Chiarotto A, Clijsen R, Fernandez-de-las-Penas C, Barbero M. Prevalence of myofascial trigger points in spinal disorders: a systematic review and meta-analysis. *Arch Phys Med Rehabil.* 2016;97(2):316-337. doi:10.1016/j.apmr.2015.09.021.

34. Lavelle ED, Lavelle W, Smith HS. Myofascial trigger points. *Anesthesiol Clin.* 2007;25(4):841-851. doi:10.1016/j.anclin.2007.07.003.

35. Huguenin LK. Myofascial trigger points: the current evidence. *Phys Ther Sport.* 2004;5(1):2-12. doi:10.1016/j.ptsp.2003.11.002.

36. Snider KT, Johnson JC, Snider EJ, Degenhardt BF. Increased incidence and severity of somatic dysfunction in subjects with chronic low back pain. *J Am Osteopath Assoc.* 2008;108(8):372-378. http://www.ncbi.nlm.nih.gov/pubmed/18723455. Accessed March 12, 2017.

37. Greenman PE. Syndromes of the lumbar spine, pelvis, and sacrum. *Phys Med Rehabil Clin North Am.* 1996;7:773-785, 40.

38. Licciardone JC, Kearns CM, Minotti DE. Outcomes of osteopathic manual treatment for chronic low back pain according to baseline pain severity: results from the OSTEOPATHIC Trial. *Man Ther.* 2013;18(6):533-540. doi:10.1016/j.math.2013.05.006.

39. Franke H, Franke J-D, Fryer G, et al. Osteopathic manipulative treatment for nonspecific low back pain: a systematic review and meta-analysis. *BMC Musculoskelet Disord.* 2014;15(1):286. doi:10.1186/1471-2474-15-286.

40. Task Force on the Low Back Pain Clinical Practice Guidelines. American Osteopathic Association guidelines for osteopathic manipulative treatment (OMT) for patients with low back pain. *J Am Osteopat Assoc.* 2010;97(2):80. doi:10.7556/JAOA.2010.110.11.653.

41. Task Force on the Low Back Pain Clinical Practice Guidelines. American Osteopathic Association guidelines for osteopathic manipulative treatment (OMT) for patients with low back pain. *J Am Osteopat Assoc.* 2016;116(8). doi:10.7556/jaoa.2016.107.

42. Prinsen J, Hensel K, Snow R. OMT associated with reduced analgesic prescribing and fewer missed work days in patients with low back pain: an observational study. *J Am Osteopath Assoc.* 2014;114(2):90-98. doi:10.7556/jaoa.2014.022.

43. 11.2.1 Cervicogenic Headache – ICHD-3 Beta The International Classification of Headache Disorders 3rd edition (Beta version). https://www.ichd-3.org/11-headache-or-facial-pain-attributed-to-disorder-of-the-cranium-neck-eyes-ears-nose-sinuses-teeth-mouth-or-other-facial-or-cervical-structure/11-2-headache-attributed-to-disorder-of-the-neck/11-2-1-cervicogenic-headache/. Accessed March 12, 2017.

44. Hall T, Robinson K. The flexion – rotation test and active cervical mobility — a comparative measurement study in cervicogenic headache. *Man Ther.* 2004;9:197-202. doi:10.1016/j.math.2004.04.004.

45. Bogduk N. The anatomical basis for cervicogenic headache. *J Manipulative Physiol Ther.* 1992;15(1):67-70. http://www.ncbi.nlm.nih.gov/pubmed/1740655. Accessed February 18, 2017.

46. Bronfort G, Assendelft WJ, Evans R, Haas M, Bouter L. Efficacy of spinal manipulation for chronic headache: a systematic review. *J Manipulative Physiol Ther.* 2001;24(7):457-466. http://www.ncbi.nlm.nih.gov/pubmed/11562654. Accessed March 12, 2017.

47. Biondi DM. Cervicogenic headache: mechanisms, evaluation, and treatment strategies. *J Am Osteopath Assoc.* 2000;100(9 suppl):S7-S14. http://www.ncbi.nlm.nih.gov/pubmed/11070659. Accessed March 12, 2017.

48. Grimshaw DN. Cervicogenic headache: manual and manipulative therapies. *Curr Pain Headache Rep.* 2001;5(4):369-375. http://www.ncbi.nlm.nih.gov/pubmed/11403741. Accessed March 12, 2017.

49. Miller J, Gross A, D'Sylva J, et al. Manual therapy and exercise for neck pain: a systematic review. *Man Ther.* 2010;15(4):334-354. http://www.ncbi.nlm.nih.gov/pubmed/20593537. Accessed March 12, 2017.

50. Binder DS, Nampiaparampil DE. The provocative lumbar facet joint. *Curr Rev Musculoskelet Med.* 2009;2(1):15-24. doi:10.1007/s12178-008-9039-y.

51. Bogduk N, Bogduk N. *Clinical and Radiological Anatomy of the Lumbar Spine.* Elsevier/Churchill Livingstone; 2012.

52. Tettambel M. Low back pain in pregnancy. In: Chila AG, et al, eds. *Foundations of Osteopathic Medicine.* 3rd ed. Baltimore, MD: Lippincott Williams & Wilkins, A Wolters Kluwer Business; 2011:967-973

53. Hastings V, McCallister AM, Curtis SA, Valant RJ, Yao S. Efficacy of osteopathic manipulative treatment for management of postpartum pain. *J Am Osteopath Assoc.* 2016;116(8):502-509.

54. Seffinger MA, Sanchez J, Fraix MP. Acute neck pain. In: Chila AG, et al, eds. *Foundations of Osteopathic Medicine.* 3rd ed. Baltimore, MD: Lippincott Williams & Wilkins, A Wolters Kluwer Business; 2011:979-989.

55. Adler-Michaelson P, Seffinger MA. Abdominal pain. In: Chila AG, et al, eds. *Foundations of Osteopathic Medicine.* 3rd ed. Baltimore, MD: Lippincott Williams & Wilkins, A Wolters Kluwer Business; 2011:999-1005.

56. Cerritelli F, Ginevri L, Messi G, et al. Clinical effectiveness of osteopathic treatment in chronic migraine: 3-armed randomized controlled trial. *Compliment Ther Med.* 2015;23(2):149-156.

57. DiGiovanna EL. The manipulative prescription. In: DiGiovanna EL, Schiowitz S, Dowling DJ, eds. *An Osteopathic Approach to Diagnosis and Treatment.* 3rd ed. Philadelphia, PA: Lippincott Williams & Wilkins; 2005:667-673.

58. Kuchera ML, Jerome JA. Adult with chronic pain and depression. In: Chila AG, et al, eds. *Foundations of Osteopathic Medicine.* 3rd ed. Baltimore, MD: Lippincott Williams & Wilkins, A Wolters Kluwer Business; 2011:903-909.

59. Nicholas AS, Nicholas EA. Balanced ligamentous tension and ligamentous articular strain techniques. In: Nicholas AS, Nicholas EA, eds. *Atlas of Osteopathic Technique.* 3rd ed. Philadelphia, PA: Wolters Kluwer; 2016:455-483.

60. Nicholas AS, Nicholas EA. Counterstrain techniques. In: Nicholas AS, Nicholas EA, eds. *Atlas of Osteopathic Technique.* 3rd ed. Philadelphia, PA: Wolters Kluwer; 2016:151-245.

61. Hohner JG, Cymet TC. Thrust (high velocity/low amplitude) approach; "the Pop". In: Chila AG, et al, eds. *Foundations of Osteopathic Medicine.* 3rd ed. Baltimore, MD: Lippincott Williams & Wilkins, A Wolters Kluwer Business; 2011:669-681.

62. Nicholas AS, Nicholas EA. High-velocity, low-amplitude techniques. In: Nicholas AS, Nicholas EA, eds. *Atlas of Osteopathic Technique.* 3rd ed. Philadelphia, PA: Wolters Kluwer; 2016:358-419.

63. O'Connell JA. Myofascial release approach. In: Chila AG, et al, eds. *Foundations of Osteopathic Medicine.* 3rd ed. Baltimore, MD: Lippincott Williams & Wilkins, A Wolters Kluwer Business; 2011:698-727

64. Nicholas AS, Nicholas EA. Myofascial release techniques. In: Nicholas AS, Nicholas EA, eds. *Atlas of Osteopathic Technique.* 3rd ed. Philadelphia, PA: Wolters Kluwer; 2016:130-150.

65. Nicholas AS, Nicholas EA. Muscle energy techniques. In: Nicholas AS, Nicholas EA. *Atlas of Osteopathic Technique.* 3rd ed. Philadelphia, PA: Wolters Kluwer; 2016:246-357.

66. Nicholas AS, Nicholas EA. Osteopathic cranial manipulative medicine. In: Nicholas AS, Nicholas EA. *Atlas of Osteopathic Technique.* 3rd ed. Philadelphia, PA: Wolters Kluwer; 2016:570-590.

25

REGENERATIVE MEDICINE

Prathap Jayaram, MD, Joslyn John, MD and Nicolas Karvelas, MD

FAST FACTS

- Platelet rich plasma (PRP) and mesenchymal stem cell (MSC) therapy are regenerative strategies for musculoskeletal injuries.
- Osteoarthritis and tendinopathy are disease processes in which regenerative strategies have demonstrated clinical value.
- Although regenerative strategies are showing promise, they should be used in conjunction with rather than replace standard treatments, including prescriptive physical therapy, adaptive equipment, and bracing.

REGENERATIVE STRATEGIES FOR MUSCULOSKELETAL INJURIES

Introduction to Regenerative Medicine

Regenerative medicine has gained increased popularity in modern medical delivery strategies. At its core, regenerative medicine aims to restore diseased tissue to a healthier physiologic baseline. In the last decade there has been an explosive application of regenerative strategies for musculoskeletal pathology. The recent literature has demonstrated certain regenerative strategies to have excellent safety profile with improved clinical outcomes in musculoskeletal injuries.[1] Osteoarthritis (OA) and tendinopathy are 2 particular disease processes that commonly present to the primary care physician and in which regenerative strategies have shown clinical value. This chapter focuses on clinical applications of platelet rich plasma (PRP) and mesenchymal stem cell (MSC) therapy as it pertains to the primary care physician. While stem cell products in orthopedic applications have the potential to treat many medical conditions, it is not fully known if such products have clear benefit or if the products are entirely safe to use at this time. Seek information directly from the Food and Drug Administration for current guidelines and the status of stem cell therapies under investigation. Also seek information from Academic Physicians who specialize in the field or are involved in Clinical Stem Cell Research.

Definition and Mechanism of Action

Platelet Rich Plasma

PRP by definition is inherently an autologous derivative blood product with a higher physiologic concentration of platelets.[2] Although PRP has been used more routinely in clinical practice, its exact mechanism in the reparative spectrum is still being explored. The common theory is that platelets house certain growth factors through its alpha granules and once degranulated are able to alter the microenvironment allowing for optimization of tissues with, otherwise, low intrinsic healing potential.[1] Specific applications and evidence of PRP will be explained in tendinopathy and osteoarthritis sections.

Mesenchymal Stem Cells

Adult MSCs are found abundantly in many tissue constructs. For orthopedic applications, adipose and bone marrow–derived MSCs have been much of the clinical focus. Adults MSCs are derived from perivascular cells, pericytes.[3] Once a pericyte has been dissociated from its native blood vessel and exposed to the surrounding environment, it becomes an MSC proper.[3] MSCs have multiple mechanisms that include anti-inflammatory, immunomodulatory, and paracrine effects.[1] Much like PRP the exact mechanism of MSC-derived therapy is still being explored and still in its infancy in terms of delineating exact mechanisms. The following text explains specific applications and evidence of MSC-derived therapy.

Common Conditions Presenting to Primary Care: Tendinopathy/Osteoarthritis and Supporting Evidence

Tendinopathy

Tendinopathy and OA are some of the more prevalent diagnoses that present to the primary care physician. Tendinopathy, a common degenerative condition, is thought to arise from a disordered healing response to an acute inflammatory episode within a tendon.[4] This initial insult is repeated chronically through tendon overload resulting in microscopic alterations at the cellular level that weaken mechanical properties of the tendon.[4] The more common anatomic presentations of tendinopathy are located in the lateral elbow (wrist extensor tendinopathy), shoulder (rotator cuff tendinopathy), hip (gluteal tendinopathy), knee (patellar tendinopathy), and ankle (Achilles tendinopathy). Rotator cuff tendinopathy accounts for 30% of shoulder-related pain,[5] and gluteal tendinopathy is the most common in the lower extremity tendinopathy, attributing to a large percentage of hip-related pathology.[6]

The earliest clinical studies for PRP applications in orthopedic injuries have been for lateral elbow tendinopathy. To date there is good evidence to support its use in chronic lateral elbow tendinopathy.[7] One of the challenges in quantifying PRP outcomes is the variability in PRP preparation and delivery. Despite the lack of standardizing PRP delivery there continues to be a growing body of literature to support its use in the above-mentioned tendinopathies. MSCs, more accurately lipoaspirate and bone marrow aspirate cell therapies, have shown a good safety profile in tendinopathy; however, more studies are needed to evaluate clinical efficacy. In a study examining patellar tendinopathy response to bone marrow–derived MSC injections, 7 of 8 patients were subjectively satisfied and showed statistical significance in clinical outcomes involving sport subscores.[8] There is recent evidence to support the use of stem cell therapy to augment surgical repair of rotator cuff tears, with one particular study showing 87% rate of intact rotator cuff compared with 44% in the control group.[9]

When dealing with acute or chronic musculoskeletal tendinopathy, it is always important to understand and treat the contributing biomechanical factors through proper ergonomic correction and prescription-guided physical/occupational therapy. A referral to a physical medicine and rehabilitation specialist can help guide prescriptive therapy, necessary adaptive equipment, braces, and injection techniques. Although regenerative strategies are showing promise, they should be used in conjunction with rather than replace the above-mentioned conservative strategies.

Osteoarthritis

OA is another disabling impairment affecting more than 80% of individuals older than 55 years.[10] Current treatment strategies for both these disabling conditions are limited to activity modification, analgesics, physical therapy, bracing, corticosteroid injections, and, in late stages, surgical intervention. Although conservative strategies have been shown to be effective, there is still an overwhelming population with continued loss of function for which a regenerative strategy may have clinical value. There are roughly 35 clinical studies that have involved PRP for OA. All studies have shown excellent safety profile with variable outcomes.[11] Variability in outcomes is in part due to variability in PRP protocols. There is certainly a growing body of evidence to support use of PRP injections; there have been studies to support its use in conjunction with other first-generation biologics.[12] There has been a surge in using cell-based therapy, namely, lipoaspirate and bone marrow concentrate for knee OA. The hypothesis is that these aspirates house important cell lines, including MSCs, that can alter paracrine activity in OA environments.[13] One of the earlier studies of bone marrow aspirate delivery showed an increase in cartilage and meniscus volume with improvements in knee range of motion and overall pain scores.[14] More recent studies, although small, have demonstrated consistent excellent safety profile with variation in objective cartilage volume improvements.[15]

The clinician, as mentioned earlier in tendinopathy section, should have a good understanding of the biomechanical factors that effect OA. Treatment should always aim at addressing these underlying factors. A referral to a physical medicine and rehabilitation specialist can help guide prescriptive therapy, necessary adaptive equipment, braces, and injection techniques. Such modalities when combined with regenerative strategies hold promise for optimizing function and enhancing quality of life.

CONCLUSIONS

Regenerative medicine is emerging as a powerful tool in combating degenerative musculoskeletal conditions. OA and tendinopathy are common disorders that present to the primary care clinician, and regenerative applications have demonstrated that they have a role in treatment. It is extremely important that, given the rising popularity of regenerative techniques, the clinical provider continues to address all contributing causes that lead to musculoskeletal impairments, which may involve multiple treatment strategies, including prescriptive therapy, bracing, and appropriate pharmacological treatments. As the field continues to expand and treatments become more sophisticated in terms of precision diagnosis and therapeutic delivery, regenerative medicine will have a place as part of the standard of care.

TABLE 25-1 Summary Points for Regenerative Medicine Strategies

1. The purpose of regenerative techniques is to restore diseased tissue to a healthier physiologic baseline.

2. Types of regenerative strategies that have shown benefit for musculoskeletal disorders include platelet rich plasma (PRP) and mesenchymal stem cells.

3. PRP has strong clinical evidence to support its benefits in chronic tendinopathies. Although stem cells have shown to have a good safety profile, further studies are needed on clinical efficacy.

4. In osteoarthritis, PRP has shown excellent safety profiles but variable outcomes. Cell-based therapies (such as lipoaspirate and bone marrow concentrate) have shown promising benefits in underlying cartilage and meniscal tissue as well as functional outcomes such as pain and range of motion. Further studies are needed to establish appropriate protocols for both strategies.

5. Regenerative strategies are a good addition to conservative care of tendinopathies and osteoarthritis. These methods are not meant to be used in isolation. Referral to a physical medicine and rehabilitation specialist can be extremely beneficial to patients suffering from chronic musculoskeletal disorders to optimize the span of conservative options.

REFERENCES

1. Malanga G, Abdelshahed D, Jayaram P. Orthobiologic interventions using ultrasound guidance. *Phys Med Rehabil Clin N Am.* 2016;27(3):717-731.

2. Mishra A, Harmon K, Woodall J, et al. Sports medicine applications of platelet rich plasma. *Curr Pharm Biotechnol.* 2012;13:1185-1195.

3. Caplan AI. All MSCs are pericytes? *Cell Stem Cell.* 2008;3(3):229-230.

4. Khan KM, Cook JL, Bonar F. Histopathology of common tendinopathies: update and implications for clinical management. *Sports Med.* 1999;27:393-408.

5. Van der Windt DA, Koes BW, de Jong BA, et al. Shoulder disorders in general practice: incidence, patient characteristics, and management. *Ann Rheum Dis.* 1995;54(12):959-964.

6. Brinks A, van Rijn RM, Willemsen SP, et al. Corticosteroid injections for greater trochanteric pain syndrome: a randomized controlled trial in primary care. *Ann Fam Med.* 2011;9(3):226-234.

7. Malanga G, Nakamura R. The role of regenerative medicine in the treatment of sports injuries. *Phys Med Rehabil Clin N Am.* 2014;25(4):881-895.

8. Pascual-Garrido C, Rolón A, Makino A. Treatment of chronic patellar tendinopathy with autologous bone marrow stem cells: a 5-year-followup. *Stem Cells Int.* 2012;2012:953510.

9. Hernigou P, Flouzat Lachaniette CH, Delambre J, et al. Biologic augmentation of rotator cuff repair with mesenchymal stem cells during arthroscopy improves healing and prevents further tears: a case-controlled study. *Int Orthop.* 2014;38(9):1811-1818.

10. Evans CH, Ghivizzani SC, Smith P, et al. Using gene therapy to protect and restore cartilage. *Clin Orthop Relat Res.* 2000;(379 suppl):S214–S219.

11. Dhillon MS, Patel S, John R. PRP in OA knee - update, current confusions and future options. *SICOT J.* 2017;3:27.

12. Lana JF, Weglein A, Sampson S, et al. Randomized controlled trial comparing hyaluronic acid, platelet-rich plasma and the combination of both in the treatment of mild and moderate osteoarthritis of the knee. *J Stem Cells Regen Med.* 2016;12(2):69-78.

13. Cianca CJ, Jayaram P. Musculoskeletal injuries and regenerative medicine in the elderly patient. *Phys Med Rehabil Clin N Am.* 2017.

14. Goldring MB. The role of the chondrocyte in osteoarthritis. *Arthritis Rheum.* 2000;43:1916-1926.

15. Centeno CJ, Al-Sayegh H, Freeman MD, et al. A multi-center analysis of adverse events among two thousand, three hundred and seventy two adult patients undergoing adult autologous stem cell therapy for orthopaedic conditions. *Int Orthop.* 2016;40:1755.

26

INTEGRATIVE PAIN MANAGEMENT

Ian J. Koebner, PhD, MSc, MAOM and Anthony DiGirolamo, DO

FAST FACTS

- Complementary medicine combines nonmainstream medical practices with conventional medical practice.
- Integrative health involves the intentional and coordinated use of complementary medicine.
- One of the most common reasons patients seek out complementary medicine is for pain.
- Several complementary and integrative health approaches to pain management are safe and effective.

INTRODUCTION

Although chronic pain is widely understood as a complex biopsychosocial phenomenon,[1-4] the degree to which pain is successfully attenuated by physiological, psychological, and/or social interventions is variable. Unfortunately, usual care for some chronic pain conditions increasingly relies on diagnostic tests and treatment options that have not been well validated in terms of safety or effectiveness[5] and abuse of opioid pain medications has become a major public health concern in the United States.[6] Since 2003, more overdose deaths have involved opioid analgesics than heroin and cocaine combined.[6] For every unintentional overdose death related to an opioid analgesic, 9 persons are admitted for substance abuse treatment, 35 visit emergency departments,

161 report drug abuse or dependence, and 461 report nonmedical uses of opioid analgesics.[6] Faced with an epidemic of chronic pain,[7] usual care that can be ineffective or unsafe,[5,8] and a health care workforce unprepared to meet these challenges,[7,9] many individuals turn toward complementary or integrative health approaches to address their pain.

Complementary health approaches encompass a wide range of procedures by licensed practitioners (e.g., acupuncturists, chiropractors, and massage therapists), self-care approaches (e.g., meditation and movement-based practices), and natural products (e.g., dietary supplements such as herbal medicines).[10] The National Institutes of Health's (NIH) lead agency for scientific research on complementary and integrative health approaches, the National Center for Complementary and Integrative Health (NCCIH), defines complementary medicine as the use of a nonmainstream practice used *together* with conventional medicine.[11] Conventional medicine refers to allopathic medicine as taught in medical schools, which generally engages the patient around a problem or a disease, focusing on disease management over health promotion.[11] Alternative medicine, the use of a nonmainstream practice *in place of* conventional medicine, is rare.[11] Although a number of definitions and constructs exist for integrative health,[12] they all involve in part the intentional and coordinated use of complementary medicine. The National Academy of Medicine describes integrative medicine as "orienting the health care process to create a seamless engagement by patients and caregivers of the full range of physical, psychological, social, preventive, and therapeutic factors known to be effective and necessary for the achievement of optimal health throughout the life span."[13]

About 30% to 40% of US adults use complementary approaches to health in a given year,[14-18] most commonly for painful health conditions.[14,15,17-19] The National Health Interview Survey of 2007, for example, demonstrated that approximately 14.3 million adults used a complementary health approach for back pain, 5.0 million adults used these approaches for neck pain, and 3.1 million adults used these approaches for arthritis.[10,14] The high utilization of complementary health approaches has created a significant cash market for these services and products. In 2007, individuals spent $8.5 billion in out-of-pocket payments on complementary health approaches to manage back pain, $3.6 billion to manage neck pain, and $2.3 billion to manage arthritis.[10,19] By comparison, individuals used complementary health approaches much less often and spent significantly less out of pocket for other chronic diseases such as depression (1.0 million adults/$1.1 billion), hypertension (0.8 million adults/$0.7 billion), diabetes (0.7 million adults/$0.3 billion), or cancer (0.4 million adults/$0.2 billion).[10,14,19]

The widespread use of complementary health approaches for pain has led to numerous mechanistic and clinical trials to assess their safety and effectiveness. For example, an evidence-based evaluation of complementary health approaches for pain management published by the NIH-NCCIH[10] explored some of the most frequently used complementary health approaches used to treat common pain conditions seen by primary care providers within the United States.[10] In 2017, the American College of Physicians (ACP) established guidelines for the noninvasive treatment of low back pain that included recommendations for several complementary therapies.[20] Over the past 5 years, the Ottawa Panel has established several guidelines supporting the use of complementary therapies to manage neck, back, and knee pain.[21-23] The results of these studies are outlined in Tables 26-1 to 26-4. A comprehensive review of all complementary health approaches for all painful conditions is beyond the scope of this chapter. Instead, details on the effectiveness and safety of several widely used complementary health approaches for common pain conditions seen in the primary care setting are presented. Biologically based therapies, including supplements, are not discussed; although individual studies have variable results, a recent systematic review of select supplements commonly used in the treatment of pain revealed insufficient evidence to support their use.[10]

ACUPUNCTURE

Although the origin of acupuncture is a subject of debate, the practice was already codified by the first century BC in the *Huang Di Nei Jing* (The Yellow Emperor's Internal Classic).[24] In 1976, the New England School of Acupuncture became the first American college of acupuncture and oriental medicine. There are approximately 65 accredited or candidacy status schools with the Accreditation Commission for Acupuncture and Oriental Medicine (ACAOM), and 42 states and the District of Columbia regulate acupuncture.[25] All candidates for a state license are required to pass the National Certification Commission for Acupuncture and Oriental Medicine (NCCAOM) examination except for California, which administers its own comprehensive examination.[26] ACAOM requires a 3-year/27-month, 1905-hour, 105-semester-credits program to receive the Master of Acupuncture degree and a 4-year/36-month, 2625-hour, 146-semester-credits program to qualify for the Master of Acupuncture and Oriental Medicine degree, which includes training in Chinese herbal medicine.[26]

TABLE 26-1 Summary of ACP Guidelines for the Use of Select Complementary Health Approaches for Low Back Pain

TYPE OF CAM	ACUTE TO SUBACUTE LOW BACK PAIN	CHRONIC LOW BACK PAIN
Acupuncture	Strong recommendation	Strong recommendation
Spinal manipulation	Strong recommendation	Strong recommendation
Massage	Strong recommendation	Insufficient evidence
Meditation[a]	Insufficient evidence	Strong recommendation
Tai chi	Insufficient evidence	Strong recommendation
Yoga	Insufficient evidence	Strong recommendation

Adapted from Qaseem A, Wilt TJ, McLean RM, Forciea MA, Clinical Guidelines Committee of the American College of Physicians. Noninvasive treatments for acute, subacute, and chronic low back pain: a clinical practice guideline from the American College of Physicians. Ann Intern Med. 2017;166.
[a]Mindfulness-based stress reduction.
ACP, American College of Physicians; CAM, complementary and alternative medicine.

Acupuncture has been shown to provide significant relief of both acute and chronic low back pain and is currently recommended by ACP guidelines.[20] There is also a body of evidence to suggest that acupuncture may provide significant improvements in knee pain in the setting of osteoarthritis.[10] Several studies have shown that acupuncture may be beneficial in reducing impact scores of chronic daily headaches[10,27] and long-term reduction in migraine recurrence.[28] Acupuncture may also provide pain relief for patients with fibromyalgia; however, better quality studies are needed.[29,30] There is a moderate level of evidence to suggest acupuncture is beneficial in the treatment of neck pain.[31] Acupuncture is generally well tolerated with low risk of adverse events; in the above-mentioned studies, adverse events were minimal and included minor pain and/or bruising at the needle site[10] and vasovagal symptoms.[29]

SPINAL MANIPULATION

Spinal manipulation dates to ancient times and has roots within most cultures of the world. Traditionally referred to as "bone setting," manipulation of the spine and peripheral joints was described by Hippocrates and has been recorded in a multitude of physician and surgical texts over the millennia.[32] For unclear reasons, bone setting fell out of favor within the US medical community in the 19th century.[32] It was during this time, however, that the 2 leading professions of spinal manipulation, osteopathic medicine and chiropractic, were born. Currently within the United States, both chiropractors

TABLE 26-2 Summary of Benefits for the Use of Complementary Health Approaches for Select Pain Conditions

TYPE OF CAM	BACK PAIN	KNEE PAIN (OA)	NECK PAIN	HEADACHES	FIBROMYALGIA
Acupuncture	Beneficial ++	Beneficial ++	Insufficient evidence	Insufficient evidence	Insufficient evidence
Spinal manipulation	Beneficial +	Insufficient evidence	Insufficient evidence	Insufficient evidence	Insufficient evidence
Massage	Beneficial +	Insufficient evidence	Beneficial ++	Insufficient evidence	Insufficient evidence
Relaxation approaches	Insufficient evidence	Insufficient evidence	Insufficient evidence	Beneficial ++	Beneficial +
Tai chi	Insufficient evidence	Beneficial ++	Insufficient evidence	Insufficient evidence	Beneficial +
Yoga	Beneficial ++	Insufficient evidence	Insufficient evidence	Insufficient evidence	Insufficient evidence

Reprinted from Nahin RL, Boineau R, Khalsa PS, Stussman BJ, Weber WJ. Evidence-based evaluation of complementary health approaches for pain management in the United States. Mayo Clin Proc. 2016;91(9):1292-1306. Copyright © 2016 Mayo Foundation for Medical Education and Research. With permission.
The above summary may be used as a guide to help the primary care provider identify possible complementary health approaches for their patients with a chronic pain condition.
(++) stronger evidence of benefit; (+) weaker evidence of benefit; CAM, complementary and alternative medicine; OA, osteoarthritis.

TABLE 26-3 Systematic Review-Based Quality of Evidence for the Use of Complementary Health Approaches in Select Pain Conditions

PAIN CONDITION	ACUPUNCTURE	SPINAL MANIPULATION	MASSAGE
Acute low back pain	Low[a]	Low[a]	Low[a]
Chronic low back pain	Mod[a]	Low[a]	Low/very low[b]
Knee pain (OA)	N/A	N/A	Low/mod[c]
Neck pain	Mod[b]	Low/mod[b,d]; mod[c,e]	Low/very low[b]
Headaches	Mod/low[b] (FTTH); mod[b] (MH)	N/A	N/A
Fibromyalgia	Low/mod[b] (EA)	N/A	N/A

Reproduced from Schünemann HJ, Schünemann AH, Oxman AD, et al; GRADE working group. Grading quality of evidence and strength of recommendations for diagnostic tests and strategies. BMJ. 2008;336(7653):1106-1110. With permission from BMJ Publishing Group Ltd.
[a]*Qaseem A, Wilt TJ, McLean RM, Forciea MA, Clinical Guidelines Committee of the American College of Physicians. Noninvasive treatments for acute, subacute, and chronic low back pain: a clinical practice guideline from the American College of Physicians. Ann Intern Med. 2017;166.*
[b]*Deare JC, Zheng Z, Xue CC, et al. Acupuncture for treating fibromyalgia. The Cochrane Library. 2013.*
[c]*Zhu L, Wei X, Wang S. Does cervical spine manipulation reduce pain in people with degenerative cervical radiculopathy? A systematic review of the evidence, and a meta-analysis. Clin Rehabil. 2016;30(2):145-155.*
[d]*Neck pain.*
[e]*Cervical radicular pain.*
EA, electroacupuncture, FTTH, frequent tension-type headache; MH, migraine headache; N/A, not assessed; OA, osteoarthritis.
Very low: "Any estimate of effect is very uncertain."
Low: "Further research is very likely to have an important impact on our confidence in the estimate of effect and is likely to change the estimate."
Mod: (moderate) "Further research is likely to have an important impact on our confidence in the estimate of effect and may change the estimate."

and osteopathic physicians continue to use spinal manipulation techniques. Within some states, spinal manipulation is also practiced in the fields of physical therapy and naturopathic medicine depending on individual state licensing and scope of practice laws.

Spinal manipulation has been researched extensively over the past several decades. Although most studies are small and have produced varying results, spinal manipulation is thought to provide relief of both acute and chronic low back pain and is currently recommended by ACP guidelines.[20] There is also a body of evidence to suggest that spinal manipulation is beneficial in the treatment of neck pain[33-35] and headaches (cervicogenic and chronic tension type).[10,36] Spinal manipulation is generally well tolerated with relatively low risk of adverse events. In the above-mentioned studies, adverse events were minimal and included muscle soreness and transient increase in pain.[20,36] However, serious adverse events have been reported in both low back[37] and cervical manipulations.[38] In one review of manipulations of the low back that screened 2046 studies and included 41 studies, the authors reported 77 cases of adverse events, including cauda equina syndrome (29 cases, 38% of total); lumbar disk herniation (23 cases, 30%); fracture (7 cases, 9%); hematoma or hemorrhagic cyst (6 cases, 8%); or other serious adverse events (12 cases, 16%), such as neurologic or vascular compromise, soft tissue trauma, muscle abscess formation, disrupted fracture healing, and esophageal rupture.[37] In a review of cervical spinal manipulations that screened 1043 studies and included 144 studies, the authors reported 227 cases of adverse events and cervical arterial dissection was the most common adverse event reported (57% of the cases).[38]

MASSAGE

Massage was first recorded in the *Huang Di Nei Jing* (The Yellow Emperor's Internal Classic) from China in the first century BC, although the practice has roots within most cultures of the world, including India, ancient

TABLE 26-4 Ottawa Panel Clinical Practice Guidelines for the Use of Complementary Health Approaches for Select Pain Conditions

MODALITY	SUBACUTE LOW BACK PAIN	CHRONIC LOW BACK PAIN	SUBACUTE NECK PAIN	CHRONIC NECK PAIN	KNEE PAIN (OA)
Massage	Recommended	Recommended	Recommended[a]	Recommended[a]	N/A
Tai chi	N/A	N/A	N/A	N/A	Recommended[b]
Yoga	N/A	N/A	N/A	N/A	Recommended

Adapted from Brosseau L, Taki J, Desjardins B, et al. The Ottawa panel clinical practice guidelines for the management of knee osteoarthritis. Part one: Introduction, and mind-body exercise programs. Clin Rehabil. 2017:0269215517691083; Brosseau L, Wells GA, Poitras S, et al. Ottawa Panel evidence-based clinical practice guidelines on therapeutic massage for low back pain. J Bodyw Mov Ther. 2012;16(4):424-455; Brosseau L, Wells GA, Tugwell P, et al. Ottawa panel evidence-based clinical practice guidelines on therapeutic massage for neck pain. J Bodyw Mov Ther. 2012;16(3):300-325.
[a]Recommended for short-term relief of symptoms; inconclusive data on long-term benefit.
[b]Both a 12-week (recommended) and a 20-week (strongly recommended) tai chi program were assessed.
The above summary may be used as a guide to help the primary care provider identify possible complementary health approaches for their patients with a chronic pain condition.
N/A, not assessed; OA, osteoarthritis.

Greece, and the Pacific islands.[32] Over the last century, massage and bodywork therapies have grown to incorporate a multitude of techniques including but not limited to osteopathic-based treatments such as myofascial release, craniosacral therapy, and visceral manipulation. According to the American Massage Therapy Association (AMTA), massage therapy is regulated and/or has licensing requirement within 46 states and is covered with increasing frequency by health insurance plans.[39]

Owing to the heterogeneity of massage techniques, assessing the benefit for chronic pain conditions is difficult and has resulted in variable findings. Massage has been shown to provide relief of symptoms in acute and subacute low back pain and is currently recommended by ACP and Ottawa panel guidelines.[20,33] Massage has also been shown to provide short-term relief of symptoms in chronic low back pain.[10,20,33,40,41] Several studies have also shown improvements in symptoms of chronic neck pain[10,33,42] in addition to frequent episodic tension-type headache and chronic tension type headache[10,43] treated with massage. A few small studies have shown improvements in knee pain associated with osteoarthritis treated with massage.[10,44-47] Fibromyalgia has been studied with varying results based on the type of massage.[10] A moderate quality of evidence[48] suggests that myofascial release-type massage is beneficial at alleviating pain, fatigue, anxiety, and depression associated with fibromyalgia.[49] Although reported data on safety of massage across conditions are limited, and rare instances of adverse events have been reported, massage by a trained therapist is typically well tolerated and safe.[10]

MEDITATION

A variety of meditation techniques have been used in the management of pain. However, mindfulness-based meditation techniques, which involve self-regulation of attention and an open, curious, and accepting orientation toward the present moment,[50] are some of the most well studied. Mindfulness meditation techniques originate from Buddhist philosophy and practices. These ancient techniques are increasingly being adapted and used in the health care setting to address a number of health-related conditions, including but not limited to pain management.

Mindfulness-based techniques have been shown to provide some level of relief for many chronic pain conditions. For example, Mindfulness Based Stress Reduction (MBSR) has been shown to reduce the symptoms of chronic low back pain and is currently recommended by the ACP.[20] MBSR is a structured 8 to 10-week group program that focuses on the development of mindfulness through mindfulness meditation practice, mindful awareness during yoga postures, and mindfulness during stressful situations and social interactions.[51] Several studies have shown mindfulness-based techniques to provide symptom improvement in patients with fibromyalgia[10,52-54] and headache disorders.[55,56] Meditation and mindfulness-based techniques are low-risk treatment options and are generally well tolerated.[10]

TAI CHI

Tai chi is an ancient Chinese Taoist internal martial art. The first written records of *tai chi* date back to the 17th century; however, the philosophy and techniques are based on qigong and other internal martial arts dating back several thousand years.[57] Sharing its roots with acupuncture, *tai chi* is based on the relationship of opposites known as *yin* and *yang*, which work in a complementary way to maintain balance. *Tai chi* movements are coordinated with the breath and performed in a relaxed, slow, and repetitive manner. Individuals across the life span can participate in *tai chi*. Considered an active movement-based form of meditation, *tai chi* can improve cardiovascular and physical fitness.[57]

Tai chi has been studied for a number of health conditions and has been shown to improve strength, balance, aerobic capacity, psychological well-being, and quality of life and, more recently, to provide significant relief of several chronic pain conditions.[57] *Tai chi* is currently recommended by ACP guidelines for chronic low back pain and has been shown to provide significant improvements in knee pain in the setting of osteoarthritis.[10,20] *Tai chi* has also been found to provide pain relief for patients with fibromyalgia.[10,52] *Tai chi* is a low-risk treatment option with no reported serious adverse effects.[10]

YOGA

Yoga is a system of mind, body, and spiritual practices that originated in India several thousand years ago. The term "*yoga*" has several translations and is most commonly referred to as "union." *Yoga* came to be known in the West in the 19th century and over the past few decades has grown dramatically in popularity.[58] Within the West, *yoga* is mostly practiced as a form of physical exercise or series of postures known as "*asana*."[59] In 2011, it was estimated that more than 20 million people within the United States had practiced *yoga*.[58] Several studies have shown *yoga* to be beneficial in alleviating symptoms associated with chronic pain conditions.[10,21]

Yoga is currently recommended by ACP guidelines for chronic low back pain and is recommended by Ottawa Panel guidelines for knee pain.[10,21] Although the different types of *yoga* used in studies of pain conditions make interpretation and generalization of results challenging, various forms of *yoga* have been found to be beneficial in the treatment of fibromyalgia, neck pain, and headaches.[60] Given the heterogeneity of *yoga* styles and practices, with significant differences in physical exertion and cardiovascular intensity, safety is variable, with the majority of injuries occurring among those older than 65 years.[58] Older adults, particularly with osteoporosis, should engage in a multicomponent exercise program that includes resistance and balance training and avoids movements with end-range flexion/extension/rotation of the spine and internal/external rotation of the hip.[61] Yoga postures emphasizing spinal alignment and extension to mid-range while standing and on the floor may be encouraged.[61] Generally, yoga classes should be facilitated by an instructor with proper training for the population they are teaching (e.g., older adults with osteoporosis), should be a noncompetitive environment, and should give attention to which postures are safe and how to transition safely.[61]

SUMMARY

Pain is a prevalent and costly public health problem in the United States,[7] yet some treatment options are unsafe or ineffective[5,6] and training in pain management for many health care providers is inadequate.[7] Perhaps in part as a result of these factors complementary health approaches are commonly used in the management of pain[14,15,17-19] and a number of recent guidelines and evidence-based evaluations have supported several approaches as safe and effective complements in the effort to relieve pain. For example, ACP guidelines recommend massage, acupuncture, and spinal manipulation for acute and subacute low back pain[20] and acupuncture, MBSR, *tai chi*, *yoga* and spinal manipulation for chronic low back pain.[20] An NIH-NCCIH review concluded that there was evidence to support the use of acupuncture and *yoga* for back pain, acupuncture and *tai chi* for knee pain associated with osteoarthritis, massage therapy for neck pain, and relaxation techniques for headache disorders.[10] This study also showed weaker evidence to support the use of spinal manipulation, osteopathic manipulation, and massage therapy for back pain and *tai chi* and relaxation techniques for fibromyalgia.[10] The Ottawa Panel has also established guidelines in support of the use of several complementary health approaches to manage neck, back, and knee pain.[21-23] Against the national backdrop of an epidemic of both chronic pain and abuse of opioid analgesics, complementary health approaches with demonstrated safety and effectiveness should be integrated when appropriate into treatment plans for individuals with pain.

REFERENCES

1. Merskey H, Bogduk N. *Task Force on Taxonomy of the International Association for the Study of Pain: Classification of Chronic Pain. Description of Pain Syndromes and Definitions of Pain Terms.* Seattle, WA: IASP Press; 1994.

2. Turk DC, Monarch ES. *Biopsychosocial perspective on chronic pain.* Psychological Approaches to Pain Management: A Practitioner's Handbook; 1996:3-32.

3. Gatchel RJ, Peng YB, Peters ML, Fuchs PN, Turk DC. The biopsychosocial approach to chronic pain: scientific advances and future directions. *Psychol Bull.* 2007;133(4):581.

4. Hadjistavropoulos T, Craig KD, Duck S, et al. A biopsychosocial formulation of pain communication. *Psychol Bull.* 2011;137(6):910-939.

5. Deyo RA, Mirza SK, Turner JA, Martin BI. Overtreating chronic back pain: time to back off? *J Am Board Fam Med.* 2009;22(1):62-68.

6. Centers for Disease Control Prevention. CDC grand rounds: prescription drug overdoses-a US epidemic. *MMWR Morb Mortal Wkly Rep.* 2012;61(1):10.

7. Institute of Medicine. *Relieving Pain in America: A blueprint for Transforming Prevention, Care, Education, and Research.* National Academies Press; 2011.

8. Okie S. A flood of opioids, a rising tide of deaths. *N Engl J Med.* 2010;363(21):1981-1985.

9. Fishman SM, Young HM, Lucas Arwood E, et al. Core competencies for pain management: results of an interprofessional consensus summit. *Pain Med.* 2013;14(7):971-981.

10. Nahin RL, Boineau R, Khalsa PS, Stussman BJ, Weber WJ. Evidence-based evaluation of complementary health approaches for pain management in the United States. *Mayo Clin Proc.* 2016;91(9):1292-1306.

11. National Center for Complementary and Integrative Health; 2017. https://nccih.nih.gov/health/integrative-health. Accessed 4 April 2017.

12. Witt CM, Chiaramonte D, Berman S, et al. Defining health in a comprehensive context: a new definition of integrative health. *Am J Prev Med.* 2017;53(1):134-137.

13. Institute of Medicine. *Integrative Medicine and the Health of the Public: A Summary of the February 2009 Summit.* National Academy of Science Press; 2009.

14. Barnes PM, Bloom B, Nahin RL. Complementary and alternative medicine use among adults and children: United States, 2007. *Natl Health Stat Report.* 2008;(12):1-23.

15. Barnes PM, Powell-Griner E, McFann K, Nahin RL. *Complementary and alternative medicine use among adults: United States, 2002. Paper Presented At: Seminars in Integrative Medicine.* 2004.

16. Clarke TC, Black LI, Stussman BJ, Barnes PM, Nahin RL. Trends in the use of complementary health approaches among adults: United States, 2002-2012. *Natl Health Stat Report.* 2015;(79):1-16.

17. Eisenberg DM, Davis RB, Ettner SL, et al. Trends in alternative medicine use in the United States, 1990-1997: results of a follow-up national survey. *JAMA.* 1998;280(18):1569-1575.

18. Eisenberg DM, Kessler RC, Foster C, Norlock FE, Calkins DR, Delbanco TL. Unconventional medicine in the United States. Prevalence, costs, and patterns of use. *N Engl J Med.* 1993;328(4):246-252.

19. Nahin RL, Stussman BJ, Herman PM. Out-of-pocket expenditures on complementary health approaches associated with painful health conditions in a nationally representative adult sample. *J Pain.* 2015;16(11):1147-1162.

20. Qaseem A, Wilt TJ, McLean RM, Forciea MA, Clinical Guidelines Committee of the American College of Physicians. Noninvasive treatments for acute, subacute, and chronic low back pain: a clinical practice guideline from the American College of Physicians. *Ann Intern Med.* 2017;166.

21. Brosseau L, Taki J, Desjardins B, et al. The Ottawa panel clinical practice guidelines for the management of knee osteoarthritis. Part one: introduction, and mind-body exercise programs. *Clin Rehabil.* 2017. doi:10.1177/0269215517691083.

22. Brosseau L, Wells GA, Poitras S, et al. Ottawa panel evidence-based clinical practice guidelines on therapeutic massage for low back pain. *J Bodyw Mov Ther.* 2012;16(4):424-455.

23. Brosseau L, Wells GA, Tugwell P, et al. Ottawa panel evidence-based clinical practice guidelines on therapeutic massage for neck pain. *J Bodyw Mov Ther.* 2012;16(3):300-325.

24. Kaptchuk TJ. Acupuncture: theory, efficacy, and practice. *Ann Intern Med.* 2002;136(5):374-383.

25. Braverman C, Baker C, Harris R. *Acupuncture and Oriental Medicine (AOM) in the United States.* Reprinted from: The American Acupuncturist. Vol. 47; 2009. http://www.aaaomonline.info/aom_in_us.pdf. Accessed 7 August 2012.

26. Braverman C, Baker C, Harris R. Acupuncture and oriental medicine (AOM) in the United States. *Am Acupuncturist.* 2009;47.

27. Linde K, Allais G, Brinkhaus B, et al. Acupuncture for the prevention of tension-type headache. *Cochrane Database Syst Rev.* 2016;4:CD007587.

28. Zhao L, Chen J, Li Y, et al. The long-term effect of acupuncture for migraine prophylaxis: a randomized clinical trial. *JAMA Intern Med.* 2017;177(4):508-515.

29. Deare JC, Zheng Z, Xue CC, et al. Acupuncture for treating fibromyalgia. *Cochrane Database Syst Rev.* 2013;(5):CD007070.

30. Vas J, Santos-Rey K, Navarro-Pablo R, et al. Acupuncture for fibromyalgia in primary care: a randomised controlled trial. *Acupunct Med.* 2016;34(4):257-266.

31. Trinh K, Graham N, Irnich D, Cameron I, Forget M. Acupuncture for neck disorders. *Cochrane Database Syst Rev.* 2016;5:CD004870.

32. Pettman E. A history of manipulative therapy. *J Man Manip Ther.* 2007;15(3):165-174.

33. Bussières AE, Stewart G, Al-Zoubi F, et al. The treatment of neck pain–associated disorders and whiplash-associated disorders: a clinical practice guideline. *J Manipulative Physiol Ther.* 2016;39(8):523-564.e527.

34. Gross A, Langevin P, Burnie SJ, et al. Manipulation and mobilisation for neck pain contrasted against an inactive control or another active treatment. *Cochrane Database Syst Rev.* 2015;(9):CD004249.

35. Zhu L, Wei X, Wang S. Does cervical spine manipulation reduce pain in people with degenerative cervical radiculopathy? A systematic review of the evidence, and a meta-analysis. *Clin Rehabil.* 2016;30(2):145-155.

36. Varatharajan S, Ferguson B, Chrobak K, et al. Are non-invasive interventions effective for the management of headaches associated with neck pain? An update of the bone and joint decade task force on neck pain and its associated disorders by the Ontario Protocol for Traffic Injury Management (OPTIMa) collaboration. *Eur Spine J.* 2016;25(7):1971-1999.

37. Hebert JJ, Stomski NJ, French SD, Rubinstein SM. Serious adverse events and spinal manipulative therapy of the low back region: a systematic review of cases. *J Manipulative Physiol Ther.* 2015;38(9):677-691.

38. Kranenburg H, Schmitt M, Puentedura E, Luijckx G, van der Schans C. Adverse events associated with the use of cervical spine manipulation or mobilization and patient characteristics: a systematic review. *Musculoskelet Sci Pract.* 2017;28:32-38.

39. Nahin RL, Barnes PM, Stussman BJ. Insurance coverage for complementary health approaches among adult users: United States, 2002 and 2012. *NCHS Data Brief.* 2016;(235):1-8.

40. Furlan AD, Giraldo M, Baskwill A, Irvin E, Imamura M. Massage for low-back pain. *Cochrane Database Syst Rev.* 2015;(9):CD001929.

41. Kumar S, Rampp T, Kessler C, et al. Effectiveness of ayurvedic massage (sahacharadi taila) in patients with chronic low back pain: a randomized controlled trial. *J Altern Complement Med.* 2017;23(2):109-115.

42. Patel KC, Gross A, Graham N, et al. Massage for mechanical neck disorders. *Cochrane Database Syst Rev.* 2012;(9):CD004871.

43. Ferragut-Garcías A, Plaza-Manzano G, Rodríguez-Blanco C, et al. Effectiveness of a treatment involving soft tissue techniques and/or neural mobilization techniques in the management of tension-type headache: a randomized controlled trial. *Arch Phys Med Rehabil.* 2017;98(2):211-219. e212.

44. Bervoets DC, Luijsterburg PA, Alessie JJ, Buijs MJ, Verhagen AP. Massage therapy has short-term benefits for people with common musculoskeletal disorders compared to no treatment: a systematic review. *J Physiother.* 2015;61(3):106-116.

45. Field T. Knee osteoarthritis pain in the elderly can be reduced by massage therapy, yoga and tai chi: a review. *Complement Ther Clin Pract.* 2016;22:87-92.

46. Field T. Massage therapy research review. *Complement Ther Clin Pract.* 2016;24:19-31.

47. Nelson NL, Churilla JR. Massage therapy for pain and function in patients with arthritis: a systematic review of randomized controlled trials. *Am J Phys Med Rehabil.* 2017.

48. Schunemann HJ, Oxman AD, Brozek J, et al; GRADE working group. Grading quality of evidence and strength of recommendations for diagnostic tests and strategies. *BMJ.* 2008;336(7653):1106-1110.

49. Yuan SLK, Matsutani LA, Marques AP. Effectiveness of different styles of massage therapy in fibromyalgia: a systematic review and meta-analysis. *Man Ther.* 2015;20(2):257-264.

50. Bishop SR, Lau M, Shapiro S, et al. Mindfulness: a proposed operational definition. *Clin Psychol.* 2004;11(3):230-241.

51. Grossman P, Niemann L, Schmidt S, Walach H. Mindfulness-based stress reduction and health benefits. A meta-analysis. *J Psychosom Res.* 2004;57(1):35-43.

52. Lauche R, Cramer H, Dobos G, Langhorst J, Schmidt S. A systematic review and meta-analysis of mindfulness-based stress reduction for the fibromyalgia syndrome. *J Psychosom Res.* 2013;75(6):500-510.

53. Theadom A, Cropley M, Smith HE, Feigin VL, McPherson K. Mind and body therapy for fibromyalgia. *Cochrane Database Syst Rev.* 2015;(4):CD001980.

54. Van Gordon W, Shonin E, Dunn TJ, Garcia-Campayo J, Griffiths MD. Meditation awareness training for the treatment of fibromyalgia syndrome: a randomized controlled trial. *Br J Health Psychol.* 2017;22(1):186-206.

55. Andrasik F, Grazzi L, D'Amico D, et al. Mindfulness and headache: a "new" old treatment, with new findings. *Cephalalgia.* 2016;36(12):1192-1205.

56. Azam MA, Katz J, Mohabir V, Ritvo P. Individuals with tension and migraine headaches exhibit increased heart rate variability during post-stress mindfulness meditation practice but a decrease during a post-stress control condition–a randomized, controlled experiment. *Int J Psychophysiol.* 2016;110:66-74.

57. Lan C, Wolf SL, Tsang WW. Tai chi exercise in medicine and health promotion. *Evid Based Complement Alternat Med.* 2013;2013.

58. Swain TA, McGwin G. Yoga-related injuries in the United States from 2001 to 2014. *Orthop J Sports Med.* 2016;4(11). doi:10.1177/2325967116671703.

59. De Michelis E. *A History of Modern Yoga: Patanjali and Western Esotericism.* A&C Black; 2005.

60. Sutar R, Yadav S, Desai G. Yoga intervention and functional pain syndromes: a selective review. *Int Rev Psychiatry.* 2016;28(3):316-322.

61. McArthur C, Laprade J, Giangregorio LM. Suggestions for adapting yoga to the needs of older adults with osteoporosis. *J Altern Complement Med.* 2016;22(3):223-226.

27

COGNITIVE BEHAVIORAL THERAPY AND ACCEPTANCE AND COMMITMENT THERAPY

Payal Mapara, PsyD and Ami Student, PsyD

Chronic pain is a significant public health concern globally with ever increasing prevalence rates and costs.[1] In the United States alone, at least 116 million people are affected by chronic pain at a cost of 560 to 635 billion dollars annually owing to direct medical care, higher rates of health care utilization, and lost productivity.[1] In addition, chronic pain is associated with decreased quality of life[2] and increased rates of depression.[3–6]

Chronic pain is complex, and understanding the cause and maintenance requires a shift from the biomedical model to the biopsychosocial model. In traditional biomedical models, mind and body are conceptualized as separate entities that function independently of one other. Historically, utilizing the dualistic model to guide treatment has proven to be inadequate across a wide range of medical disorders. This has been particularly true for chronic pain, where psychosocial factors such as emotional distress significantly impact symptom reporting and treatment response.[7] The biopsychosocial model frames chronic pain as a complex output of biological factors, psychosocial factors, and environmental factors interacting in a dynamic and reciprocal fashion. Each of these factors contributes to the development, experience, and maintenance of pain and response to treatment.[8,9]

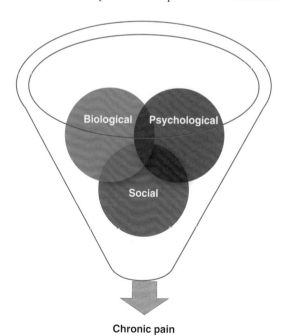

Chronic pain

From the biopsychosocial perspective, ideal chronic pain treatment is multimodal, with treatment plans incorporating several interventions for chronic pain. Potential interventions include but are not limited to pharmacology, manual therapies, procedural therapies, and psychological interventions. This chapter focuses on 2 widely used psychological interventions for chronic pain: cognitive behavioral therapy (CBT) and acceptance and commitment therapy (ACT).

COGNITIVE BEHAVIORAL THERAPY FOR CHRONIC PAIN

CBT, adapted and studied to treat a wide range of problems (e.g., substance use disorders, insomnia, somatoform disorders, and mood disorders)[10] across diverse populations, is based on the premise that cognitions cause and maintain negative emotional states and maladaptive behavioral patterns. More simply put, how individuals think influences how they feel and what they do in response. CBT is short term and goal oriented with the expectation that the patient is an active participant; the therapeutic relationship is marked by collaboration. CBT focuses on how maladaptive cognitive thinking styles (e.g., all or nothing thinking, mind reading, and overgeneralization) and behaviors manifest and the impact that these patterns have on current emotions and functioning. Interventions include goal setting, disputing distorted (or maladaptive) thoughts through Socratic questioning, and behavioral experiments in which individuals trial different coping strategies and record outcomes.

CBT for chronic pain, or CBT-CP, is one of the most widely used and empirically supported psychosocial interventions for chronic pain. CBT-CP incorporates the pain experience into the traditional CBT model: the way an individual thinks, feels, and acts influences pain, and pain in turn impacts thoughts, emotions, and behaviors.

Several meta-analyses have examined the efficacy of CBT for a multitude of chronic pain conditions, including chronic low back pain,[11] fibromyalgia,[12] arthritis, and orofacial pain.[13] The consensus across these studies is that CBT *is* an efficacious treatment of a multitude of chronic pain conditions. CBT for chronic pain has demonstrated "positive effects" on pain intensity, quality of life, depression, and physical functioning when compared with treatment as usual (TAU) or waitlist.[11] Williams, Eccleston, and Morely[14] completed a systematic review comparing CBT with both *other* behavioral treatments and TAU for chronic pain. When compared with behavioral treatments (defined as "treatments that are purely behavioural technologies such as biofeedback") and TAU, CBT demonstrated small to moderate *significant* improvements in pain intensity, disability, mood, and catastrophizing.[14] From a biopsychosocial perspective, the most robust treatment would be multimodal, with simultaneous interventions targeting different areas of functioning. For example, one would expect that CBT in addition to physical therapy and pharmacotherapy would result in better outcomes than any intervention alone.[15]

The treatment focus in CBT-CP is on improving self-efficacy, increasing functioning, and improving overall quality of life. Note that identifying the cause of a patient's pain and finding a "cure" or "fix" for chronic pain are not focal points in treatment, although many report a decrease in pain scores. This is an important distinction for several reasons. The first is that this approach promotes an internal locus of control versus external locus of control (i.e., "Only surgery can help me"). Second, it reinforces active coping and self-management strategies. Third, this approach promotes improvement on measurable, functional goals rather than subjective pain scores. Last, this approach promotes self-efficacy and a focus on how to live life in a valued and functional way.[16]

Active Coping

A primary goal in CBT-CP is the development and strengthening of active coping for pain, which is defined as managing pain through one's own resources. Examples of active coping include exercise, use of relaxation techniques, and increasing engagement in valued activities. Many patients with chronic pain seen in medical settings engage in passive coping, defined as managing pain through a reliance on external factors and/or behaviors that reflect perceived helplessness.[17] Passive coping includes guarding, excessive rest, activity avoidance, and use of pain medications. Reliance solely on passive coping strategies is associated with higher rates of disability, increased pain, and greater medication utilization.[18–20] Active coping, on the other hand, is associated with decreased disability[19] and higher self-efficacy beliefs.[17] Utilizing active strategies can disrupt the passive pain coping cycle often seen in patients with chronic pain. A comprehensive chronic pain care plan includes both passive and active coping strategies.

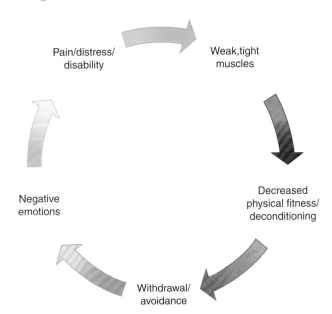

Interventions

Common CBT interventions used for chronic pain are listed in Table 27-1.

Goal Setting

Goal setting is an integral part of CBT-CP. Setting well-developed, individualized goals helps patients engage in treatment and providers tailor pain care plans and interventions. Goals should be specific and behavioral and avoid vagueness or focusing on pain score reductions. Although reductions in pain scores can be a by-product of CBT-CP, the primary objectives in CBT-CP are to increase pain self-management skills and to improve functioning and quality of life. Pain scores are not always reliable or accurate measures of functioning on their own. When setting goals, it is helpful to use the SMART goal model[21]:

S—Specific
M—Measurable
A—Achievable
R—Relevant and personally meaningful
T—Time bound

Providers can elicit SMART goals by asking questions such as, "How do you know if you are meeting your goal?" "What would that look like?" "What would you like to get back to or be doing more of if your pain were better managed?" An example of a SMART goal is "I will walk for ten minutes every morning for the next two weeks." As patients meet their goals, they build confidence in their abilities to engage in important activities and ultimately develop more substantial goals. If patients are unable to meet goals, it provides good clinical information that helps providers work with patients to problem-solve challenges and also adjust goals to reflect the patient's current level of functioning.

Relaxation Training

The stress response is a sympathetic nervous system response comprising cognitive, emotional, and physiological components, colloquially referred to as "fight or flight." Signs of the stress response are increased heart rate, shallow breathing, muscle tension, anxiety, and negative beliefs about a particular activity or situation. Chronic pain, as a chronic stressor, can result in a prolonged stress response.

Relaxation training engages the parasympathetic nervous system by targeting the physiological arousal of the stress response and working to calm the body. Relaxation techniques are a direct way to intervene and slow down or stop the stress response. There are several different types of relaxation techniques, with diaphragmatic breathing, progressive muscle relaxation, and guided imagery being the most commonly used for chronic pain. Relaxation techniques offer a direct and purposeful method for patients to experience their body and pain differently. This can be a very powerful experience for patients with chronic pain who hold the belief that they have no control over their bodies or pain. As patients become more adept at eliciting the relaxation response, they can decrease the frequency and intensity of the stress response and their reliance on passive pain management strategies.

Time-Based Pacing

Patients with chronic pain often experience frustration and distress over their reduced activity level over time. They may describe themselves as cycling through "good days and bad days" or an up and down cycle characterized by a perceived lack of control and inevitability of pain flares. The result is a profound negative impact on an individual's confidence in their ability to engage in even the most basic of activities, such as preparing meals or completing chores at home. It often leads to avoidance of activities, increased social isolation, and a higher frequency of pain flares.

Among patients with chronic pain, a common pattern of activity is that individuals will ignore early pain signals and "push through" pain until it is too intense to continue or the activity is complete. This often triggers a pain flare, which can last from hours to days. As this pattern continues to occur, the brain lowers the pain threshold for the activity in an effort to reduce the frequency of flares and stress on the body. Over time, this increased pain sensitivity results in lower amounts of activity, triggering more intense flares and a subsequent overall lower level of general activity.

Time-based pacing involves taking a thoughtful approach to activities and working "smarter not harder" by alternating periods of activity with breaks.[21]

TABLE 27-1 Common CBT Interventions Used for Chronic Pain

INTERVENTION	COMMENTS
Goal setting	Should concentrate on functional goals. Use SMART format
Relaxation training	Diaphragmatic breathing, progressive muscle relaxation, and guided imagery are most common techniques
Time-based pacing	Work "smarter not harder" by alternating periods of activity with breaks to avoid pain flares
Cognitive restructuring	Explore and challenge negative thoughts and create and generate an alternative, more balanced thought
Flare planning	Create coping plan with specific behaviors ahead of time to implement in the event of a pain flare

CBT, cognitive behavioral therapy.

Individuals create a baseline activity level calculated by identifying how long an activity takes before significant pain, and reduce that time by 20%. For example, if an individual identifies that 10 minutes of walking results in a flare, then they would walk for 8 minutes, take a break, and walk again for 8 minutes, and so on. The goal is to stay below the pain threshold. Between periods of activity, patients are asked to take breaks and engage in relaxing activities that calm the body and lower the stress response. Over time, as individuals are able to engage in more activities with a lower frequency of flares, they become less sensitive to pain. As their pain thresholds increase, periods of rest decrease and we see an overall upward trend in activity level.

Cognitive Restructuring

Identifying and challenging negative cognitions is a powerful intervention for patients with chronic pain. Negative cognitions are associated with disability, pain intensity, depression, interference with daily activities, and beliefs about one's ability to cope with pain.[16,22–24] Cognitions play an important role in motivation to engage and exert effort in treatment and perception of treatment efficacy. For example, pain catastrophizing, defined as ruminating about worst-case scenarios, has been associated with poorer physical and psychological outcomes, even when controlling for pain.[13] Although it is known that chronic pain is not simply "in the head," the beliefs that we hold about our pain and ability to cope have a significant impact on pain experience and treatment outcomes.

Cognitive restructuring is a multistep process, with the first being the identification of negative thoughts. Negative emotions often serve as reliable cues for finding such cognitions. Once the thought is identified, the second step is to explore and challenge the thought by examining facts and looking for alternative perspectives. When challenging beliefs, it is helpful to ask several different questions to better assess the accuracy and validity of the belief, such as "Is this 100% accurate?" "Is there any evidence to contradict this thought?" "Is this thought helpful or harmful to me?" The last step is to generate an alternative, or more balanced, thought. Alternative thoughts should be realistic and unbiased, offering an accurate and healthy perspective on how one interprets experiences.

Flare Planning

Pain flares are defined as times pain increases from its average intensity level to a higher level and remains at that higher level for a prolonged period of time (ranging from hours to weeks). Pain flares are a common phenomenon in chronic pain, and although many patients with pain can significantly decrease the frequency of flares through a variety of behavioral techniques, pain flares can still occur periodically. Planning ahead is essential when it comes to managing pain flares. Flare plans should utilize a variety of coping strategies from multiple categories. These may include

relaxation techniques, coping statements, distraction activities, ice or heat therapies, and gentle stretches. The purpose of the plan is to provide the patient with a variety of coping strategies for sustaining through the flare in a safe manner without inadvertently prolonging it. For many patients with pain, it is difficult to generate a plan in the midst of a flare. Preparing a flare plan builds confidence within the patient that they have the skills necessary to address a flare should it arise. Moreover, a flare plan can reduce reliance on maladaptive behaviors, such as dangerously escalating usage of opioid pain medications or using illicit drugs or alcohol to address a severe increase in pain intensity.

Case Example

Mr. S is a 46-year-old married man. He has a history of lower back pain and right knee pain. He reports his pain as insidious in onset with a worsening course over time. His primary care physician referred him after 2 surgeries were only mildly successful at reducing his pain.

He has completed a course of physical therapy with some moderate functional gains. Mr. S is currently prescribed 6 oxycodone 5 mg/325 acetaminophen per day. He manages pain with medication and rest. He reports constipation and fatigue as side effects to pain medications.

Although he was employed for many years in helicopter maintenance, he has not worked in 5 years because of his pain, which has caused his family significant financial stress. He also reports symptoms of depression.

He enjoys being active, spending time with his family, and going to church. He has not been able to go to family functions or church because he cannot sit for long periods of time and does not want to have to explain his pain to others, stating, "nobody understands."

Mr. S used to enjoy bowling, hunting, and fishing but now spends the majority of his time watching television or playing computer games. He reports that he tried going back to bowling with his friends, but after one night it left him "laid out" for 2 days.

In the following section, we outline a representative 6-session CBT-CP plan for Mr. S that incorporates active coping through these interventions.

Session 1: Assessment and Goal Setting

In session 1, the focus is on assessment and goal setting. Pain assessment includes identification of functional goals and personal values; impact of pain on physical, emotional, and interpersonal functioning; assessment of quality of life; pain coping; and lastly, assessment of diversity factors that may impact treatment. Goal setting involves modifying functional goals into SMART goals. The following is an excerpt from session 1.

Therapist: Mr. S you have shared a lot about how pain impacts your life and how you have been coping. Let me summarize to make sure I got everything. Your goals are to be more active and to improve your physical health so that you can go back to work. Spending time with your family is very important to you, but you have not been able to because the pain gets in the way, especially if you have to do anything that requires sitting or standing too long. When you try to help around the house or be more active, you end up being "laid out" for days at a time, so you spend a lot of time avoiding activities that may hurt. The pain makes you feel frustrated and depressed, which makes it hard to be around other people especially since it's stressful to explain your pain to other people. So far you found a few things to help with the pain, mainly resting, pain meds, and watching TV Does that about sum it up?

Mr. S: Yes, I think you got it all.

Therapist: Let's spend some time talking more about the goals that you had mentioned earlier. Goals help guide our treatment and give us specific behaviors to work toward. When setting goals, we use a SMART goal format. Are you familiar?

Mr. S: No, I haven't heard of that.

Therapist: SMART goals are specific, measurable, achievable, personally relevant, and on a timeline. We can set short-term goals to work on in therapy and long-term goals to work toward with the new skills you will learn. You had mentioned going back to work, walking outside, going to church, and spending time with your family. Which of these are your top priority in the short term?

Mr. S: Walking more and spending time with my family.

Therapist: Let's set one or two goals that you would like to work on in the next two weeks. We will check in on goals each week and track your progress. What would you like to start with?

Mr. S: I would like to walk more.

Therapist: Let's use the SMART goal format to help us be more specific.

Mr. S: I will walk for 10 minutes every Monday, Wednesday, and Friday for the next two weeks.

Therapist: That is a great goal. We will check in on this goal next week. We will meet for five more sessions. Each session we will check in around goals, learn a new skill, and practice relaxation exercises. I will be asking you to practice in-between sessions. We know that repetition and practice are the best ways to learn a new behavior. We can solve any challenge that comes up with new skills together.

Session 2–3: Relaxation Training and Time-Based Pacing

Session 2 focuses on providing education about the reciprocal relationship between chronic pain and stress and introducing the relaxation response and relaxation training. The following is an excerpt from session 2 with Mr. S on how to introduce relaxation techniques.

Therapist: Now that we have talked about how stress and pain are related and how we use the relaxation response to treat stress, how do you experience stress in your body?

Mr. S: Well, my muscles get tense, my pain increases, and I can feel my heart beat faster.

Therapist: How do you know you pain is increasing?

Mr. S: I start to have a sharp stabbing feeling in my back.

Therapist: Anything else you notice?

Mr. S: I hold my breath when that happens, and get stiff.

Therapist: How do you feel when this happens, and what do you do?

Mr. S: I get irritable and depressed. Normally I go to my bedroom to play video games so that I don't snap at anyone.

Therapist: And how do you know when you are feeling relaxed? What are the physical signs of relaxation for you?

Mr. S: I definitely don't hold my breath and by body feels looser.

Therapist: And what is your mood like?

Mr. S: My mood is better, I can talk to my family, and I don't worry about getting mad for no reason.

Therapist: Today we are going to learn how to purposefully elicit the relaxation response on our own. Have you performed relaxation techniques before?

Mr. S: No. I don't think it will work because I always get distracted.

Therapist: It's common to get distracted when learning a new skill. As you practice more, you will find that your ability to relax comes more easily. Today we will start with a simple five-minute deep breathing exercise. Practice your deep breathing exercises for five minutes every day. We will check in on deep breathing next week.

Session 3 introduces time-based pacing and provides rationale for "working smarter not harder." The goal of this session is to complete a pacing plan and problem-solve challenges that may arise in implementing the plan. The following is an excerpt from session 3 with Mr. S as we develop a pacing plan.

Therapist: Now that we have talked about why we use pacing to help build up activity levels and decrease pain flares, let's make a pacing plan together. What activity would you like to pace?

Mr. S: Since I can't work, I would like to help more around the house. I can try to do something like clean the floors.

Therapist: How long do you think you can clean before your pain "alarm bells" get really loud?

Mr. S: I think I could go for five minutes.

Therapist: And how much focused relaxation time do you need for your body to calm down?

Mr. S: Five minutes. But if I try to clean that way, it will take too long. I don't like to start and stop...I want to finish what I start.

continued

Therapist: Let's think about time. How long do you think it will take you to clean the floors without taking a break?

Mr. S: 30 minutes.

Therapist: And what would happen if you were to work for 30 minutes straight?

Mr. S: Well, it would get done but I would also be laid out for at least four hours.

Therapist: So without pacing, you would spend 30 minutes working and four hours resting. The total time you spend will be about four and a half hours total with a pain flare. If you pace, you will spend one hour total and you won't have a flare. Which method do you think is more consistent with your goals and values?

Sessions 4–5: Cognitive Restructuring

Cognitive restructuring is a core skill in CBT, and sessions 4 and 5 will address this. The following is an excerpt highlighting cognitive restructuring with Mr. S.

Therapist: So it sounds like when your pain increases suddenly, you have the thought "There is nothing I can do for my pain. I'll never feel better." That thought leads to feeling depressed and angry. You respond by snapping at your family and playing video games alone. Is this thought helpful or harmful in the moment?

Mr. S: I think this is a harmful thought because it makes me feel worse.

Therapist: Is your thought 100% accurate?

Mr. S: No. There are definitely things I can do about my pain.

Therapist: So we know it is harmful and not accurate. Is there any evidence against this thought?

Mr. S: Well, yeah. I know that my pain goes up and down, and that I will probably feel better in a few hours.

Therapist: Any other evidence that contradicts the belief there is nothing you can do?

Mr. S: Yes, I can practice my breathing exercises—that usually helps the pain.

Therapist: Is there another more realistic and balanced way of looking at this?

Mr. S: Well, I could tell myself that, even though I have more pain, I can practice some relaxation exercises and I know that the pain will go down again.

Therapist: How do you think you would feel if you said that to yourself instead of "There is nothing you can do and the pain will never get better."

Mr. S: I think I would feel more hopeful and definitely less stressed.

Session 6: Flare Planning

The following is an excerpt from session 6 with Mr. S as we develop a flare plan.

Therapist: Now that we have reviewed all the different skills you have learned let's spend some time making a flare plan. Why do you think it is important to make a flare plan?

Mr. S: It is a good reminder of what I can do during a flare, especially when I have thoughts like there is nothing I can do about my pain and I start to feel helpless and frustrated.

Therapist: That is a really good reason and good insight into how a pain flare can impact how you feel. Let's make a plan together. Remember, we want to have strategies that are safe and won't prolong the flare. Let's think of different types of coping techniques. Let's start with skills you have learned in therapy.

Mr. S: I can do my breathing exercises since they have been very helpful. I can also challenge negative thoughts that come up. I can tell myself that I've gotten through flares before.

Therapist: Those are great strategies. How about pacing?

Mr. S: Yes, I can pace my activities that I have to do.

Therapist: Let's think of some other strategies that can help distract you during a flare.

Mr. S: I can watch a funny movie and listen to some music. I can also use my ice packs or take a hot shower.

Therapist: Is there anyone you can talk to?

Mr. S: I can let my wife know I am in a flare so she understands that my pain is worse.

Therapist: Any other strategies?

Mr. S: I can take a walk or do some stretching.

Therapist: This is a great flare plan. Remember to write it down and keep it somewhere easily accessible so you don't have to look for it.

ACCEPTANCE AND COMMITMENT THERAPY FOR CHRONIC PAIN

ACT is considered a newer "third wave" behavioral treatment, following in the steps of its "second wave" cousin CBT. Research has demonstrated ACT's strengths in treating diverse mental health concerns, including depression, anxiety, and substance use problems.[25,26]

ACT has also proven itself with individuals struggling with chronic pain.[27] Studies of ACT demonstrated significant utility at reducing the interference of pain on an individual's functioning and well-being, exhibiting moderate effect sizes immediately post treatment and large effect sizes 2 to 6 months later.[27] In addition, ACT has shown moderate effect sizes at later follow-up for anxiety, depression, and quality of life. As ACT is focused on reducing the *interference* caused by struggling with one's pain, and not concerned directly with a reduction in pain sensation, ACT and other mindfulness-based pain interventions have unsurprisingly demonstrated only small to moderate effects on pain intensity.[28]

The ACT approach is rooted in functional contextualism, which posits that the symptom of pain is not itself a problem that can be solved; instead, it is how individuals relate to their pain and how it functions in their life, which is the cause of their difficulties.[29] Although ACT certainly views pain as an incredibly uncomfortable part of an individual's lived experience, it distinguishes the sensation of pain from the suffering that frequently comes along with its introduction.

As patients live with pain, they frequently begin to identify with rigid beliefs and rules about their experience that dominate their behavioral choices. They also frequently start making vigilant attempts to avoid pain sensations. In doing so, they inadvertently narrow the scope and scale of their lives, decreasing functioning and well-being across multiple domains. It is this process that ACT views as suffering: the struggle to "solve" the unsolvable pain—at the cost of vitality (defined as being fully engaged in one's life in the here-and-now). ACT aims to develop a more psychologically flexible approach to living with pain. Psychological flexibility is defined as an ability to remain in the present moment with awareness and openness to our experience while pursuing actions that are driven by values.[29,30] Harris further simplifies the definition as "the ability to 'be present, open up, and do what matters.'"[31] For an individual with chronic pain, this may entail being open to the experience of pain and any accompanying anxiety, fear, or frustration so that one has room to be present to their full lived experience, and can make active choices about how one lives, so as to build a life of fulfillment and meaning. This counters a narrative of psychological inflexibility, which sees individuals living in active avoidance of their pain and directed by unhelpful cognitions about their capabilities and options, such that they are rarely focused on the present experience of the world around them. From an inflexible stance, one is stuck waiting until pain resolves to build a life worth living.

ACT cultivates psychological flexibility through 6 processes: defusion, acceptance, contact with the present moment, self-as-context, values, and committed action.[29] Although each of these processes is considered a core aspect of flexibility, ACT takes a functional approach to their application. Instead of steadfast techniques for success, ACT acknowledges that at times reducing one's pain, anxiety, or distress may be a workable option toward a more thriving life, whereas at others an impediment; the aim is a flexible approach to one's internal experience such that one is free to actively choose a thriving life.

The power of ACT is that it does not require patients to decrease their pain before they begin living again. Moreover, they do not need to change their thinking to live well. Instead they are asked to change their *relationship* to their affective, cognitive, and sensory experiences so they do not dominate and direct their behavioral choices. With that new perspective they reconnect with their agency, reminding themselves they are in the driver seat and can choose the direction they drive.

ACT therapy relies heavily on experiential exercises and metaphor in building a patient's dexterity with the 6 processes. Each process overlaps and connects to the other processes in the "hexaflex"—a visual representation of the core elements of psychological flexibility.[29]

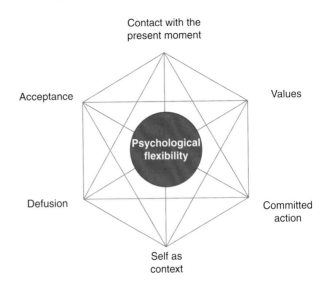

Copyright Steven C. Hayes. Used by permission.

Processes

We have outlined each of the processes to better understand their impact on patients' learning to live with their pain.

Defusion

Cognitive defusion is the process of distinguishing between one's thoughts and the content of their descriptions. Thoughts such as "my life is over with pain," "I can't work while I'm in pain," or "I cannot take a break because if I do I'm a failure" are all cognitions that one can come to believe with 100% certainty, such that they dominate behavioral choices at the cost of vitality. Defusion helps individuals see their thoughts as language created by their mind, and as a result not dictating of their actions. If they no longer take these thoughts as literal reality, they can respond to their environment based on functional and value-driven goals as opposed to those prompted by unhelpful cognitions. Although traditional CBT asks an individual to restructure the contents of their thinking, ACT disentangles the thinker from the thought content such that an individual can chose how and whether to respond based on their values.

Acceptance

Experiential acceptance aims to build an allowance of uncomfortable thoughts, feelings, memories, and somatic sensations (such as pain). Humans have a tendency toward avoiding discomfort, but if people's lives are dictated by this aim, they are frequently bound and constrained in life choices. Experiential avoidance may vary for different people in pain: some may greatly limit their activities, others may vigilantly seek cures, others may ignore their pain when they should rest, and yet others may demand increasingly powerful medications that dull their pain, cognition, and senses. When avoiding pain means loss of vitality then it becomes a problem. ACT posits that willingness to experience pain provides flexibility in choosing how one lives.

Contact With the Present Moment

When individuals spend much of their time focused on the past ("my life was so much better before my pain"), the future ("I bet next week's work trip is going to be a disaster for my pain"), or a singular aspect of their experience ("my shoulder pain is all there is"), they miss out on the present. They are so concerned about addressing and problem-solving pain-related concerns that they miss the experience of living as it is happening. ACT works to help patients expand their awareness to include their current lived experiences so they can respond to the immediate needs of their environment and make behavioral choices in line with their goals and values.

Self-As-Context

A hallmark of psychological inflexibility is the conflation of self with the content of internal experiences whether they are thoughts, feelings, memories, or sensations such as pain. When we are fused to our internal content, our behaviors can become directed by this content. In addition, we can cling to a collection of these internal experiences, what one might call a "conceptualized self," such that we begin to selectively engage the world based on these experiences. For instance, one might begin to see himself/herself as a "victim," an "invalid," or a "failure."

A more flexible stance involves seeing oneself as the context in which these internal experiences are occurring. In so doing, one can see oneself as greater than any individual cognition, emotion, memory, sensation, or concept of self. From such a stance it is easier to accept distressing internal experiences without needing to fix or avoid them. Moreover, internal experiences such as

physical pain or pain-related beliefs are no longer seen as dictating of one's actions. Finally, from such a stance one can recognize that the self is intact regardless of the ever-changing content (including pain) experiences.

Values

A consequence of an inflexible stance toward pain is that one becomes disconnected from what is important to oneself. ACT's ultimate aim is to help a person build a life worth living by choosing behaviors consistent with one's values. ACT defines values as "freely chosen, verbally constructed consequences of ongoing, dynamic, evolving patterns of activity, which establish predominant reinforcers for that activity which are intrinsic in engagement in the valued behavioral pattern itself" (Ref. 32, p. 66). This definition is best understood through an example: if one values being a loving and supportive friend, this is something that is chosen regardless of external or internal expectations such as society or guilt. Appreciating the quality of being loving with one's friends emerges from living one's life in a certain way, such that one experiences purpose and vitality while acting on that value. As such, values are not goals—goals have specific and achievable end points, whereas values are global, ongoing, and accessible through one's actions at any point. ACT treatments work to help clarify one's values, identify if one is engaging them regularly, and help patients reconnect with them in their activities and behaviors.

Committed Action

Individuals with chronic pain may resort to vitality-draining behaviors prompted by avoidance of pain, such as isolating oneself socially, misusing substances, or lashing out at others in frustration. Ultimately, living a valued life not only requires knowing what is important but also committing to enacting behaviors consistent with those values, even when pulled in other directions.

Case Example

The following case outlines an ACT approach to chronic pain over 10 sessions, specifically illustrating the use of the 6 processes.

Session 1: Creative Hopelessness

Treatment with ACT frequently begins with an intervention known as "creative hopelessness." Patients are asked to identify the strategies they have used to manage pain and the costs and benefits of each strategy in both short and long terms. The aim is to draw out the agenda of trying to control, eliminate, or avoid pain and then collaboratively evaluate the efficacy of such an approach. Frequently, individuals may find their employed strategies successful in reducing or avoiding pain in the short term, but the strategies may have negative consequences in the long term toward an individual's functioning and vitality.

By completing this process in an exhaustive manner, patients can begin to feel a sense of hopelessness that none of their efforts to eliminate their pain have worked long term; furthermore, the strategies may have contributed to functional losses or additional suffering. Indeed, patients may have jumped from one strategy to the next, putting their lives on hold until the pain is successfully eliminated or reduced. Creative hopelessness illuminates the unworkable consequences of this approach, with the aim of offering an alternative one, *acceptance* of pain, and *commitment* to a valued life with it.

Therapist: Mr. S, I would like to start off by seeing how you've been working with your pain and difficult emotions. I want to see if we can lay out what you've been using to address them, and then see how those strategies have been working for you. (Therapist pulls out creative hopelessness worksheet). Let's take a look at this worksheet. On the left I was hoping we could list all of the types of pain you experience.

CREATIVE HOPELESSNESS WORKSHEET

PAIN SENSATIONS	MANAGEMENT STRATEGY or TREATMENT	BENEFITS		COSTS	
		Short-Term	Long-Term	Short-Term	Long-Term

Mr. S: I have all sorts of pains, but mostly it's my back and knee that hurt. Sometimes it's a dull ache in my back, but it can be really sharp sometimes if I twist. The knee just gets worse throughout the day; it starts with a soreness at the beginning of the day, and by the end I can barely walk.

Therapist: Would you write those descriptions on the left side under "Pain Sensations?" Thank you. Ok, let's move to the next column. What sort of strategies have you used to manage your pain?

Mr. S: Well I use my medications.

Therapist: Ok, please add that to the second column.

Mr. S: And I try to rest when it gets really bad.

Therapist: Please add that too. Ok, what else have you tried?

Mr. S: Well I guess I tried those surgeries...but they didn't do the trick.,,, (He writes "surgeries" in the second column).

Therapist: I get the sense based on what you told me at our intake that you have also tried "pushing through" your pain, like when you went bowling that time?

Mr. S: Yeah. That didn't go so well. Sometimes I still push through it when I have to get something done.

Therapist: I guess another strategy you mentioned might be that you avoid doing things that you think might make your pain worse, so you spend most of your time on the couch watching TV or playing video games.

Mr. S: Yeah, I wouldn't have called those strategies, but I guess they are a way I try to keep my pain at bay.

Therapist: Would you please add "pushing through," "avoiding activity," and "distracting myself with TV and video games" in that second column?

Mr. S: Oh, and I tried physical therapy—that helped a bit.

Therapist: Great! Yes, put that down too. Ok, let's move to the next few columns. I want to take a step back

and look at these strategies, and evaluate their short and long-term costs and benefits in your life.

Mr. S: Ok, well I can tell you right now that the surgeries were really helpful in the short term, but the benefit didn't last in the long term. And it cost me a lot of time and money to get those done.

Therapist: Let's take each of your strategies and evaluate them that way. How about the medications?

Mr. S: Well they work in the short term to pull down my pain. And probably in the long term, although I keep needing more because they stop working after a while.

Therapist: How about the benefits and costs to your quality of life?

Mr. S: In the short term they seem to make things a bit better because the pain subsides, but they also make me tired and constipated.

Therapist: So in the long term, not the best on your quality of life? Please write that down as well. How about the strategy of staying away from others and avoiding activities by watching TV and playing video games all day?

Mr. S: Well it definitely keeps my mind off the pain.

Therapist: Ok, so in the short term it helps distract you from the pain.

Mr. S: Yeah, but in the long term it has meant my life is basically just those two things...there's not much else.

Therapist: Kind of like you are stuck with an option of either ignoring your pain or living your life?

Mr. S: Yes that's about right.

(The therapist then proceeds through the rest of the listed strategies with Mr. S.)

Therapist: It looks like you have tried a lot of things in order to get this pain under control. Although some helped in the short term, most have not remained helpful in the long-term, and they've almost all had

continued

negative effects on your ability to live a full life. The pain itself has caused problems, but the strategies you've used to try and control the pain have caused their own suffering in the end. It makes a lot of sense that you've tried to control your pain, but I think what we're seeing is that controlling pain may not be the best answer if you want to live well.

Mr. S: Yeah, but what other option do I have? I get what you are saying, but where does that leave me? Do you want me to just give up?

Therapist: Good question! I can see why you might feel that way after what we've reviewed today. I definitely don't want you to give up...but I do think we've discovered controlling your pain isn't working either. I have an alternative in mind, and would love to explore it with you next week if that would be ok?

Mr. S: I'm willing to give it a try, but honestly not sure there is anything else to try.

Therapist: Well thank you for being willing to give it a try even if you aren't sure.

Session 2–3: Acceptance

The hexaflex is a model of processes, with no prescribed order or protocol in mind. Depending on a patient's presentation and needs, one may start and progress through each of the processes in a different order. In fact, many times a therapist may work on more than one process at a time, as they are all deeply connected and can even overlap in practice.

Excerpt from session 2:

Therapist: Last week we went through a number of the strategies you have used to control your pain, and after exploring the costs and benefits, came to some conclusion that controlling your pain sometimes leaves you more focused on the very thing you are trying to avoid. In fact, trying to control it appears to have left your life extremely narrow and limited. I'd like to share a metaphor that reminds me of the situation you've found yourself in, because I think it might also provide a good way to see alternative approaches that might be more helpful.

Mr. S: Ok.

Therapist: I want you to imagine you're hosting a barbecue for the 4th of July. You have planned the barbecue for weeks and invited all your friends and family to the event. You invited friends to play live music to entertain the guests, and you also set up a sprinkler for the kids to play in. Imagine that a little way into the afternoon you hear a knock at the door, and on opening it you see Jerry the neighbor from across the street. Without being asked, he barges past you, saying "I see you're having a barbecue! You must have forgotten to send me an invitation! Good thing I figured out what was going on." He proceeds to head out to your backyard. You had actually purposefully left Jerry off the invite list because he's a bit of a challenging guy to be around: he's incredibly rude with people, is always criticizing

and gossiping about others, makes a mess of things and never picks up after himself. Mr. S, what might you do in that situation?

Mr. S: Well, I'd ask him to leave.

Therapist: At first you do try to get Jerry to leave, but Jerry simply ignores your pleas and demands.

Mr. S: Well, then I might watch him and make sure he doesn't cause problems with my guests.

Therapist: That's a reasonable option. Let's say you do try running around after Jerry to contain and manage the problems he creates. You might try to smooth over any uncomfortable moments he has with friends, or clean up the table after he leaves a mess. The problem is Jerry is so active you are likely to spend your whole party focused on managing Jerry, and you won't get to enjoy the party at all. You could also try to ignore him by keeping busy and distracting yourself at the party; you might even try to drink excessively to block him out; however, both options also leave you disengaged from your friends and family, and not really focused on enjoying your party. There is one more option...

Mr. S: Not sure I see one.

Therapist: What if you actively accepted Jerry at the party—just as he is—smelly, rude, messy, and frustrating to be around.

Mr. S: Why would anyone do that?

Therapist: I think the reason to do it would be so that you could actually be present for the party you've been looking forward to all these months; the one you spent all this energy and time planning. If you allow Jerry to simply be at the party as he is, you can focus on enjoying your time there.

Mr. S: I think your point here is that Jerry is like my pain? I don't want him, but nothing I am doing is working. It's like I'm trying to kick Jerry out or manage him all the time. You want me to find a way to be at my "party."

Therapist: Exactly! And just like with Jerry, that may mean truly accepting your pain as it is—without trying to get rid of it or control it all the time.

Once Mr. S has an idea of what acceptance might look like, the therapist takes him through some exercises aimed at identifying his pain and meeting it with a stance of acceptance.

Session 4–5: Defusion

Excerpt from session 4:

Therapist: Mr. S, I have the sense that your mind has been quite active at telling you about your pain and its role in your life.

Mr. S: Oh my mind is always going on about my pain.

Therapist: Sometimes our mind can really hook us in and boss us around a bit. One type of thought that tends to *really* hook us are the thoughts that are actually rules. I'm curious what sort of rules your mind sends you regarding your pain.

Mr. S: Rules?

Therapist: Well you mentioned one thing that sounded like a rule to me when you said you "can't speak to your friends about your pain because they wouldn't understand." When your mind brings you that thought what do you end up doing?

Mr. S: Honestly, I avoid spending time with people because I don't want them to start asking questions about my difficulty walking or standing.

Therapist: So believing that rule leads you to withdraw socially. Ok, let's think of some other rules your mind brings you. What does your mind tell you about your pain and your ability to enjoy your life?

Mr. S: Well unless my pain gets better life is going to be pretty terrible.

Therapist: When your mind shows you that thought, what do you end up doing?

Mr. S: Well first I get pretty upset, and then I end up sitting at home and watching TV all day to distract myself. Sometimes I get on the internet and start looking for new ways to treat my pain.

Therapist: So by getting hooked by those thoughts you either end up spending your day distracting yourself or searching for more answers. It doesn't sound like those thoughts lead you toward building a more full life. How often does your mind give you those thoughts?

Mr. S: Pretty frequently. My mind also tells me my pain is going to cause the end of my marriage since I can't work or take care of my kids.

Therapist: When that thought starts running the show I bet things seem pretty dire.

Mr. S: Oh yeah.

For homework the therapist asks Mr. S to log his thoughts about his pain and the emotional and behavioral consequences of buying into those thoughts. In the next session, the therapist employs a defusion exercise to help him approach his thoughts as an observer, instead of getting caught up in them.

Session 5: Contact With the Present Moment

Excerpt from session 5:

Therapist: Have you noticed what happens to your mind when you are in pain?

Mr. S: Well I don't do much of anything but focus *on* the pain when it's bad.

Therapist: Would it be fair to say your attention gets caught up in the pain so fully that everything else in your life fades into the background?

Mr. S: Oh definitely!

Therapist: When you're caught up in the pain or how it's affecting your life, how easy is it to focus on being the father or husband you want to be? Or put energy into living your life fully?

Mr. S: Next to impossible.

Therapist: It's almost like you become disconnected with what's happening in the here-and-now, as though the world narrows to this one thing. Well I'd like to introduce a process called "mindfulness" to

our work. Mindfulness is a practice of noticing what is happening in the moment. With pain we can get so caught up that we miss the moment and start making decisions for the pain instead of doing what's important to us. Mindfulness is simply practicing observing what is happening without trying to make changes to it. Would it be ok if we try an exercise to get a sense of how mindfulness works?

Mr. S: Sure.

The therapist then guides Mr. S through a mindfulness exercise, focusing first on awareness of his internal experience in the moment. The therapist asks Mr. S to observe his breathing, and then his thoughts and feelings—all with an emphasis on just watching without acting or changing in reaction to his observations. Over time the therapist may ask him to focus on his pain, learning to observe it from a position of noticing and examining without acting to change it or becoming overly attached to it. The provider then may guide Mr. S to observe the present moment of the world around him, having him focus through each of his five senses one after the other. Ultimately, there are many ways to build flexible attention to the present moment, but they almost all involve an active experiential component and regular practice.

Session 6–7: Self-As-Context

Excerpt from session 6:

Therapist: I have a sense that sometimes there is a battle going on inside of you—between the uncomfortable thoughts, feelings, and sensations and the "good" ones trying to mask, solve, fix, and beat those uncomfortable ones into submission.

Mr. S: Oh, I feel like I'm always struggling against my pain. I get upset about it all the time and then try to make myself stop being upset and move on.

Therapist: And then what happens?

Mr. S: Well usually that works for a while, and then the pain gets bad or something else upsets me and I'm back in it.

Therapist: I'd like you to imagine for a moment that your life is like a game of chess (therapist takes out a chessboard). Imagine each of the pieces represents a thought, feeling, or sensation. The silver pieces are the unsettling ones like frustrations about your pain, worries about the future, the pain sensations themselves, fatigue, and more. The gold pieces represent the positive ones like optimism, hope, excitement about seeing a friend, feeling rested, etc. They are in a game that goes on and on, one side always trying to outsmart the other side. In fact, the game never really ends. I'd like to ask an odd question...Who are *you* in this game?

Mr. S: Well I guess I'm all of those pieces!

Therapist: Which pieces in particular are you? Are you the silver ones or the gold ones?

Mr. S: Both!

Therapist: You are both sides of the battle? So you are ultimately battling yourself?

Mr. S: I guess...

Therapist: Who else might you be in this scenario?

Mr. S: The players?

Therapist: Again, I wonder which player are you? Are you playing yourself in this game? If you are both sides, couldn't you just stop playing the game? Or beat yourself by purposefully losing the negative side?

Mr. S: Hmm...good point.

Therapist: Anything else you could be in this scenario? How about the board?

Mr. S: The board?

Therapist: The board is in contact and aware of the battle, but not the battle itself. You are like an observer. If I ask you to detail the game you could do that for me right?

Mr. S: Oh yeah, that game is back and forth all day in my head.

Therapist: So the board is greater than any individual piece, move, or play on the board; it can watch the whole thing. Also notice that the board can move around regardless of the current status of the game going on (moves the board up and down and forward and back). The other thing about the board is that it is remains solid, no matter what happens with the pieces. It can experience them without being them or being directed by them.

Mr. S: I can see that being the board is kind of freeing.

Therapist: It can be useful to live from the place of being the board. I call this the "observer self." The observer self can notice and make contact with all the difficult thoughts, feelings, and sensations that present themselves—like your worries, frustrations, and pain sensations...but there's a "you" who's bigger than any one of them (points to board), that is whole and solid, and able to make decisions independent of the game.

Mr. S: Are you saying I'm not my pain or my feelings?

Therapist: I'm saying there's a "you" who's greater than any individual pain or feeling, who is able to notice them and describe them. And that "you" is not beholden to them.

In session 7 the therapist moves from the chessboard metaphor to experiential exercises that aim to help Mr. S view his internal experience from the perspective of the board ("the observing self") and experience the freedom and agency such a perspective provides.

Session 8–9: Values Clarification

Excerpt from session 8:

Therapist: One of the things you've mentioned that has happened in your chronic pain experience is that you've found yourself quite checked out of your life. You've also said that it can be hard to even know what you want from your life now that you are managing chronic pain. I have an exercise that can sometimes be useful at getting down to basics...figuring out what is important to you at a fundamental level. If you're up for it maybe we can go through that exercise in a minute?

Mr. S: Fine by me.

Therapist: Excellent. What I'm aiming for here is determining what you value. I see values like directions on a compass. If you decide to use a compass to head north, you never reach a place that *is* north. Instead, you can always head north from any point just like you can always head your life in the direction of a value at any point. On the other hand, goals are like needing to ford a stream or scale a wall to head north. Goals have end points—once you've scaled the wall the goal has been accomplished. What directions for your life are important in your relationships, your work, your leisure time, etc.? What values are your *north*?

Mr. S: I see what you mean by values, but I'm not sure what *I* value.

The therapist then walks Mr. S through an exercise aimed at clarifying his personal values. Once identified, the therapist helps the patient assess how fully he is living each of his values with his chronic pain. Those values he finds himself distant from in his actions are those that the therapist will target in the remaining appointments.

Session 9–10: Committed Action

Excerpt from session 9:

Therapist: Remember how you identified a number of values that you find important but have had difficulty living day-to-day with your pain?

Mr. S: Yes.

Therapist: One of those that you described was being loving with your family. I wonder if you'd be willing to commit to choosing that valued direction this next week a bit in your actions?

Mr. S: I'd love to, and I try, but my pain just gets in the way sometimes.

Therapist: Ahh...notice how the mind is sending you reasons why you can't commit to living the way you want to live.

Mr. S: Oh yeah, there's my mind again.

Therapist: Would you mind taking a second and just noticing and labeling your thought as a thought.

Mr. S: Yeah I'm letting it "run my show" a bit...

The therapist briefly repeats a defusion exercise with patient on this interfering thought.

Therapist: Now that you're back in charge of your life, would you be willing to commit to being more loving with your family this week?

Mr. S: Yes.

Therapist: What one or two specific things could you do this week that would be in line with this value?

Mr. S: I could give my kids and wife hugs and tell them I love them more.

Therapist: Great idea! When could you do that?

Mr. S: Maybe in the evening when each of them comes home from school or work.

Therapist: I love this idea. How often would you think is realistic to do this?

Mr. S: Oh I could definitely try it nightly.

Therapist: I wonder if you'd be willing to commit to doing this—as opposed to simply *trying* to do it?

Mr. S: I'd be willing.

Therapist: Excellent! Sometimes it can help to almost formally commit in these situations—give it the gravitas it deserves. Would you mind standing and looking me in the eye and speaking your commitment out loud?

Mr. S: Sure, but that's a little weird?

Therapist: Exactly—because it's a little out of the ordinary it's likely to make an impression!

Mr. S: (Stands, looks therapist in the eye) I commit to give my kids and wife a hug and tell them I love them each night when I get home.

The next session is then used to review Mr. S's progress with enacting his value-consistent goal. If he had difficulties, it is likely because of fusion, experiential avoidance, or choosing an action that is not consistent with his values. The therapist would then help him, using previously explored processes to address these challenges and try again.

FUTURE DIRECTIONS IN PRIMARY CARE

Research findings over the past 30 years have established the general efficacy of CBT-CP. A new body of research is emerging in the integration of CBT-CP into primary care with promising initial findings. Lamb et al.[33] completed a randomized control trial in which they trained a variety of health providers in CBT-CP. Significant differences were found at 12-month follow-up between CBT and control groups in regard to pain intensity and quality of life. Trafton et al.[34] compared 12 weeks of CBT-CP and TAU in public HIV primary care clinics. Trafton and colleagues also found participation in CBT-CP in primary care was significantly associated with lower pain intensity scores, decreased anxiety, and improved pain-related functioning. Although these initial studies are promising, future research is needed to evaluate whether treatment can generalize to a variety of pain conditions and if there is a specific effective dose of CBT-CP in primary care and to identify underlying mechanisms of change in CBT-CP.

As with other psychological treatments, primary care adaptations for ACT are also fairly new. There is little research yet on adjusting such treatments for the briefer, condensed frame of such settings. That said, investigative and pilot studies have shown promise, both transdiagnostically[35] and specifically with pain.[36,37]

CONCLUSION

Chronic pain is an incredibly difficult and overwhelming experience. Indeed, the lived experience of chronic pain is much more than a sensory phenomenon as it is intimately influenced by and influencing of one's psychosocial well-being.

It is not surprising that many individuals work vigilantly to try and cure or greatly reduce their pain. Although such an approach makes logical sense, our current medical options cannot always produce the desired results or do so in a safe, consistent, or side-effect-free manner. Psychology has worked to address this reality by making its primary focus on decreasing pain interference, improving functioning, and building self-efficacy, encouraging patients to start rebuilding their lives without first needing to defeat their pain. As a result, adding psychological interventions to a patient's treatment plan can prove incredibly helpful to their recovery.

REFERENCES

1. Institute of Medicine (IOM). *Relieving Pain in America: A Blueprint for Transforming Prevention, Care, Education, and Research.* Washington, DC: The National Academies Press; 2011

2. Lovejoy TI, Dobscha SK, Cavanagh R, et al. Chronic pain treatment and health service utilization of veterans with hepatitis C virus infection. *Pain Med.* 2012;13:1407-1416.

3. Campbell LC, Clauw DJ, Keefe FJ. Persistent pain and depression: a biopsychosocial perspective. *Biol Psychiatry.* 2003;54:399-409.

4. Dersh J, Polatin PB, Gatchel RJ. Chronic pain and psychopathology: research findings and theoretical considerations. *Psychosom Med.* 2002;64:773-786.

5. Fishbain DA, Cutler R, Rosomoff HL, et al. Chronic pain-associated depression: antecedent or consequence of chronic pain? A review. *Clin J Pain.* 1997;13(2):116-137.

6. McWilliams LA, Cox BJ, Enns MW. (2003). Mood and anxiety disorders associated with chronic pain: an examination in a nationally representative sample. *Pain.* 2003;106:127-133.

7. Gatchel RJ, Peng YB, Peters ML, et al. The biopsychosocial approach to chronic pain: scientific advances and future directions. *Psychol Bull.* 2007;33(4):581-624.

8. Turk DC, Okifuji A. Psychological factors in chronic pain: evolution and revolution. *J Consult Clin Psychol.* 2002;70(3):678-690.

9. Morasco BJ, Lovejoy TI, Turk DC, et al. Biopsychosocial factors associated with pain in Veterans with the hepatitis C virus. *J Behav Med.* 2014;37:902-911.

10. Hoffman SG, Asnaani A, Vonk IJJ, et al. The efficacy of cognitive behavioral therapy: a review of meta-analyses. *Cognit Ther Res.* 2012;36:427-440.

11. Hoffman BM, Papas RK, Chatkoff DK, et al. Meta-analysis of psychological interventions for chronic low back pain. *Health Psychol.* 2007;26(1):1-9.

12. Glombiewski JA, Sawyer AT, Guttermann J, et al. Psychological treatments for fibromyalgia: a meta-analysis. *Pain.* 2010;151:280-295.

13. Ehde DM, Dillworth TM, Turner JA. Cognitive-behavioral therapy for individuals with chronic pain: efficacy, innovations, and directions for research. *Am Psychol.* 2014;69(2):153-166.

14. Williams AC, Eccleston C, Morely S. Psychological therapies for the management of chronic pain (excluding headache) in adults (review). *Cochrane Database Syst Rev.* 2012;11:1-109.

15. Gatchel RJ, Rollings KH. Evidence-informed management of chronic low back pain with cognitive behavioral therapy. *Spine J.* 2008;8(1):40-44.

16. Grant LD, Havercamp BE. A cognitive-behavioral approach to chronic pain management. *J Couns Dev.* 1995;74:25-32.

17. Turner JA, Ersek M, Kemp C. Self-efficacy for managing pain is associated with disability, depression, and pain coping among retirement community residents with chronic pain. *J Pain.* 2005;6(7):471-479.

18. Ramond A, Bouton C, Richard I, et al. Psychosocial risk factors for chronic low back pain in primary care—a systematic review. *Fam Pract.* 2011;28:12-21.

19. Barry LC, Kerns RD, Guo Z, et al. Identification of strategies used to cope with chronic pain in older persons receiving primary care from a veterans affairs medical center. *J Am Geriatr Soc.* 2004;52(6):950-956.

20. Peppin J, Cheatle MD, Kirsh KL, et al. The complexity model: a novel approach to improve chronic pain care. *Pain Med.* 2015;16:653-666.

21. Murphy JL, McKellar J, Raffa SD, et al. *Cognitive Behavioral Therapy for Chronic Pain Among Veterans: Therapist Manual.* Washington, DC: U.S. Department of Veterans Affairs; 2015.

22. Jensen MP, Turner JA, Romano JM. Changes in beliefs, catastrophizing, and coping are associated with improvement in multidisciplinary pain treatment. *J Consult Clin Psychol.* 2001;69(4):655-662.

23. Jensen MP, Turner JA, Romano JM, et al. Coping with chronic pain: a critical review of the literature. *Pain.* 1991;47:249-283.

24. De Rooij A, de Boer MR, Van der Leeden M, et al. Cognitive mechanisms of change in multidisciplinary treatment of patients with chronic widespread pain: a prospective cohort study. *J Rehabil Med.* 2014;46:173-180.

25. Lee EB, An W, Levin ME, Twohig MP. An initial meta-analysis of acceptance and commitment therapy for treating substance use disorders. *Drug Alcohol Depend.* 2015;155:1-7.

26. A-Tjak JGL, Davis ML, Morina N, et al. A meta-analysis of the efficacy of acceptance and commitment therapy for clinically relevant mental and physical health problems. *Psychother Psychosom.* 2015;84:30-36.

27. Veehof MM, Trompetter HR, Bohlmeijer ET, Schreurs KMG. Acceptance- and mindfulness-based interventions for the treatment of chronic pain: a meta-analytic review. *Cogn Behav Ther.* 2016;45(1):5-31.

28. Reiner K, Tibi L, Lipsitz JD. Do mindfulness-based interventions reduced pain intensity? A critical review of literature. *Pain Med.* 2013;14:230-242.

29. Hayes SC, Strosahl KD, Wilson KG. *Acceptance and Commitment Therapy: The Process and Practice of Mindful Change.* New York, NY: The Guilford Press; 2012.

30. McCracken LM, Morley S. The psychological flexibility model: a basis for integration and progress in psychological approaches to chronic pain management. *J Pain.* 2014;15(3):221-234.

31. Harris R. *ACT Made Simple.* Oakland, CA: New Harbinger Publications; 2009.

32. Wilson KG, Dufrene T. *Mindfulness for Two: An Acceptance and Commitment Therapy Approach to Mindfulness in Psychotherapy.* Oakland, CA: New Harbinger; 2009.

33. Lamb SE, Hansen Z, Lall R, et al. Group cognitive behavioural treatment for low-back pain in primary care: a randomised controlled trial and cost-effectiveness analysis. *Lancet.* 2010;375:916-923.

34. Trafton JA, Sorrell JT, Holodniy M, et al. Outcomes associated with a cognitive-behavioral chronic pain management program implemented in three public HIV primary care clinics. *J Behav Health Serv Res.* 2012;39(2):158-173.

35. Glover NG, Sylvers PD, Shearer EM, et al. The efficacy of focused acceptance and commitment therapy in VA primary care. *Psychol Serv.* 2016;13(2):156-161.

36. McCracken LM, Sato A, Taylor GJ. A trial of brief group-based form of acceptance and commitment therapy (ACT) for chronic pain in general practice: pilot outcome and process results. *J Pain.* 2013;14(11):1398-1406.

37. Wetherell JL, Afari N, Rutledge T, et al. A randomized, controlled trial of acceptance and commitment therapy and cognitive-behavioral therapy for chronic pain. *Pain.* 2011;152:2098-2107.

28

BIOFEEDBACK APPLICATIONS FOR THE MANAGEMENT OF MEDICAL, PSYCHIATRIC, AND NEUROCOGNITIVE CONDITIONS IN THE PRIMARY CARE SETTING

Amir Ramezani, PhD, Mark Johnson, PhD,
Christopher Gilbert, PhD and Ravi Prasad, MD

FAST FACTS

- Biofeedback is the process by which an individual's physiological activity, such as muscle tension or brain activity, is presented to the individual in the form of a computerized game, graphic, auditory, tactile, or visual display in real time.
- In chronic conditions, biofeedback training can increase patients' sense of control over their condition, instilling greater confidence in their ability to self-regulate and gain better control over their symptoms.

- Cognitive-, mindfulness-, compassion-, and acceptance-based therapies teach individuals skills to develop healthy, realistic, value-based and compassionate ways of mentally relating to their pain.

INTRODUCTION

Biofeedback is one of the longest established, nonpharmacological treatments available since the 1960s. Biofeedback makes invisible stress-related physiological activity visible.[1] With advances in wireless technology and wearable devices, biofeedback has become easier to implement in a fast-paced environment, such as the primary care setting.

Biofeedback is the process by which an individual's physiological activity, such as muscle tension or brain activity, is presented to the individual in the form of a computerized game, graphic, auditory, tactile, or visual display in real time. This process helps the individual to "see" their body's activity, moment-to-moment, to learn how to change their physiological activities through trial-and-error learning (e.g., operant conditioning). This leads to increased self-regulation of the physiological activity that is being recorded[2] and "fed back" to the individual. This leads to better self-management of medical and psychiatric conditions.

Leading biofeedback, psychophysiology, and neuroscience organizations representing the field of biofeedback have developed the following standard definition:

"Biofeedback is a process that enables an individual to learn how to change physiological activity for the purposes of improving health and performance. Precise instruments measure physiological activity such as brainwaves, heart function, breathing, muscle activity, and skin temperature. These instruments rapidly and accurately 'feed back' information to the user. The presentation of this information—often in conjunction with changes in thinking, emotions, and behavior—supports desired physiological changes. Over time, these changes can endure without continued use of an instrument"[3] (Association for Applied Psychophysiology and Biofeedback [AAPB], Biofeedback Certification International Alliance [BCIA], International Society for Neurofeedback and Research [ISNR]).

This chapter discusses the significance of biofeedback for pain management and comorbid psychological and emotional conditions; the importance of integrating biofeedback treatment with adjunctive psychological modalities; restoration of functional impairment to improve activities of daily living/quality of life, and a summary of the research and evidential support for the application of biofeedback for pain. Case approach methods/protocols will also be presented to demonstrate practical applications in a primary care environment.

BIOFEEDBACK APPLICATIONS

Yucha and Montgomery (2008) outlined the criteria for levels of efficacy of psychophysiological interventions[4] and categorized them as "not empirically supported" (level 1), "possibly efficacious" (level 2), "probably efficacious" (level 3), "efficacious" (level 4), and "efficacious and specific" (level 5).[4] The term "efficacy levels" refers to outcome studies with higher standards of research (e.g., randomization, placebo/sham control groups). It should be noted that a categorical rating of less than efficacious does not necessarily mean the intervention is not effective, but rather that there may be insufficient evidence to make such a determination at the time.[5] See Table 28-1 for a list of evidence-based applications of biofeedback.

Primary care medical settings have great potential for biofeedback given that many patients in these settings have poorly understood conditions.[6] Patients who over-utilize health services are sometimes labeled as "difficult" or psychosomatic. Newer diagnoses have reconceptualized medically unexplained disorders as functional disorders that include fibromyalgia, chronic fatigue syndrome, irritable bowel syndrome, chemical sensitivity, chronic pain disorder, and anxiety with somatic symptoms.[6] These disorders are also gradually being remedicalized as central sensitivity syndromes and autonomic dysregulation syndromes (i.e., disorders of the central and peripheral nervous system where persistent pain and other overlapping symptoms are prominent features) in which biofeedback has good potential to effect autonomic and central response and treat these symptoms.

COST-EFFECTIVENESS

Behavioral treatments such as biofeedback are front-loaded. After a number of initial self-regulation training sessions, treatment benefits last for years. For example,

---

TABLE 28-1 Evidence-Based Applications of Biofeedback[4,30]

Comorbid Physical and Psychiatric Condition in Pain *(Efficacy levels 4 and 5)*

- Fecal incontinence (balloon manometer, rectal EMG, ultrasound sensor)
- Erectile dysfunction (pelvic floor EMG)
- Attention and attention deficit disorders (ADHD) (EEG)
- Major depressive disorder (EEG: alpha asymmetry, fMRI upregulation, HRV)
- Epileptic seizures: (EEG: sensorimotor rhythm, slow cortical potential)
- Glycemic control (forehead EMG, hand temperature)
- Anxiety disorders (EMG, HRV, breathing)
- Essential hypertension—including preeclampsia (thermal, breathing, HRV)
- Raynaud's disease (thermal)

Pain Primarily *(efficacy levels 3, 4, and 5)*

- Adult and pediatric headache, migraine and tension-type (EEG, EMG, thermal, BVP)
- Pain related to the following (fMRI, EEG, EMG, breathing, HRV):
  Level 4: jaw and facial pain, noncardiac chest pain, posture-related pain, chronic and experimentally induced pain;
  Level 3: low-back, pelvic, phantom limb, patellofemoral, cancer pain
- Irritable bowel syndrome (HRV)
- TMJ dysfunction (EMG, hand temperature)
- Arthritis (EMG, breathing, thermal, GSR)
- Fibromyalgia (EMG)

Note: BVP, blood volume pulse; EEG, electroencephalography; EMG, electromyography; fMRI, functional magnetic resonance imaging; HRV, heart rate variability; GSR, galvanic skin response.
Clinical judgment should be exercised when making decision and may override the above suggestions.

---

in the management of chronic headaches, over the course of a one-year period of treatment, minimal contact treatment (i.e., training in biofeedback with home practice) cost $500 less than pharmacological treatment.[7] Biofeedback is considered a cost-effective treatment for reducing symptoms and symptom severity of irritable bowel syndrome[8,9] and for reducing stress, anxiety and depression.[10,11] A review of multicomponent behavioral medicine studies in the treatment of psychosomatic illness and pain suggested that biofeedback and relaxation training were cost-effective in the majority of dimensions of healthcare costs including reductions in physician visits and/or use of medication, reduced medical costs to patients, reduced hospital stays and/or rehospitalizations, reduced mortality, and enhanced quality of life.[12]

Although biofeedback is cost-effective for a number of disorders, access to services is often a barrier. Reimbursement for biofeedback is inconsistent and unpredictable. It is recommended that a consultation with a board-certified biofeedback specialist be undertaken to appropriately bill services (e.g., CPT codes for medical coverage include health and behavior codes while mental health coverage has stand-alone biofeedback and biofeedback and therapy procedures codes).

REASONS FOR REFERRAL AND ASSESSING SUITABILITY

Patients in primary care settings may be referred for biofeedback as an alternative or adjunctive treatment for a variety of presenting issues. Reasons for referral may include a lack of positive response to current treatment, disinterest in medication, pharmaceutical contraindication (e.g., pregnancy, breast-feeding), or stress being a major component of the patient's presentation.[13] In chronic conditions, biofeedback training can increase patients' sense of control over their condition, instilling greater confidence in their ability to self-regulate and gain better control over their symptoms. Before initiating biofeedback or psychophysiological monitoring/training or a referral, it is important to recognize clear contraindications and to determine if the individual is a suitable biofeedback candidate (see Table 28-2).

STAGES OF TRAINING

There are four general stages of training (see Figure 28-1). These include

1. Education: providing the patient with education on biofeedback, the stress-response, hyper- or hypoarousal states, self-regulation of physiological functioning, sensor placement, and devices used for nondiagnostic and training purposes to name a few;
2. Psychophysiological assessment (PPA): assessing cognitive and emotional influence on physiological activities;
3. Biofeedback training: tailoring the training to the PPA, practicing cognitive/behavioral skills, and practicing mastery of body attunement and self-regulation; and
4. Generalization training: turning off the feedback or any other assistance and allowing the individual to self-regulate.

The PPA is carefully administered in a controlled environment. This allows the practitioner to clearly identify multiple cognitive, affective, and physical factors that affect arousal. This procedure also serves as an intervention.[14]

The PPA has multiple dimensions, but there are four primary aspects of the PPA phases to which we will limit discussion to the following: prebaseline phase, anticipatory phase, stressors/performance phase, and postbaseline phase.[15,16] These phases help to determine how the person's physiology is responding and coping when there is a disruption (e.g., stressor or task to be performed) to his/her nervous system's homeostasis. Table 28-3 lists the different types of response that can be assessed during these phases.

At the heart of the PPA is the ability to assess, analyze, and determine influences of physiological change in real time with the individual and link this to the cognitive, emotional, and sensory aspects of the chronic pain condition. This initial assessment helps determine what additional behavioral interventions may be warranted as adjunctive treatment.

TABLE 28-2 Candidacy for Biofeedback Training
Good Candidate

- Muscle tension associated with pain
- Head, jaw, neck, shoulder, and back pain.
- Peripheral neuropathy or complex regional pain syndrome
- Peripheral limb temperature changes
- Increased arousal or physiological reactivity impacting pain (e.g., stress, hypervigilance, or anxiety worsening pain)
- Patient wants to learn pain-coping skills
- Urinary incontinence
- Pelvic floor muscle problems
- Attention, executive function, or mild-moderate cognitive problems

Fair or Not a Good Candidate

- Severe mental health conditions:
  - Psychotic disorders, personality disorders, factitious disorders, illness anxiety (hypochondriasis), malingering
  - Severe and active substance use, bipolar, and obsessive compulsive disorder
- Individuals with illness anxiety (hypochondriasis) and functional neurological syndrome (conversion disorders) should avoid physiological monitoring devices/biofeedback to prevent reinforcing the belief that their somatic presentation has a biological basis.
- Dermatological conditions (allergic reactions) to medical tape (e.g., eczema, dermatitis)
- Allergy to the electrode or contact material (medical tape/gel)
- Patients who are unable to understand or respond to the instructions of the therapist (e.g., delirium or severe dementia)
- Epilepsy (patients may experience an adverse response to the visual display of flashing lights or computer screen).

Note: psychological evaluation is helpful to make the above determination particular as some situations may not neatly fit in the above suggestions.
Clinical judgment should be exercised when making decision and may override the above suggestions.

BEHAVIORAL INTERVENTIONS

Cognitive Behavioral Therapy and Biofeedback

Chronic pain conditions vary considerably in presentation: some are characterized by episodic flare-ups with pain-free periods in between, whereas others are marked by constant baseline pain with acute exacerbations. One commonality across all chronic pain conditions is the lack of a definitive end point; thus, treatment paradigms typically emphasize management principles rather than a focus on finding a cure. Regardless of the etiology of such chronic conditions, behaviors (e.g., sleep habits, substance use, activity patterns, etc.), and emotional states (e.g., depression, anxiety, anger, etc.) can directly and indirectly affect the overall physiological reactivity and sensory experience of pain. Helping individuals understand the interrelationships among these factors and how to modify them to achieve positive outcomes lies at the core of cognitive–behavioral approaches to pain management.

Cognitive behavioral therapies (CBT) involve teaching individuals strategies and techniques that specifically address maladaptive thoughts and behaviors that perpetuate pain conditions. It has demonstrated efficacy in addressing disability, altering mood, and catastrophizing

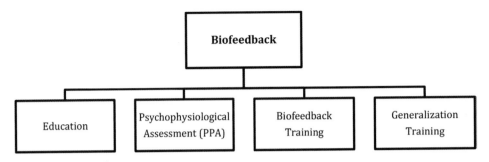

FIGURE 28-1 Four stages of biofeedback training. From Khazan IZ. *The Clinical Handbook of Biofeedback: A Step-by-Step Guide for Training and Practice with Mindfulness.* Malden, MA: John Wiley and Son; 2013 and Arena M, Schwartz M. *Psychophysiological Assessment and Biofeedback: A Primer.* In: Schwartz M, Andrasik F. New York, NY: Guilford Press; 2003.

TABLE 28-3 Psychophysiological Assessment[14,15]	
PHYSIOLOGICAL PRINCIPLES	**RESPONSE**
Autonomic imbalance	Dysregulation or imbalance of the sympathetic and parasympathetic nervous systems
Stimulus response specificity	Does the task or stressor produce the expected response? Is there flexibility in the system (e.g., reasonable return to baseline functioning following a stressor)?
Individual response stereotype	What unique or paradoxical responses are present during a task or stressor?
Homeostasis time	The length of time it takes to return to the prestimulus baseline. Is the patient affected by negative feedback to return to balance or positive feedback to increase or maintain vigilance?
Recovery	Is there a return to first baseline. For example, is there a return to 5% of EMG and temperature. Heart rate within 2 bmp

EMG, electromyography.

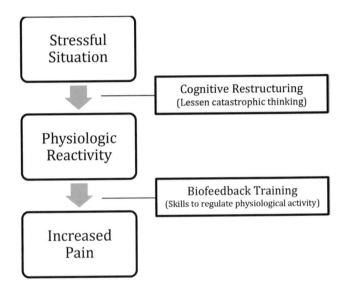

FIGURE 28-2 Combined cognitive behavioral therapy and biofeedback.

situation-specific and future-oriented potential negative outcomes and can alter the brain's responses to repeated pain exposure.[17-20] CBT can be combined with biofeedback in a multimodal nonpharmacologic approach to managing pain that addresses both immediate and longer term outcomes. Biofeedback training can help individuals become aware of, and regulate, physiological responses to emotionally threatening yet physically benign stimuli in real time and thereby minimize any impact that the arousal would have on the sensory experience of pain. CBT strategies specifically target the cognitive appraisals that initially lead to the physiologic reactivity. The end goal of CBT and biofeedback training would be that the same inciting stressor no longer creates the same physiological response pattern (Figure 28-2). This ultimately translates to less physiological and psychological reactivity in response to pain and stress, which can improve flare-ups and constant baseline pain.

Mindfulness, Compassion, and Acceptance

Primary care providers can benefit from having familiarity with mindfulness and acceptance-based approaches. The practices of mindfulness, compassion, and acceptance aim to bring attention to sensations, emotions, and thoughts in a curious, nonjudgmental, and kind way. This attitude is an antidote to "fight-off pain" or to change the pain.[21] Studies support the practice of mindfulness to improve anxiety and depression, stress-related disorders, and acute and chronic pain conditions.[21,22] Training in mindfulness and acceptance both aim to expand psychological flexibility to include increased openness, awareness, and ability to change attention and attitudes.[21]

Biofeedback training is complementary to these goals and allows the body's response to mindfulness and acceptance practice to be seen and learned. These complementary goals include learning to monitor body variables such as breathing, muscle tension, and heart rate. To master or become attuned to such physical reactions, the individual needs to be in a state of openness to ongoing fluctuations and changes. Trying too hard to control such things usually activates the sympathetic nervous system therefore increasing arousal and emotionality. Noting sensations but remaining attuned, accepting, and even cultivating curiosity will produce a more calming autonomic balance. Learning and using biofeedback helps one to remain nonreactive to disruptions, including pain, and the success in this mental maneuver is rendered visible through the displayed biofeedback signals.

Other Behavioral Skills

In addition to the application of mindfulness, acceptance, and CBT skills as adjunctive interventions to biofeedback, a multitude of other interventions have also yielded beneficial results to improve physical functioning and pain.[23,24] These applications include the following:

- Postural adjustment during electromyography (EMG) biofeedback
- Autogenic training to increase skin temperature
- Progressive muscle relaxation to reduce EMG biofeedback
- Breathing retraining for heart rate variability (HRV) and respiration
- Mindful attunement of physiological response and sensations related to pain
- Body scan to reduce arousal and muscle tension
- Home practice devices
- Exposure therapy–based protocols
- Generalization: Practicing self-regulation and skills in different environments

PROTOCOLS FOR BACK, NECK, SHOULDER, AND HEAD PAIN

It can be helpful for providers to review a sample of a case involving myofascial pain conditions. Regarding back pain, lumbar paraspinal muscles can be monitored with surface EMG to develop a more accurate awareness of muscle tension with behavioral interventions. With respect to managing neck and head pain, several biofeedback modalities (electroencephalography [EEG], EMG, thermal, slow cortical potential [SCP], hemoencephalograghy [HEG]) are used in children and adults, and studies have shown effective results, particularly when biofeedback is combined with other methods such as behavioral changes and tracking of headache triggers.[25-27] Please see following for a list of biofeedback protocols and adjunctive interventions:

Using Electromyography and Thermal

- Assess and improve habitual posture, jaw, upper trapezius, masseter, forehead, and neck muscles tension when in normal versus emotional tension
- Reduce fear of movement with CBT, posture adjustment, and mindful movements[29]
- Increasing accurate muscle tension awareness and discrimination of muscle relaxation[28]
- Use visual and auditory feedback to discriminate muscle tension and correlate felt negative emotions with tension and pain

- Mindful awareness of local muscle bracing and relaxing muscles via progressive muscle relaxation
- Decreasing muscle tension via behavioral relaxation strategies
- Spikes of arousal or muscle tension in a relaxation baseline may suggest that the patient experienced an unhelpful thought that increases arousal. The clinician can use real-time CBT skills to help the patient recognize unhelpful thinking and the influence on their body. The clinician can further teach the patient to see what their body's arousal would look like if they had more helpful and adaptive thinking in real-time
- Visual and audio feedback along with hand-warming imagery, recall of relaxing memories, mindfulness, and slowed breathing, while watching for an increase in finger/hand temperature
- Hand-warming homework practice

TRAINING AND QUALIFICATIONS

Given that there are clinical and nonclinical applications of biofeedback (e.g., athletic performance, peak performance, rehabilitation, stress management, coaching, psychiatric treatment, and cognitive and physical training), a variety of professionals (e.g., psychologists, physical therapists, counselors, physicians, nonlicensed professionals, researchers, bioengineers, educators) practice biofeedback. As a result, biofeedback education and training standards have been developed and accepted upon by national and international psychophysiology and neuroscience associations.

The Biofeedback Certification International Alliance (BCIA) sets and promotes specific standards of education and training to establish entry-level qualifications for practitioners who seek to provide biofeedback training. The guidelines and standards are intended to protect the consumer and the provider by asserting the knowledge and experience level needed for entry-level competence. Individuals who practice biofeedback in a primary care setting may wish to consult the BCIA (www.bcia.org) to optimize their practice and to adhere to training guidelines.[30] Finally, when choosing equipment, consult with biofeedback or psychophysiology specialists first to avoid nonconforming or pseudoscientific devices.

SUMMARY

Biofeedback training is an established nonpharmacological approach that translates invisible psychophysiological activity into observable and teachable activity. The advent of newer and affordable technologies has increased its cost-effectiveness and accessibility for clinical and nonclinical applications toward the prevention and treatment of a variety of neuromusculoskeletal disorders, co-occurring mood disorders, and disorders associated with autonomic dysregulation and/or central sensitization. Criteria for levels of clinical-based efficacy of psychophysiological interventions are available to guide practitioners in their use of evidence-based, or evidence-informed, applications. Trained and qualified biofeedback practitioners should assess suitability and contraindications, guide patients through stages of training, and incorporate concomitant cognitive/behavioral interventions as indicated and applicable.

REFERENCES

1. Harvey R, Pepper E. I thought I was relaxed: the use of SEMG biofeedback for training awareness and control. In: Edmonds , Tenenbaum G, eds. *Case Studies in Applied Psychophysiology: Neurofeedback and Biofeedback Treatments for Advances in Human Performance*. West Sussex, UK: Wiley-Blackwell; 2012:144-159.

2. Schwartz N, Schwartz M. *Definition of Biofeedback and Applied Psychophysiology*. In: Schwartz M, Andrasik F, eds. New York, NY: Guilford Press; 2003.

3. Association for Applied Psychophysiology and Biofeedback. Retrieved from the World Wide Web on 31 March 2017. www.AAPB.org.

4. Yucha C, Montgomery D. *Evidence-Based Practice in Biofeedback and Neurofeedback*. Wheat Ridge: Association for Applied Psychophysiology and Biofeedback; 2008.

5. Bohart AC. Evidence-based psychotherapy means evidence-informed, not evidence-driven. *J Contemp Psychother*. 2005;35:39. doi:10.1007/s10879-005-0802-8.

6. Gevirtz R. Applied psychophysiology/biofeedback in primary care medicine. *Biofeedback*. 2006;34(4):145-147.

7. Schafer AM, Rains JC, Penzien DB, Groban L, Smitherman TA, Houle TT. Direct costs of preventive headache treatments: comparison of behavioral and pharmacologic approaches. *Headache*. 2011;51(6):985-991. doi:10.1111/j.1526-4610.2011.01905.x.

8. Dobbin A, Dobbin J, Ross SC, Graham C, Ford MJ. Randomised controlled trial of brief intervention with biofeedback and hypnotherapy in patients with refractory irritable bowel syndrome. *J R Coll Physicians Edinb*. 2013;43:15-23.

9. Leahy A, Epstein O. Non-pharmacological treatments in the irritable bowel syndrome. *World J Gastroenterol*. 2001;7(3):313-316. doi:10.3748/wjg.v7.i3.313.

10. Ratanasiripong P, Kaewboonchoo O, Ratanasiripong N, Hanklang S, Chumchai P. Biofeedback intervention for stress, anxiety, and depression among graduate students in public health nursing. *Nurs Res Pract*. 2015.

11. Ratanasiripong P, Sverduk K, Hayashino D, Prince J. Setting up the next generation biofeedback program for stress and anxiety management for college students: a simple and cost-effective approach. *Coll Stud J*. 2010;44:97-100.

12. Schneider CJ. Cost effectiveness of biofeedback and behavioral medicine treatments: a review of the literature. *Biofeedback Self Regul*. 1987;12(2):71-92.

13. Frank DL, Khorshid L, Kiffer JF, Moravec CS, McKee MG. Biofeedback in medicine: who, when, why and how? *Mental Health Fam Med*. 2010;7(2):85-91.

14. Khazan IZ. *The Clinical Handbook of Biofeedback: A Step-by-Step Guide for Training and Practice with Mindfulness*. Malden, MA: John Wiley and Son; 2013.

15. Arena M. and Schwartz M. *Psychophysiological Assessment and Biofeedback: A Primer*. In: Schwartz M, Andrasik F. New York, NY: Guilford Progress; 2003.

16. Sandweiss JH, Wolf SL. *Biofeedback and Sports Sciences*. New York, NY: Plenum Press; 1985.

17. Morley S, Williams A, Eccleston C. Examining the evidence of psychological treatments for chronic pain: time for a paradigm shift? *Pain*. 2013;154:1929-1931.

18. Williams AC, Eccleston C, Morley S. Psychological therapies for the management of chronic pain (excluding headache) in adults. *Cochrane Database Syst Rev*. 2012;11:CD007407.

19. Salomons TV, Moayedi M, Erpelding N, Davis KD. A brief cognitive-behavioural intervention for pain reduces secondary hyperalgesia. *Pain*. 2014;155(8):1446-1452.

20. Kucyi A, Salomons TV, Davis KD. Cognitive behavioral training reverses the effect of pain exposure on brain network activity. *Pain*. 2016;157(9):1895-1904. doi: 10.1097/j.pain.0000000000000592.

21. Kabat-Zinn J. *Full Catastrophe Living: Using the Wisdom of Your Body and Mind to Face Stress, Pain, and Illness*. New York, NY: Dell Pub., a division of Bantam Doubleday Dell Pub. Group; 1991.

22. Scott W, Hann KEJ, McCracken LM. A comprehensive examination of changes in psychological flexibility following acceptance and commitment therapy for chronic pain. *J Contemp Psychother*. 2016;46:139-148. doi:10.1007/s10879-016-9328-5.

23. Whelan J, Mahoney M, Meyers A. Performance enhancement in sport: a cognitive-behavioral domain. *Behav Ther*, 1991;22:307-327.

24. Qaseem A, Wilt TJ, McLean RM, Forciea MA; Clinical Guidelines Committee of the American College of Physicians. Noninvasive treatments for acute, subacute, and chronic low back pain: a clinical practice guideline from the American College of Physicians. *Ann Intern Med*. 2017:1-17.

25. Nestoriuc Y, Martin A, Rief W, Andrasik F. Biofeedback treatment for headache disorders: a comprehensive efficacy review. *Appl Psychophysiol Biofeedback*. 2008;33(3):125-140.

26. Verhagen AP, Damen L, Berger MY, Passchier J, Koes BW. Behavioral treatments of chronic tension-type headache in adults: are they beneficial? *CNS Neurosci Ther*. 2009;15:183-205. doi:10.1111/j.1755-5949.2009.00077.x.

27. Andrasik F. Biofeedback in headache: an overview of approaches and evidence. *Cleveland Clin J Med*. 2010;77(3):S72-S76.

28. Flor H, Fürst M, Birbaumer N. Deficient discrimination of EMG levels and overestimation of perceived tension in chronic pain patients. *Appl Psychophysiol Biofeedback*. 1999;24:55-66.

29. Neblett R. Surface electromyographic (SEMG) biofeedback for chronic low back pain. *Healthcare*. 2016;4(2):27.

30. Tan G, Shaffer F, Lyle R, Teo I. *Evidence-based Practice in Biofeedback & Neurofeedback*. 3rd ed. Wheat Ridge, CO: Association for Applied Psychophysiology and Biofeedback; 2016.

NON-PHARMACOLOGIC OPTIONS FOR THE TREATMENT OF NEUROPATHIC PAIN

Naileshni Singh, MD, Jon Zhou, MD and Samir J. Sheth, MD

FAST FACTS

- Neuropathic pain (NP) has a significant impact on function and quality of life.
- Owing to the multiple etiologies of NP, it often is not straightforward to diagnose and can be difficult to treat.
- NP is best treated with a careful, stepwise approach that utilizes a biopsychosocial model.

INTRODUCTION

Neuropathic pain (NP) is a difficult to diagnose and treat medical condition that affects millions of people worldwide. Adequately caring for those suffering from NP can be challenging because of its complex pathophysiology and multidimensional nature. This chapter reviews the mechanisms, assessment, and treatment of a variety of NP pain conditions.

DEFINITIONS AND MECHANISMS

Neuropathic pain is defined by the International Association for the Study of Pain (IASP) as "pain caused by a lesion or disease of the somatosensory nervous system." In contrast, nociceptive pain is defined as "pain that arrives from actual or threatened damage to non-neural tissue and is due to activation of nociceptors." The need for a "lesion" in the nervous system in the definition of neuropathic pain may be difficult to assess for, even with diagnostic studies. Many neuropathic pain conditions may not have demonstrable lesions or a known "disease" that makes the diagnosis largely determined by clinical information. The presence and level of severity of NP has significant levels of morbidity, higher depression, higher anxiety, compromised sleep, higher health care utilization, poorer quality of life, lost productivity, and increased health care costs as compared with the general population.[1-4]

Neuropathic pain can present in a variety of different ways, and the prevalence and incidence of neuropathic pain conditions vary with each syndrome. For conditions such as diabetes, painful diabetic peripheral neuropathy (DPN) can occur in up to 30% of diabetics. The prevalence of phantom limb pain ranges from 40% to 80% of amputations but is based on patient-related factors and the site of the amputation.[5] Postsurgical pain is common after surgeries such as mastectomies and thoracotomies because of either direct or indirect nerve injury. See Table 29-1 for a description of the prevalence and incidence of common neuropathic pain conditions.[6]

The research literature describes a variety of mechanisms that can lead to the experience of neuropathic pain. The theories regarding causes of neuropathic pain start peripherally and spread centrally in the nervous system. Specifically, mechanisms focus on abnormal firing of nerves, abnormal amplification or propagation of nerve signals, or altered inhibition of pain pathways.[6] Spontaneous neuronal activity from an injured primary afferent neuron such as a neuroma or lesion in the dorsal horn of the spinal cord, thalamus, or other supraspinal structures may cause pain. Upregulation of receptors such as voltage-gated sodium channels (Nav. 1.8) and

TABLE 29-1 Prevalence and Incidence of Neuropathic Pain Conditions

NEUROPATHIC PAIN CONDITION	PREVALENCE (BEST ESTIMATE)	INCIDENCE
Painful diabetic neuropathy (DPN)	15%	15.3/100,000
Postherpetic neuralgia (PHN)	7%-27%	11-40/100,000
HIV neuropathy	35%	Unknown
AIDS neuropathy	50%	Unknown
Central poststroke pain	8%-11%	Unknown
Multiple sclerosis (MS) pain	23%	Unknown
Spinal cord injury (SCI) pain	40%-70%	Unknown
Phantom limb pain	53%-85%	Unknown
Trigeminal neuralgia	Unknown	5-8/100,000

Adapted from Sadosky A, McDermott A, Brandenberg N. A review of the epidemiology of painful diabetic peripheral neuropathy, postherpetic neuralgia, and less commonly studied neuropathic pain conditions. Pain Pract. 2008;8(1):45-56. Copyright © 2008 World Institute of Pain. With permission of John Wiley & Sons, Inc.

transient receptor potential vanilloid (TRPV1) on nerves known to modulate neuropathic pain has been demonstrated. Demyelination of nerves may cause abnormal signaling between pain fibers and other nonpain fibers. For example, ectopic discharges from damaged and demyelinated nerves may cause ephaptic crosstalk (i.e., communication) between nerves that typically propagate pain and ones that typically do not such as sympathetic fibers. Nonephaptic crosstalk through repetitive firing that releases neurotransmitters that activate nearby nonnoxious fibers may also occur.[6] Furthermore, functional reorganization of receptive fields, known as sprouting, occurs in spinal cord dorsal horn neurons such that sensory input from surrounding intact nerves emphasizes or aggravates input from the initial area of injury. Sprouting into the dorsal horn or dorsal root ganglion (DRG) causes increased activity to both noxious and nonnoxious stimuli. Additionally, loss of segmental inhibition or descending inhibition in the spinal cord may contribute to neuropathic pain.[7] For instance, pain can occur if A beta fibers (touch, pressure, and vibration) fail to modulate input from unmyelinated C fibers and myelinated A delta fibers.

Neurotransmitters and neuropeptides have action on specific receptors that are involved in pain pathways. Understanding the interactions of these molecules in the propagation or attenuation of pain signals is important in choosing medications. Many neuropathic pain medications and treatments will alter or enhance one or more neurotransmitters. For example, glutamate and aspartate along with the neuropeptide substance P are known to transmit pain. Substance P, along with other local mediators released by primary afferent neurons, may interact with C fibers to cause the perpetuation of pain chronically.[7] Endorphins and opioids are known to target both the ascending and descending pain pathways to inhibit pain. GABA and glycine are the main inhibitory neurotransmitters in the nervous system that modulate pain, whereas serotonin is an inhibitory neurotransmitter involved in mood and emotion. Norepinephrine is involved in the descending inhibitory pain pathways.[7] Owing to neurotransmitter and neuropeptide profiles, relevant drug targets may include the GABA pathways or agents that release norepinephrine and serotonin such as duloxetine. See chapter 2: *Pain Anatomy and Physiology* for further reference.

The phenomenon of central and peripheral sensitization as it relates to neuropathic pain is of interest when considering the chronicity of many pain conditions, which often exceeds the initial injury. Neuroinflammatory mediators such as substance P, cytokines, prostaglandins, and histamine can stimulate or sensitize pain fibers to cause peripheral sensitization of the nervous system. Through repetitive stimulation of pain fibers, molecular and anatomical changes occur in the central nervous system called central sensitization. Central sensitization occurs through multiple mechanisms that include abnormal signaling or altered inhibition from the peripheral nervous system.[6]

Neuropathic pain conditions such as postherpetic neuralgia (PHN) or painful DPN have mechanisms that are complicated and specific to the condition. PHN is caused by reactivation of the varicella zoster virus latent in the dorsal columns of spinal cord sensory neurons after an initial infection. The virus causes focal necrosis of neuronal cell bodies, decrease in epidermal nerve fiber density, neurogenic inflammation, and demyelination of neurons in the dorsal root ganglion (DRG) and peripheral nervous system.[8] The virus may be reactivated in the elderly or immunocompromised leading to a severe pain condition. DPN has a mechanism of pain related to hyperglycemia causing nerve damage, sprouting and hyperexcitability of nerves, and the release of inflammatory mediators. Neurovascular changes causing hypoxia or sympathetic nervous system sprouting in the DRG are also thought to contribute to the pain experience in diabetics.[9] Mechanical pain associated with chronic nerve compression such as in trigeminal neuralgia (TN) or carpal tunnel syndrome may be relieved by decompression. Direct nerve injury and sensitization may occur during common surgical procedures such as mastectomy, inguinal herniorrhaphy, or thoracotomy.[10] Patients who undergo chemotherapy may experience pain because of neurotoxic therapeutic agents, such as platinum agents, vinca alkaloids, and taxanes. Radiation-induced nerve injury is believed to be related to fibrotic compression of nerves, injury to the vascular supply, and direct axonal injury and demyelination from X-rays.[11] Sympathetically maintained pain in causalgia or complex regional pain syndrome (CRPS) is hypothesized to be related to dysfunction of the sympathetic nervous system along with neurogenic inflammation and sensitization of nociceptors; however, neuroplastic changes and autoimmune mechanisms have not been ruled out.[12]

The myriad of conditions along with the differing pain mechanisms makes the treatment and diagnosis of NP challenging for clinicians and frustrating to patients.

CLINICAL PRESENTATION

The presentation of neuropathic pain may be variable and specific to the underlying clinical condition. Patients who experience neuropathic pain may describe the pain as "burning," "numbness," "itchy," "sharp," and "shooting," or "electric." The pain may be evoked or spontaneous. In DPN, the pain occurs in a "stocking glove pattern" sensitive to touch and typically in the lower extremities. Patients with radiculitis may report pain radiating to the extremities from the lumbar or cervical spine in a dermatomal pattern. Patients who suffer from TN may experience pain along any of the 3 dermatomal regions innervated by cranial nerve V, which is the trigeminal nerve. A thorough history may reveal a recent surgery, procedure, stroke, injury, worsening diabetes or other metabolic disorder, new medications, or use of chemotherapy agents. However, in many cases, it may be idiopathic.

Physical examination and diagnostic testing may assist with the diagnosis of neuropathic pain. The physical examination involves a detailed neurological examination with special attention paid to neurologic deficits and/or gains. Unique physical examination maneuvers include measuring the affected body part for atrophy and sensory testing for vibration/temperature, among others. Table 29-2 details physical examination maneuvers and diagnostic testing that may provide evidence for many common and uncommon NP conditions. Responses to physical examination may be illustrated through pain descriptors such as allodynia, hyperalgesia, or paresthesia, which are common in NP disorders (Table 29-3). Additionally, being familiar with and referring to neuropathic pain screening and assessment tools may assist with describing the experience of pain and tracking response to treatments. See Table 29-4 for a list of NP clinical screening and assessment tools.[13] Validated tool and surveys can assess the quality of pain, severity of symptoms, exacerbating and alleviating factors, affective manifestations, and physical examination signs and other factors that may assist patients and clinicians in recognizing and treating NP.

INTRODUCTION TO TREATMENTS

The treatment of neuropathic pain conditions can be generally described as conservative or nonconservative. Conservative measures typically include physical therapy modalities, integrative therapies, and medications. Nonconservative measures may include interventional procedures, implanted devices, and surgery. Generally, the evidence for medication treatments includes first-line, second-line, and third-line recommendations. The research and evidence-based guidelines on treatments options are usually divided by the specific pain condition.

TABLE 29-2 Physical Examination and Diagnostic Testing for Neuropathic Pain

PHYSICAL EXAMINATION	DIAGNOSTIC TESTING
Touch	Comprehensive metabolic panel
Pinprick	Complete blood count
Pressure	Sedimentation rate
Cold	Folic acid
Heat	Thyroid function test
Vibration	Hgb A1c and fasting glucose
Temporal summation	Infectious Disease Panel including HIV, hepatitis, and Lyme disease titer
Measure affected areas for loss of mass	MRI
Motor strength	CT
Cranial nerves	EMG/NCS
Gait	Skin biopsy
Reflexes	Vitamin B_{12} level
Skin changes	Heavy metal serum
Atrophy	Serum electrophoresis and immunofixation
Rash	Antinuclear antibody
Temperature	Rheumatoid factor
Upper motor neuron signs	Sjogren titers
Palpation of masses or lymph nodes	Cryoglobulins
	CSF study
	Orthostatic vital signs
	Urine or serum toxicology

Adapted from Kerstman E, Ahn A, Battu S, et al. Neuropathic pain. Handb Clin Neurol. 2013;110:175-187. Copyright © 2013 Elsevier. With permission.

CONSERVATIVE, INTEGRATIVE, AND ALTERNATIVE MODALITIES

Physical therapy (PT) modalities are often the first-line conservative treatment for most painful conditions. Exercise reduces neuropathic pain symptoms in both experimental studies and clinical studies of DPN. Balance, mobility, strength, decreased inflammation, decreased allodynia, and increased hypoalgesia are some of the improvements seen with exercise therapy in peripheral neuropathic conditions such as DPN.[14] In

TABLE 29-3 Screening and Assessment Tools for Neuropathic Pain.

SCREENING TOOLS	ASSESSMENT TOOLS
Leeds Assessment of Neuropathic Symptoms and Signs (LANSS)	Neuropathic Pain Scale (NPS)
Neuropathic Pain Questionnaire (NPQ)	Neuropathic Pain Symptom Invent
Douleur Neuropathique 4 Questions (DN4)	Short-Form McGill Pain Questionnaire 2 (SF-MPQ-2)
painDETECT	
ID Pain	
Standardized Evaluation of Pain	

Adapted by permission from Springer Jones RC 3rd, Backonja MM. Review of neuropathic pain screening and assessment tools. Curr Pain Headache Rep. 2013;17(9):363. Copyright © 2013 Springer Science+Business Media New York.

TABLE 29-4 Pain Nomenclature and Definitions.

PAIN NOMENCLATURE	DEFINITION
Allodynia	Pain due to a stimulus that does not normally provoke pain, lowered threshold stimulus and response differ
Anesthesia dolorosa	Pain in an area or region that is anesthetic
Dysesthesia	An unpleasant abnormal sensation, whether spontaneous or evoked
Hyperalgesia	Increased pain to a normally painful stimulus
Hyperesthesia	Increased sensitivity to stimulation, excluding the special senses
Hyperpathia	Abnormally painful reaction to a stimulus, especially a repetitive stimulus
Hypoalgesia	Decreased pain in response to a normally painful stimulus
Neuralgia	Pain in the distribution of a nerve or nerves
Neuritis	Inflammation of a nerve or nerves
Neuropathy	A disturbance of function or pathological change in a nerve(s)
Paresthesia	An abnormal sensation, whether spontaneous or evoked

This table has been reproduced with permission of the International Association for the Study of Pain® (IASP). The table may not be reproduced for any other purpose without permission.

CRPS, range of motion exercises are thought be a cornerstone of treatment that prevents loss in bone density and muscle atrophy and can reduce the symptoms of chronic pain. If PT and other movement-based or active therapies fail, other modalities can be considered.

Passive modalities for patients with NP may include transcutaneous electrical nerve stimulation (TENS), devices that are applied externally to painful areas that reduce action potentials and increase pain thresholds in the peripheral nervous system. TENS can be used for neuropathic pain including DPN, TN, stump pain, phantom limb pain, radiculopathy, HIV neuropathy, CRPS, entrapment neuropathy, spinal cord injury, postlaminectomy, cancer-related neuropathic pain, poststoke, and central pain where efficacy has been demonstrated.[15] Along with TENS, ultrasound and manual therapy may also be prescribed.

Acupuncture has a basis in Eastern Medicine and relies on carefully placed aseptic needles on points that elicit *deqi*, which is the sensation responsible for the therapeutic results. Acupuncture has been studied in clinical situations and is effective in back and neck pain and postoperative nausea and vomiting.[16] Acupuncture can decrease pain in PDH, Bell palsy, HIV neuropathy, spinal cord injury, and carpal tunnel syndrome.[17] Because the risk of acupuncture intervention is low and the possible benefit is high, acupuncture can be a useful first-line treatment option.

PSYCHOLOGICAL MODALITIES

A multitude of psychological modalities and therapies can offer pain reduction and improved functioning in patients with neuropathic pain. Cognitive behavioral therapy (CBT) addresses the negative thinking that causes distress and increased levels of pain in patients. CBT addresses pain catastrophizing, which is defined as an exaggerated response to pain or "overappraisal" of the sensation of pain.[18] CBT assists patients by teaching tools to counter negative and irrational thinking. Patients are asked to consciously address behaviors and thoughts that are counterproductive to the management of pain. To date, evidence suggests efficacy for the use of CBT in HIV neuropathy and spinal cord injury.[19]

Mindfulness-based strategies including mindfulness-based stress reduction (MBSR), mindfulness meditation, and mindfulness-based cognitive therapy are meditative schools of thought centered on awareness and attention in the moment without judgment. MBSR is typically a process that is taught in an 8- to 12-week session, but shorter mindfulness interventions have been described in the literature. Mindfulness has been used for decades to treat varied pain conditions such as PHN and chronic low back pain, resulting in improved functioning and decreased disability. Lifestyle issues that exacerbate pain such as stress, poor sleep, poor interpersonal interactions, and lack of exercise may be addressed through meditative modalities centered on mindfulness.[20-22] There is also some evidence that reduction in the depression and anxiety can be achieved with mindfulness.[22]

MEDICATION-BASED MODALITIES

"See chapter 34".

Neuromodulation

Neuromodulation refers to the broad array of technologies that may alter the nervous system to decrease and improve the experience of pain for patients with neuropathic pain conditions. This relies on the use of electrical energy that is applied near the spinal cord and dorsal horn that alters the pain pathways through multiple central and peripheral mechanisms. Neuromodulation is typically an invasive modality and used when other conservative therapies, including medications, fail.

The field of neuromodulation includes the technologies of spinal cord stimulation (SCS), peripheral field stimulation or peripheral nerve stimulation, deep brain stimulation (DBS), and motor cortex stimulation (MCS). These advanced therapies are used when conservative measures have been exhausted and patients have passed a thorough psychological evaluation to assess their appropriateness and preparedness for neuromodulation therapies. Patients with uncontrolled depression, anxiety, substance abuse, psychosis, pain catastrophizing, and inability to cope have poorer outcomes with spinal cord stimulation.[23,24] As an advanced technique, pain interventionalists and surgeons may offer this technology using fluoroscopic guidance. Wireless and injectable SCS systems are on the horizon, which may make neuromodulation more readily available to other types of providers.

Spinal cord stimulation is the most common of the neuromodulation therapies and uses electrodes placed in the epidural space to cause paresthesias that are experienced by the patient. The proposed mechanism of SCS includes spinal modulation, attenuation of dorsal horn neurons, action on A beta fibers, and alteration of neurochemistry of the dorsal columns.[25] SCS is FDA approved for CRPS and failed back surgery syndrome (FBSS) but has been successfully used for many types of neuropathic and vascular pain conditions including peripheral neuropathy, DPN, peripheral vascular disease, and angina.[26] Typically, patients undergo percutaneous placement of leads with multiple electrodes into the epidural space using fluoroscopy. The dorsal columns of the spinal cord are stimulated and mapped during the 1-week trial to cover all the patient's pain locations. Patients may use a variety of preprogrammed options that offer combinations of amplitudes and frequencies of stimulation to see which experience provides the most pain relief and increased functioning. Some patients may be good candidates for high-frequency SCS, which is a paresthesia-free option using high-frequency parameters to modulate pain.[27] Patients are also asked to monitor activity levels and functional goals to assess whether to proceed to the implantation of the SCS system and pulse generator. If SCS trial is difficult because of inability to place the percutaneous leads, then paddle leads, which have multiple imbedded leads in a "paddle" shape, may be placed by a surgeon through a laminotomy. SCS implantation is typically an outpatient procedure done in a surgical setting.

Other variations of neuromodulation have been found to be successful in pain conditions. High-cervical SCS has been shown to be effective for intractable migraines or facial pain, and stimulation of the DRG is as beneficial as traditional SCS.[28,29] Stimulation of the DRG, which is at the junction of the central and peripheral nervous system, has been successful for FBSS and other neuropathic pain conditions.[29] Peripheral nerve field stimulation, where leads are placed over the area of a nerve subcutaneously, has been showed to be effective for illioinguinal neuritis and greater occipital neuritis through an A beta fiber pathway.[30] Peripheral nerve field stimulation uses leads typically placed in a nerve distribution and can be helpful for TN, head pain, face pain, and thoracic neuropathic pain.[31,32] Peripheral neuromodulation has highlighted some initial efficacy in phantom limb pain and stump pain.[33] The type of neuromodulation system will largely depend on the patient's pain area and symptoms. Risks of neuromodulation include failure to manage pain, bleeding, infection, spinal cord injury, migration of the leads, equipment failure, urinary retention, and tolerance.

Deep brain stimulation is FDA approved for movement disorders intractable to conservative measures such as Parkinson disease and essential tremor. DBS has been used successfully for pain control in neuropathic pain conditions such as CRPS, poststroke pain, spinal cord injury, facial pain, FBSS, and peripheral nerve plexus injury. DBS delivers constant electrical stimulation to areas of the brain, typically the thalamus and/or periventricular areas; however, this technology can be offered in many locations.[34] Similarly, motor cortex stimulation appears to be beneficial for phantom limb pain, TN or facial pain, and poststroke pain.[34] The invasiveness of these treatment modalities needs to be considered when assessing for patient appropriateness. Noninvasive transcranial magnetic stimulation over the primary somatosensory area or the premotor cortex using a high frequency that activates neurons has been used successfully for short-term pain management.[35]

Lastly, intrathecal therapies that deliver low-dose medications into the CSF may be a last resort modality for neuropathic pain conditions. Opioids, baclofen, and ziconitide are FDA-approved medications for intrathecal therapy. Ziconitide is a calcium channel blocker that has been used for refractory neuropathic pain.[36] The side effect profile of mood changes, ataxia, nausea, dizziness, sedation, altered mentation, and urinary retention may make this medication challenging to tolerate. However, lower doses of ziconitide can be combined with other intrathecal medications such as opioids or local anesthetics to be used for neuropathic pain conditions.

Nerve and Spinal Cord Ligation

Stump pain due to a neuroma is often a consequence of amputations and is a separate entity from phantom limb pain or phantom limb sensations. Patients may present with point tenderness at the stump and neuropathic pain qualities such as numbness. Surgical neuroma excision and steroid injections performed perineurally (surrounding the neuroma) are effective in treating stump pain.[37,38]

Dorsal root entry zone (DREZ) lesioning of the spinal cord causes deafferentation of pain fibers and has had successes in facial pain, refractory TN, spinal cord injury, phantom limb pain, and brachial plexus avulsion.[39,40] This involves surgically placed lesions in the spinal cord that disrupt the dorsal columns. A more targeted approach for central pain management may also be accomplished by gamma knife surgical techniques that use focused doses of radiation in conditions such as TN.[41] Gamma knife may be performed prior to microvascular decompression as a less invasive modality for TN and can be repeated if the pain reoccurs.

Nerve Blocks and Ablation

A variety of nerves can be "blocked" temporarily or permanently by local anesthetic, local anesthetics plus steroids, or nerve degenerative solutions such as phenol or glycerol, or ablated using high-level thermal energy (80°C) or low-level pulsing energy (pulse dose radiofrequency at lower temperature but longer treatment time). There is evidence for steroid and local anesthetic blocks of the greater and lesser occipital nerve for occipital neuralgia and other headache disorders.[42] Headache and facial pain can also be treated by blocks of the third occipital, supraorbital, auriculotemporal, supratrochlear nerves, and the sphenopalatine ganglion.[43,44] Gasserian ganglion radiofrequency (RF) thermal lesioning and neurolytic lesioning has been shown to be effective for facial pain due to TN.[45] Pulsed RF is efficacious in TN, facial pain, postthoracotomy pain, radicular pain, joint pain, peripheral neuropathy, and myofascial pain.[46] The intercostal nerves (or the corresponding dorsal root ganglion) may undergo cryoablation, pulsed or thermal radiofrequency ablation, or even surgical neurectomy to relieve postthoracotomy pain.[47] Sympathetically maintained pain conditions such as causalgia and CRPS types I and II can be diagnosed and treated with blockade of the sympathetic nervous system.[48-50] Chronic pelvic pain, coccydynia, or perineal pain may be relieved by an impar ganglion, which is the most distal aspect of the sympathetic chain.[50] Lastly, patients with intractable abdominal pain from malignancy may benefit from a neurolytic celiac plexus block or hypogastric block with alcohol, phenol, or glycerol.[51]

Botulinum Toxin

Botulinum toxin A has been used for dystonia, spasticity, and migraines as well as peripheral neuropathic pain. However, the evidence behind its efficacy for decreasing neuropathic pain is equivocal with botulinum being recommended as a third-line medication for peripheral neuropathic pain.[52] The antinociceptive effects of botulinum toxin A are attributed to the inhibition of inflammatory mediators from peripheral sensory nerves, including substance P, glutamate, and calcitonin gene–related peptide (CGRP). There are no guidelines for the ideal dosage of botulinum toxin A for neuropathic pain, but most studies evaluated used 50 to 200 units at the site of pain.[53] Smaller trials have shown efficacy in decreasing DPN pain with injections directly into the patient's feet when compared with placebo.[54] Botulinum toxin A has a low side effect profile with the most common side effect listed as neck pain, injection site pain, and muscular weakness. Overall, smaller trials show efficacy with use of botulinum toxin A for TN, DPN, but others show no improvement in occipital neural pain or CRPS. The true potential of this medication for peripheral neuropathy requires more research as most studies have small enrollment numbers and have varying doses of toxin given.

Neuropathic Pain Conditions

A few of the most common neuropathic pain conditions will be described in detail below. A more complete list of conditions is shown in Table 29-5.

Trigeminal Neuralgia

TN, which is also called *tic douloureux*, is a chronic neuropathic pain status that primarily affects the fifth cranial nerve, the trigeminal nerve. The disease typically presents in patients older than 50 years and is more common in women. The presentation of TN is an evoked, severe, and burning pain that may last from several seconds to a few minutes located in the dermatomes of the trigeminal nerve. Patients may have dozens of these episodes in a day. An atypical presentation is a lower-intensity neuropathic pain state that lasts longer than the time frame of the typical presentation.[55] The diagnosis of TN is mainly through the physical examination and patient history, but most patients require MRI imaging to rule out tumor, vascular impingement, or multiple sclerosis as the primary cause. A fine cut high-resolution MRI will follow the course of the trigeminal nerve to see if there is mechanical impingement as the nerve exits the neural foramen and enters the face. A trial of antiepileptic or neuropathic medications may help diagnosis TN.

There are various causes of TN, one of which may be vascular in origin where an aberrant branch of the superior cerebellar artery applies pressure onto the trigeminal nerve causing myelin sheath irritation and injury. Central nervous system disorders such as multiple sclerosis may also cause degradation of the myelin that causes TN pain. Other less common causes may include tumors, facial trauma, jaw pain, dental-related pain, Bell palsy, stroke, and ear, nose, or throat diseases or malignancies that may produce TN pain.

Treatment options are primarily pharmacologic, with microvascular surgery reserved for intractable TN pain from a vascular impingement. Medications used first line include sodium channel blockers and calcium channel blockers such as gabapentin and carbamazepine and tricyclic antidepressants such as amitriptyline. Owing to the neuropathic nature of TN, mu agonists such as opioids

TABLE 29-5 Neuropathic Pain Conditions and Diagnoses

TYPE OF NEUROPATHY	CLINICAL CONDITIONS
Peripheral neuropathy	Phantom pain, stump pain, nerve injury, nerve root avulsion, neuroma, posttraumatic neuralgia, entrapment syndrome, Morton neuralgia, painful scar, herpes zoster (acute and chronic), diabetic neuropathy, diabetic amyotrophy, ischemic neuropathy, borreliosis, vasculitis or connective tissue disease, neuralgic amyotrophy, peripheral nerve tumor, radiation-induced neuropathy, plexus neuritis, trigeminal neuralgia, glossopharyngeal neuralgia, vagus neuralgia, pudendal neuralgia, vascular compression syndrome, postsurgical pain (postmastectomy or postthoracotomy)
Generalized neuropathy	Metabolic or nutritional: diabetes, alcoholism, amyloidosis, hypothyroidism, beri beri, pellagra
	Drug related: examples are chemotherapy agents and antiretrovirals
	Toxin-related: examples are arsenic and thallium
	Hereditary: amyloid neuropathy, Fabry disease, Charcot-Marie-Tooth disease, hereditary autonomic and sensory neuropathy
	Malignant: paraneoplastic neuropathy, myeloma
	Infectious or immune related: acute or inflammatory polyradiculoneuropathy (Guillain-Barre syndrome), borreliosis, HIV neuropathy, syphilis
	Other or unknown: idiopathic small fiber neuropathy, trench foot, erythromelalgia
Central pain syndromes	Vascular lesions in the brain and spinal cord, multiple sclerosis, traumatic spinal cord injury, traumatic brain injury, atypical facial pain, syringomyelia and syringobulbia, tumor and abscess (depends on location), myelitis, epilepsy, Parkinson disease
Sympathetically maintained pain	Chronic regional pain syndrome (types I and II)
Mixed pain syndromes or unknown	Low back or neck pain with radiculitis or radiculopathy, malignant plexus invasion, functional abdominal pain, coccydynia, orofacial dystonia, burning mouth syndrome

Adapted from Baron R, Binder A, Wasner G. Neuropathic pain: diagnosis, pathophysiological mechanisms, and treatment. Lancet Neurol. 2010;9(8):807-819. Copyright © 2010 Elsevier. With permission.

are not reliably effective and thus not recommended as the first-line pharmacologic agent. If the patient suffers relapse despite medications, other neurosurgical procedures such as gamma knife stereotactic radiotherapy or ablation are available to treat the symptoms from trigeminal nerve injury. The risks involved in surgery include damage to other nerves and cerebrospinal fluid leak.

Diabetic Neuropathy

DPN is a neuropathic condition associated with diabetes mellitus and is often the result of microvascular injury due to the chronic hyperglycemic state. DPN affects all the peripheral nerves including the small pain fibers, the autonomic system, and even motor neurons. DPN presents as a symmetrical, length-dependent sensorimotor polyneuropathy. The pathophysiology of the diabetic neuropathy is multifactorial, with microvascular narrowing of vessels that supply the peripheral nerves as one of the main causes. Elevated levels of glucose may cause increased inflammatory states, thus worsening of DPN. EMG/nerve conduction testing will typically show reduced functioning of peripheral nerves by demonstrating positive sharp waves, decreased amplitudes, slower conduction velocity, and spontaneous discharges.[56]

Patients with severe DPN may have decreased sensation in their extremities, often described as a glove-stock distribution with numbness and dysesthesia. Diagnosis is primarily based on physical examination of the patient showing decreased sensation and/or pain in the extremities and impaired or lost reflexes. Small fiber neuropathy can be assessed with pinprick and temperature sensation, whereas large fiber neuropathy can be assessed with proprioception maneuvers and the use of a 128-Hz tuning fork for vibration sense.[57] Autonomic manifestations of DPH should also be evaluated such as heart rate abnormalities with Valsalva maneuver and standing, R-R interval variation, orthostatic hypotension, gastroparesis, tachycardia, sudomotor dysfunction, and erectile dysfuction.[58] Patients are at an elevated risk of injuring themselves when ambulating and developing ulcers and infections in the lower extremity, which may lead to amputation, falls, and fractures. Other disorders should be considered in the differential such as prediabetes, thyroid disease, vasculitis, vitamin deficiency, alcohol abuse, drugs related, heavy metal poisoning, chronic inflammatory demyelinating polyradiculoneuropathy, or HIV neuropathy when making the diagnosis of DPN.[57]

Treatment for DPN includes pharmacologic agents that are used to treat many other neuropathic conditions including anticonvulsants, tricyclic antidepressants, and topical agents. The 3 FDA-approved medications for DPN are the calcium channel blocker, pregabalin, the serotonin-norepinephrine reuptake inhibitor duloxetine, and tapentadol extended release. Tapentadol is a centrally acting mu opioid agonist and a norepinephrine reuptake inhibitor, with a similar mechanism of action to tramadol. The use of pure mu agonist opioids for DPN is controversial because of long-term side effects of opioids including dependence, constipation, and opioid-induced hyperalgesia. Other nonpharmacologic agents include acupuncture and capsaicin for DPN although further research needs to be conducted to establish efficacy. Long-term treatment of DPN depends on improved glucose control through lifestyle management.

Postherpetic Neuralgia

PHN is a pain condition stemming from the reactivation of herpes zoster virus that may result in a chronic condition with a significant amount of morbidity. The course of the disease starts with an initial contagious infection (chickenpox) with varicella zoster virus, often in childhood. The virus then becomes latent in the dorsal column sensory ganglia and reactivates decades later to produce neuropathic pain and a rash in a dermatomal pattern. In contrast, zoster sine herpete is another version of the disease manifestation but without a rash. Studies vary but as many as half of individuals who present with herpes zoster (HZ) may develop the chronic painful condition. The skin manifestation presents as a maculopapular rash in a unilateral dermatomal pattern typically in the thoracic spine, high lumbar spine, and rarely in the distribution of cranial nerve V. Patients present with allodynia, dysesthesia, sensitivity to thermal stimuli, and hyperalgesia.[59] Those with facial symptoms (herpes zoster ophthalmicus) in the ophthalmic branch of the facial nerve are at risk of blindness due to retinal damage and should be treated right away.

The shingles vaccine with live attenuated varicella zoster virus may prevent the development of HZ and PHN for individuals aged 60 years or more.[60] Those with the acute phase of the infection should be treated with opioid therapy, oral or ophthalmic steroids, and a 7- to 10-day course of antiviral agents such as acyclovir, famciclovir, or valacyclovir, which can decrease the viral load and the severity of HZ.[61] Those who are immunocompromised and elderly are at higher risk of developing HZ. The chronic disease of pain that persists longer than 30 days after the disease onset is termed PHN. PHN can be treated with a multiple of options including calcium channel agents, lidocaine patches or topical agents, capsaicin, and TCAs.

Treating Neuropathic Pain in Patients With Comorbid Conditions

Individuals with neuropathic pain may also have multiple medical comorbidities that can complicate treatment. An awareness of pharmacokinetics and pharmacodynamics along with drug-drug interactions should be considered when offering polypharmacy. Adverse drug reactions from neuropathic agents can be life-threatening such as in cases with increased suicidal thoughts, prolonged QTc, Stevens-Johnson syndrome with antiepileptic drugs (AEDs), and serotonin syndrome. Anticholinergic medications, such as TCAs, should be avoided in those being treated with anticholinesterase drugs such as in Alzheimer disease or have acute angle glaucoma. Many interactions are due to isoenzymes of the hepatic cytochrome P450 (CYP) system. Some medications may induce or mitigate the effect of other medications through the CYP system. For example, carbamazepine may reduce the serum levels of TCAs or the anticoagulation effects of warfarin.[62] Codeine and tramadol are medications for which actions depend on the CYP system and therefore effects can be variable depending on whether the patient is a rapid metabolizer or does not bio-transform the medication.[62]

Patients with liver or kidney disease will need their medications carefully monitored and dosed appropriately. Gabapentin is excreted unchanged in the urine but will need to be renally dosed in the setting of kidney disease. NSAIDs will also need to be used sparingly in those with renal disease, but topical NSAIDs may be a better option in this setting. Neurotoxic metabolites of morphine may accumulate in those with renal failure. Liver cirrhosis may cause alterations in drug metabolism, plasma protein binding, elimination, and distribution. TCAs, duloxetine, carbamazepine, and opioids should be used with extreme caution in those with liver disease.[62] MAO inhibitors are contraindicated in patients on norepinephrine-modulating medications such as venlafaxine or duloxetine. Furthermore, hypertension can be a side effect of venlafaxine and duloxetine or NSAIDs. ECG changes such as prolonged QTc can be seen with methadone and TCAs. Weight gain and congestive heart failure have been described with pregabalin, especially in the elderly. Opioids may also effect the cardiovascular system by causing hypotension or hypertension, bradycardia, sleep apnea, and respiratory depression. Respiratory depression occurs more frequently at higher opioid doses and when combined with benzodiazepines or alcohol. AEDs, which are often teratogenic, should be avoided in those planning on getting pregnant. The first trimester is crucial in avoiding medications that may cause complications for the mother and fetus. The lowest effective dose should be recommended along with supplementation with folic acid.[62] Most neuropathic agents, except gabapentin and high-dose opioids, pass into breast milk sparingly or without clinical effect.

The elderly is a group susceptible to NP owing to progression of comorbid conditions, overwhelming polypharmacy, or risk of developing PHN and other illnesses. NP is overrepresented in those who are elderly with high levels of morbidity.[4,63] There are challenges in treating this group of individuals that include their ability to communicate pain or show signs of classical clinical presentations. Additionally, fall risk and subsequent injury make the use of medications or other aggressive treatments challenging. Aging itself alters pharmacokinetics and pharmacodynamics of water-soluble and fat-soluble medications along with changes in the metabolic liver pathways. A practical approach where adverse drug effects are screened for frequently and the lowest effective doses are used is likely the best treatment plan for elderly patients in preserving independence and functionality.

CONCLUSIONS

The assessment and treatment of patients with NP remains a challenge for providers, but the high levels of morbidity and suffering cannot be discounted. The multitude of pharmacologic, nonpharmacologic, and interventional-based treatments for NP offers clinicians and patients treatment options that fit personal goals.

REFERENCES

1. Doth AH, Hansson PT, Jensen MP, Taylor RS. The burden of neuropathic pain: a systematic review and meta-analysis of health utilities. *Pain*. 2010;149(2):338-344.

2. Schaefer C, Sadosky A, Mann R, et al. Pain severity and the economic burden of neuropathic pain in the United States: BEAT Neuropathic Pain Observational Study. *Clinicoecon Outcomes Res*. 2014;6:483-496.

3. Schaefer C, Mann R, Sadosky A, et al. Burden of illness associated with peripheral and central neuropathic pain among adults seeking treatment in the United States: a patient-centered evaluation. *Pain Med*. 2014;15(12):2105-2119.

4. McDermott AM, Toelle TR, Rowbotham DJ, Schaefer CP, Dukes EM. The burden of neuropathic pain: results from a cross-sectional survey. *Eur J Pain*. 2006;10(2):127-135.

5. Luo Y, Anderson TA. Phantom limb pain: a review. *Int Anesthesiol Clin*. 2016;54(2):121-139.

6. Kerstman E, Ahn S, Battu S, Tariq S, Grabois M. Neuropathic pain. *Handb Clin Neurol*. 2013;110:175-187.

7. Benzon HT, Raja SN, Liu SS, Fishman SM, Cohen SP. *Essentials of Pain Medicine*. 3rd ed. Philadelphia, PA: Elsevier; 2011.

8. Opstelten W, McElhaney J, Weinberger B, Oaklander AL, Johnson RW. The impact of varicella zoster virus: chronic pain. *J Clin Virol*. 2010;48(suppl 1):S8-S13.

9. Aslam A, Singh J, Rajbhandari S. Pathogenesis of painful diabetic neuropathy. *Pain Res Treat*. 2014;2014:412041.

10. Rashiq S, Dick BD. Post-surgical pain syndromes: a review for the non-pain specialist. *Can J Anaesth*. 2014;61(2):123-130.

11. Delanian S, Lefaix JL, Pradat PF. Radiation-induced neuropathy in cancer survivors. *Radiother Oncol*. 2012;105(3):273-282.

12. Tajerian M, Clark JD. New concepts in complex regional pain syndrome. *Hand Clin*. 2016;32(1):41-49.

13. Jones RC, 3rd, Backonja MM. Review of neuropathic pain screening and assessment tools. *Curr Pain Headache Rep*. 2013;17(9):363.

14. Cooper MA, Kluding PM, Wright DE. Emerging relationships between exercise, sensory nerves, and neuropathic pain. *Front Neurosci*. 2016;10:372.

15. Johnson MI, Bjordal JM. Transcutaneous electrical nerve stimulation for the management of painful conditions: focus on neuropathic pain. *Expert Rev Neurother*. 2011;11(5):735-753.

16. Tang Y, Yin HY, Rubini P, Illes P. Acupuncture-induced analgesia: a neurobiological basis in purinergic signaling. *Neuroscientist*. 2016;22(6):563-578.

17. Dimitrova A, Murchison C, Oken B. Acupuncture for the treatment of peripheral neuropathy: a systematic review and meta-analysis. *J Altern Complement Med*. 2017.

18. Severeijns R, Vlaeyen JW, van den Hout MA, Weber WE. Pain catastrophizing predicts pain intensity, disability, and psychological distress independent of the level of physical impairment. *Clin J Pain*. 2001;17(2):165-172.

19. Jones RC, Lawson E, Backonja M. Managing neuropathic pain. *Med Clin North Am*. 2016;100(1):151-167.

20. Meize-Grochowski R, Shuster G, Boursaw B, et al. Mindfulness meditation in older adults with postherpetic neuralgia: a randomized controlled pilot study. *Geriatr Nurs*. 2015;36(2):154-160.

21. Poulin PA, Romanow HC, Rahbari N, et al. The relationship between mindfulness, pain intensity, pain catastrophizing, depression, and quality of life among cancer survivors living with chronic neuropathic pain. *Support Care Cancer*. 2016;24(10):4167-4175.

22. Creswell JD. Mindfulness Interventions. *Ann Rev Psychol* 2017;68:491-516.

23. Sparkes E, Duarte RV, Mann S, Lawrence TR, Raphael JH. Analysis of psychological characteristics impacting spinal cord stimulation treatment outcomes: a prospective assessment. *Pain Phys*. 2015;18(3):E369-E377.

24. Fama CA, Chen N, Prusik J, et al. The use of preoperative psychological evaluations to predict spinal cord stimulation success: our experience and a review of the literature. *Neuromodulation*. 2016;19(4):429-436.

25. Meyerson BA, Linderoth B. Mechanisms of spinal cord stimulation in neuropathic pain. *Neurol Res*. 2000;22(3):285-292.

26. Verrills P, Sinclair C, Barnard A. A review of spinal cord stimulation systems for chronic pain. *J Pain Res*. 2016;9:481-492.

27. Bicket MC, Dunn RY, Ahmed SU. High-frequency spinal cord stimulation for chronic pain: pre-clinical overview and systematic review of controlled trials. *Pain Med*. 2016;17(12):2326-2336.

28. Lambru G, Trimboli M, Palmisani S, Smith T, Al-Kaisy A. Safety and efficacy of cervical 10 kHz spinal cord stimulation in chronic refractory primary headaches: a retrospective case series. *J Headache Pain*. 2016;17(1):66.

29. Liem L. Stimulation of the dorsal root ganglion. *Prog Neurol Surg*. 2015;29:213-224.

30. Chakravarthy K, Nava A, Christo PJ, Williams K. Review of recent advances in peripheral nerve stimulation (PNS). *Curr Pain Headache Rep*. 2016;20(11):60.

31. Mitchell B, Verrills P, Vivian D, DuToit N, Barnard A, Sinclair C. Peripheral nerve field stimulation therapy for patients with thoracic pain: a prospective study. *Neuromodulation*. 2016;19(7):752-759.

32. Verrills P, Rose R, Mitchell B, Vivian D, Barnard A. Peripheral nerve field stimulation for chronic headache: 60 cases and long-term follow-up. *Neuromodulation*. 2014;17(1):54-59.

33. Soin A, Fang ZP, Velasco J. Peripheral neuromodulation to treat postamputation pain. *Prog Neurol Surg*. 2015;29:158-167.

34. Honey CM, Tronnier VM, Honey CR. Deep brain stimulation versus motor cortex stimulation for neuropathic pain: a minireview of the literature and proposal for future research. *Comput Struct Biotechnol J*. 2016;14:234-237.

35. O'Connell NE, Wand BM, Marston L, Spencer S, Desouza LH. Non-invasive brain stimulation techniques for chronic pain. *Cochrane Database Syst Rev*. 2014;(4):cd008208.

36. Rauck RL, Wallace MS, Burton AW, Kapural L, North JM. Intrathecal ziconotide for neuropathic pain: a review. *Pain Pract*. 2009;9(5):327-337.

37. Domeshek LF, Krauss EM, Snyder-Warwick AK, et al. Surgical treatment of neuromas improves patient-reported pain, depression, and quality of life. *Plast Reconstruct Surg*. 2017;139(2):407-418.

38. Hung YH, Wu CH, Ozcakar L, Wang TG. Ultrasound-guided steroid injections for two painful neuromas in the stump of a below-elbow amputee. *Am J Phys Med Rehabil*. 2016;95(5):e73-e74.

39. Haninec P, Kaiser R, Mencl L, Waldauf P. Usefulness of screening tools in the evaluation of long-term effectiveness of DREZ lesioning in the treatment of neuropathic pain after brachial plexus injury. *BMC Neurol.* 2014;14:225.

40. Chivukula S, Tempel ZJ, Chen CJ, Shin SS, Gande AV, Moossy JJ. Spinal and nucleus caudalis dorsal root entry zone lesioning for chronic pain: efficacy and outcomes. *World Neurosurg.* 2015;84(2):494-504.

41. Regis J, Tuleasca C, Resseguier N, et al. Long-term safety and efficacy of Gamma Knife surgery in classical trigeminal neuralgia: a 497-patient historical cohort study. *J Neurosurg.* 2016;124(4):1079-1087.

42. Choi I, Jeon SR. Neuralgias of the head: occipital neuralgia. *J Korean Med Sci.* 2016;31(4):479-488.

43. Blumenfeld A, Ashkenazi A, Napchan U, et al. Expert consensus recommendations for the performance of peripheral nerve blocks for headaches–a narrative review. *Headache.* 2013;53(3):437-446.

44. Robbins MS, Robertson CE, Kaplan E, et al. The sphenopalatine ganglion: anatomy, pathophysiology, and therapeutic targeting in headache. *Headache.* 2016;56(2):240-258.

45. Peters G, Nurmikko TJ. Peripheral and gasserian ganglion-level procedures for the treatment of trigeminal neuralgia. *Clin J Pain.* 2002;18(1):28-34.

46. Chua NH, Vissers KC, Sluijter ME. Pulsed radiofrequency treatment in interventional pain management: mechanisms and potential indications-a review. *Acta Neurochir.* 2011;153(4):763-771.

47. Cohen SP, Sireci A, Wu CL, Larkin TM, Williams KA, Hurley RW. Pulsed radiofrequency of the dorsal root ganglia is superior to pharmacotherapy or pulsed radiofrequency of the intercostal nerves in the treatment of chronic postsurgical thoracic pain. *Pain Phys.* 2006;9(3):227-235.

48. Imani F, Hemati K, Rahimzadeh P, Kazemi MR, Hejazian K. Effectiveness of Stellate Ganglion Block under fluoroscopy or ultrasound guidance in upper extremity CRPS. *J Clin Diagn Res.* 2016;10(1):Uc09-Uc12.

49. van Eijs F, Stanton-Hicks M, Van Zundert J, et al. Evidence-based interventional pain medicine according to clinical diagnoses. 16. Complex regional pain syndrome. *Pain Pract.* 2011;11(1):70-87.

50. Walters A, Muhleman M, Osiro S, et al. One is the loneliest number: a review of the ganglion impar and its relation to pelvic pain syndromes. *Clin Anat.* 2013;26(7):855-861.

51. Mercadante S, Klepstad P, Kurita GP, Sjogren P, Giarratano A. Sympathetic blocks for visceral cancer pain management: a systematic review and EAPC recommendations. *Crit Rev Oncol Hematol.* 2015;96(3):577-583.

52. Finnerup NB, Attal N, Haroutounian S, et al. Pharmacotherapy for neuropathic pain in adults: a systematic review and meta-analysis. *Lancet Neurol.* 2015;14(2):162-173.

53. Oh HM, Chung ME. Botulinum toxin for neuropathic pain: a review of the literature. *Toxins.* 2015;7(8):3127-3154.

54. Chen WT, Yuan RY, Chiang SC, et al. OnabotulinumtoxinA improves tactile and mechanical pain perception in painful diabetic polyneuropathy. *Clin J Pain.* 2013;29(4):305-310.

55. Cruccu G, Finnerup NB, Jensen TS, et al. Trigeminal neuralgia: new classification and diagnostic grading for practice and research. *Neurology.* 2016;87(2):220-228.

56. Bagai K, Wilson JR, Khanna M, Song Y, Wang L, Fisher MA. Electrophysiological patterns of diabetic polyneuropathy. *Electromyogr Clin Neurophysiol.* 2008;48(3-4):139-145.

57. Pop-Busui R, Boulton AJ, Feldman EL, et al. Diabetic neuropathy: a position statement by the American Diabetes Association. *Diab Care.* 2017;40(1):136-154.

58. Vinik AI, Maser RE, Mitchell BD, Freeman R. Diabetic autonomic neuropathy. *Diab Care.* 2003;26(5):1553-1579.

59. Mallick-Searle T, Snodgrass B, Brant JM. Postherpetic neuralgia: epidemiology, pathophysiology, and pain management pharmacology. *J Multidiscip Healthcare.* 2016;9:447-454.

60. Gagliardi AM, Andriolo BN, Torloni MR, Soares BG. Vaccines for preventing herpes zoster in older adults. *Cochrane Database Syst Rev.* 2016;3:cd008858.

61. Whitley RJ, Volpi A, McKendrick M, Wijck A, Oaklander AL. Management of herpes zoster and post-herpetic neuralgia now and in the future. *J Clin Virol.* 2010;48(suppl 1):S20-28.

62. Haanpaa ML, Gourlay GK, Kent JL, et al. Treatment considerations for patients with neuropathic pain and other medical comorbidities. *Mayo Clin Proc.* 2010;85(3 suppl):S15-S25.

63. Schmader KE, Baron R, Haanpaa ML, et al. Treatment considerations for elderly and frail patients with neuropathic pain. *Mayo Clin Proc.* 2010;85(3 suppl):S26-S32.

64. http://www.iasp-pain.org/Taxonomy. Accessed March, 22nd 2017.

Part **2**

PHARMACOLOGIC THERAPIES

30

MEDICOLEGAL ESSENTIALS AND BEST PRACTICES IN OPIOID PRESCRIBING

Scott Stayner, MD, PhD

OVERVIEW
INTRODUCTION
FEDERAL LAWS AND POLICIES THAT GOVERN THE USE OF OPIOIDS FOR PAIN MANAGEMENT
THE ROLE OF THE DRUG ENFORCEMENT ADMINISTRATION
STATE LAWS AND POLICIES THAT GOVERN THE USE OF OPIOIDS FOR PAIN MANAGEMENT
PRESCRIPTION DRUG MONITORING PROGRAMS
PATIENT AND PROVIDER AGREEMENTS WHEN USING OPIOID MEDICATIONS TO MANAGE CHRONIC PAIN
URINE DRUG SCREEN TESTING
CONCLUSION
    References

FAST FACTS

- In 2015, 12.5 million people in the United States misused opioid medications[1] and 33,000 died from complications associated with opioid overdose.[2]
- The Centers for Disease Control (CDC)[3] and Federation of State Medical Boards (FSMB)[4] released updated opioid medication guidelines to reduce the risk of harm to patients who may benefit from opioids medications to help manage chronic pain.
- Physicians who invest the time and effort to learn about the full regulatory requirements for prescribing opioid medications will help provide the best care possible for their patients.

INTRODUCTION

In the late 1990s, the American Pain Society advocated assessing pain more frequently[5] and the Veteran's Administration subsequently initiated the "Pain as the 5th Vital Sign" initiative.[6] Concurrently, relatively poorly designed studies of patients who received opioid medications to manage pain showed little risk of addiction.[7,8] As a result of the increased emphasis on pain management, many pain experts used these and other similar studies to justify escalation of opioid medications for the management of chronic pain.[9]

In spite of the liberalization of opioid use for chronic pain management, it is estimated that over 100 million people in the United States suffer from chronic pain and often turn to their primary care physician for treatment.[10] However, morbidity and mortality from opioid-related overdose has grown with the increase in opioid prescriptions. In 2015, 12.5 million people in the United States misused opioid medications[1] and 33,000 died from complications associated with opioid overdose.[2] In fact, at the time of this publication, opioid overdose is now the leading cause of accidental death in the United States[2]

Roughly 50% of the deaths were attributed to overdose of prescription medications. However the 2009 National Survey on Drug Use and Health (NSDUH) reported that one-third of individuals older than 12 years who misused any drug started by abusing prescription medications.[11] In essence, prescription medications have been implicated as a "gateway" drug for those who abuse other controlled substances that often result in significant morbidity and mortality.[2]

Federal and state laws and regulations govern the prescribing and distribution of opioids and other medications used in pain management. The language contained in legislation written to govern opioid distribution tends to be general rather than specific. The regulatory agency assigned to enforce these laws is tasked with interpreting broad language in these laws.

The Centers for Disease Control (CDC)[3] and Federation of State Medical Boards (FSMB)[4] released updated opioid medication guidelines to reduce the risk of harm to patients who may benefit from opioids medications to help manage chronic pain. These guidelines also outline recommendations for optimal physician and patient opioid pain agreements. Adherence to these recommendations will help prescribers practice within the standard of care when prescribing opioids and other scheduled medications. Well-written opioid agreements can also be used to document that the patient has been educated regarding the risks and benefits of chronic opioid therapy as well as certain provider expectations such as appropriate use of opioids, refills, and monitoring when opioid medications are prescribed for chronic pain.

FEDERAL LAWS AND POLICIES THAT GOVERN THE USE OF OPIOIDS FOR PAIN MANAGEMENT

The principal federal law that governs the prescribing of controlled substances is the Controlled Substance Act (CSA), a subset of the Comprehensive Drug Abuse Prevention and Control Act of 1970.[12,13] The CSA stipulates that licensed medical practitioners can prescribe controlled substances for legitimate medical purposes in accordance with accepted standard medical practice. The CSA also assigned controlled substances to five classifications, with differing penalties for unlawful uses, based on the potential for misuse. Schedule I substances have an extremely high potential for abuse, are deemed to have no medicinal benefit, and cannot be prescribed. Drugs in this class include the opioid heroin and nonopioid drugs such as marijuana, gamma-hydroxybutyric acid (GHB), and lysergic acid diethylamide (LSD). Schedule II drugs also have an extremely high potential for abuse yet are deemed to have medicinal benefit in limited circumstances. Such substances include the opioids fentanyl, codeine, hydromorphone, meperidine, methadone, morphine, and oxycodone. When the CSA was developed, schedule III drugs were believed to have less abuse potential than schedule II drugs, and include opioids such as dihydrocodeine, or codeine, in combination with non-steroidal anti-inflammatory drugs (NSAIDs) or acetaminophen. Schedule IV drugs are those that have less abuse potential than schedule III drugs and include the weak opioid pentazocine and benzodiazepine drugs such as clonazepam, diazepam, and alprazolam.

Schedule V drugs are those with lowest abuse potential among the controlled substances within the CSA and include compounds with limited quantities of opioids such as codeine or opium used in preparations for cough or diarrhea, respectively.

The CSA does not regulate medical practice, as state governments hold this authority. However, the CSA specifically stipulates that controlled substances must be made available for medical purposes. This is accomplished through a quota system that attempts to balance the medical need for these medications while discouraging overproduction, which could lead to diversion. The CSA also does not limit the dose or the length of time that patients may use controlled substances for legitimate medical purposes. In fact, specific language contained in the CSA addressed the issue of extended opioid use for the treatment of intractable pain.[14]

THE ROLE OF THE DRUG ENFORCEMENT ADMINISTRATION

Within the United States, the Drug Enforcement Agency (DEA) has been designated by the US Department of Justice to ensure that controlled substances are prescribed, administered, and dispensed by licensed practitioners solely for legitimate medical purposes.[15] Legitimate medical purpose has been further interpreted to mean that practitioners act in the "usual course of professional practice" when prescribing such medications for their patients.[16] To fulfill this role, licensed clinicians who wish to prescribe controlled substances must be registered with the DEA.[14] Although the DEA does not have the legal authority to regulate medical practice, it does have the authority to investigate practitioners who do not comply with laws regarding controlled substance prescribing practices. The DEA has stated that it uses court rulings and legal precedent when evaluating whether a practitioner is prescribing opioid medications in accordance with the CSA. In the Supreme Court Case *Gonzales v. Oregon*, the definition of legitimate medical purpose is clarified. The ruling states that the CSA "ensures patients use controlled substances under the supervision of a doctor to prevent addiction and recreational use." Furthermore the court stated: "as a corollary, the provision also bars doctors from peddling to patients who crave the drugs for those prohibited uses."[16,17] The DEA has cited these statements when describing how it determines whether or not physicians are prescribing opioids for a legitimate legal purpose. The DEA has outlined common behaviors that result in the revocation of DEA registration: issuing prescriptions for controlled substances without a bona fide physician–patient relationship, issuing prescriptions in exchange for sex, issuing several prescriptions at once for a highly potent combination of controlled substances, charging fees commensurate with drug dealing rather than providing medical services, issuing prescriptions using fraudulent names, and self-abuse by practitioners.[16,18]

The DEA has also said that there are no specific parameters that would lead to the conclusion that a physician is practicing outside the norms of professional practice citing legal precedent that the evidence of reasonable guilt must be decided on a case-by-case basis.[19] According to reporting data available through 2005, in any given year less than 0.01% of physicians in the United States lose their controlled substance registrations based on a DEA investigation. Additionally, most investigations of physicians suspected of substandard prescribing practices that result in the revocation of DEA registration are initiated by state medical boards.[16]

STATE LAWS AND POLICIES THAT GOVERN THE USE OF OPIOIDS FOR PAIN MANAGEMENT

State governments share the responsibility of governing the prescribing and dispensing of controlled substances with the federal government. However, States also have the sole responsibility of regulating the health care practice of physicians, pharmacists, nurses, and other health care professionals. State licensing boards establish minimum standards of practice for any profession as well as for the use of controlled substances. They also have the authority to discipline practitioners who fail to adhere to these minimum standards. States have now turned to the state medical boards to assist with the control of opioid distribution by authorizing them to issue regulatory health guidelines. By allowing the State Medical Boards to shoulder this responsibility, the hope was that regulatory guidelines would be more congruent with recent scientific findings and medical interventions than laws passed by legislative bodies. This was done to promote better pain management and address provider fears of investigation and disciplinary action.[20] In 1998, the Federation of State Medical Boards adopted a policy template entitled Model Guideline for the Use of Controlled Substances for the Treatment of Pain (Model Policy).[21] This template was introduced with the intention of promoting consistent policy across state medical boards with regards to pain medication regulations for clinicians. An update to the policy was introduced in 2004, and the current policy was updated in 2013.[4,22]

Recent reports in the popular press regarding the opioid epidemic in the United States and the release of the CDC Guidelines for Opioid Prescribing in 2016[3] have prompted several states to pass laws restricting opioid prescribing for chronic and acute pain. Many of these new laws mirror the guidelines set forth by the CDC or similar guidelines.[23–25] Additionally, many states now require that practitioners who prescribe schedule II substances participate in approved Continuing Medical Education (CME) courses that address the risks and benefits of opioid medication use for chronic pain treatment.[26]

PRESCRIPTION DRUG MONITORING PROGRAMS

Prescription drug monitoring programs (PDMPs) have been in existence since the middle of the 20th Century, with California and Hawaii implementing PDMPs in the 1940s. Such programs collect prescription data at the state level to monitor the flow of controlled medication prescriptions. As of 2017, all 50 states, with the exception of Missouri, and the US Territory Guam have functional PDMPs.[27] For a PDMP to be fully functional, data on a prescribed controlled substance must be entered into the system. Most states have mandatory reporting policies, usually through data input from the pharmacist, though some states only strongly encourage pharmacies and physicians to report these data. New York enacted a law requiring that physicians supply controlled substance prescription information to the state PDMP at the time a prescription is written. Furthermore, pharmacists are also required to update the database as soon as such prescriptions are filled. Similar laws have been passed or are under consideration in other states.[28,29]

In addition to timely reporting, the data need to be centrally stored and processed. In the early days, these data were stored in the form of duplicate or triplicate copies of prescriptions, with one copy being sent to the state for cataloging. Current PDMPs store these data electronically for easy access by authorized users. Data from a PDMP must be protected and used carefully. A set of rules must be established regarding who can access the data. In this regard, there is considerable variability among different states. Generally, pharmacists and physicians can obtain PDMP data for their own patients. In some states, other agencies or regulatory boards, such as licensing boards and law enforcement, either have direct access or can access the data for official investigations. In some cases, access may even require a subpoena.[30]

The effectiveness of PDMPs on producing tangible outcomes has been a source of controversy. One recent study failed to show that states with PDMPs had significantly lower rates of drug overdose, opioid overdose–related mortality, or rates of consumption of opioid drugs.[31] It has postulated that this finding is due to grouping together well-developed state PDMP programs with those that are not yet as effective as they may be in the future. Secondly, it also reflects a lack of physician awareness of PDMPs, difficulty accessing the data, or unfamiliarity with how to utilize the PDMP data when writing opioid prescriptions.[32] There is a need for appropriately designed studies that account for these potential confounding factors to assess the efficacy of PDMP databases in curtailing opioid misuse. PDMP databases are helpful in assisting physicians assess the risks and benefits of prescribing opioids for pain management on a case-by-case basis.

Many states are struggling to find funding sources to support their PDMP. Funding for PDMPs has been a combined effort of state and more recently federal funds. Programs can be costly to run, and states with increasingly tight budgets are under pressure to reduce funding further. However, states can get initial seed money to begin PDMPs via the Harold Johnson Prescription Monitoring Program, which was initiated in 2002,[33] and the National All Schedules Prescription Electronic Reporting Act (NASPER), initially signed in 2005.[34] However, at present, funding for the NASPER program has not been reauthorized by Congress, and its future is uncertain in spite of ongoing efforts to renew funding.[35]

One issue of concern with PDMPs is that until recently there was little sharing of data across state borders. This occurred either because of administrative differences or that neighboring states did not have a functional PDMP. The NASPER program attempts to address this issue by language that requires the sharing of opioid prescription information with other states, especially bordering states. Additionally, recently the Harold Johnson Monitoring Program has also mandated that states receiving funding share data with neighboring states.[33] Practical implementation of this requirement has been slow, and so the issue of potential doctor shopping for opioid medications in neighboring states still exists.

In spite of the challenges and weaknesses of current state PDMPs, these programs offer a promising tool for helping physicians know where and from whom their patients are receiving controlled substances. As more states adopt and implement PDMPs as well as facilitate the sharing of data across state borders, the effectiveness of this tool should increase dramatically and enhance patient safety.

PATIENT AND PROVIDER AGREEMENTS WHEN USING OPIOID MEDICATIONS TO MANAGE CHRONIC PAIN

In 2013, the FSMB updated its model policy on opioid prescribing for pain management,[4] and similar recommendations were recently published by the CDC.[3] The FSMB policy instructs physicians to discuss the risks and benefits of any pain treatment plan with the patient or appropriate surrogate or guardian. Additionally, it recommends that a written informed consent and treatment agreement be signed by both the physician and the patient then placed in the patient's medical record. It is wise to update and review such agreements with patients periodically, perhaps as frequently as yearly. Such an agreement, though not technically legally binding, helps establish expectations for the patient and is a tool to help demonstrate that the patient has been informed of the risks and benefits and wishes to proceed with opioid-based treatment therapies. Such documents are often referred to as "opioid treatment agreements."

The FSMB policy states that informed consent documents typically include the following:

- Potential risks and benefits of chronic opioid therapy including potential long- and short-term side effects.
- Specifically state the following risks: tolerance and physical dependence, impaired motor skills, drug interactions and oversedation, misuses, dependence, addiction, and overdose
- Limited evidence regarding benefit of long-term opioid therapy
- Physician's prescribing polices and expectations such as number and frequency of refills, policy on early refills, and replacement of lost or stolen medication
- Specific reasons for which the drug therapy may be changed or discontinued (i.e., violation of the policies spelled out in the treatment agreement)

The FSMB policy further recommends that a treatment agreement address the joint responsibilities of the physician and patient when opioid or other abusable medications are used:

- Goals of treatment: pain management and functional improvement
- Patient responsibility for safe medication us including concomitant use of alcohol or other sedating substances, medication overuse, secure storage of medication, safe disposal of unused medication
- Patient must obtain medication from one physician or practice
- Patient consent for monitoring of medication use by periodic drug testing and random drug testing
- Physician or practice responsibility to be available to address unforeseen problems and prescribe scheduled refills

The FSMB policy also suggests that the informed consent and treatment agreements may be combined into a single document for convenience. A sample opioid treatment agreement along with recommendations for implementation of the agreement written by the National Institute of Drug Abuse is available free of charge.[36]

If a patient does not achieve functional improvement after a trial of opioid medications or the patient violates the terms in the opioid agreement, it may be necessary to discontinue treatment of pain with opioid medications. The FSMB policy states that even the presence of persistence of debilitating pain does not justify escalation or continuation of opioid-based treatments. In such situations, it can be helpful to refer to the initial opioid agreement to remind the patient of the expectations agreed upon before initiation or assuming prescribing of opioid medications.

URINE DRUG SCREEN TESTING

In a retrospective study with one million chronic pain patients, it was reported that 75% of those patients did not use their pain medications as prescribed.[37] Current opioid prescribing medication guidelines recommend the use of random UDT as part of a comprehensive opioid medication management program.[3,4,21,22,38] Federal law does not specifically mandate that such testing be performed for patients receiving opioid medications; however, the DEA has cited: "a departure from, or the failure to conform to, minimal standards of care of similar practitioners" as justification for revoking privileges to prescribe opioid medications.[39] Some states have also incorporated mandatory UDT for clinicians who prescribe opioid medications for chronic pain.[23,25,29] It seems that clinicians who prescribe medications for chronic use should incorporate a UDT program to help avoid potential medicolegal problems.

There are two types of UDT: a relatively inexpensive immunoassay that provides a result within minutes and a more costly confirmatory test that utilizes mass spectrometry and gas chromatography but may take up to 2 weeks for a result report. Although the point-of-care immunoassay provides a quick result, this test often produces false positive and false negative results. Additionally, the immunoassay test does not always specify which opioid is present or detect the presence of all substances that might be of concern. It is often recommended that the more expensive confirmatory testing be performed, especially for high risk patients, as it can detect virtually any substance and/or its metabolite in the sample (see Tables 30-1 and 30-2).

Confirmatory UDT, though more reliable than the immunoassay test, can fail to provide an accurate assessment of appropriate opioid medication use. Some patients purposely try to evade detection of prescription medication misuse, concomitant illicit substance use, or diversion. This can result in a false sense of security regarding appropriate opioid medication use. Such patients may dilute urine with tap water, bring in another person's urine, or try to alter the assay results using glutaraldehyde,[43] niacin,[44] or other substances.[45] Therefore, it is best to document that UDT has been used as a tool in conjunction with other supporting information such as physical examination, diagnostic imaging, risk stratification, and improvement in function with regard to the decision to initiate, continue or discontinue opioid therapy.

TABLE 30-1 Urine Detection Times of Some Common Drugs of Abuse[40]

DRUG	SCREENING CUTOFF CONCENTRATIONS ng/mL URINE	CONFIRMATION CUTOFF CONCENTRATIONS ng/mL (NONREGULATED)	CONFIRMATION CUTOFF CONCENTRATIONS ng/mL (FEDERALLY REGULATED)	URINE DETECTION TIME
Opioids				
Morphine	300	50	2000	3-4 d
Codeine	300	50	2000; 300	1-3 d
Hydrocodone	300	50	2000	1-2 d
Oxycodone	100	50	2000	1-3 d
Methadone	300	100	2000	2-4 d
Benzodiazepines	200	20-50	NA	Up to 30 d
Cocaine	300	50	150	1-3 d
Marijuana	50	15	15	1-3 d for casual use; up to 30 d for chronic use
Amphetamine	1000	100	500	2-4 d
Methamphetamine	1000	100	500	2-4 d
Heroin[a]	10	10	NA	1-3 d
Phencyclidine	25	10	25	2-7 d for causal use; up to 30 d for chronic use

[a] *6-MAM, the specific metabolite is detected only for 6 hours.*
More comprehensive lists are available from specific laboratories.[41]

TABLE 30-2 Metabolites of Common Opioid Substances[40,42]

OPIATE	METABOLITES	COMMENT
Hydrocodone	Hydromorphone	If codeine to hydrocodone ratio <10, codeine is not the sole source
	Dihydrocodine	Level generally lower than its hydrocodone source and below detection if only codeine was ingested
	Normorphine	
	Norhydrocodone	
	Hydrocodol	
	Hydromorphol	
Oxycodone	Oxymorphone	
	Noroxycodone	
	Oxycodols and their respective oxide	
Morphine	Hydromorphone (minor)	If codeine to morphine ration <6, codeine is likely not the sole source
	Morphine-3-glucuronide	Level generally lower than its hydrocodone source and below detection if only codeine was ingested
	Morphine-6-glucuronide	
	Normorphine	
Methodone	2-Ethylidene-1,5-dimethyl-3, 3-diphenylpyrrolidine 2-ethyl-5-methyl-3, 3-diphenylpyrrolidine	
Hydromorphone	Dihydromorphine Hydromorphone-3-glucuronide	Level generally lower than its hydrocodone source and below detection if only codeine was ingested
Oxymorphone	Oxymorphone-3-glucuronide oxymorphol	
Codeine	Hydrocodone (minor)	If codeine to hydrocodone ration <10, codeine is not the sole source
	Norcodeine	If codeine to morphine ration <6, codeine is likely not the sole source
	Morphine	Level generally lower than its hydrocodone source and below detection if only codeine was ingested
Propoxyphene	Norpropoxyphene	
Fentanyl	Norfentanyl	
Tarmadol	O-desmethyl-tramadol Nortramadol	
Butrophanol	Hydroxybutorphanol Norbutrophanol	
Bupernorphine	Norbuprenorphine	
	Norbuprenorphine-3-glucuronide	
	Buprenorphine-3-glucuronide	
Heroin	Morphine codeine (contaminant) 6-Monoacetylmorphine	

CONCLUSION

Current federal and state law regulations attempt to promote balanced approaches to the management of pain. In light of data revealing increasing risks associated with prescription opioids, it is imperative that physicians maintain heightened awareness of the risks as well as the benefits of using controlled medications to treat pain. This requires periodic review of current treatment guidelines as well as recent changes in policy and law. A well-crafted Opioid Treatment Agreement can be used as a tool to educate patients regarding risks and benefits of opioid medications in chronic pain management and set expectations for continued use of opioid-based treatments. Such agreements also establish clear parameters for discontinuation of opioid-based treatments if functional goals are not met or the patient violates the tenets outlined in the agreement. Physicians who invest the time and effort to learn about the full regulatory requirements for prescribing opioid medications will help provide the best care possible for their patients.

REFERENCES

1. Walsh L. *Reports and Detailed Tables From the 2015 National Survey on Drug Use and Health (NSDUH)*; 2016. https://www.samhsa.gov/samhsa-data-outcomes-quality/major-data-collections/reports-detailed-tables-2015-NSDUH. Accessed 6 July 2017.

2. Rudd RA, Seth P, David F, Scholl L. Increases in drug and opioid-involved overdose deaths – United States, 2010–2015. *MMWR Morb Mortal Wkly Rep.* 2016;65(5051):1445-1452. doi:10.15585/mmwr.mm655051e1.

3. Dowell D, Haegerich TM, Chou R. CDC guideline for prescribing ppioids for chronic pain – United States, 2016. *MMWR Recomm Rep.* 2016;65(1):1-49. doi:10.15585/mmwr.rr6501e1.

4. Federation of State Medical Boards of the United States Inc. *Model Policy for the Use of Opioid Analgesics in the Treatment.* Federation of State Medical Boards of the United States Inc; 2013. http://www.fsmb.org/pdf/pain_policy_july2013.pdf.

5. Quality improvement guidelines for the treatment of acute pain and cancer pain. American Pain Society Quality of Care Committee. *JAMA.* 1995;274(23):1874-1880.

6. Veterans Health Administration. *Pain as the 5th Vital Sign Toolkit*; October 2000. http://www.va.gov/painmanagement/docs/toolkit.pdf. Accessed 24 November 2018.

7. Portenoy RK, Foley KM. Chronic use of opioid analgesics in non-malignant pain: report of 38 cases. *Pain.* 1986;25(2):171-186.

8. Porter J, Jick H. Addiction rare in patients treated with narcotics. *N Engl J Med.* 1980;302(2):123.

9. Rosenthal E. *Patients in Pain Find Relief, Not Addiction, in Narcotics.* The New York Times; 1993. http://www.nytimes.com/1993/03/28/us/patients-in-pain-find-relief-not-addiction-in-narcotics.html. Accessed 8 July 2017.

10. Institute of Medicine of the National Academies. *Relieving Pain in America: A Blueprint for Transforming Prevention, Care, Education, and Research.* Vol. 2012. 2011.

11. Population Data/NSDUH/data/population-data-nsduh. Accessed 8 July 2017.

12. *Controlled Substances Act.* Vol Pub L No. 91-513, 84 Stat 1242; 1970.

13. U.S. House of Representatives, Interstate and Foreign Commerce Committee. 1970. Comprehensive Drug Abuse Prevention and Control Act of 1970 Report No. 91–1444, 91st Congress, 2nd Session (September 10).

14. Title 21 – Food and Drugs, Chapter II – Drug Enforcement Administration, Department of Justice, Part 1306 – Prescriptions, General Information. 24 April 1971.

15. Title 21. Food and Drugs; Chapter 13. Drug Abuse Prevention and Control; Control and Enforcement. Vol Chapter 13. Drug Abuse Prvention and Control; 2011.

16. Department of Justice, Drug Enforcement Administration. *Dispensing Controlled Substances for the Treatment of Pain, Part V.* Vol. 71; 2006.

17. *Gonzales v. Oregon, 126 S. Ct. 904.* Vol. 04-623; 2006.

18. *United States v. Morton Salt Co.* Vol. 273; 1950.

19. *United States v. August.* Vol. 91-2331; 1992.

20. Gilson AM, Maurer MA, Joranson DE. State policy affecting pain management: recent improvements and the positive impact of regulatory health policies. *Health Policy.* 2005;74(2):192-204.

21. Federation of State Medical Boards of the United States Inc. *Model Guidelines for the Use of Controlled Substances for the Treatment of Pain.* Euless, TX, USA: Federation of State Medical Boards of the United States Inc; 1998.

22. Federation of State Medical Boards of the United States Inc. *Model Policy for the Use of Controlled Substances for the Treatment of Pain.* Dallas, TX, USA: Federation of State Medical Boards of the United States Inc; 2004.

23. *New Indiana Law Imposes a Seven-Day Limit on Opioid Prescriptions | Health Care Law Firm in the USA | Hall Render. Law Firm | Health Care Law Firm in the USA | Hall Render*; 2017. http://www.hallrender.com/2017/06/21/new-indiana-law-imposes-a-seven-day-limit-on-opioid-prescriptions/. Accessed 19 November 2017.

24. Fla. Gov. Announces Proposed 3-Day Limit on Opioid Prescriptions. US News & World Report. 26 September 2017. https://www.usnews.com/news/national-news/articles/2017-09-26/fl-gov-announces-3-day-limit-on-opioid-prescriptions. Accessed 19 November 2017.

25. New Prescribing Law for Treatment of Acute and Chronic Pain | NJAFP. 15 February 2017. https://www.njafp.org/content/new-prescribing-law-treatment-acute-and-chronic-pain. Accessed 19 November 2017.

26. GRPOL_CME_Overview_by_State.pdf. https://www.fsmb.org/Media/Default/PDF/FSMB/Advocacy/GRPOL_CME_Overview_by_State.pdf. Accessed 19 November 2017.

27. Green S. *Compilation of Prescription Monitoring Program Maps.* Harrisburg, PA: National Alliance for Model State Drug Laws; 1 September 2016. http://www.namsdl.org/library/CAE654BF-BBEA-211E-694C755E16C2DD21/. Accessed 9 July 2017.

28. Larkin WJ. *Senate Passes "I-Stop" to Reduce Prescription Drug Abuse | New York State Senate.* Vol. 2012; 2012.

29. Weiss D. New York State Set to Crack Down on Painkiller Abuse. Vol. 2012. 2012.

30. Wang J, Christo PJ. The influence of prescription monitoring programs on chronic pain management. *Pain Physician.* 2009;12(3):507-515.

31. Paulozzi LJ, Kilbourne EM, Desai HA. Prescription drug monitoring programs and death rates from drug overdose. *Pain Med.* 2011;12(5):747-754. doi:10.1111/j.1526-4637.2011.01062.x.

32. Fishman SM. Prescription drug monitoring programs serve a vital clinical need. *Pain Med.* 2011;12(6):845. doi:10.1111/j.1526-4637.2011.01161.x.

33. Bureau of Justice Assistance. Prescription Drug Monitoring Program. 2002. https://www.bja.gov/ProgramDetails.aspx?Program_ID=72#horizontalTab2.

34. Public Law 109-60 [H.R. 1132]; *National All Schedules Prescription Electronic Reporting Act of 2005*; 2005.

35. American Society of Interventional Pain Physicians. National All Schedules Prescription Electronic Reporting Act (NASPER). 11 August 2005. http://nasper.org/. Accessed 10 July 2017.

36. National Institute on Drug Abuse. *Other Opioid Prescribing Resources*; 2017. https://www.drugabuse.gov/nidamed-medical-health-professionals/tool-resources-your-practice/other-opioid-prescribing-resources. Accessed 10 July 2017.

37. Couto JE, Romney MC, Leider HL, Sharma S, Goldfarb NI. High rates of inappropriate drug use in the chronic pain population. *Popul Health Manag.* 2009;12(4):185-190. doi:10.1089/pop.2009.0015.

38. Manchikanti L, Kaye AM, Knezevic NN, et al. Responsible, safe, and effective prescription of opioids for chronic non-cancer pain: American Society of Interventional Pain Physicians (ASIPP) guidelines. *Pain Physician.* 2017;20(2S):S3-S92.

39. Villavicencio JRS. *Decision and Order*; 2015. https://www.deadiversion.usdoj.gov/fed_regs/actions/2015/fr0123.htm. Accessed 19 November 2017.

40. Christo PJ, Manchikanti L, Ruan X, et al. Urine drug testing in chronic pain. *Pain Physician.* 2011;14(2):123-143.

41. Drugs of Abuse: Approximate Detection Times–Mayo Medical Laboratories. https://www.mayomedicallaboratories.com/test-info/drug-book/viewall.html. Accessed 19 November 2017.

42. Smith HS. Opioid metabolism. *Mayo Clin Proc.* 2009; 84(7):613-624.

43. George S, Braithwaite RA. The effect of glutaraldehyde adulteration of urine specimens on syva EMIT II drugs-of-abuse assays. *J Anal Toxicol.* 1996;20(3):195-196.

44. Centers for Disease Control and Prevention (CDC). Use of niacin in attempts to defeat urine drug testing–five states, January-September 2006. *MMWR Morb Mortal Wkly Rep.* 2007;56(15):365-366.

45. Wu AH. Integrity of urine specimens for toxicological analysis–adulteration, mechanisms of action, and laboratory detection. *Forensic Sci Rev.* 1998;10(1):47-65.

31

BUPRENORPHINE USE IN THE PRIMARY CARE SETTING

Nathan Bryant, PharmD and Mark Holtsman, PharmD

OVERVIEW
NATURE AND SIGNIFICANCE OF THE MEDICATION
MECHANISM OF ACTION
INDICATIONS
CONTRAINDICATIONS
    Pharmacokinetics
SPECIAL POPULATIONS
TOXICITY (CLINICAL MANIFESTATION)
BUPRENORPHINE MISCONCEPTIONS
DOSING
    References

FAST FACTS

- Buprenorphine is a unique molecule that may have certain advantages over other opioids.
- Buprenorphine is a partial agonist at the mu receptor as well as an antagonist at the kappa receptor. These receptor pharmacodynamics help to explain the advantages that buprenorphine may have over conventional opioids.
- Buprenorphine is mainly associated with medication-assisted treatment, but can also be very useful for pain management.

NATURE AND SIGNIFICANCE OF THE MEDICATION

Buprenorphine is an opioid analgesic with unique pharmacologic properties that can serve as a powerful tool for pain management in the primary care setting. It appears to possess antihyperalgesic qualities, and rotating therapy to buprenorphine from other high-dose opioids has been demonstrated to result in improved pain control.[1,2] Constipation also appears to be less of an issue.[3] Buprenorphine has a ceiling effect for respiratory depression,[4] making it potentially safer—though not risk free[5-7]—for individuals with respiratory comorbidities. Buprenorphine is available for administration via sublingual, buccal, and transdermal routes, which makes it an attractive option for those who have difficulty swallowing, unreliable intestinal absorption, or malignant bowel obstruction. There is still abuse potential,[8] and therefore similarly to other medications, only the minimum effective dose that provides a functional benefit should be used after careful analysis of the risks and benefits.

The possibility of reduced immunosuppression has been raised based on animal models[9] as well as the finding in human trials involving heroin abusers that both buprenorphine and methadone maintenance improves immune function relative to active heroin abuse[10] and matches functional markers found in healthy controls.[11]

Buprenorphine has been purported to have less of an effect on testosterone levels and sexual function based on a single study comparing it to methadone.[12] We consider this to be an unresolved clinical question as the expected potency of the mean buprenorphine dose was significantly lower than the mean methadone dose used in the comparison. However, it is worth noting that the testosterone levels of the buprenorphine-treated subjects were within the reported reference range despite being on a dose we would consider quite high in most chronic noncancer pain contexts.

MECHANISM OF ACTION

Buprenorphine is an interesting molecule because of its distinctive receptor binding profile: in regard to its opioid receptor binding behavior, it acts as a partial agonist at the mu receptor and as an antagonist at the kappa receptor[13]. It appears to have further agonist activity at the nociceptin receptor,[14] the clinical impact of which remains unclear but may have a role in terms of both analgesia and reducing reward pathway activation.

When binding to the mu receptor, buprenorphine produces a number of effects including analgesia, respiratory depression, and euphoria—just like any other opioid. Where its clinical effects depart from other opioids is the presence of an apparent ceiling dose for some effects. After a certain dose is reached, there is no further increase in the observed effect on the patient. This phenomenon is most well-described for respiratory depression[4] but appears to hold true for euphoria as well.[15] Studies demonstrating a ceiling effect were largely limited to opioid addiction settings, which may have led to extrapolation of the observed plateau in the drug's effect to analgesia. It is important to note that while buprenorphine clearly behaves as a partial mu agonist at the receptor level, the observed *clinical* effect varies between that of a partial agonist and full agonist depending on the affected organ system and efficacy endpoint.[13,16] In terms of analgesia, convincing evidence of a ceiling effect for analgesia in humans has not been demonstrated.[17-19]

The antagonist activity at the kappa receptor is a possible explanation for the antihyperalgesic qualities of buprenorphine, at least in part. Opioid administration stimulates expression of dynorphin, a kappa receptor agonist that has been implicated in the development of pain sensitization[20]. That said, this is certainly an oversimplification of a complex process that is not fully understood. It is also important to note that neither the kappa receptor antagonist nor the partial mu receptor agonist properties prevent the successful use of other opioids for breakthrough pain, as multiple human trials have demonstrated.[18,21] If a patient on buprenorphine requires acute pain management (e.g., in the event of trauma or surgery), they can expect to respond to therapy in a manner similar to other patients on prior opioid therapy.

INDICATIONS

Table 31-1 shows the FDA indications and formulations for buprenorphine. Buprenorphine is FDA approved for treatment of opiate dependence. When buprenorophine is prescribed for this indication, the physician must have a separate X-designated DEA registration, which can only be obtained after formal training in medication-assisted therapy.

Labeled indications for buprenorphine vary by formulation. Although all formulations can be appropriately

prescribed for pain management without a separate X-designated DEA registration, recognize that prescriptions for the sublingual films and tablets should indicate they are being prescribed off-label for pain management. Insurance formulary limitations further complicate product selection, as some companies will insist that only formulations used on-label are eligible for coverage. Given the dynamic nature of insurance formularies, be prepared to switch to an alternative formulation until you are familiar with the local insurance landscape.

CONTRAINDICATIONS

Buprenorphine is contraindicated if there is a history of anaphylaxis or hypersensitivity reaction after previous exposure to any drug in its structural class. Note that buprenorphine shares the same characteristic 3-ring phenanthrene structure found in morphine and its derivatives. Buprenorphine should not be used in the case of a true allergy to this structural class and vice versa.

The buprenorphine/naloxone combination products should not be used in patients with severe hepatic dysfunction (e.g., Child Pugh Class C). Whereas the naloxone component has extremely low bioavailability due to extensive first-pass metabolism to the point of being negligible in patients with normal liver function,[22] those with severe hepatic impairment experience 10-fold higher naloxone exposure, which may be sufficient to impair analgesic efficacy.[23]

Pharmacokinetics

Buccal and sublingual buprenorphine reaches peak plasma concentrations approximately 1 hour after administration (range 40 min-3.5 h) and has a half-life of around 24 hours (range 19-35 h).[24]

The bioavailability of sublingual buprenorphine in tablet form appears to be on the order of ~15% to 25%.[24,25] There are conflicting reports on sublingual bioavailability as a result of the varying conditions under which the bioavailability studies were performed. Early studies utilized a sublingual *solution* formulation and found ~30% to 50% bioavailability.[24] Subsequent studies on the tablet formulation focused on bioavailability *relative to the solution*,[25] which may account for misinterpretation of older studies.

SPECIAL POPULATIONS

Renal dysfunction: Although buprenorphine excretion is not affected by renal function, the weakly active metabolite, norbuprenorphine, has potential to accumulate in renal dysfunction. Although this does not appear to be problematic at low doses,[13] its impact at higher doses is unknown.

Hepatic dysfunction: Because buprenorphine undergoes hepatic metabolism, largely to inactive components, consider reducing the initial dose to account for increased buprenorphine exposure.[23]

TABLE 31-1 Buprenorphine Delivery Methods	
FORMULATION PRODUCT	**LABELED INDICATION**
Sublingual tablet (with or without naloxone)	Treatment of opioid dependence
Sublingual film (with naloxone)	Treatment of opioid dependence
Buccal film	Pain management
Transdermal patch	Pain management

Elderly: The safety and efficacy of transdermal buprenorphine was found to be no different in the elderly when compared with younger patients.[26]

TOXICITY (CLINICAL MANIFESTATION)

In the event of an overdose, recognize that the unique receptor binding of buprenorphine has consequences for the effective use of naloxone. Naloxone works as a competitive opioid receptor antagonist, with varying binding affinities depending on the receptor subtype. In order for naloxone to successfully outcompete buprenorphine and its exceptionally high binding affinity, a 2- to 3-fold higher dose than normal is required to achieve reversal.[27] 2 to 4 mg of naloxone IV bolus followed by a 4 mg/h infusion has been demonstrated to be an effective strategy for full reversal. Interestingly, the same study found a bell-shaped dose-response curve, with bolus doses of 5 mg and greater showing less reversal efficacy than lower doses.[27]

Although buprenorphine has demonstrated promise as a potentially safer option than other opioid analgesics, it still shares the same risk considerations as any other opioid. Respiratory depression remains a concern,[6] and patients should be advised against drinking alcohol while on buprenorphine because of the real risk of accidental overdose death. Concurrent benzodiazepine use should also generally be avoided and treated with the same level of extreme caution as with other opioids.[7,24]

A mild QT prolonging effect of buprenorphine has been shown in some clinical trials of the transdermal formulation, with a mean 11 ms increase in the QT interval noted at a dose of 40 µg/hour. A subsequent study demonstrated a small mean QT interval increase on the order of 6 ms[28] in healthy subjects. The clinical significance of the increases seen in these studies appears to be slight; even high daily doses of buprenorphine (32 mg SL) did not result in overt QT prolongation, as opposed to a 32% occurrence with equipotent methadone dosing.[29] While these studies are reassuring, electrocardiographic (ECG) monitoring may continue to be reasonable in certain patients (e.g., elevated baseline QT or concurrent use of known QT prolonging agents).

Of the minor adverse drug reactions, nausea is the most commonly reported across dosage forms and occurs at a rate of ~10% (vs. 7% for placebo)[30,31] with stable dosing. Nausea was reported far more frequently (50%) during initial dose titration in opioid-naïve patients.[30] Application site itching and redness is specific to the transdermal delivery product and occurs at a rate of 10% to 12%.[31]

BUPRENORPHINE MISCONCEPTIONS

A number of misconceptions about buprenorphine persist as a result of both its complex pharmacology, of which a complete mechanistic picture has admittedly not been fully described, and early products' labeling for opioid dependence. These mischaracterizations are addressed directly based on published human clinical trial experience:

1. Buprenorphine blocks the effects of other opioids.
   - While not directly relevant to the primary care settings, patients and/or colleagues may express concern about future management of acute pain in the event of serious injury or surgery. Clinical practice has seen that buprenorphine can be successfully used with other opioids in acute pain situations and is thus the assertion that buprenorphine blocks the effects of other opioids is demonstrably false. However, breakthrough dosing will need to be customized to account for their chronic opioid use—a reality that is unchanged whether they are maintained on buprenorphine, oxycodone, or any other opioid.

2. When being used for opioid dependence, buprenorphine can only be prescribed by practitioners who possess an X-DEA registration.
   - While prescribing the currently approved sublingual buprenorphine products for pain is an off-label use, no special DEA registration is required. The indication for chronic pain should be specified on the prescription so the dispensing pharmacist is aware of the intended use.

3. In the United States, buprenorphine was meant for opioid addiction treatment, but can also be very helpful in pain management.
   - It is true that the long half-life of the drug makes it useful in the addiction setting because it allows for once-daily dosing, but its efficacy in treating pain has also been clearly demonstrated in peer-reviewed literature. These 2 divergent uses of the same drug do require a different dosing strategy, because similarly to methadone, the duration of action for analgesia is typically only 6 to 8 hours for most patients. So, while large single doses make sense for addiction management, an appropriate pain management strategy will make use of relatively smaller doses more frequently to maintain analgesia.

DOSING

Published equianalgesic conversion data for buprenorphine are limited and likely incomplete, with seemingly contradictory results that lend further evidence to the idea that the full picture has yet to be revealed.

The most robust data currently available come from transdermal formulation studies and allow for a reasonable estimate of a 70 to 115 mg:1 mg ratio between oral morphine and transdermal buprenorphine in opioid-tolerant patients[32]. However, a study in opioid-naïve patients receiving a low-dose formulation of 0.4 mg SL buprenorphine for acute pain found analgesic efficacy equal to 5 mg of IV morphine[33] (or ~15 mg PO morphine). This study would suggest a potency ratio of 150 to 250 mg:1 mg in opioid-naïve patients, assuming bioavailability is unchanged. It is possible that the bioavailability

TABLE 31-2 Extrapolated Equianalgesic Dose When Converting to Buprenorphine From Other High-Dose Opioids

PRODUCT	DOSE	BIOAVAILABILITY	APPROXIMATE SYSTEMICALLY AVAILABLE DOSE	POSSIBLE ORAL MORPHINE EQUIVALENTS
Sublingual tablet (8 mg strength)	8 mg	15%-25%	1200-2000 μg	85-230 mg
Transdermal patch	20 μg/h	N/A	480 μg (24-h total)	35-55 mg
Buccal film	150 μg	46%-65%	70-100 μg	Very limited data (5-25 mg)

increases at lower doses (which may explain the unexpectedly high bioavailability of the buccal film), the potency is higher in opioid-naïve patients (similar to fentanyl), or some other variable is driving this difference. In the case of opioid-naïve patients, initial dosing guidelines and titration schedules are provided in the package inserts for the various buprenorphine products.

The most difficult and poorly described situations involve switching a patient on high-dose opioids to buprenorphine. Although the drug manufacturers provide some guidance for switching patients from doses as high as 160 mg oral morphine equivalents (OME), it comes with the caveat that these patients must first be tapered to 30 mg OME or less before initiating buprenorphine therapy. There are many ways to taper down to 30 mg OME.[34]

Transitioning to buprenorphine involves cessation of high-dose opioid therapy 12 to 24 hours before the first dose of a sublingual formulation of buprenorphine, which is usually administered in the clinic setting. Failure to do this may lead to acute, precipitated withdrawal symptoms upon taking the buprenorphine.

Selecting an appropriate dose of buprenorphine is the next challenge. Large variations in bioavailability have been found at the population level, so it is advisable to begin dosing at the conservative end of the scale and titrating the dose upward if needed. An extrapolated equivalent dose for the sublingual tablet formulation based on the reported bioavailability range and the relatively well-defined equianalgesic potency of transdermal buprenorphine is provided for illustrative purposes only (Table 31-2). To be sure, in our practice, we use an approximate conversion formula of 8 mg SL buprenorphine = 100 mg OME.

REFERENCES

1. Daitch J, Frey ME, Silver D, Mitnick C, Daitch D, Pergolizzi J. Conversion of chronic pain patients from full-opioid agonists to sublingual buprenorphine. *Pain Physician.* 2012;15(3 suppl):ES59-ES66.
2. Malinoff HL, Barkin RL, Wilson G. Sublingual buprenorphine is effective in the treatment of chronic pain syndrome. *Am J Ther.* 2005;12(5):379-384.
3. Mercadante S, Casuccio A, Tirelli W, Giarratano A. Equipotent doses to switch from high doses of opioids to transdermal buprenorphine. *Support Care Cancer.* 2009;17(6):715-718.
4. Dahan A, Yassen A, Bijl H, et al. Comparison of the respiratory effects of intravenous buprenorphine and fentanyl in humans and rats. *Br J Anaesth.* 2005;94(6):825-834.
5. Farney RJ, McDonald AM, Boyle KM, et al. Sleep disordered breathing in patients receiving therapy with buprenorphine/naloxone. *Eur Respir J.* 2013;42(2):394-403.
6. Toce MS, Burns MM, O'Donnell KA. Clinical effects of unintentional pediatric buprenorphine exposures: experience at a single tertiary care center. *Clin Toxicol (Phila).* 2017;55(1):12-17.
7. Bardy G, Cathala P, Eiden C, Baccino E, Petit P, Mathieu O. An unusual case of death probably triggered by the association of buprenorphine at therapeutic dose with ethanol and benzodiazepines and with very low norbuprenorphine level. *J Forensic Sci.* 2015;60(suppl 1):S269-S271.
8. Middleton LS, Nuzzo PA, Lofwall MR, Moody DE, Walsh SL. The pharmacodynamic and pharmacokinetic profile of intranasal crushed buprenorphine and buprenorphine/naloxone tablets in opioid abusers. *Addiction.* 2011;106(8):1460-1473.
9. Martucci C, Panerai AE, Sacerdote P. Chronic fentanyl or buprenorphine infusion in the mouse: similar analgesic profile but different effects on immune responses. *Pain.* 2004;110(1-2):385-392.
10. Neri S, Bruno CM, Pulvirenti D, et al. Randomized clinical trial to compare the effects of methadone and buprenorphine on the immune system in drug abusers. *Psychopharmacology (Berl).* 2005;179(3):700-704.
11. Sacerdote P, Franchi S, Gerra G, Leccese V, Panerai AE, Somaini L. Buprenorphine and methadone maintenance treatment of heroin addicts preserves immune function. *Brain Behav Immun.* 2008;22(4):606-613.
12. Bliesener N, Albrecht S, Schwager A, Weckbecker K, Lichtermann D, Klingmuller D. Plasma testosterone and sexual function in men receiving buprenorphine maintenance for opioid dependence. *J Clin Endocrinol Metab.* 2005;90(1):203-206.
13. Pergolizzi J, Aloisi AM, Dahan A, et al. Current knowledge of buprenorphine and its unique pharmacological profile. *Pain Pract.* 2010;10(5):428-450.
14. Huang P, Kehner GB, Cowan A, Liu-Chen LY. Comparison of pharmacological activities of buprenorphine and norbuprenorphine: norbuprenorphine is a potent opioid agonist. *J Pharmacol Exp Ther.* 2001;297(2):688-695.
15. Walsh SL, Preston KL, Stitzer ML, Cone EJ, Bigelow GE. Clinical pharmacology of buprenorphine: ceiling effects at high doses. *Clin Pharmacol Ther.* 1994;55(5):569-580.
16. Raffa RB, Ding Z. Examination of the preclinical antinociceptive efficacy of buprenorphine and its designation as full- or partial-agonist. *Acute Pain.* 2007;9(3):145-152.

17. Ciccozzi A, Angeletti C, Baldascino G, et al. High dose of buprenorphine in terminally ill patient with liver failure: efficacy and tolerability. *J Opioid Manag.* 2012;8(4):253-259.

18. Mercadante S, Ferrera P, Villari P. Is there a ceiling effect of transdermal buprenorphine? Preliminary data in cancer patients. *Support Care Cancer.* 2007;15(4):441-444.

19. Leppert W, Kowalski G. Long-term administration of high doses of transdermal buprenorphine in cancer patients with severe neuropathic pain. *Onco Targets Ther.* 2015;8:3621-3627.

20. Vanderah TW, Gardell LR, Burgess SE, et al. Dynorphin promotes abnormal pain and spinal opioid antinociceptive tolerance. *J Neurosci.* 2000;20(18):7074-7079.

21. Mercadante S, Villari P, Ferrera P, et al. Safety and effectiveness of intravenous morphine for episodic breakthrough pain in patients receiving transdermal buprenorphine. *J Pain Symptom Manage.* 2006;32(2):175-179.

22. Chiang CN, Hawks RL. Pharmacokinetics of the combination tablet of buprenorphine and naloxone. *Drug Alcohol Depend.* 2003;70(2 suppl):S39-S47.

23. Nasser AF, Heidbreder C, Liu Y, Fudala PJ. Pharmacokinetics of sublingual buprenorphine and naloxone in subjects with mild to severe hepatic impairment (child-pugh classes A, B, and C), in hepatitis C virus-seropositive subjects, and in healthy volunteers. *Clin Pharmacokinet.* 2015;54(8):837-849.

24. Elkader A, Sproule B. Buprenorphine: clinical pharmacokinetics in the treatment of opioid dependence. *Clin Pharmacokinet.* 2005;44(7):661-680.

25. Nath RP, Upton RA, Everhart ET, et al. Buprenorphine pharmacokinetics: relative bioavailability of sublingual tablet and liquid formulations. *J Clin Pharmacol.* 1999;39(6):619-623.

26. Likar R, Vadlau EM, Breschan C, Kager I, Korak-Leiter M, Ziervogel G. Comparable analgesic efficacy of transdermal buprenorphine in patients over and under 65 years of age. *Clin J Pain.* 2008;24(6):536-543.

27. van Dorp E, Yassen A, Sarton E, et al. Naloxone reversal of buprenorphine-induced respiratory depression. *Anesthesiology.* 2006;105(1):51-57.

28. Darpo B, Zhou M, Bai SA, Ferber G, Xiang Q, Finn A. Differentiating the effect of an opioid agonist on cardiac repolarization from micro-receptor-mediated, indirect effects on the QT interval: a randomized, 3-way crossover study in healthy subjects. *Clin Ther.* 2016;38(2):315-326.

29. Wedam EF, Bigelow GE, Johnson RE, Nuzzo PA, Haigney MC. QT-interval effects of methadone, levomethadyl, and buprenorphine in a randomized trial. *Arch Intern Med.* 2007;167(22):2469-2475.

30. Rauck RL, Potts J, Xiang Q, Tzanis E, Finn A. Efficacy and tolerability of buccal buprenorphine in opioid-naive patients with moderate to severe chronic low back pain. *Postgrad Med.* 2016;128(1):1-11.

31. Likar R, Kayser H, Sittl R. Long-term management of chronic pain with transdermal buprenorphine: a multi-center, open-label, follow-up study in patients from three short-term clinical trials. *Clin Ther.* 2006;28(6):943-952.

32. Likar R, Krainer B, Sittl R. Challenging the equipotency calculation for transdermal buprenorphine: four case studies. *Int J Clin Pract.* 2008;62(1):152-156.

33. Jalili M, Fathi M, Moradi-Lakeh M, Zehtabchi S. Sublingual buprenorphine in acute pain management: a double-blind randomized clinical trial. *Ann Emerg Med.* 2012;59(4):276-280.

34. Mahajan G, Sheth S, Holtsman M, Major opioids in pain management. In: Benzon HT, Raja SN, Liu SS, Fishman SM, Cohen SP, eds. *Essentials of Pain Medicine and Regional Anesthesia.* Philadelphia: Elsevier Churchill Livingstone; 2011:85-96.

32

ROLE OF NALOXONE IN PAIN MANAGEMENT

Kathleen Nowak, PharmD, BCACP, AAHIVP and Mark Holtsman, PharmD

FAST FACTS

- Unintentional overdose with opioids accounts for a significant amount of deaths in the United States.
- Major prevention strategies are being used for patients taking opioids, including checking prescription drug monitoring programs, urine drug tests, and dispensing naloxone.
- Naloxone has been shown to be effective in reducing death due to unintentional overdose.

NATURE AND SIGNIFICANCE

Rates of overdose deaths due to use of opioids have risen steadily since 1999. Although illicit substances, such as heroin and illegally manufactured synthetic opiates, are increasingly recognized as major contributors to increases in opioid overdose mortality since 2013, prescription opioids still account for the largest proportion (nearly 50%) of opioid overdose deaths.[1-3] In addition, prior use of prescription opioids, and particularly misuse, is strongly correlated with initiation of heroin use, and opioid prescribing rates have mirrored the increasing rates of opioid-related deaths, highlighting the important role of prescription opioids in fueling this epidemic.[4,5] Nonfatal overdoses also account for innumerable preventable health care expenses, morbidity, and emotional suffering.

In recognition of opioid overdose deaths as a major public health concern, the US Department of Health and Human Services has identified 3 priority areas to address the opioid crisis: prescriber education and training, expanding access to medication-assisted treatment for opioid use disorder, and increasing community access to naloxone.[6]

Naloxone has long been utilized by emergency medical personnel in suspected opioid overdoses, primarily intravenously. However, the majority of opioid-related fatalities occur in nonmedical facilities, typically in the patient's home.[7] In 1996, community-based opioid overdose prevention programs began providing naloxone to community members as a strategy to reduce overdose deaths.[8] Distribution of naloxone continued to increase over the following 15 years, and many states have now adopted laws and regulations aimed at increasing access to naloxone as a community-provided overdose reversal agent. Two new formulations of naloxone were approved by the US Food and Drug Administration (FDA) in 2014 and 2015, which are designed for ease of use by laypersons. Growing evidence supporting naloxone use in this capacity has led to widespread adoption of community-based programs and recommendations for prescribing naloxone in the Centers for Disease Control and Prevention (CDC) Guidelines for Prescribing Opioids for Chronic Pain.

MECHANISM OF ACTION

Naloxone is a pure opioid antagonist. Through competitive antagonism at the mu, kappa, and sigma receptor sites in the central nervous system (CNS), with primary affinity for mu receptors, naloxone reverses the effects of opioids, including respiratory depression, sedation, and hypotension.[9] It has also demonstrated reversal of psychotomimetic and dysphoric effects produced by some agonist-antagonist opioids, such as pentazocine.[9] Naloxone has essentially no pharmacologic activity when administered in usual dosages in the absence of opioids.[9]

INDICATIONS

Naloxone hydrochloride injectable solutions (excluding the preformulated autoinjector) are indicated for complete or partial reversal of opioid-induced CNS and respiratory depression caused by natural and synthetic opioids, as well as certain agonist-antagonists (pentazocine, butorphanol, nalbuphine, cyclazocine).[9] These injectable solutions are also indicated for the diagnosis of suspected acute opioid overdose.[9] The autoinjector and prepackaged nasal spray formulations are indicated for emergency treatment of known or suspected opioid overdose, manifested by respiratory and/or CNS depression in adults and pediatric patients, and are intended for immediate administration in emergency situations in which opioid use may be present.[10,11]

CONTRAINDICATIONS

Naloxone is contraindicated only in patients known to have a hypersensitivity to naloxone or any other component of the formulation.[9-11]

TOXICITY

In studies of healthy volunteers who were exposed to a 4-mg dose of the preformulated nasal spray, the most commonly reported adverse effects were increased blood pressure, musculoskeletal pain, headache, nasal dryness, nasal edema, nasal congestion, and nasal inflammation.[10] The most common adverse effects reported by healthy subjects who were exposed to naloxone via autoinjector (at 0.4-, 0.8-, or 2-mg doses) were dizziness and injection site erythema.[11] Agitation, disorientation, confusion, and anger have also been reported with use of the autoinjector in postmarketing studies.[11]

In opioid-dependent patients, administration of naloxone may precipitate acute opioid withdrawal, characterized by body aches, nausea, vomiting, diarrhea, abdominal cramping, tachycardia, piloerection, sweating, yawning, rhinorrhea, shivering, tremor, irritability, restlessness, and increased blood pressure. Abrupt postoperative reversal of opioid-induced CNS depression with naloxone has been reported to cause the following: hypotension, hypertension, tachycardia, seizures, ventricular tachycardia and fibrillation, pulmonary edema, and cardiac arrest. Serious events such as coma, encephalopathy, or death have been reported as a result of these adverse effects, primarily in patients with a history of cardiovascular disease or who were receiving medications with similar adverse cardiovascular effects.[9-11]

There are limited data available on overdose with naloxone. A small study in healthy volunteers did not demonstrate toxicity at doses of 0.2 to 0.4 mg/kg (24 mg/70 kg).[9,12] In another study of 36 patients with acute stroke who received naloxone at much higher doses (4-mg/kg loading dose followed by a continuous infusion of 2 mg/kg/h for 24 h), 23 patients reported adverse events and 7 discontinued naloxone use owing to adverse effects, including seizures, severe hypertension, hypotension, and bradycardia.[9,12] Adverse effects have also been reported in healthy subjects exposed to these higher doses (2 mg/kg), including anxiety, irritability, tension, sadness, difficulty concentrating, decreased appetite, dizziness, nausea, abdominal pain, and sweating.[9] Behavioral symptoms have been reported to persist for up to 2 to 3 days. Treatment of naloxone overdose primarily includes supportive care and close monitoring.

SUMMARY OF REGULATIONS ON NALOXONE

Although the FDA has recently approved 2 easy-to-use formulations of naloxone that are intended to be administered in emergency situations by individuals who may not be medically trained, there are currently no over-the-counter products available. Federally, naloxone is approved to be dispensed only as a prescribed medication. However, efforts by harm reduction organizations, in addition to the American Medical Association and National Association of Boards of Pharmacy, have led many states to adopt laws and regulations that increase access to naloxone in the community. Nearly all states have adopted laws that allow for naloxone to be prescribed to people other than that person for whom use is intended (referred to as third-party prescribing) or to be dispensed by a retail pharmacy under a standing order, removing the need for a patient to see the prescriber before receiving the medication.[13]

Most states have also passed overdose "Good Samaritan" laws, which provide some protection for lay individuals who report an overdose from arrest and prosecution for drug-related charges. These laws also provide immunity for laypersons who administer naloxone and medical professionals who dispense or prescribe the medication.[13] Refer to individual state laws and regulations for details.

A recent report from the National Bureau of Economic Research indicates that adoption of naloxone access laws is associated with a 9% to 11% reduction in opioid overdose deaths. Adoption of Good Samaritan laws was associated with a similar reduction in mortality; however, this outcome did not reach statistical significance. In addition, neither law was found to be associated with an increase in recreational use of prescription opioids.[14]

NALOXONE IN CLINICAL PRACTICE

The majority of evidence available supporting layperson use of naloxone for opioid overdose rescue is in patients who are using illicit opioids. In this population, opioid overdose education and naloxone distribution programs (OEND) have demonstrated significant reductions in overdose fatalities.[15,16] A modeling study has also demonstrated that naloxone distribution to heroin users is cost-effective.[17] In 2013, a network of primary care clinics in San Francisco implemented a program to prescribe naloxone to patients who were being prescribed long-term opioids for chronic pain. The program included prescriber education on indications and rationale for naloxone prescribing, patient education strategies, and pharmacy/payer coverage.[18] Support was also available for prescribers encountering logistical problems, including pharmacy issues with ordering or billing for naloxone. The decision to prescribe naloxone was then left to providers. Of the 1985 patients who were prescribed long-term opioids for pain, 38% were prescribed naloxone during the study period. Patients prescribed higher doses of opioids or with an opioid-related emergency department (ED) visit within the preceding 12 months were more likely to receive prescriptions for naloxone. This program demonstrated a 63% reduction in opioid-related ED visits over 1 year (incident rate ratio 0.37 [confidence interval, 0.22,0.64]; $P < .001$), highlighting the risk associated with prescribing long-term opioids and the importance of providing risk mitigation strategies, such as naloxone for overdose rescue.[18]

The CDC Guideline for Prescribing Opioids for Chronic Pain recommends considering providing a prescription for naloxone to patients who are at an increased risk for overdose, including patients with a history of substance use disorder, those taking benzodiazepines concomitantly with opioids, patients with a history of overdose, patients taking high-dose opioids (50 mg MME or higher), and patients at risk due to periods of abstinence resulting in loss of tolerance (e.g., postincarceration or completion of substance abuse treatment program).[19] The prudent clinician should also consider prescribing naloxone to illicit opioid users, patients with friends or relatives who use opioids, and those with other high-risk features, including sleep apnea, renal or hepatic insufficiency, age 65 years or older, or mental health disorder (e.g., anxiety or depression). The American Society of Addiction Medicine recommends that naloxone be prescribed to all patients who are undergoing treatment of opioid use disorder as well as their family members and significant others.[20]

The recommended dose of naloxone administered by formulations intended for layperson use has been debated and is not standardized. In medical settings, the recommended initial dose is wide ranging, from 0.4 to 2 mg intravenous (IV)/intramuscular (IM)/subcutaneous (SQ).[9] Typically, the initial dose given is on the lower end of the dosing range, with additional boluses titrated to patient response. If a patient is apneic or near-apneic, it is recommended to provide the 2-mg dose initially, regardless of patient history. Lower doses are used initially owing to the risk for acute opioid withdrawal syndrome in opioid-dependent patients with abrupt reversal. In addition, target plasma levels vary significantly based on multiple, and often unknown, drug and patient-specific factors, including specific opioid, dose

and formulation taken, other concurrent drug ingestions, underlying illnesses, and opioid tolerance. Indeed, it has been demonstrated that higher doses and often repeat doses are required with more potent opioid analgesics, such as fentanyl, and with partial agonists, such as buprenorphine.[21,22] This strategy of administering lower initial doses with close monitoring and titration based on patient response is appropriate in a medical setting. However, potential bystanders in the community rarely have the necessary training or resources to provide effective care in this manner. Given that the benefit of administering an effective dose greatly outweighs the risk for adverse effects related to acute opioid withdrawal, an FDA advisory committee recommends that any naloxone formulations that are being prescribed or distributed to the community be designed to administer the equivalent of 2 mg IV/IM/SQ per dose.[7] Based on these recommendations, the manufacturer of the autoinjector has discontinued manufacturing of the 0.4-mg/dose device and will continue to produce only the 2-mg/dose device. In addition, it is recommended that 2 doses be provided with each dispensed prescription to allow for repeat dosing in the event of partial effect/ineffectiveness with the first dose or misadministration or device failure.

Multiple formulations of naloxone are available for prescribing for layperson use (see Table 32-1). Both generic injectable formulations are much cheaper than the brand name single-use devices, but they also require extensive patient education regarding correct assembly and administration of the dose. The injectable vial and syringe also have the added risk of transmission of infectious diseases in the event of a needle stick injury and requires proper sharps disposal. Many harm reduction organizations distributing naloxone to community members utilize the prefilled injectable syringe plus nasal atomizer owing to the lower cost. Most of these organizations are providing the medication at no cost to the community members. However, most insurance companies now cover one of the brand name single-use devices (typically the preformulated nasal spray) when dispensed pursuant to a prescription. Many states allow for pharmacists to dispense naloxone without a prescription from a provider or pursuant to a standing order, but this method of dispensing may not allow for insurance coverage.

When prescribing or dispensing naloxone for opioid overdose rescue, it is essential to provide counseling and education on recognizing opioid overdose, emergency response, and appropriate use of the naloxone formulation prescribed. Although there is currently no standardized curriculum for providing naloxone education and counseling, Table 32-2 provides elements that are commonly included in OEND programs. Most OEND programs also provide counseling on prevention of opioid overdoses, including recognizing risk factors for overdose, in addition to medication and overdose response education. A randomized controlled trial demonstrated significant reductions in overdose risk behaviors with use of motivational interviewing techniques compared with usual care, highlighting the importance of including prevention counseling to reduce risky behaviors.[23]

TABLE 32-1 Comparison of Naloxone Formulations[9-11]

FORMULATION	STRENGTH	DOSING INSTRUCTIONS	PRESCRIBING DETAILS	PRICE	CONSIDERATIONS
Generic single or multidose vial for injection	0.4 mg/1 mL single-dose vial 4 mg/10 mL multidose vial	Inject 1 mL (0.4 mg) into shoulder or thigh. Repeat dose every 2-3 min if no or minimal response	Prescribe #2 single-dose[a] or #1 multidose vials *plus* Syringes: 3 mL, 23-25 gauge, 1-1.5 in IM needle, #2-4	$	• Requires assembly • Risk for exposure to infectious diseases • Used needles require proper disposal • Allows for dose titration • Off-label use
Generic prefilled syringe for nasal administration	2 mg/2 mL needleless prefilled syringe	Spray 1 mL (1/2 syringe) into each nostril. Repeat dose after 2-3 min if no or minimal response	Prescribe #2 prefilled syringes *plus* 2 nasal atomizers	$	• Requires assembly • Many pharmacies do not stock nasal atomizers • Atomizers may not be covered by patient's insurance • Limited efficacy and PK data • Off-label use
Narcan Nasal Spray	4 mg/0.1 mL 2 mg/0.1 mL[b]	Spray 0.1 mL (full device) into one nostril. Repeat dose in other nostril with second device after 2-3 min if no or minimal response	Each kit contains #2 single-use intranasal devices Prescribe #1 kit or #2 intranasal devices	$$	• No assembly required • 4 mg intranasal roughly equivalent to 2 mg IM[10] • Kit includes emergency response instruction card
Evzio Auto-Injector	0.4 mg/0.4 mL[c] 2 mg/0.4 mL	Inject the contents of 1 device into outer thigh as directed by voice prompt system.[d] Repeat dose with second device after 2-3 min if no or minimal response	Each kit contains #2 single-use autoinjector devices *plus* #1 trainer device Prescribe #1 kit or #2 autoinjectors	$$$[e]	• No assembly required • Needle enclosed in plastic housing, reducing risk of needle stick injury • Kit includes a trainer device that can be reused over 1000 times • Kit includes emergency response instruction card

[a]*Allows for up to 0.8-mg dose. Consider providing #5 vials for full 2-mg dose.*
[b]*The 2 mg/0.1 mL formulation has been FDA approved but has not been released.*
[c]*No longer being manufactured.*
[d]*If the voice prompt system does not function properly, the device will still deliver the dose when administered properly. Follow the written instructions provided with the kit.*
[e]*Patient assistance programs are available to offset out-of-pocket costs. See manufacturer website for details.*

RISK STRATIFICATION

Strong evidence for the accuracy and effectiveness of risk prediction tools, such as the Opioid Risk Tool (ORT) or Screener and Opioid Assessment for Patients in Pain, for predicting opioid abuse or misuse is lacking.[19] Currently, the CDC guidelines do not recommend use of these screening tools owing to limited data, but instead recommend utilizing prescription drug monitoring program (PDMP) data, urine drug testing, and review of patient medical and social history to identify patients who are at risk for opioid-related harms, including overdose.[19] Many of the indications for naloxone prescribing, as recommended in the CDC guidelines, can be identified from reviewing PDMP data, including high-dose opioids (50 mg MME or higher), concomitant benzodiazepine prescribing, and periods of abstinence resulting in reduced opioid tolerance. As of October 2016, only one state (Missouri) has yet to implement a PDMP.[24] Other

risk factors can be identified through review of medical records and from the patient interview (e.g., history of substance use disorder, mental health disorder, renal or hepatic dysfunction). Tools such as the ORT may be useful for identifying risk factors during the patient interview but should not be the only method of assessment for opioid-related risk.

Example

A 54-year-old man with past medical history significant for type 2 diabetes, hypertension, depression, generalized anxiety disorder, and degenerative disc disease presents to establish care with a new primary care provider.

A review of PDMP data indicates that the patient is prescribed hydrocodone/acetaminophen 10/325 mg, 6 tablets per day every 30 days and lorazepam 1 mg, 2 tablets per day every 30 days. No suspicious activity is noted, including using multiple prescribers or multiple pharmacies.

TABLE 32-2 Recommended Counseling Points When Prescribing Naloxone

Overdose Counseling

Recognition	• Definition and examples of opioids • Signs and symptoms of overdose: shallow breathing or not breathing at all, snoring/gurgling sounds, unconscious/unable to wake, pale, clammy skin, blue lips and/or fingernails, heartbeat slows or stops
Emergency response	• Administer naloxone • Call 911 immediately, give clear address • Follow 911 operator instructions, may include rescue breathing and/or chest compressions (CPR) • Monitor response to naloxone • Repeat dose if no or minimal effect after 2-3 min or if person responds but relapses into respiratory depression • Stay with person until emergency medical personnel arrive
Prevention	• Risk factors for overdose: using opioids alone, mixing opioids with other sedating substances (including alcohol), reduced tolerance after period of abstinence (incarceration, inpatient drug treatment program), changes in drug potency or purity, high-dose opioids

Medication Education

• Education and demonstration on assembly (if required) and dose administration[a]
• Naloxone is effective *only* in opioid overdose, no effect with other substances
• Minimal risk for harm if administered to a person who has not taken opioids[b]
• Short duration of action (30-90 min), return of respiratory and CNS depression is likely[c]
• Patients dependent on opioids are likely to experience withdrawal symptoms (nausea, vomiting, diarrhea, sweating, tremor, body aches, irritability, etc.) and may become agitated
• Other side effects are rare; however, hypersensitivity (hives, swelling of face, mouth, etc.) can occur

[a]*Recommended to provide a brochure or patient handout with diagram detailing administration.*
[b]*Recommended to review state-specific Good Samaritan and naloxone access laws.*
[c]*Important to reiterate that the responder must call 911.*

During the patient interview, the patient reports that his anxiety has been worsening lately and he has been taking more lorazepam than prescribed. A review of his prior medical records indicates a history of substance abuse (methamphetamine use, abstinent for 10 y).

Given the multiple high-risk features in this patient, including high-dose opioids (>50 mg MME), concomitant benzodiazepine prescribing, recent self-titration of benzodiazepine dose, and history of substance use disorder, he is an appropriate candidate for naloxone prescribing. CDC guidelines also recommend that safety concerns be discussed, including respiratory depression and overdose, in high-risk patients. This discussion is often a perfect introduction to the concept of naloxone. Counseling should include recognizing risk factors for opioid overdose, recognizing opioid overdose signs and symptoms, appropriate emergency response, and administration of naloxone, as outlined in Table 32-2.

SUMMARY

In recent years, there has been an alarming increase in deaths due to unintentional overdose from opioids. The introduction and subsequent adoption of naloxone as a risk mitigation strategy has been successful not only in terms of decreasing the death rate but also by giving the provider an opportunity to discuss risks/benefits of opioids before dispensing naloxone. Naloxone is available without a prescription in some states, but may not by covered by certain insurances if dispensed without a prescription. Naloxone is safe but can precipitate adverse reactions in patients who have pre-existing cardiopulmonary conditions.

REFERENCES

1. Rudd RA, Aleshire N, Zibbell JE, Gladden RM. Increases in drug and opioid overdose deaths – United States, 2000–2014. *MMWR Morb Mortal Wkly Rep.* 2016;64(50-51):1378-1382.
2. Rudd RA, Seth P, David F, Scholl L. Increases in drug and opioid-involved overdose deaths – United States, 2010–2015. *MMWR Morb Mortal Wkly Rep.* 2016;65(50-51):1445-1452.
3. Centers for Disease Control and Prevention. Prescription Opioid Overdose Data. 2017. Updated 1 August 2017. Available at: https://www.cdc.gov/drugoverdose/data/overdose.html. Accessed 7 August 2017.
4. Jones CM, Logan J, Gladden RM, Bohm MK. Vital signs: demographic and substance use trends among heroin users – United States, 2002–2013. *MMWR Morb Mortal Wkly Rep.* 2015;64(26):719-725.
5. Frenk SM, Porter KS, Paulozzi LJ. Prescription opioid analgesic use among adults: United States, 1999–2012. *NCHS Data Brief, No 189.* Hyattsville, MD: National Center for Health Statistics. 2015.
6. *HHS Takes Strong Steps to Address Opioid-Drug Related Overdose, Death, and Dependence;* March 26, 2015. Available at: https://wayback.archive-it.org/3926/20170127185704/https://www.hhs.gov/about/news/2015/03/26/hhs-takes-strong-steps-to-address-opioid-drug-related-overdose-death-and-dependence.html. Accessed 7 August 2017.
7. *FDA Advisory Committee on the Most Appropriate Dose or Doses of Naloxone to Reverse the Effects of Live-Threatening Opioid Overdose in the Community Settings.* Advisory Committee Briefing Materials; September 2, 2016. Available at: https://www.fda.gov/downloads/AdvisoryCommittees/CommitteesMeetingMaterials/Drugs/AnestheticAndAnalgesicDrugProductsAdvisoryCommittee/UCM522688.pdf. Accessed 13 August 2017.
8. Centers for Disease Control and Prevention. Community-based opioid overdose prevention programs providing naloxone- United States, 2010. *MMWR Morb Mortal Wkly Rep.* 2012;61(6):101-105.

9. *Naloxone Hydrochloride Injection, USP [package insert].* Lake Forest, IL: Hospira, Inc.; 2007.

10. *NARCAN® (Naloxone Hydrochloride) Nasal Spray [package insert].* Radnor, PA: Adapt Pharma, Inc.; 2015.

11. *EVZIO® (Naloxone Hydrochloride) Auto-Injector for Intramuscular or Subcutaneous Use [package insert].* Richmond, VA: Kaleo, Inc.; 2016.

12. Hazardous Substances Data Bank [Internet]. *Naloxone; Hazardous Substances Databank Number: 3279.* Bethesda, MD: National Library of Medicine (U.S.). 1994. Updated 25 October 2016. Available at: https://toxnet.nlm.nih.gov/cgi-bin/sis/htmlgen?HSDB. Accessed 8 August 2017.

13. The Network for Public Health Law. Legal Interventions to Reduce Overdose Mortality: Naloxone Access and Overdose Good Samaritan Laws. 2016. Updated May 2017. Available at: https://www.networkforphl.org/_asset/qz5pvn/network-naloxone-10-4.pdf. Accessed 12 August 2017.

14. Rees DI, Sabia JJ, Argys LM, Latshaw J, Dave D. *With a Little Help From My Friends: The Effects of Naloxone Access and Good Samaritan Laws on Opioid-Related Deaths.* NBER Working Paper No. 23171; February 2017. Available at: http://www.nber.org/papers/q23171. Accessed 12 August 2017.

15. Walley AY, Xuan Z, Hackman HH, et al. Opioid overdose rates and implementation of overdose education and nasal naloxone distribution in Massachusetts: interrupted time series analysis. *BMJ.* 2013;346:f174.

16. Fischbacher C, Barnsdale L, Graham L. Effectiveness of Scotland's national naloxone programme. *Addiction.* 2016;111(7):1304.

17. Coffin PO, Sullivan SD. Cost-effectiveness of distributing naloxone to heroin users for lay overdose reversal. *Ann Intern Med.* 2013;158(1):1-9.

18. Coffin PO, Behar E, Rowe C, et al. Nonrandomized intervention study of naloxone coprescription for primary care patients receiving long-term opioid therapy for pain. *Ann Intern Med.* 2016;165(4):245-252.

19. Dowell D, Haegerich TM, Chou R. CDC guideline for prescribing opioids for chronic pain – United States, 2016. *JAMA.* 2016;315(15):1624-1645.

20. Kampman K, Jarvis M. American Society of Addiction Medicine (ASAM) national practice guideline for the use of medications in the treatment of addiction involving opioid use. *J Addict Med.* 2015;9(5):358-367.

21. Dahan A, Aarts L, Smith TW. Incidence, reversal, and prevention of opioid-induced respiratory depression. *Anesthesiology.* 2010;122(1):226-238.

22. Kim HK, Nelson LS. Reducing the harm of opioid overdose with the safe use of naloxone: a pharmacologic review. *Expert Opin Drug Saf.* 2015;14(7):1137-1146.

23. Bohnert AS, Bonar EE, Cunningham R, et al. A pilot randomized clinical trial of an intervention to reduce overdose risk behaviors among emergency department patients at risk for prescription opioid overdose. *Drug Alcohol Depend.* 2016;163:40-47.

24. Prescription Drug Monitoring Program Training and Technical Assistance Center. *Status of Prescription Drug Monitoring Programs (PDMPs);* October 2016. Available at: www.pdmpassist.org/pdf/PDMPProgramStatus.pdf. Accessed 15 August 2017.

33

NONSTEROIDAL ANTI-INFLAMMATORY DRUGS

Arjun Sharma, MD, Erielle Anne P. Espina, PharmD and Charity Hale, PharmD

FAST FACTS

- Nonsteroidal anti-inflammatory drugs (NSAIDs) can be useful for acute and chronic inflammatory pain conditions as well as fever.
- NSAIDs should be used at the lowest dose possible for the shortest time needed and evaluated frequently.
- NSAIDs can cause significant gastrointestinal, cardiovascular, and renal side effects.
- Some NSAIDs confer less risk than others, especially with regard to gastrointestinal (GI) and cardiovascular (CV) complications. However, all non-ASA NSAIDs increase the chance of myocardial infarction or cerebrovascular accident.

INTRODUCTION

Nonsteroidal anti-inflammatory drugs (NSAIDs) are widely used medications to help treat acute and chronic pain conditions. Although NSAIDs are very effective for many of our patients, they are not without risk. Use of NSAIDs can be associated with kidney damage, GI bleeding, and cardiovascular risk. Understanding such risks will allow the practitioner to decide whether it is appropriate to use NSAIDs, given a patient's comorbid conditions. Likewise, the practitioner may consider options to mitigate some of the side effects of NSAIDs. For example, alternating daily between an NSAID and acetaminophen can decrease chronic exposure of NSAIDs, reduce the risk of GI bleed, prevent kidney damage, and provide satisfactory analgesia. Similar risk reduction strategies for the use of pain medications are further discussed in chapter 5 *Rational Analgesic Poly Pharmacotherapy*.

INDICATIONS AND MECHANISM OF ACTION

NSAIDs are indicated to treat fever and multiple types of pain including mild to moderate, acute, dental, musculoskeletal (e.g., sprains and strains), and inflammatory (e.g., bone pain, joint pain, ankylosing spondylitis, rheumatoid arthritis, and osteoarthritis), as well as dysmenorrhea.

Inflammatory prostaglandins are synthesized from arachidonic acid via the cyclooxygenase-2 (COX-2) pathway. These prostaglandins serve an important role in recruiting inflammatory cells, sensitizing pain receptors, and regulating hypothalamic temperature control. Nonselective agents and celecoxib inhibit the COX-2 pathway, decreasing inflammation, pain, and fever.[1] Because NSAIDs also reduce fever, it is important to understand that if treating a painful condition, an underlying infection may be masked particularly during the postsurgical period. Therefore, it is essential to integrate clinical acumen in determining appropriate use while accounting for temporal impact.

Cytoprotective prostaglandins are synthesized from arachidonic acid via the cyclooxygenase-1 (COX-1) pathway. These prostaglandins regulate renal blood flow, protect gastrointestinal mucosa, and aid in platelet activation and aggregation. Nonselective NSAIDs inhibit COX-1 enzymes potentially leading to renal dysfunction, GI complications, and cardiovascular events.[2] Unlike nonselective agents, celecoxib (a selective COX-2 inhibitor) does not affect platelet function.[3]

CONTRAINDICATIONS AND PRECAUTIONS

Cardiovascular Complications

NSAIDs increase the risk of cardiovascular thrombotic events, myocardial infarction, and stroke and are contraindicated following coronary artery bypass graft surgery per the Food and Drug Administration (FDA). These complications may occur early during NSAID therapy and increases with prolonged use. Although certain NSAIDs appear to confer lower overall CV risk than others, recent reviews have found that all NSAID therapies carry some risk, and in general, careful consideration should be given before recommending NSAIDs in patients with cardiovascular comorbities.[4,5]

Furthermore, 20% to 25% of patients use both low-dose aspirin for secondary prevention and an additional NSAID for pain management. It appears that nonselective NSAIDs may impair the antiplatelet activities of aspirin. This interaction is more evident when nonselective agents are administered before the aspirin dose.[6,7] This is potentially due to the reversible binding properties of all NSAIDs apart from aspirin. With this being said, discontinuation of low-dose aspirin increases the risk of cardiovascular events more than 3-fold and by 90-fold in patients with intracoronary stents.[7-9]

GI Complications

More than 30 million people use NSAIDs every day, and over 40% of patients consume more than the recommended dose of over-the-counter (OTC) analgesics including NSAIDs and acetaminophen.[7,10-12] Endoscopic gastrointestinal (GI) lesions including hemorrhages, erosions, and ulcerations are seen in 30% to 50% of chronic NSAID users. Generally, these lesions have no clinical significance and are not symptomatic. It appears that the GI mucosa adapts to the presence of NSAIDs, and the lesions often reduce or disappear with chronic NSAID use.[11,13,14]

Nearly 40% of NSAID users are symptomatic most frequently presenting as gastroesophageal reflux disease, heartburn, belching, epigastric discomfort, bloating, early satiety, and postprandial nausea.[11,14] Serious complications including bleeding, perforation, and obstruction are seen in 1% to 2% of patients.[11] There are 7000 to 10,000 deaths associated with NSAID-induced GI complications each year.[10,15-17] These risks appear to be highest within the first month of therapy and remain elevated for up to 2 months after discontinuation.[11,18]

There are over 100,000 hospitalizations due to NSAID-induced GI complications each year.[10,15-17] Eighty-six percent of hospitalized patients with lower GI bleeds reported using NSAIDs or aspirin for a short duration, 7 days or less. Furthermore, the reported mortality rate due to bleeding associated with peptic ulcers is 5%.[11,19-23]

NSAIDs increase the risk of developing peptic ulcers by 4 to 5 times.[11,18,24,25] Additional risk factors that increase the likelihood of GI complications include age greater than 65 years, history of peptic ulcer disease or GI bleed, severe illness, concomitant therapy with more than one NSAID, antiplatelet agents, anticoagulants, corticosteroids, SSRIs (selective serotonin reuptake inhibitors), and SNRIs (selective norepinephrine reuptake inhibitors) as well as the synergistic combination of *Helicobacter pylori* and NSAIDs.[11,25,26]

Ibuprofen may be a safer option because of lower doses needed to achieve adequate analgesia. Nonselective agents with a higher selectivity for COX-2 (nabumetone, meloxicam, and etodolac) also appear to cause less GI harm.[15,27] On the other hand, agents with longer half-lives (ketorolac, piroxicam, and sulindac) provide longer exposure to the GI mucosa increasing the risk for complications.[11,15,28]

Although NSAIDs inhibit mucosal prostaglandin synthesis along the entire GI system, there are pathological differences between the proximal and distal tract. The upper GI tract contains acidic secretions that play a role in GI mucosal damage, whereas the lower GI tract contains bacteria and bile. Therefore, proton pump inhibitors (PPIs) provide protection against NSAID-induced damage in the upper GI system by blocking the production of acidic secretions. Because the lower GI system does not have these acidic secretions, PPIs do not provide protection past the duodenum.[7,29,30] Lower GI complications account for 40% of serious GI events.[11,31] Recent publications show decreasing trends for upper GI bleeds and increasing trends for lower GI bleeds.[7,32] This is potentially due to an increased use of PPIs for GI protection as well as advanced imaging for diagnostic purposes.

Whereas enteric-coating NSAIDs, buffering NSAIDs, and sucralfate have not been shown to be effective in preventing GI mucosal damage associated with NSAID use, misoprostol and PPIs appear to be significantly more effective than H2RAs (histamine 2 receptor antagonists) at preventing GI mucosal damage.[15,33-37] PPIs seem to be more effective than misoprostol in preventing duodenal ulcers and equally effective in preventing gastric ulcers. When comparing PPIs and misoprostol at a more tolerable dose (200 µg BID), PPIs seem to be more effective. However, higher and potentially more effective doses of misoprostol (200 µg QID) are often not well-tolerated because of significant abdominal cramping and diarrhea.[15,23,38-46] Therefore, PPIs seem to be the most favorable option for GI mucosal protection from NSAIDs.

It appears that celecoxib is associated with significantly less mucosal harm, bleeds, perforations, and obstructions throughout the entire GI system than seen with nonselective agents.[11,47] Therefore, it may be reasonable to consider celecoxib in combination with a PPI for high-risk patients.

For patients taking low-dose aspirin for secondary prevention, it appears that standard doses of celecoxib at 200 mg or naproxen are a safer option for pain management than nonselective agents. However, it must be stressed that it is best to avoid all NSAIDs in patients at high risk for CV events.[7]

Renal Dysfunction

NSAIDs block the production of prostaglandins responsible for maintaining renal blood flow, which may lead to renal insufficiency. This risk is greater in patients with existing renal dysfunction, dehydration, hypovolemia, heart failure, hepatic dysfunction, and concomitant nephrotoxic drugs including diuretics and angiotensin-converting enzyme (ACE) inhibitors.[2,48] Renal function should be monitored in patients taking NSAIDs.

TOPICAL NSAIDS

Topical NSAIDs are used as first- to second-line therapy for pain related to osteoarthritis (OA) and rheumatoid arthritis (RA). Topical agents concentrate in the synovial fluid decreasing systemic exposure, side effects, and the need for systemic NSAIDs by 40%.[49] Currently, diclofenac gel, solution, and patch formulations are commercially available. Additional agents such as diclofenac spray, ibuprofen gel, and ketoprofen gel may be compounded at select pharmacies but are often not covered by insurance providers. Topical agents are also indicated for acute pain such as sprains and strains.

CONCLUSIONS

NSAIDs effectively reduce fever and inflammation and relieve pain. They are frequently prescribed for acute or chronic conditions, such as moderately painful musculoskeletal conditions, moderate to severe osteoarthritis, and rheumatoid arthritis.

As health care practitioners, it is essential to assess any medication risks and benefits before use as part of a comprehensive treatment program. This requires careful consideration of comorbid conditions such as renal and heart disease or risk factors for heart disease such as smoking, diabetes, hypertension, and hypercholesterolemia. Additionally, consider prescribing NSAIDs only after physical examination, review of X-rays/blood tests, and determination of other acute medical conditions because these will affect the treatment plan.

Use the lowest dose possible for the shortest time needed and meet periodically with the patient to monitor for any harmful side effects. Interval evaluation may include complete blood count, basic metabolic panel, and kidney function tests.

Cardiovascular complications including hypertension that may be caused by NSAIDs typically happen within the first weeks of use and may happen more frequently with higher doses or with long-term use. NSAIDs should not be used right before or after heart bypass surgery, and they may increase the chances of gastrointestinal ulceration and bleeding particularly in the elderly. The GI side effects can occur without warning signs.

Rarely, NSAIDs can cause allergic reactions. There are 2 main categories of allergic reactions (1) allergic reactions (i.e., anaphylaxis) and (2) pseudoallergic reactions. Allergic reactions are believed to be immunoglobulin E (IgE) mediated and involve anaphylaxis, urticaria, or angioedema. Pseudoallergic reactions are related to the inhibition of COX-1. These reactions can occur with NSAIDs, which preferentially inhibit COX-1 and cross-react with aspirin such as diclofenac, ibuprofen, indomethacin (ketorolac), naprosyn, and sulindac.[50] Such reactions are usually seen in patients with certain preexisting conditions such as asthma, nasal polyps, and chronic rhinosinusitis or urticarial.[51]

When used properly, NSAIDs can help relieve pain for acute and chronic inflammatory pain conditions See Table 33-1 for a quick reference guide to the various NSAIDs (Table 33-1).

TABLE 33-1 Common Oral NSAIDs						
NSAID	DURATION OF ACTION FOR ORAL DOSING	DAILY DOSE TOTAL (MG)	COX SELECTIVITY	CARDIOVASCULAR RISK	GASTROINTESTINAL RISK	RENAL RISK[a]
Celecoxib	12 h	Low dose: <200 mg; high dose: >200 mg	COX-2 selective	Moderate cardiovascular risk at low and high doses (pooled RR 1.17)	Lowest risk of all NSAIDs; however, risk still exists for gastrointestinal complications (pooled RR 1.5)	No increased risk of AKI
Ibuprofen	4-6 h	Low dose: <1200 mg; high dose: >1200 mg	Mixed COX-1 and COX-2 selectivity	Low dose is associated with low to moderate risk (pooled RR 1.18), whereas higher dose is associated with increased risk	Lower risk of gastrointestinal complications (pooled RR 1.8)	Increased risk of AKI

TABLE 33-1 Common Oral NSAIDs (Continued)						
NSAID	**DURATION OF ACTION FOR ORAL DOSING**	**DAILY DOSE TOTAL (MG)**	**COX SELECTIVITY**	**CARDIOVASCULAR RISK**	**GASTROINTESTINAL RISK**	**RENAL RISK[a]**
Diclofenac	8-12 for hours IR, 24 h for ER	Low dose: <100 mg; high dose: >100 mg	Greater COX-2 selectivity than COX-1	PO Diclofenac has highest cardiovascular risk among the NSAIDs (pooled RR 1.4)	Moderate risk of gastrointestinal complications (pooled RR 3.3)	No increased risk of AKI
Meloxicam	Up to 24 h	5-15 mg	Greater COX-2 selectivity than COX-1	Moderate cardiovascular risk among NSAIDs (pooled RR 1.2)	Moderate risk of gastrointestinal complications (pooled RR 3.5)	No increased risk of AKI
Naproxen	8-12 h	Low dose: <750 mg; high dose: >750 mg	Slightly greater COX-1 than COX-2 selectivity	No cardiovascular risk associated with high- or low-dose naproxen (pooled RR 1.09)	Moderate to higher risk of gastrointestinal complications (pooled RR 4.1)	Increased risk of AKI
Indomethacin	4-6 h for IR, 12 h for ER	50-200 mg for IR formulation, 75-150 mg for ER formulation	Greater COX-1 than COX-2 selectivity	Higher cardiovascular risk among NSAIDs (pooled RR 1.3)	Moderate to higher risk of gastrointestinal complications (pooled RR 4.1)	Increased risk of AKI
Ketorolac	4-6 h	10-40 mg	Greater COX-1 than COX-2 selectivity	Similar risk profile to other NSAIDs with regard to cardiovascular risk	Highest risk of gastrointestinal complications (pooled RR 11.5)	Increased risk of AKI
Piroxicam	40-60 h	10-20 mg	Mixed COX-1 and COX-2 selectivity	Lower risk profile for cardiovascular risk	Higher risk of gastrointestinal complications	Increased risk of renal toxicity
Sulindac	12 h	300-400 mg	Slightly greater COX-2 than COX-1 selectivity	Higher risk profile for cardiovascular risk	Moderate risk of gastrointestinal complications	Increased risk of renal toxicity
Etodolac	5-6 h for IR, 12-24 h for ER	600-1000 mg	Greater COX-2 selectivity than COX-1	Higher risk profile for cardiovascular risk among NSAIDs (pooled RR 1.55)	Lower risk of gastrointestinal complications	Increased risk of renal toxicity, may be short term and reversible
Nabumetone	24 h	1000-2000 mg	Mixed COX-1 and COX-2 selectivity	Lower risk profile for cardiovascular risk	Lower risk of gastrointestinal complications	Increased risk of renal toxicity, although may be less than other NSAIDs
Ketoprofen	6 h for IR, 24 h for ER	100-200 mg	Greater COX-1 than COX-2 selectivity	Lower risk profile for cardiovascular risk	Higher risk of gastrointestinal complications	Increased risk of renal toxicity

[a]*All NSAIDs have escalating risk of AKI as dose increases in elderly population.*
AKI, acute kidney injury.

REFERENCES

1. Gong L, Thorn CF, Bertagnolli MM, Grosser T, Altman RB, Kleina TE. Celecoxib pathways: pharmacokinetics and pharmacodynamics. *Pharmacogenet Genom.* 2012;22(4):310-318.

2. Hunter LJ, Wood DM, Dargan PI. The patterns of toxicity and management of acute nonsteroidal anti-inflammatory drug (NSAID) overdose. *Open Access Emerg Med.* 2011;3:39-48.

3. Leese PT, Hubbard RC, Karim A, Isakson PC, Yu SS, Geis GS. Effects of celecoxib, a novel cyclooxygenase-2 inhibitor, on platelet function in healthy adults: a randomized, controlled trial. *J Clin Pharmacol.* 2000;40(2):124-132.

4. Bally M, Dendukuri N, Rich B, et al. Risk of acute myocardial infarction with NSAIDs in real world use: bayesian meta-analysis of individual patient data. *BMJ.* 2017;357:j1909.

5. Nissen SE. Cardiovascular safety of celecoxib, naproxen, or ibuprofen for arthritis. *N Engl J Med.* 2017;376(14):1390.

6. Anzellotti P, Capone ML, Jeyam A, et al. Low-dose naproxen interferes with the antiplatelet effects of aspirin in healthy subjects: recommendations to minimize the functional consequences. *Arthritis Rheum.* 2011;63(3):850-859.

7. Scarpignato C, Lanas A, Blandizzi C, et al. Safe prescribing of non-steroidal anti-inflammatory drugs in patients with osteoarthritis–an expert consensus addressing benefits as well as gastrointestinal and cardiovascular risks. *BMC Med.* 2015;13:55.

8. Biondi-Zoccai GG, Lotrionte M, Agostoni P, et al. A systematic review and meta-analysis on the hazards of discontinuing or not adhering to aspirin among 50,279 patients at risk for coronary artery disease. *Eur Heart J.* 2006;27(22):2667-2674.

9. Maulaz AB, Bezerra DC, Michel P, Bogousslavsky J. Effect of discontinuing aspirin therapy on the risk of brain ischemic stroke. *Arch Neurol.* 2005;62(8):1217-1220.

10. Singh G. Gastrointestinal complications of prescription and over-the-counter nonsteroidal anti-inflammatory drugs: a view from the ARAMIS database. Arthritis, rheumatism, and aging medical information system. *Am J Ther.* 2000;7(2):115-121.

11. Sostres C, Gargallo CJ, Lanas A. Nonsteroidal anti-inflammatory drugs and upper and lower gastrointestinal mucosal damage. *Arthritis Res Ther.* 2013;15(suppl 3):S3.

12. Wilcox CM, Cryer B, Triadafilopoulos G. Patterns of use and public perception of over-the-counter pain relievers: focus on nonsteroidal antiinflammatory drugs. *J Rheumatol.* 2005;32(11):2218-2224.

13. Lanas A, Hunt R. Prevention of anti-inflammatory drug-induced gastrointestinal damage: benefits and risks of therapeutic strategies. *Ann Med.* 2006;38(6):415-428.

14. Larkai EN, Smith JL, Lidsky MD, Graham DY. Gastroduodenal mucosa and dyspeptic symptoms in arthritic patients during chronic nonsteroidal anti-inflammatory drug use. *Am J Gastroenterol.* 1987;82(11):1153-1158.

15. Lanza FL, Chan FK, Quigley EM. Guidelines for prevention of NSAID-related ulcer complications. *Am J Gastroenterol.* 2009;104(3):728-738.

16. Singh G, Triadafilopoulos G. Epidemiology of NSAID induced gastrointestinal complications. *J Rheumatol Suppl.* 1999;56:18-24.

17. Wolfe MM, Lichtenstein DR, Singh G. Gastrointestinal toxicity of nonsteroidal antiinflammatory drugs. *N Engl J Med.* 1999;340(24):1888-1899.

18. Hernandez-Diaz S, Rodriguez LA. Association between nonsteroidal anti-inflammatory drugs and upper gastrointestinal tract bleeding/perforation: an overview of epidemiologic studies published in the 1990s. *Arch Intern Med.* 2000;160(14):2093-2099.

19. Lanas A, García-Rodríguez LA, Polo-Tomás M, et al. Time trends and impact of upper and lower gastrointestinal bleeding and perforation in clinical practice. *Am J Gastroenterol.* 2009;104(7):1633-1641.

20. Lanas A, Perez-Aisa MA, Feu F, et al. A nationwide study of mortality associated with hospital admission due to severe gastrointestinal events and those associated with nonsteroidal antiinflammatory drug use. *Am J Gastroenterol.* 2005;100(8):1685-1693.

21. Lanas A, Sekar MC, Hirschowitz BI. Objective evidence of aspirin use in both ulcer and nonulcer upper and lower gastrointestinal bleeding. *Gastroenterology.* 1992;103(3):862-869.

22. Lanas A, Serrano P, Bajador E, Esteva F, Benito R, Sáinz R. Evidence of aspirin use in both upper and lower gastrointestinal perforation. *Gastroenterology.* 1997;112(3):683-689.

23. Sadic J, Borgström A, Manjer J, Toth E, Lindell G. Bleeding peptic ulcer - time trends in incidence, treatment and mortality in Sweden. *Aliment Pharmacol Ther.* 2009;30(4):392-398.

24. Gutthann SP, Garcia Rodriguez LA, Raiford DS. Individual nonsteroidal antiinflammatory drugs and other risk factors for upper gastrointestinal bleeding and perforation. *Epidemiology.* 1997;8(1):18-24.

25. Huang JQ, Sridhar S, Hunt RH. Role of Helicobacter pylori infection and non-steroidal anti-inflammatory drugs in peptic-ulcer disease: a meta-analysis. *Lancet.* 2002;359(9300):14-22.

26. Sostres C, Gargallo CJ, Arroyo MT, Lanas A. Adverse effects of non-steroidal anti-inflammatory drugs (NSAIDs, aspirin and coxibs) on upper gastrointestinal tract. *Best Pract Res Clin Gastroenterol.* 2010;24(2):121-132.

27. Simon LS, Mills JA. Drug therapy: nonsteroidal anti-inflammatory drugs (first of two parts). *N Engl J Med.* 1980;302(21):1179-1185.

28. Castellsague J, Riera-Guardia N, Calingaert B, et al. Individual NSAIDs and upper gastrointestinal complications: a systematic review and meta-analysis of observational studies (the SOS project). *Drug Saf.* 2012;35(12):1127-1146.

29. Scarpignato C, Hunt RH. Nonsteroidal antiinflammatory drug-related injury to the gastrointestinal tract: clinical picture, pathogenesis, and prevention. *Gastroenterol Clin North Am.* 2010;39(3):433-464.

30. Scarpignato C, Pelosini I. Prevention and treatment of non-steroidal anti-inflammatory drug-induced gastro-duodenal damage: rationale for the use of antisecretory compounds. *Ital J Gastroenterol Hepatol.* 1999;31(suppl 1):S63-S72.

31. Laine L, Curtis SP, Langman M, et al. Lower gastrointestinal events in a double-blind trial of the cyclo-oxygenase-2 selective inhibitor etoricoxib and the traditional nonsteroidal anti-inflammatory drug diclofenac. *Gastroenterology.* 2008;135(5):1517-1525.

32. Zhao Y, Encinosa W. *Hospitalizations for Gastrointestinal Bleeding in 1998 and 2006: Statistical Brief #65, in Healthcare Cost and Utilization Project (HCUP) Statistical Briefs.* Rockville, MD: Agency for Healthcare Research and Quality (US); 2006,

33. Agrawal NM, Roth S, Graham DY, et al. Misoprostol compared with sucralfate in the prevention of nonsteroidal anti-inflammatory drug-induced gastric ulcer. A randomized, controlled trial. *Ann Intern Med.* 1991;115(3):195-200.

34. Derry S, Loke YK. Risk of gastrointestinal haemorrhage with long term use of aspirin: meta-analysis. *BMJ.* 2000;321(7270):1183-1187.

35. Lanza F, Peace K, Gustitus L, Rack MF, Dickson B. A blinded endoscopic comparative study of misoprostol versus sucralfate and placebo in the prevention of aspirin-induced gastric and duodenal ulceration. *Am J Gastroenterol.* 1988;83(2):143-146.

36. Lanza FL, Royer GL, Nelson RS. Endoscopic evaluation of the effects of aspirin, buffered aspirin, and enteric-coated aspirin on gastric and duodenal mucosa. *N Engl J Med.* 1980;303(3):136-138.

37. McCarthy DM. Sucralfate. *N Engl J Med.* 1991;325(14):1017-1025.

38. Aadland E, Fausa O, Vatn M, Cohen H, Quinlan D. Protection by misoprostol against naproxen-induced gastric mucosal damage. *Am J Med.* 1987;83(1a):37-40.

39. Bardhan KD, Bjarnason I, Scott DL, et al. The prevention and healing of acute non-steroidal anti-inflammatory drug-associated gastroduodenal mucosal damage by misoprostol. *Br J Rheumatol.* 1993;32(11):990-995.

40. Elliott SL, Yeomans ND, Buchanan RR, Smallwood RA. Efficacy of 12 months' misoprostol as prophylaxis against NSAID-induced gastric ulcers. A placebo-controlled trial. *Scand J Rheumatol.* 1994;23(4):171-176.

41. Graham DY, Agrawal NM, Roth SH. Prevention of NSAID-induced gastric ulcer with misoprostol: multicentre, double-blind, placebo-controlled trial. *Lancet.* 1988;2(8623):1277-1280.

42. Graham DY, White RH, Moreland LW, et al. Duodenal and gastric ulcer prevention with misoprostol in arthritis patients taking NSAIDs. Misoprostol Study Group. *Ann Intern Med.* 1993;119(4):257-262.

43. Lanza FL. A double-blind study of prophylactic effect of misoprostol on lesions of gastric and duodenal mucosa induced by oral administration of tolmetin in healthy subjects. *Dig Dis Sci.* 1986;31(2 suppl):131s-136s.

44. Lanza FL, Fakouhi DRubin A, et al. A double-blind placebo-controlled comparison of the efficacy and safety of 50, 100, and 200 micrograms of misoprostol QID in the prevention of ibuprofen-induced gastric and duodenal mucosal lesions and symptoms. *Am J Gastroenterol.* 1989;84(6):633-636.

45. Raskin JB, White RH, Jackson JE, et al. Misoprostol dosage in the prevention of nonsteroidal anti-inflammatory drug-induced gastric and duodenal ulcers: a comparison of three regimens. *Ann Intern Med.* 1995;123(5):344-350.

46. Raskin JB, White RH, Jaszewski R, et al. Misoprostol and ranitidine in the prevention of NSAID-induced ulcers: a prospective, double-blind, multicenter study. *Am J Gastroenterol.* 1996;91(2):223-227.

47. Moore RA, Derry S, Makinson GT, McQuay HJ. Tolerability and adverse events in clinical trials of celecoxib in osteoarthritis and rheumatoid arthritis: systematic review and meta-analysis of information from company clinical trial reports. *Arthritis Res Ther.* 2005;7(3):R644-65.

48. Clive DM, Stoff JS. Renal syndromes associated with nonsteroidal antiinflammatory drugs. *N Engl J Med.* 1984;310(9):563-572.

49. Rannou F, Pelletier JP, Martel-Pelletier J. Efficacy and safety of topical NSAIDs in the management of osteoarthritis: Evidence from real-life setting trials and surveys. *Semin Arthritis Rheum.* 2016;45(4 suppl):S18-S21.

50. Stevenson DD. Aspirin and NSAID sensitivity. *Immunol Allergy Clin North Am.* 2004;24(3):491-505, vii.

51. Kowalski ML, Makowska JS, Blanca M, et al. Hypersensitivity to nonsteroidal anti-inflammatory drugs (NSAIDs) - classification, diagnosis and management: review of the EAACI/ENDA(#) and GA2LEN/HANNA*. *Allergy.* 2011;66(7):818-829.

34

NEUROPATHIC PAIN MEDICATIONS

Naileshni Singh, MD, Jon Zhou, MD and Samir J. Sheth, MD

FAST FACTS

- There are a variety of different types of medications that can be used to treat neuropathic pain.
- Many of the medications are antiseizure or antidepressant medications.
- The treatment of neuropathic pain with pharmacologic interventions can lead to substantial pain relief when dosed correctly, but the adverse effects from these medications can prevent patients from reaching their therapeutic dose.

Many classes of medications are thought to be effective and are evidence based for neuropathic pain. These include antiseizure and antidepressant medications, which may work in both the central and peripheral nervous systems. Class, initial dosing, and dosing of medications researched for effectiveness in treating neuropathic pain are detailed in Tables 34-1 and 34-2. There is also evidence that combination therapy, from multiple classes, is more efficacious than placebo or the single medication by itself. For example, there is evidence that opioids or TCAs combined with gabapentinoid medications are more effective than either medication alone for painful diabetic peripheral neuropathy (DPN) and postherpetic neuralgia (PHN).[1] Dosages for combinations medication therapies may be lower than usual, which will also decrease side effects.

ANTISEIZURE MEDICATIONS

Medications typically considered "antiseizure" treatments act as sodium channel blockers or calcium channel blockers or both. Sodium channel blockers inhibit initiation, maintenance, and propagation of neural discharges. Medications such as carbamazepine and local anesthetics such as lidocaine are examples of sodium channel blockers. Calcium channel blockers, such as gabapentin, bind to the alpha 2 delta subunit of L-type calcium channel, which causes decreases in glutamate and substance P and increases norepinephrine and GABA in pain pathways. Both sodium and calcium channel blockers have known efficacy in the treatment of neuropathic pain.[2]

Topiramate is FDA approved for the treatment of seizures and migraine prophylaxis. This medication has been used for bipolar disorder, weight loss, eating disorders, alcohol and drug dependence, headaches, posttraumatic stress disorder (PTSD), DPN, PHN, and complex regional pain syndrome (CRPS). The mechanism of action involves both the sodium and calcium channels to enhance GABA activity. Side effects of nephrolithiasis and ocular glaucoma are related to its effects as a carbonic anhydrase inhibitor, which lowers bicarbonate and should be monitored with electrolytes. Other effects included weight loss, sedation, and metabolic acidosis. Patients on topiramate and some other antiepileptic drugs (AEDs) need to be counseled regarding the potential for fetal birth defects.[3] Bicarbonate levels and liver function tests may also need to be assessed during treatment.

Carbamazepine is FDA approved for seizures, trigeminal neuralgia (TN), and bipolar disorder. There is evidence for efficacy in PHN, DPN, and poststroke pain.[4] Carbamazepine selectively blocks abnormally active C fibers and A delta fibers through voltage-gated sodium channels. Additionally, it acts as a GABA agonist and works both peripherally and centrally. Side effects include Stevens-Johnson syndrome, aplastic anemia, or other changes in the hematopoietic system, ataxia, dizziness, bitemporal heminanopsia, hormonal abnormalities, lipid abnormalities, and toxic epidermal necrolysis.[5] Oxcarbazepine, a structural variant of carbamazepine,

TABLE 34-1 Efficacy of Medications for Neuropathic Pain Conditions							
	TRICYCLIC ANTIDEPRESSANTS	**DULOXETINE**	**VENLAFAXINE**	**GABAPENTIN**	**PREGABALIN**	**OPIOIDS**	**LIDOCAINE PATCH**
Painful diabetic neuropathy	+	+	+	+/−	+/−	+	n/a
Postherpetic neuropathy	+	n/a	−	+	+/−	+	+
Painful polyneuropathy	+	n/a	+	+	n/a	+	+
Postmastectomy pain	+	n/a	−	n/a	n/a	n/a	n/a
Chronic lumbar root pain	−	n/a	n/a	n/a	n/a	−	n/a
Central poststroke pain	+	n/a	n/a	n/a	+	n/a	n/a
Spinal cord injury	−	n/a	n/a	+	+	n/a	n/a
Phantom limb pain	−	n/a	n/a	n/a	+/−	+	n/a
Neuropathic cancer pain	−	n/a	n/a	+	n/a	n/a	n/a
Complex regional pain syndrome (type 1)	n/a	n/a	n/a	−	n/a	n/a	n/a
Chemotherapy-induced neuropathy	−	n/a	n/a		n/a	n/a	n/a
HIV neuropathy	−	n/a	n/a	−	n/a	n/a	n/a

Adapted from O'Connor AB, Dworkin RH. Treatment of neuropathic pain: an overview of recent guidelines. Am J Med. 2009;122(10 Suppl):S22-S32. Copyright © 2009 Elsevier. With permission.
+ = ≥1 Trial showed statistically significant pain relief for the primary outcome compared with placebo.
− = ≥1 Trial showed no statistically significant pain relief for the primary outcome compared with placebo.
n/a = unavailable data.

has less side effects and is better tolerated.[6] This alternative is FDA approved for seizures and bipolar disorder and its main side effect is hyponatremia. These medication therapies should be monitored with electrolytes, blood counts, and liver function tests before initiation and then with subsequent periodic follow-up.

Lamotrigine is FDA approved for bipolar disorder and seizures. It is used for treatment of TN, DPN, polyneuropathy, and central pain.[7] This medication's proposed mechanism of action includes sodium channel blockade that prevents the release of glutamate. The side effect profile includes rash and Stevens-Johnson syndrome, blood dyscrasias, dermatitis, alopecia, nausea, and vomiting. The medication needs to be discontinued immediately for patients who present with a rash.

Local anesthetics are commonly used to treat neuropathic pain and are available in multiple formulations such as lidocaine ointments or creams and lidocaine transdermal patches. As a sodium channel blocker, lidocaine is the most commonly available local anesthetic for pain management. Pain conditions treated with lidocaine include PHN, meralgia parasthetica, intercostal

neuralgia, and postthoracotomy neuralgia. There is evidence that intravenous application of lidocaine can be effective for neuropathic pain conditions such as TN, chemotherapy-induced neuropathy, PHN, DPN, and postoperative pain through repeated treatments.[8] The intravenous application of lidocaine is typically done at specialized pain centers.

Gabapentin is FDA approved for PHN, seizure, and restless legs syndrome, whereas pregabalin is FDA approved for DPN, PHN, partial onset seizures, and fibromyalgia. These medications bind voltage-gated calcium channels that modify firing of neurons and cause release of GABA.[9] Side effects for gabapentin include somnolence, dizziness, nausea, edema, and myoclonus. Side effects for pregabalin are similar and include somnolence, dizziness, dry mouth, altered mentation, weight gain, blurry vision, constipation, and swelling. The main differences between gabapentin and pregabalin are in the pharmacodynamics and pharmacokinetics. Gabapentin has a nonlinear pharmacokinetic profile, is variably absorbed in the gastrointestinal system, and is less bioavailable at higher doses. In contrast, pregabalin

TABLE 34-2 Neuropathic Pain Medication Effective Dosages and Indications

DRUG CLASS	MEDICATION	EFFECTIVE DOSAGE	INDICATION
TCAs	Nortriptyline Desipramine	25 mg to start to 150 mg/d	Central and peripheral NP
SNRI	Duloxetine	60-120 mg/d	DPN, musculoskeletal pain
SNRI	Venlafaxine	37.5 mg-225 mg/d or bid	DPN
Multiple mechanisms including calcium channel inhibition	Pregabalin	75-600 mg/d in divided doses tid or bid	DPN, PHN, SCI
Multiple mechanisms including calcium channel inhibition	Gabapentin	300-3600 mg/d in divided doses tid	DPN, PHN, cancer-related neuropathy
Multiple mechanisms including calcium channel inhibition	Extended release gabapentin	300-1800 mg/d	PHN
Multiple mechanisms including sodium channel blocker	Carbamazepine	100-800 mg/d in divided doses	TN
Sodium channel blocker	Lidocaine patch	1-3 patches per day, 12 h on and 12 h off	PHN
TRPV1 channel agonist	Capsaicin patch	1 patch to the painful area for 30-60 min every 3 mo	HIV neuropathy, PHN
TRPV1 channel agonist	Capsaicin cream	0.025%-1% to the affected area tid-qid	Peripheral NP
Opioid mu receptor agonist	Strong opioids such as morphine and oxycodone	Depends on patient	DPN, PHN, phantom pain, radiculopathy
Opioid mu receptor agonist	Weak opioids such as tramadol	Depends on patient	DPN, phantom pain, SCI, cancer-related pain
Cannabinoid receptor	Cannabis	Depends on patient, oral or inhaled	Peripheral and central NP

Adapted from Jones RC 3rd, Lawson E, Backonja M. Managing neuropathic pain. Med Clin North Am. 2016;100(1):151-167. Copyright © 2016 Elsevier. With permission.

DPN, painful diabetic peripheral neuropathy; NP, neuropathic pain; PHN, postherpetic neuralgia; SCI, spinal cord injury; TN, trigeminal neuralgia.

has a linear profile and is well absorbed with consistent bioavailability across dosages.[9] Clinical effects from gabapentin are achieved at higher doses, whereas benefits from pregabalin might be discerned quicker. Neither medication has drug-drug interactions nor effects on the liver or kidneys but must be renally dosed in those with kidney disease.[2] Both pregabalin and gabapentin are first-line treatments for neuropathic pain.[10] Gabapentin at doses between 1800 and 3600 mg is effective for pain from PHN and diabetic neuropathy.[4] Pregablin is thought to provide pain relief at doses of 300, 450, and 600 mg.[11] Side effect profiles for these medications may limit use.

ANTIDEPRESSANT MEDICATIONS

Antidepressants have been used for neuropathic pain for decades. The most well studied are the classes of tricyclic antidepressants (TCAs) such as amitriptyline, nortriptyline, desipramine, and imipramine. These medications work by inhibiting serotonergic and noradrenergic neurotransmitter reuptake in the synaptic cleft near neurons. Side effects include those that are both anticholinergic and antihistaminic: constipation, dry mouth, blurry vision, glaucoma, urinary retention, paralytic ileus, visual problems, lower seizure threshold, and prolongation of the QT interval.[12] Patients should have a baseline ECG beforc initiating therapy.[13] Patients should avoid abrupt cessation of TCAs owing to withdrawal symptoms such as fever, diaphoresis, headaches, nausea, dizziness, and akathisia. TCAs are FDA approved for depression, obsessive compulsive disorder, and enuresis, and considered off label for panic disorder, bulimia, phantom limb pain, chronic itching, migraine, tension headaches, myofascial pain, anxiety, burning mouth syndrome, smoking cessation, attention deficit-hyperactivity (ADD or ADHD) disorder, PTSD, central pain, diabetic neuropathy, and PHN. TCAs are first-line treatments for neuropathic pain.[10]

Medications that favor noradrenergic pathways such as duloxetine and venlafaxine have been used for a variety of pain conditions including fibromyalgia. Duloxetine is FDA approved for use in depression, anxiety, DPN, fibromyalgia, and chronic musculoskeletal pain with evidence for efficacy in arthritis and low back pain.[14] Side effects may include anxiety, fatigue, nausea, xerostomia, dizziness, constipation, hepatic and sexual dysfunction.

Doses of 60 to 120 mg of duloxetine have been found to be beneficial.[15] Venlafaxine is FDA approved for depression, generalized and social anxiety disorder, pain disorder and off label or investigational for PTSD, migraine prophylaxis, fibromyalgia, tension-type headache, DPN, chronic pain and fatigue, irritable bowel syndrome, ADD and ADHD, bipolar depression, and premenstrual dysphoric disorder. Side effects include hypertension, so cardiac disease needs to be assessed before initiation.[16] Venlafaxine may also cause sexual dysfunction, similar as other serotonergic medications. Duloxetine and venlafaxine are generally considered first-line treatment for neuropathic pain, but there may be less evidence for venlafaxine.[10,17,18]

Antidepressants, regardless of class, may also increase the risk of suicidality in children and young adults and therefore should be closely monitored when initiated.[19] There are FDA black box warnings for antidepressants because of this issue. Depression and pain often appear to go together; those with higher levels of depression report more pain and are a challenge to treat. This may be the reason certain SSRI medications, such fluvoxamine, fluoxetine, and escitalopram, improve pain symptomatology through mood regulation.[20] SSRIs inhibit the reuptake of serotonin in the synaptic cleft and have roles in both nociception and mood regulation. However, in general, we would not recommend SSRI medications for nondepressed patients in pain. The side effect profile of SSRIs may make these classes of medications typically better tolerated than TCAs. Common side effects of SSRIs include sexual dysfunction, urinary retention, agitation, drowsiness, nausea, insomnia, and dry mouth.[21] Clinicians should be vigilant in identifying patients using several serotonergic medications at once. Serotonin syndrome may result from increased levels of serotonin when patients take one or more SSRIs or SNRIs or combine treatment with other serotonin releasing medications such as tramadol or antiemetic medications. Patients may experience elevated body temperature, agitation, hyperreflexia, diaphoresis, diarrhea, tremor, and seizures. Treatment consists of cessation of the offending medication(s) and providing supportive care.[22]

Opioids

Opioid medications have been used for treatment of neuropathic pain conditions, but concern for addiction and unintentional death with chronic and high-dose therapy may limit its uses. Opioid medications bind to a variety of opioid receptors including mu, kappa, and delta that cause hyperpolarization of neurons, thus reducing action potential and neurotransmitter release. Opioid receptors are found throughout the peripheral pre- and postsynaptic nervous system and central nervous system including the thalamus, brainstem, midbrain, and cortex. Alternatively, methadone is a unique opioid that releases norepinephrine and serotonin and binds to N-methyl D aspartate (NMDA) receptors and muscarinic receptors to modulate pain, but the complexity of the pharmacokinetics of methadone makes it difficult to dose and accordingly has been implicated in a disproportionate amount of unintentional overdose deaths.[23] Opioid mechanisms of action are postulated to be through both the ascending pain transmission pathways and descending inhibition pathways.

Research has shown that opioid agonists have variable effects on neuropathic pain.[24] Use of opioids acutely and for short time frames such as less than 24 hours appears to decrease neuropathic pain when compared with placebo.[24] Opioids seem to be effective for spontaneous neuropathic pain but do not improve emotional experience or physical functioning. The IASP's guidelines do include the use of tramadol and stronger opioids for neuropathic pain but with weak recommendations. Tramadol is considered second line, and stronger opioids (sustained release oxycodone or morphine) are considered third-line treatments.[10] A careful risk-benefit analysis needs to be completed when initiating opioid therapies.

Cannabinoids

The use of cannabis sativa as a treatment modality for neuropathic pain has had a renewed interest in pain medicine; however, the FDA has yet to formally approve any product containing cannabis for a neuropathic condition. Cannabinoids target the endocannabinoid signaling system including cannabinoid receptors and endogenous ligands. Activation of the cannabinoid receptors suppresses calcium conductance and decreases neuronal excitability, which may lead to decreased inflammatory pain states. Cannabinoids have been examined in clinical trials for their suppression of neuropathic pain with positive evidence to support its efficacy. Studies evaluating the use of dronabinol, a synthetic cannabinoid, showed improvements in multiple sclerosis–related neuropathic pain in patients.[25] Although pain was better controlled, the most frequently reported side effects were dizziness, impairment of balance, and sedation. Other side effects of marijuana use include visual and auditory hallucinations and even acute psychosis in certain patients.[26] There is also concern with the medical community that cannabinoids may be a gateway drug with a relationship to the use of other illicit drugs.[27] Other studies on MS using a variety of cannabinoid formulations have demonstrated efficacy.[28] Several studies have demonstrated a 30% decrease in HIV neuropathy pain with the use of smoked cannabis as compared with placebo.[29] Other studies have shown efficacy in neuropathic pain, fibromyalgia, and rheumatoid arthritis with good tolerability.[30] During the last two decades, research articles have demonstrated the efficacy of synthetic cannabinoids in decreasing neuropathic pain and the quality of hyperalgesia. Although proven as an appetite stimulant and antiemetic, larger randomized control trials are needed to further elucidate the efficacy and safety profile of cannabinoids for neuropathic pain.[31] Overall, cannabinoids and marijuana remain a controversial topic and at the time of this book's publication, it was a schedule I medication.

Clonidine

Clonidine is an α2-adrenergic receptor agonist, originally used as an oral product for treatment of hypertension, with central and peripheral analgesic properties. Activation of central and peripheral α2-adrenergic receptors leads to downregulation of nociceptors, which may decrease allodynia and neuropathic pain. Clonidine is FDA approved for the treatment of hypertension, while the intrathecal form is FDA approved for intractable cancer pain. There is no current FDA approval for the use of oral or topical clonidine for neuropathic pain despite studies showing analgesic effects. Typical dosing interval for clonidine patch is twice a day, 0.1 to 0.8 mg/day. Case reports have demonstrated pain relief from disabling neuropathic leg pain with oral clonidine and pain relief with topical clonidine cream in the treatment of orofacial pain.[32,33] One larger randomized control trial looked at topical 0.1% clonidine gel for diabetic neuropathy of the feet and showed improved pain scores after 12 weeks of daily use compared with placebo.[34] The most common side effects include dry mouth, sedation, and headache, although topical clonidine may have an improved side effect profile. Smaller clinical trials using clonidine (oral and topical) show some efficacy for neuropathic pain.

Muscle Relaxants

Despite a wide variety of muscle relaxants in the marketplace, only baclofen has been studied for its use in neuropathic pain control. Baclofen is a GABA-B receptor agonist, used as a muscle relaxant for myofascial pain and spasticity. There is no current FDA approval for use of baclofen for neuropathic pain specifically, although it is approved for intrathecal use for spasticity. A small case series and one clinical trial of 10 patients showed decreased pain from TN compared with placebo.[35] Side effects with baclofen include muscle weakness, fatigue, and light-headedness. Typical daily dose is twice a day to three times a day, with doses between 20 and 200 mg/day. Based on the current evidence, baclofen is a second- or third-line alternative for controlling neuropathic pain states.[35] Other muscle relaxers such as cyclobenzaprine, carisoprodol, tizanidine, methocarbamol, and benzodiazepines have conflicting reports on short-term efficacy.[2]

Ketamine

Ketamine, an NMDA antagonist agent, has seen a resurgence of late in the control of chronic pain. Hyperactivity of NMDA receptors may be one of the factors in potentiating central neuropathic pain. Ketamine in a low dose produces opioid sparing and analgesic effects by the enhancement of anti-inflammatory effects at central sites of action. It is often administered as a short-term IV infusion for neuropathic pain, with some studies showing prolonged effects for up to 3 months following infusion. Intravenous administration of ketamine can be done in specialized care centers and required continuous monitoring. Ketamine has psychedelic side effects of hallucinations, somnolence, vivid dreams, and nausea.

In clinical settings, ketamine is well tolerated when benzodiazepines are used to decrease the psychotropic side effects and vomiting. Oral ketamine may play a role as an agent for patients experiencing neuropathic pain outside of the inpatient or hospital setting. Smaller case series have highlighted ketamine to be efficacious as an adjunct for patients who are at maximum tolerable doses of opioids.[36] As an oral agent, the most common reason for cessation of therapy was frequent and intolerable side effects, mainly psychomimetics effects.[37] Additionally, owing to nystagmus, ketamine is not recommended for individuals who wish to continue to drive, which may make this therapy further limiting. Oral ketamine is a controlled substance and needs to be compounded, so this may not be a readily available product for patients. In summary, ketamine may be an adjunct for neuropathic pain control when used orally, but patients should be monitored and cautioned in regard to psychomimetic reactions from the medication.

Topical Analgesics

Topical analgesics are a group of agents including topical lidocaine, low- and high-dose capsaicin creams, and compounding agents that are a mixture of low-dose medications used to alleviate neuropathic pain. These locally acting agents are beneficial because of their focused site of action and minimal systemic side effects. They are typically used as adjuncts to oral systemic agents to alleviate neuropathic pain. Lidocaine patch 5% can decrease pain in PHN without any increase in systemic side effects.[38] There are 2 topical analgesics FDA approved for use in PHN: 5% lidocaine patch and capsaicin 8% patch. Adverse events from the lidocaine patch include skin rashes from the site of application. The dosage for the lidocaine patch is typically 1 to 3 patches for a 12-hour period, alternating with 12 hours of cessation, to prevent local anesthetic toxicity.

Capsaicin is an ingredient found naturally in spicy peppers, and its use for neuropathic pain has been an area of focus recently. A typical formulation is a low-concentration (0.075%) topical agent that is applied to the affected area up to 4 times a day. Low-dose capsaicin has a favorable side effect profile, with mainly skin irritation and burning sensation as symptoms. Topical capsaicin is efficacious for several neuropathic pain states including postsurgical neuropathic pain.[39] One newer type of capsaicin is a highly concentrated 8% patch, which may have prolonged pain relief following a single application. It is the first pure, concentrated, synthetic capsaicin-containing prescription medication developed and FDA approved for treatment of PHN. The safety profile is low risk with typically localized pain and burning sensation in the region of application. The patch is applied to the skin by a physician after application of topical local anesthetics and opioid or sedating medications and left in place for 30 to 60 minutes. A recent meta-analysis of all completed randomized control studies of capsaicin 8% showed a meaningful (>30%) pain reduction after one treatment in 45% of PHN patients.[40] In one study of over 1000 patients, the researcher found the patch to reduce pain intensity, improve sleep, and decrease use of opioids and antiepileptics medications in those with a variety of peripheral neuropathies while reporting mostly mild adverse effects of skin irritation.[41] Capsaicin 8% has not been fully evaluated for other neuropathic pain states such as phantom limb pain and CRPS. There is one case report of the capsaicin patch decreasing chronic phantom limb pain and opioid use by 50% in 2 patients.[42] Other studies have shown benefit postmastectomy pain, HIV-neuropathy, and DPN along with improvement in quality-of-life measures.[40,43] In summary, the high dose capsaicin 8% patch is FDA approved for PHN with some evidence supporting its use in other neuropathic pain states.

Combination therapies have also been used for neuropathic pain, in which a specialized compounding pharmacy mixes a combination of local anesthetics, capsaicin, anti-inflammatory agents, and topical anticonvulsants into one mixture for patients to apply. This concoction offers low-dose medications that can be applied topically. Results for compounding agents are mixed, and unfortunately, many medical insurances may not provide coverage for compounded experimental treatments. Agents included in research trials of compounding agents include clonidine, ketamine, amitriptyline, and lidocaine in various combinations. However, most clinical trials were small (<50 per group) and each study had varying doses and combinations.[44] Despite the research limitations, one study evaluated amitriptyline 4%/ketamine 2% cream versus placebo in 251 patients with PHN and demonstrated superior analgesia compared with a lower concentration of the therapy and placebo.[45] Another trial evaluated topical baclofen 10 mg, amitriptyline HCL 40 mg, and ketamine 20 mg combination compared with placebo for treatment of chemotherapy-induced peripheral neuropathic with significant improvements in NP.[46] Although there are smaller studies showing efficacy of lidocaine 5%, capsaicin, and combination topical agents, further studies may be needed before recommending any particular topical as first-line therapy. There is increased interest in the use of topical agents to treat neuropathic pain that is localized to specific areas. There is a significant body of evidence that topical lidocaine (5%) is beneficial in some types of neuropathic pain, whereas limited evidence for benefit from combination compounding medications.

CONCLUSIONS

There are a variety of different neuropathic pain medications with unique mechanisms of actions. When treating patients with neuropathic pain, consideration of medications along with other conservative therapies should be highly considered. Limitations of these medications are often due to side effects. Even when effective, patients complain of lack of mental clarity and being "in a fog". Careful monitoring of side effects, and in some cases, blood work, is necessary when prescribing these medications. Many treatment failures stem from rapid dose escalation. It is important to ask the patient, even

when failing the medication in the past, how they were administered the medication, and how quickly they were escalated in order to reach a therapeutic dosage. In addition to antiseizure and antidepressant medications, ketamine and topical medications offer unique alternatives in patients who have failed conventional first-line treatments. Finally, further research is needed for marijuana and opioids before definitive recommendations can be made.

REFERENCES

1. Dworkin RH, O'Connor AB, Audette J, et al. Recommendations for the pharmacological management of neuropathic pain: an overview and literature update. *Mayo Clin Proc.* 2010;85(3 suppl):S3-S14.

2. Benzon HT, Raja SN, Liu SS, Fishman SM, Cohen SP. *Essentials of Pain Medicine.* 3rd ed. Philadelphia, PA: Elsevier; 2011.

3. Meador KJ, Loring DW. Developmental effects of antiepileptic drugs and the need for improved regulations. *Neurology.* 2016;86(3):297-306.

4. Wiffen PJ, Derry S, Moore RA, Kalso EA. Carbamazepine for chronic neuropathic pain and fibromyalgia in adults. *Cochrane Database Syst Rev.* 2014;(4):Cd005451.

5. Pellock JM. Carbamazepine side effects in children and adults. *Epilepsia.* 1987;28(suppl 3):S64-S70.

6. Nasreddine W, Beydoun A. Oxcarbazepine in neuropathic pain. *Expert Opin Investig Drugs.* 2007;16(10):1615-1625.

7. Wiffen PJ, Derry S, Moore RA. Lamotrigine for chronic neuropathic pain and fibromyalgia in adults. *Cochrane Database Syst Rev.* 2013;(12):cd006044.

8. Przeklasa-Muszynska A, Kocot-Kepska M, Dobrogowski J, Wiatr M, Mika J. Intravenous lidocaine infusions in a multidirectional model of treatment of neuropathic pain patients. *Pharmacol Rep.* 2016;68(5):1069-1075.

9. Bockbrader HN, Wesche D, Miller R, Chapel S, Janiczek N, Burger P. A comparison of the pharmacokinetics and pharmacodynamics of pregabalin and gabapentin. *Clinical pharmacokinetics.* 2010;49(10):661-669.

10. Finnerup NB, Attal N, Haroutounian S, et al. Pharmacotherapy for neuropathic pain in adults: a systematic review and meta-analysis. *Lancet Neurol.* 2015;14(2):162-173.

11. Moore RA, Straube S, Wiffen PJ, Derry S, McQuay HJ. Pregabalin for acute and chronic pain in adults. *Cochrane Database Syst Rev.* 2009(3):cd007076.

12. Gillman PK. Tricyclic antidepressant pharmacology and therapeutic drug interactions updated. *Br J Pharmacol.* 2007;151(6):737-748.

13. Funai Y, Funao T, Ikenaga K, Takahashi R, Hase I, Nishikawa K. Use of tricyclic antidepressants as analgesic adjuvants results in nonhazardous prolongation of the QTc interval. *Osaka City Med J.* 2014;60(1):11-19.

14. Pergolizzi JV, Raffa RB, Taylor R, Rodriguez G, Nalamachu S, Langley P. A review of duloxetine 60 mg once-daily dosing for the management of diabetic peripheral neuropathic pain, fibromyalgia, and chronic musculoskeletal pain due to chronic osteoarthritis pain and low back pain. *Pain Pract.* 2013;13(3):239-252.

15. Lunn MP, Hughes RA, Wiffen PJ. Duloxetine for treating painful neuropathy, chronic pain or fibromyalgia. *Cochrane Database Syst Rev.* 2014;(1):cd007115.

16. Whiskey E, Taylor D. A review of the adverse effects and safety of noradrenergic antidepressants. *J Psychopharmacol.* 2013;27(8):732-739.

17. Gallagher HC, Gallagher RM, Butler M, Buggy DJ, Henman MC. Venlafaxine for neuropathic pain in adults. *Cochrane Database Syst Rev.* 2015;(8):Cd011091.

18. Aiyer R, Barkin RL, Bhatia A. Treatment of neuropathic pain with venlafaxine: a systematic review. *Pain Med.* 2016.

19. Miller M, Pate V, Swanson SA, Azrael D, White A, Sturmer T. Antidepressant class, age, and the risk of deliberate self-harm: a propensity score matched cohort study of SSRI and SNRI users in the USA. *CNS Drugs.* 2014;28(1):79-88.

20. Patetsos E, Horjales-Araujo E. Treating chronic pain with SSRIs: what do we know? *Pain Res Manag.* 2016;2016:2020915.

21. Kennedy SH, Rizvi S. Sexual dysfunction, depression, and the impact of antidepressants. *J Clin Psychopharmacol.* 2009;29(2):157-164.

22. Buckley NA, Dawson AH, Isbister GK. Serotonin syndrome. *BMJ.* 2014;348:g1626.

23. Faul M, Bohm M, Alexander C. Methadone prescribing and overdose and the association with medicaid preferred drug list policies - United States, 2007-2014. *MMWR Morb Mortal Wkly Rep.* 2017;66(12):320-323.

24. McNicol ED, Midbari A, Eisenberg E. Opioids for neuropathic pain. *Cochrane Database Syst Rev.* 2013;(8):cd006146.

25. Svendsen KB, Jensen TS, Bach FW. Does the cannabinoid dronabinol reduce central pain in multiple sclerosis? Randomised double blind placebo controlled crossover trial. *BMJ.* 2004;329(7460):253.

26. Kilmer B. Recreational cannabis - minimizing the health risks from legalization. *New Engl J Med.* 2017;376(8):705-707.

27. Nkansah-Amankra S, Minelli M. "Gateway hypothesis" and early drug use: additional findings from tracking a population-based sample of adolescents to adulthood. *Prev Med Rep.* 2016;4:134-141.

28. Iskedjian M, Bereza B, Gordon A, Piwko C, Einarson TR. Meta-analysis of cannabis based treatments for neuropathic and multiple sclerosis-related pain. *Curr Med Res Opin.* 2007;23(1):17-24.

29. Abrams DI, Jay CA, Shade SB, et al. Cannabis in painful HIV-associated sensory neuropathy: a randomized placebo-controlled trial. *Neurology.* 2007;68(7):515-521.

30. Lynch ME, Campbell F. Cannabinoids for treatment of chronic non-cancer pain; a systematic review of randomized trials. *Br J Clin Pharmacol.* 2011;72(5):735-744.

31. Volkow ND, Compton WM, Weiss SR. Adverse health effects of marijuana use. *New Engl J Med.* 2014;371(9):879.

32. Tan YM, Croese J. Clonidine and diabetic patients with leg pains. *Ann Intern Med.* 1986;105(4):633-634.

33. Epstein JB, Grushka M, Le N. Topical clonidine for orofacial pain: a pilot study. *J Orofac Pain.* 1997;11(4):346-352.

34. Campbell CM, Kipnes MS, Stouch BC, et al. Randomized control trial of topical clonidine for treatment of painful diabetic neuropathy. *Pain.* 2012;153(9):1815-1823.

35. Fromm GH, Terrence CF, Chattha AS. Baclofen in the treatment of trigeminal neuralgia: double-blind study and long-term follow-up. *Ann Neurol.* 1984;15(3):240-244.

36. Kannan TR, Saxena A, Bhatnagar S, Barry A. Oral ketamine as an adjuvant to oral morphine for neuropathic pain in cancer patients. *J Pain Symptom Manage.* 2002;23(1):60-65.

37. Enarson MC, Hays H, Woodroffe MA. Clinical experience with oral ketamine. *J Pain Symptom Manage.* 1999;17(5):384-386.

38. Finnerup NB, Otto M, McQuay HJ, Jensen TS, Sindrup SH. Algorithm for neuropathic pain treatment: an evidence based proposal. *Pain.* 2005;118(3):289-305.

39. Ellison N, Loprinzi CL, Kugler J, et al. Phase III placebo-controlled trial of capsaicin cream in the management of surgical neuropathic pain in cancer patients. *J Clin Oncol.* 1997;15(8):2974-2980.

40. Derry S, Rice AS, Cole P, Tan T, Moore RA. Topical capsaicin (high concentration) for chronic neuropathic pain in adults. *Cochrane Database Syst Rev.* 2017;1:cd007393.

41. Maihofner C, Heskamp ML. Prospective, non-interventional study on the tolerability and analgesic effectiveness over 12 weeks after a single application of capsaicin 8% cutaneous patch in 1044 patients with peripheral neuropathic pain: first results of the QUEPP study. *Curr Med Res Opin.* 2013;29(6):673-683.

42. Moses BA, Brewer DB, Panula TL, Goff BJ. Eight percent capsaicin patch (Qutenza) for chronic phantom limb pain. *Pain Med.* 2012;12(2):329-330.

43. Moses BA, Brewer DB, Panula TL, Goff BJ. Eight percent capsaicin patch (Qutenza) for chronic post-mastectomy pain. *Pain Med.* 2012;13(2):329.

44. Zur E. Topical treatment of neuropathic pain using compounded medications. *Clin J Pain.* 2014;30(1):73-91.

45. Everton D, Bhagwat D, Damask M. (787): A multicenter, double-blind, randomized, placebo controlled study of the efficacy/safety of two doses of amitriptyline/ketamine topical cream in treating post-herpetic neuralgia (PHN). *J Pain.* 2007;8(4):S47.

46. Barton DL, Wos EJ, Qin R, et al. A double-blind, placebo-controlled trial of a topical treatment for chemotherapy-induced peripheral neuropathy: NCCTG trial N06CA. *Support Care Cancer.* 2011;19(6):833-841.

35

COMPOUNDED TOPICAL ANALGESICS

Amode Tembhekar, BS, Christopher Migdal, BS and Martin AC Manoukian, BS

FAST FACTS

- Topical analgesics and anesthetics may include patches, creams, ointments, or gels prepared for local delivery to the skin, targeting sensory nerve endings and tissues after dermal penetration.
- Topical administration allows effective delivery of medications while reducing systemic side effects.
- Topical analgesics can improve patient adherence and acceptance.

INTRODUCTION

The use of compounded pain medications has long been used in pain management to increase drug efficacy while simultaneously decreasing toxicity. Recently, this method of pharmaceutical delivery has gained increasing popularity owing to a greater understanding of the adverse effects, addiction potential, and abuse of currently prescribed oral analgesics. Many physicians prefer to use compounded topical medications owing to perceived improvements in efficacy and a resultant decreased narcotic prescribing.[1] In particular, compounded topical analgesics have been demonstrated to be effective tools for treating various types of pain, including musculoskeletal pain, fibromyalgia, peripheral neuropathic pain, diabetic neuropathy, postherpetic neuralgia, and vulvodynia.[2] Although there are a plethora of options and formulations, this chapter will provide a concise summary of commonly used compounding medications and the principles behind their use. There are numerous advantages to using compounding medications, chief among them their ability to produce local, targeted effects while avoiding the undesirable systemic effects of oral dosing, thereby resulting in improved patient adherence.[2,3]

DELIVERY TO TARGET TISSUE

To be effective, compounded topical analgesics must be able to traverse the skin to reach their site of action at the nerve endings located within the dermis. To do so they must either enter the dermis via the skin appendages or diffuse through the epidermis. Although entry via the skin appendages is less selective, these appendages are not uniformly distributed throughout the body, and the drug can be sequestered in the hair follicles.[4] Drugs that reach the dermis via diffusion must first cross stratum corneum, a layer of dead keratinocytes that contains intracellular lipids and is covered by a lipid film.[4] To effectively cross this lipophilic barrier, drugs must follow Lipinski's rule of five, which states that drugs must weigh less than 500 daltons, must have a log P of less than 5 (a measure of lipophilicity), must have less than 5 hydrogen bond donors, and must have less than 10 hydrogen bond acceptors.[5] Next, compound topical analgesics must cross the layers of the epidermis, which from superficial to deep are the stratum lucidum, stratum granulosum, stratum spinosum, and stratum basale, each of which are aqueous layers of keratinocytes at successive stages of differentiation.[6] The final barrier is the basement membrane, a charged layer of connective tissue, anchoring fibrils, and glycoproteins that is mostly permeable to cationic molecules.[7] Upon traversing the basement membrane, drugs then enter the dermis, which contains the sensory nerve endings that are the targets for compounded analgesics. The dermis is also highly vascularized, allowing for the delivery of drug to local downstream tissue (Figure 35-1). However, if too much drug enters the dermal vasculature, it is possible for the drug to reach detectable levels systemically.[8]

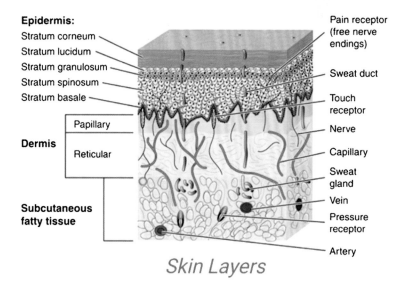

FIGURE 35-1 The skin layers.

FORMULATIONS

Multiple formulations of compounded analgesics exist, and selection should be based on the etiology of a particular pain condition. For example, for a patient with neuropathic pain a regimen may include Ketamine 10%, Gabapentin 6%, and Clonidine 0.2%.[9] Baclofen 2% and Amitriptyline 2% may be supplemented as deemed appropriate. For mechanical or inflammatory pain associated with muscle spasms, another analgesic compounded combination of Ketoprofen, Lidocaine, and Cyclobenzaprine would be favorable. Capsaicin is another promising topical analgesic that has been effective in treating postherpetic neurlagia.[10] The mechanisms of action of these drugs are summarized in Table 35-1. These analgesics are delivered in the form of creams, gels, and ointments that may have limited efficacy when used alone. Thus, compounded topical analgesics are usually delivered with transdermal bases such as Pluronic lecithin organogel, Speed Gel, VanPen, DemiGel, Lipoderm, or LipodermActiveMax to enhance permeation and absorption.[3,11,12] Keep in mind that multiple mechanisms and potential targets exist for therapeutic pharmacologic intervention for both acute and chronic pain. Careful assessment should guide treatment strategy.

INDICATIONS

Compounded topical analgesics are an excellent alternative for patients who cannot tolerate oral analgesics, such as patients prone to nonsteroidal anti-inflammatory drug (NSAID)–induced gastrointestinal bleeding or for those who want to avoid potential addiction and abuse, as seen with opioids.[13,14] Compounded topical analgesics can also improve patient adherence, eliminate first-pass metabolism, and provide localized access to the targeted

TABLE 35-1 Drug Mechanisms of Action	
DRUG	**MECHANISM OF ACTION**
Ketamine	Predominantly NMDA receptor antagonism
Gabapentin	Inhibits voltage-gated calcium channels
Clonidine	Alpha-2 receptor agonist
Baclofen	Activates GABA-B receptors
Amitriptyline	Inhibition of norepinephrine and serotonin reuptake
Nifedapine	Calcium channel blocker (primarily L-type)
Opioids	Agonism of beta-endorphin, enkephalin, and dynorphin opioid receptors
Lidocaine	Blockage of sodium channels
Cyclobenzaprine	Muscle relaxant
Ketoprofen	Inhibition of prostaglandin formation
Capsaicin	Cellular depolarization via vanilloid receptor subtype 1 receptor

GABA, gamma-aminobutyric acid; NMDA, N-methyl-D-aspartic acid.

site of pain.[3] Furthermore, compounded medications give clinicians the ability to use several drugs in one compound, targeting various receptors and pathways, potentially yielding additive or synergistic effects while limiting toxic potential. They are particularly effective in treating neuropathic pain but can also be used for musculoskeletal, arthritic, and postoperative pain when traditional oral medications have been unsuccessful or are not tolerated.[15]

CONTRAINDICATIONS AND TOXICITY

Owing to their localized nature, compounded topical analgesics have fewer contraindications than their oral counterparts. The primary contraindications are dermatologic, as it is not uncommon for these medications to cause irritant contact dermatitis or allergic contact dermatitis.[3] Thus, it is important to ask patients about their dermatologic history and warn patients of these potential adverse effects.

Although the contraindications are primarily dermatologic, it is important to note that compounded topical analgesics can infiltrate the systemic circulation and cause systemic side-effects. Notably, the FDA submitted a warning in 2006 regarding two patient deaths linked to lidocaine toxicity from compounding creams.[16] Various case reports demonstrate safety hazards resulting from the use of compounded topical analgesics. Some of the adverse effects include interstitial nephritis, severe central nervous system (CNS) depression in a pediatric patient and hypertensive emergency.[17-20] Furthermore, systemic side effects of topical amitriptyline have also been noted.[21] Although relatively rare, systemic side effects should always be considered and discussed when prescribing compounding medications.

CONCLUSION

Compounded topical analgesics exist in a vast array of formulations to treat certain pain conditions. Beyond these formulations, physicians should observe the following principle: keep the total percentages of ingredients under 30% and molecular weight of each ingredient <500 g/mol to maximize absorption. In addition, individual components should be dosed as they would be orally when new formulations are being first prescribed. Permeation enhancers should be included in formulations, with no significant differences in absorption exist between major types. Compounded topical analgesics offer a superior safety profile to oral analgesics, with the most likely side effect being contact dermatitis. However, absorption of topical agents can rarely result in high systemic concentrations, leading to serious adverse effects. By adhering to these guidelines, physicians working with qualified and competent pharmacists can adjust both medications and doses in compounded topical analgesics to create an individualized, targeted therapy for a variety of pain conditions.

EFFECTIVE DRUGS IN PAIN CONTROL	OPIOD	NSAID	CORTICOSTEROID	ANTIDEPRESSANT	ANTICONVULSANT	ANTISPASMODIC	LOCAL ANESTHETIC
Types of pain							
Visceral/soft tissue pain	+	+	+	+	+	+	+
Bone pain	+	+	–	–	–	–	–
Nerve compression	+	–	+	+	+	–	+
Neuropathic pain	–	+	+	+	+	–	+
Muscle spasm	–	+	–	–	–	+	–

NSAID, nonsteroidal anti-inflammatory drug.

REFERENCES

1. Warner M, Tuder D. A brief survey on prescriber beliefs regarding compounded topical pain medications. *Int J Pharm Compd.* 2014;18(3):182-188.
2. Branvold A, Carvalho M. Pain management therapy: the benefits of compounded transdermal pain medication. *J Gen Pract.* 2014;2:188.
3. Cline AE, Turrentine JE. Compounded topical analgesics for chronic pain. *Dermatitis.* 2016;27(5):263-271.
4. Boer M, Duchnik E, Maleszka R, Marchlewicz M. Structural and biophysical characteristics of human skin in maintaining proper epidermal barrier function. *Postepy Dermatol Alergol.* 2016;33(1):1-5.
5. Lipinski CA, Lombardo F, Dominy BW, Feeney PJ. Experimental and computational approaches to estimate solubility and permeability in drug discovery and development settings. *Adv Drug Deliv Rev.* 2001;46(1-3):3-26.
6. Nitsche JM, Kasting GB. A microscopic multiphase diffusion model of viable epidermis permeability. *Biophys J.* 2013;104(10):2307-2320.
7. Kazama T, Yaoita E, Ito M, Sato Y. Charge-selective permeability of dermo-epidermal junction: tracer studies with cationic and anionic ferritins. *J Invest Dermatol.* 1988;91(6):560-565.
8. Lawlor KT, Kaur P. Dermal contributions to human interfollicular epidermal architecture and self-renewal. *Int J Mol Sci.* 2015;16(12):28098-28107.

9. McNulty JP, Muller G. Update on managing neuropathic pain. *Int J Pharm Compd.* 2009;13(3):182.

10. Irving GA, Backonja M, Rauck R, Webster LR, Tobias JK, Vanhove G. NGX-4010, a capsaicin 8% dermal patch, administered alone or in combination with systemic neuropathic pain medications, reduces pain in patients with postherpetic neuralgia. *Clin J Pain.* 2012;28(2):101-107.

11. Bassani AS, Banov D. Evaluation of the percutaneous absorption of ketamine HCl, gabapentin, clonidine HCl, and baclofen, in compounded transdermal pain formulations, using the franz finite dose model. *Pain Med.* 2016;17(2):230-238.

12. Franckum J, Ramsay D, Das N, Das S. Pluronic lecithin organogel for local delivery of anti-inflammatory drugs. *Int J Pharm Compd.* 2004;8(2):101-105.

13. Evans JM, McMahon AD, McGilchrist MM, et al. Topical non-steroidal anti-inflammatory drugs and admission to hospital for upper gastrointestinal bleeding and perforation: a record linkage case-control study. *BMJ.* 1995;311(6996):22-26.

14. Anitescu M, Benzon HT, Argoff CE. Advances in topical analgesics. *Curr Opin Anaesthesiol.* 2013;26(5):555-561.

15. Zur E. Topical treatment of neuropathic pain using compounded medications. *Clin J Pain.* 2014;30(1):73-91.

16. Young D. Student's death sparks concerns about compounded preparations. *Am J Health Syst Pharm.* 2005; 62(5):450-452.

17. Andrews PA, Sampson SA. Topical non-steroidal drugs are systemically absorbed and may cause renal disease. *Nephrol Dial Transplant.* 1999;14(1):187-189.

18. O'Callaghan CA, Andrews PA, Ogg CS. Renal disease and use of topical non-steroidal anti-inflammatory drugs. *BMJ.* 1994;308(6921):110-111.

19. Ross S, Ryzewski M, Holland MG, Marraffa JM. Compounded ointment results in severe toxicity in a pediatric patient. *Pediatr Emerg Care.* 2013;29(11):1220-1222.

20. Pomerleau AC, Gooden CE, Fantz CR, Morgan BW. Dermal exposure to a compounded pain cream resulting in severely elevated clonidine concentration. *J Med Toxicol.* 2014;10(1):61-64.

21. Kopsky DJ, Hesselink JM. High doses of topical amitriptyline in neuropathic pain: two cases and literature review. *Pain Pract.* 2012;12(2):148-153.

INDEX

Note: Page numbers followed by "f" indicate figures, "t" indicate tables and "b" indicate boxes.